Major herbs of ***Ayurveda***

For Churchill Livingstone:

Publishing Manager: Inta Ozols
Project Manager: Jane Dingwall
Design Direction: Judith Wright

Major herbs of
Ayurveda

Compiled by **The Dabur Research Foundation**
and **Dabur Ayurvet Limited**, Ghaziabad, India

Edited by **Elizabeth M Williamson** BSc PhD MRPharmS FLS
Senior Lecturer in Pharmacognosy and Phytotherapy,
The School of Pharmacy, University of London, London, UK
Editor-in-chief of *Phytotherapy Research*
Member of the Herbal Drugs Committees for
The British Pharmacopœia and The *European Pharmacopœia*

Foreword by **Professor Malcolm Hooper** PhD BPharm CChem MRIC
Emeritus Professor of Medicinal Chemistry,
School of Sciences, University of Sunderland, Sunderland, UK

CHURCHILL
LIVINGSTONE

CHURCHILL LIVINGSTONE
An imprint of Elsevier Science Limited

First published 2002
ISBN 0 443 07203 5

British Library Cataloguing in Publication Data
A catalogue record for this book is available from the British Library

Library of Congress Cataloging in Publication Data
A catalog record for this book is available from the Library of Congress

Note
Medical knowledge is constantly changing. As new information becomes available, changes in treatment, procedures, equipment and the use of drugs become necessary. The editors, contributors and the publishers have taken care to ensure that the information given in this text is accurate and up to date. However, readers are strongly advised to confiirm that the information, especialy with regard to drug usage, complies with the latest legislation and standards of practice.

Printed in China

Contents

Contributors vii
The Dabur Research Foundation viii
Foreword xi
Preface xiii
Colour plate section
Introduction: the principles of Ayurveda 1
Abrus precatorius 6
Acacia catechu 13
Acorus calamus 16
Adhatoda vasica 20
Aegle marmelos 25
Allium sativum 30
Andrographis paniculata 40
Aristolochia indica 46
Asparagus racemosus 51
Azadirachta indica 56
Bacopa monniera 64
Berberis aristata 69
Boerhaavia diffusa 76
Boswellia serrata 79
Caesalpinia bonducella 83
Carica papaya 88
Cedrus deodara 99
Centella asiatica 102
Cissus quadrangularis 106
Commiphora mukul 110
Crataeva nurvala 114
Curcuma longa 117
Cyperus rotundus 122
Eclipta alba 126
Embelia ribes 129
Eucalyptus globulus 134
Euphorbia hirta 141
Ficus religiosa 145
Fumaria indica 150
Gardenia gummifera 154
Glycyrrhiza glabra 157
Gossypium herbaceum 163
Gymnema sylvestre 167
Holarrhena antidysenterica 172
Leptadenia reticulata 175
Mangifera indica 178
Momordica charantia 182
Mucuna pruriens 190
Nigella sativa 196
Ocimum sanctum 201
Paederia foetida 206
Phyllanthus emblica 210
Phyllanthus niruri 215
Picrorrhiza kurroa 220
Piper longum 225
Piper nigrum 231
Plantago ovata 236
Plumbago zeylanica 239
Polygonum aviculare 244
Punica granatum 247
Ricinus communis 251
Rubia cordifolia 257
Salmalia malabarica 261
Semecarpus anacardium 263
Solanum nigrum 268
Solanum xanthocarpum 271
Swertia chirata 274
Symplocos racemosa 277

Syzygium cumini 279
Tamarindus indica 283
Terminalia arjuna 290
Terminalia belerica 294
Terminalia chebula 298
Tinospora cordifolia 302
Trachyspermum ammi 306
Tribulus terrestris 311
Trigonella foenum-graecum 315
Withania somnifera 321
Woodfordia fruticosa 326
Zingiber officinale 329

Therapeutic guide to plants 334
Glossary 342
Index 347

Contributors

Dabur Research Foundation

DB Ananthanarayana MPharm PhD
Director of R&D
Dabur Research Foundation
Ghaziabad, India

NB Brindavanam BAMS FES
Manager of Medical Services
and Clinical Research
Dabur Research Foundation
Ghaziabad, India

Rajendra M Dobriyal MSc
Scientist, Dabur Research Foundation
Ghaziabad, India

Dabur Ayurvet Limited

Mohan Saxena BSc BPharm MPharm
General Manager
Dabur Ayurvet Limited
Ghaziabad, India

K Ravikanth MPharm
Manager R&D
Dabur Ayurvet Limited
Ghaziabad, India

Vandita Srivastava MSc PhD
Senior Scientist
Dabur Ayurvet Limited
Ghaziabad, India

The Dabur Research Foundation

The DRF was founded in 1979 as a non-profit making organisation for the purpose of conducting scientific research on health care for both humans and animals. The main focus is on the ancient medical system called Ayurveda, which is not only still relevant but also becoming popular all over the world. The Foundation is now an important research organisation, recognised by the Department of Scientific and Industrial Research, Ministry of Science and Technology, Government of India. The DRF is affiliated to several government research institutes, universities and regulatory agencies.

Objectives

Research and development covers:

- exploration and investigation of the principles of Ayurveda
- providing scientific validation for existing traditional knowledge
- development of new formulations with improved levels of safety and efficacy
- cultivation and propagation of medicinal plants
- oncology and biotechnology research
- new drug research and new drug delivery systems for oncologic drugs
- consumer understanding for product development.

Activities

Multidisciplinary research work is carried out in the following areas:

- Ayurvedic medicines
- health supplements
- allopathic drugs
- herbal veterinary formulations
- phytochemicals/phytopharmaceuticals
- cosmetics, foods, oils and fats
- oncology–screening and development of new anticancer drugs
- new drug delivery systems for anticancer drugs
- technology development for phytochemicals
- studies on peptidomimetics
- bio-informatics
- clinical research for both botanical-based products and anticancer drugs.

Manpower

The Foundation works under the overall vision and guidance of Dr Anand C Burman MS, PhD (USA). The foundation is headed by Dr DBA Narayana MPharm, PhD. There is a pool of over 130 scientists and technologists from different scientific disciplines, many with PhD and MD qualifications, together with information experts. All are engaged in full-time interdisciplinary research and development of health-care products, mainly based on Ayurveda and other traditional systems. Oncology and biotechnology research is headed by Dr Rama Mukherjee and phytochemical technology development is carried out under the direction of Dr PS Srinivasan.

Facilities

The DRF has established independent laboratories including a well-equipped instrumentation centre consisting of nuclear magnetic resonance, infrared and ultraviolet spectroscopy, high-pressure liquid chromatography, gas chromatography and high-performance thin-layer chromatography, atomic absorption spectrophotometer, peptide synthesiser, fermenter, programmable furnaces, pilot facilities and stability test chambers. It has established state-of-the-art molecular biology and screening labs. For food products, sensory evaluation labs have been set up. The Foundation also has a modern and comprehensive library, subscribing to many print and electronic media journals and with access to over 200 databases.

Networking

The Foundation has networking arrangements with over 35 institutions in India, including universities, laboratories, Ayurvedic and conventional hospitals, medical and pharmacy colleges, which help to build technological and scientific bridges.

Funding

The DRF is a non-profit making organisation, receiving contributions from companies sponsoring various research programmes.

Annual budget

The annual R&D expenditure of the DRF is about $2.5 million.

Further information

Please contact:

Dabur Research Foundation
22, Site IV, Sahibabad
Ghaziabad – 201010
India

Websites: www.dabur.com
www.ayurvet.com

Dabur Ayurvet Limited

Dabur Ayurvet Limited is an extension of Dabur's status as a pioneer in herbal medicines, so as to include the animal population in the gamut of its healthcare operations. Dabur Ayurvet Limited is 'Dedicated to improve animal health through the wisdom of traditional knowledge and modern research'.

Foreword

I warmly welcome this interesting collection of monographs on the more common plants/herbs used in Ayurvedic medicine, an ancient and living system of medicine that uses herbo-mineral preparations. It shares with Chinese herbal medicine, which is equally ancient, the distinction of providing a comprehensive system of complementary medicine, developed over thousands of years, yet still today is widely used and practised, in the sub-continent and elsewhere. Ayurveda continues to exist alongside allopathic, western, medicine and undoubtedly offers medical treatment to many more people, particularly away from the urban centres where the more expensive allopathic medicine is largely practised.

In many parts of India, Ayurvedic practitioners, colleges and hospitals are found alongside more familiar allopathic colleges and schools of medicine, pharmacy, and teaching hospitals. The philosophy of Ayurveda provides an holistic understanding of health and disease that is both challenging and curious to the western allopathic mind. Body, mind and spirit are understood as integral to human health and addressed by the medicines and concepts used. In agreement with the holistic understanding of Ayurveda some of the plants are used as foods (e.g. papaya, turmeric, tamarind) and spices (e.g. pepper, ginger) whilst others are associated with worship in the household and community (e.g. Holy Basil, the tree of Shiva, and *Ficus religiosa*) as well as medicinal purposes. This points to the holistic nature of all life and emphasises the need for a healthy and responsible diet and lifestyle that is an essential part of Ayurvedic philosophy and practice – a message the west is only just beginning to recognise as important for individual and communal health.

It is interesting that Ayurveda has no category of infectious diseases, taking the view that if the immune system is functioning properly then infections, cancers, rheumatoid arthritis, asthma and other chronic disorders can be corrected by the judicious use of herbo-mineral preparations that modulate the immune response. This is very much in agreement with contemporary ideas about the immune system.

The monographs present information in an attractive and systematic manner that makes reading and comparison easy and informative. The general layout covers nomenclature, habitat and a brief botanical description of the plant and the parts used, traditional and modern usage, ethnoveterinary usage, major chemical constituents, medicinal and pharmacological activities, safety profile and toxicology, dosage and Ayurvedic properties. The chemical constituents cover all the major chemical groups, alkaloids, different types of glycosides, various categories of flavanoids, quinones, different classes of terpenes and terpenoids, phenols and phenolic derivatives, steroidal compounds, proteins, carbohydrates, fatty and organic and amino acids, minerals, trace elements and vitamins. The information on toxicology is a very important aspect of the monographs. The naïve, but not uncommon, attitude that any natural material is safe will find no support in these pages. Some natural materials are very toxic. Finally, recommendations for further reading and a list of references covering mainly medicinal and pharmacological information are provided. Many of the references describe work carried out in the Central Drug Research

Institute at Lucknow and are testimony to the many Indian scientists who have explored Ayurveda.

The reader will need to look elsewhere for detailed botanical information, essential for identification, but this is available in herbal pharmacopoeias that are referenced. No structures of the many compounds are provided and some chemistry is not referenced, for example the outstanding study on azadirachtin by Ley and colleagues. Information of this nature is provided by other sources that specialise in natural product and medicinal chemistry.

The most significant and unique feature of this book is the bringing together in a readily accessible form information that is of tremendous interest to anyone involved in contemporary and complementary medicine – including veterinary medicine, pharmacology, and drug development and design.

The modern drug industry is very adept at developing potent and effective medicines from a lead compound. This volume is bursting with information on possible lead compounds that address important contemporary health concerns. Immunomodulatory compounds, modulators of memory, cognition, and central executive functions, antidiabetic compounds, anti-cancer and antimutagenic substances, modifiers of lipid and cholesterol metabolism, antiinflammatory molecules, antiviral (including hepatitis B) and other anti-microbial agents, adaptogens, antiulcer and antistress compounds, antiallergic and anti-anaphylactic substances, nootropic drugs, hepatoprotective molecules, radioprotective and radiosensitising compounds, antioxidants, antifertility compounds for use by men and women, and even a treatment for crooked teeth are among the long list of biological activities. Every human organ and system is covered. For this reason alone, this volume should be on the shelves of medical scientists and practitioners who are concerned with medicine and drugs in any way. Drug formulation and delivery is also touched upon in some monographs (tamarind).

Some drugs from Ayurveda, which address modern disorders, have already reached the market place such as, 'gugul lipid', see *Commiphora mukul* and guggulsterone, and curcumin from turmeric. More challenging is the information about the modulation of the biological activity, including synergism, of one compound by another. This is an area which poses demanding scientific challenges and contrasts with the problems associated with the polypharmacy that often develops in the treatment of many western patients.

There is a useful *Therapeutic Guide* and some informative plates of the crude drug preparations that will delight pharmacists and pharmacognocists and remind them of their earlier education.

There are some interesting surprises. Sweet flag, *Alores calamus,* a European plant has a place here, indicating the eclectic nature of Ayurveda. Where the plants listed are used in other parts of the world such as Africa and South America then this information is also provided – doubly authenticating their clinical value.

The Dabur Foundation and the editor Elizabeth Williamson are to be congratulated on producing such a fascinating and informative book that makes accessible an ancient wisdom that will provide inspiration and ideas for all concerned with the health and well-being of people and communities. I recommend it unreservedly.

Malcolm Hooper

Preface

Ayurveda is the traditional healing system of India, with its origins firmly rooted in the culture of the Indian subcontinent, but its popularity is now increasing all over the world, like other forms of holistic medicine. This is partly due to a dissatisfaction with modern medicine, which appears to treat illness as an isolated malfunctioning in the body, rather than a weakness or imbalance in the complex interaction between mind, body and the environment. In Ayurveda, the human organism is considered to be a microcosm, or individual universe, within the macrocosm, or external cosmos. Over 5000 years ago, the great *rishis* or seers observed the 'fundamentals of life' and organised them into a system: Ayurveda was the result, not only an oral tradition passed down from generation to generation but a well-documented health-care philosophy revised over the years. It has evolved to accommodate modern science and research and growth are not only permitted but encouraged; the results of some of these scientific investigations are documented in this book The background and principles will be explained briefly in the next chapter but for a greater understanding the references and Further Reading lists at the end of each monograph should be consulted.

Western thinking tends to generalise populations and consider as 'normal' that which applies to the majority, whereas Ayurveda and other forms of holistic medicine view the patient as unique and 'normality' for them is whatever is most appropriate for that person. Another vital difference is that the Western mind prizes objectivity but Eastern thought views subjectivity as at least as important and, in fact, as going a step further, which can make acceptance and understanding difficult for some Westerners. However, although the principles may be abstruse, there is no doubt that many of the herbs of Ayurveda have a scientific rationale for their effects and this book is an attempt to show these and bring them to a wider audience. Treatment is, of course, not confined to medication with herbs but includes breathing exercises, meditation, massage, fasting and yoga, but they are outside the scope of this book.

In a continent as large and diverse as Asia there are various forms of Ayurveda, such as Jammu in Indonesia, and very many different plants are used. It would be impossible to include all of them so a selection of the most widely used has been chosen. They include food plants such as ginger (*Zingiber officinale*) and turmeric (*Curcuma longa*), common plants such as nut grass (*Cyperus rotundus*) and snakeweed (*Euphorbia hirta*) and more specialised plants including arjuna (*Terminalia arjuna*) and tellicherry (*Holarrhena antidysenterica*). There is a wealth of information on some plants, for example neem (*Azadirachta indica*), and very little on others, such as the silk cotton tree (*Salmalia malabarica*). Asian medicinal plants are being increasingly used throughout the rest of the world, examples being ashwaghanda (*Withania somnifera*) and Indian pennywort (*Centella asiatica*, also known as gotu kola), and there is also the worrying case of Indian birthwort (*Aristolochia indica*). This has been found to be toxic, causing fatalities in parts of Europe, but is included despite the ban on sale in some countries since it is still found elsewhere and information on it may be useful. Recently, regulatory bodies in the West have become concerned about reports of toxicity associated with Asian and Oriental herbs. In many cases these are due to contamination rather than intrinsic toxicity of the herb itself (Aristolochia being an exception) and sometimes misidentification of the plant has taken place. It is important that these problems are addressed to prevent an undeserved reputation for toxicity being associated with such herbs, some of which have a great potential for healing.

Health-care practitioners trained in the West know very little about Ayurvedic medicines, despite the fact that their patients include ethnic groups who may prefer to use familiar products imported from Asia. Americans and Europeans are also becoming interested in these remedies and often self-medicate, in addition to consulting a practitioner of complementary medicine. It is therefore essential that information is more easily available to both patients and professionals. The monographs cover the historical and mythological aspects of the herbs only briefly and concentrate on the phytochemical constituents and medicinal uses, supported by references to the scientific literature. There is mention of ethnoveterinary usage since farmers and householders in Asia also treat livestock and pets with these remedies; however, as with human use, we do not advocate administration to animals without professional advice. Safety data and doses are given where known but it is always wise to initiate therapy under the guidance of a qualified expert. Each monograph gives briefly the Ayurvedic characteristics of the herb to aid those interested in the philosophy; however, our aim is to provide evidence to support the safe and effective use of these herbs, whether they are being used according to Ayurvedic principles or not.

Elizabeth M Williamson

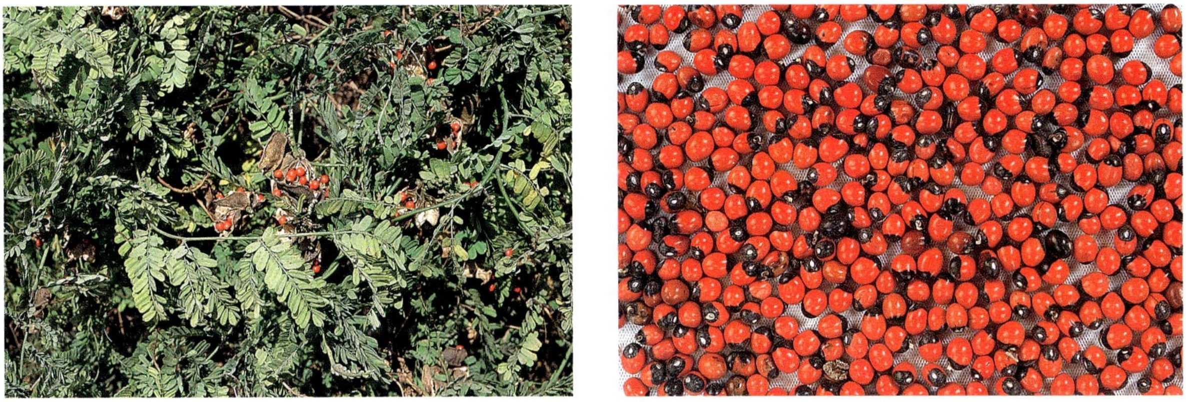

Plate 1 Abrus precatorius. (a) Fresh. (b) Dried.

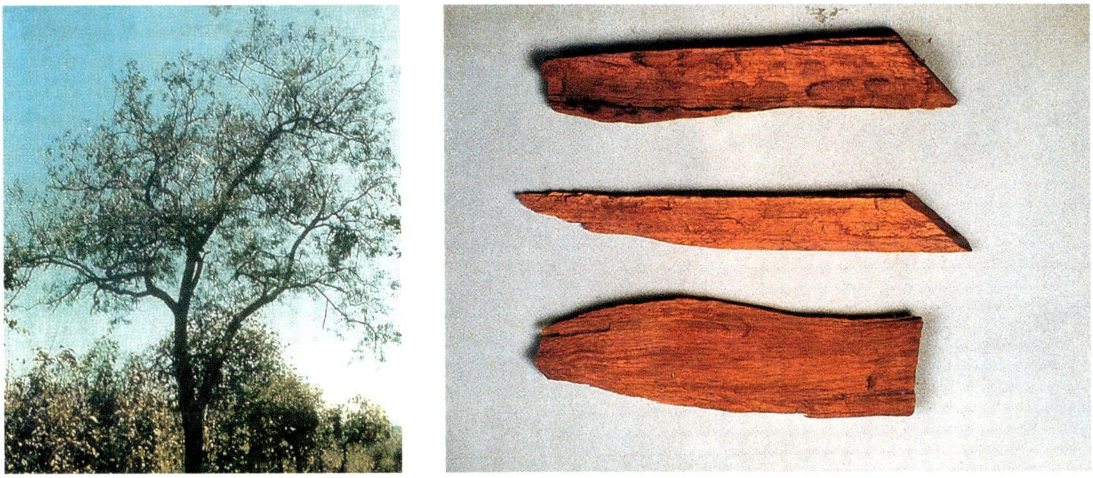

Plate 2 Acacia catechu. (a) Fresh. (b) Dried.

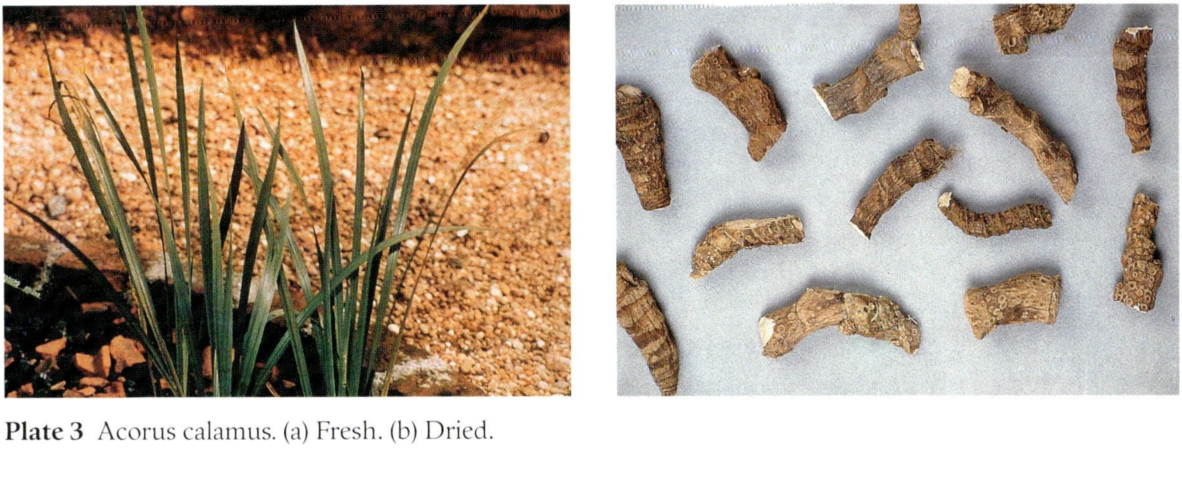

Plate 3 Acorus calamus. (a) Fresh. (b) Dried.

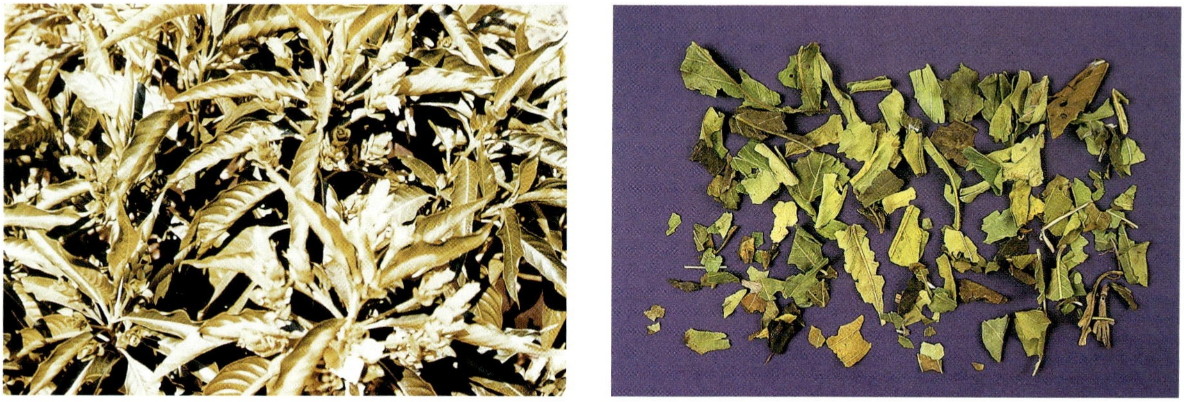

Plate 4 Adhatoda vasica. (a) Fresh. (b) Dried.

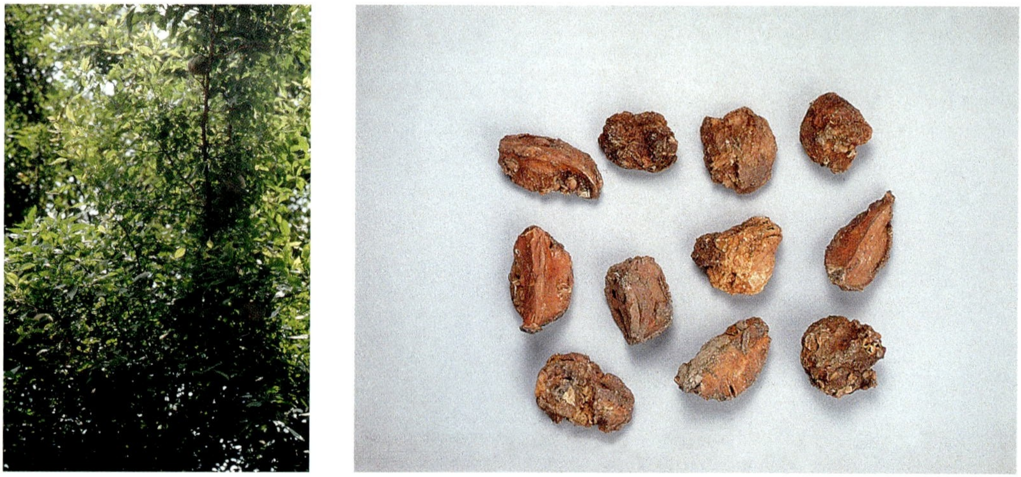

Plate 5 Aegle marmelos. (a) Fresh. (b) Dried.

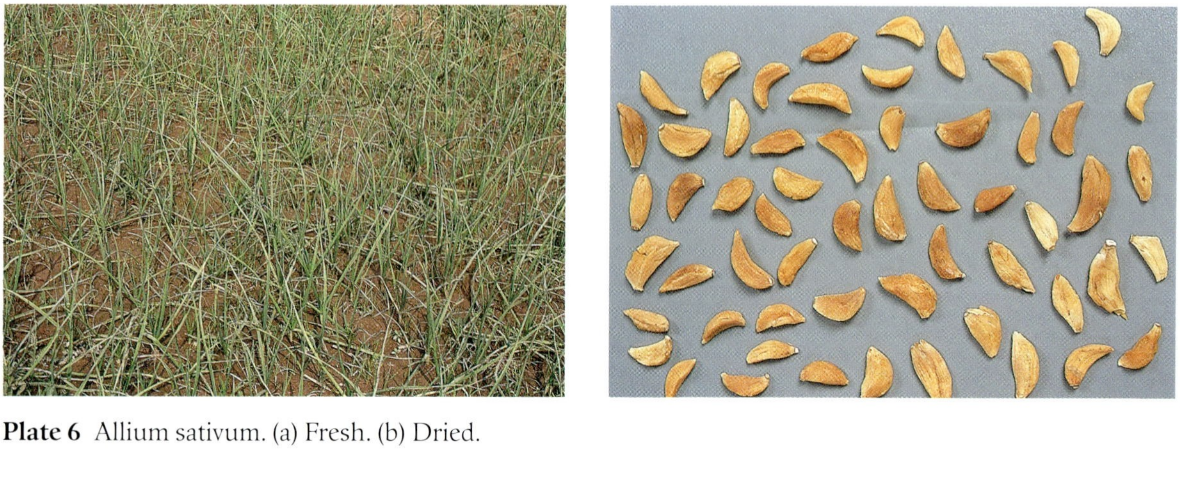

Plate 6 Allium sativum. (a) Fresh. (b) Dried.

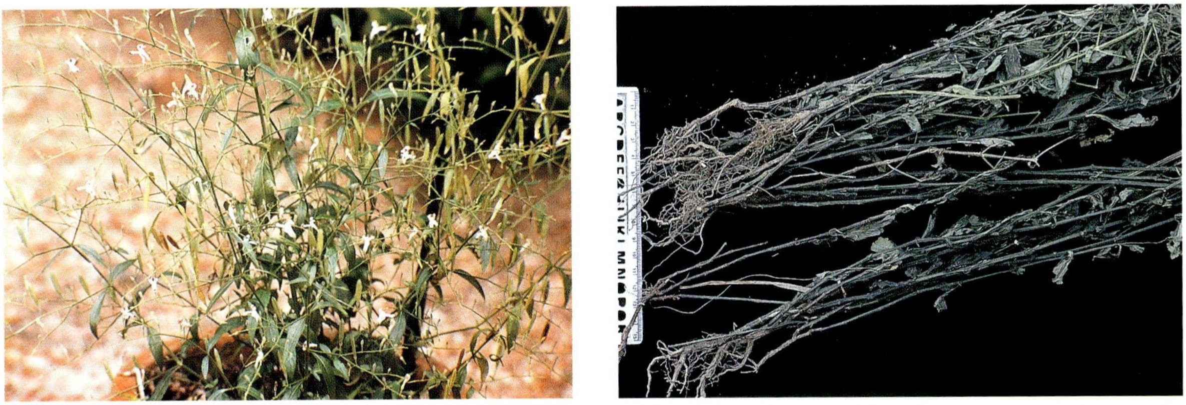

Plate 7 Andrographis paniculata. (a) Fresh. (b) Dried.

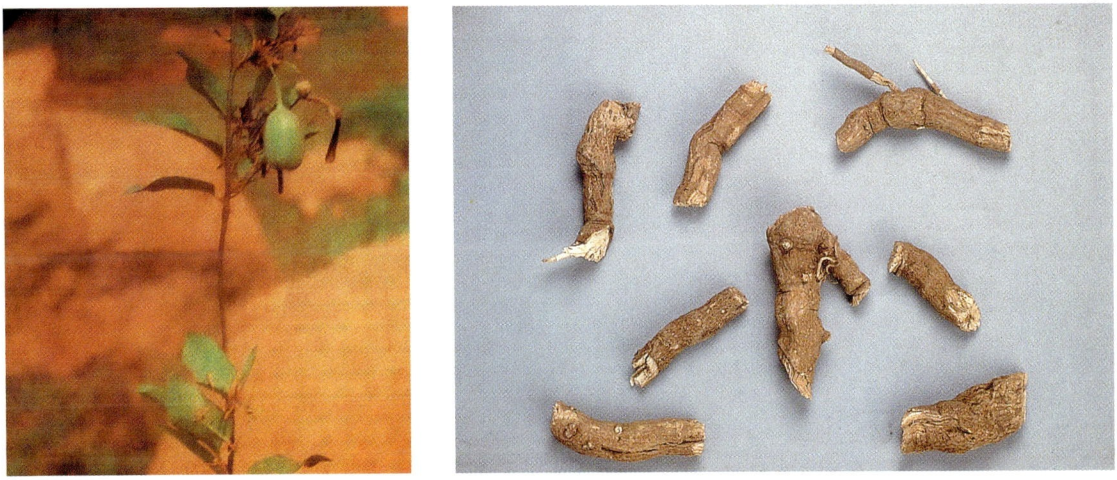

Plate 8 Aristolochia indica. (a) Fresh. (b) Dried.

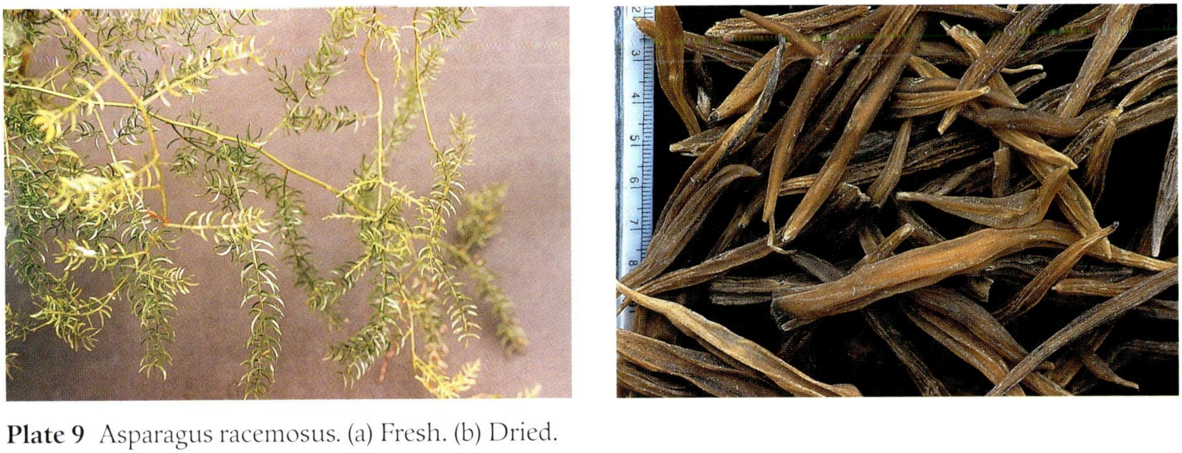

Plate 9 Asparagus racemosus. (a) Fresh. (b) Dried.

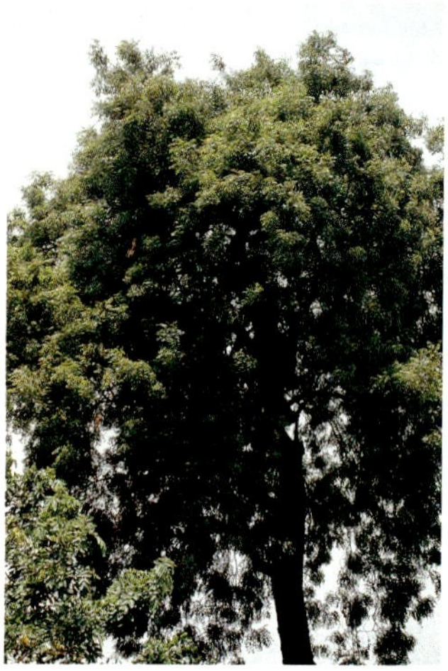
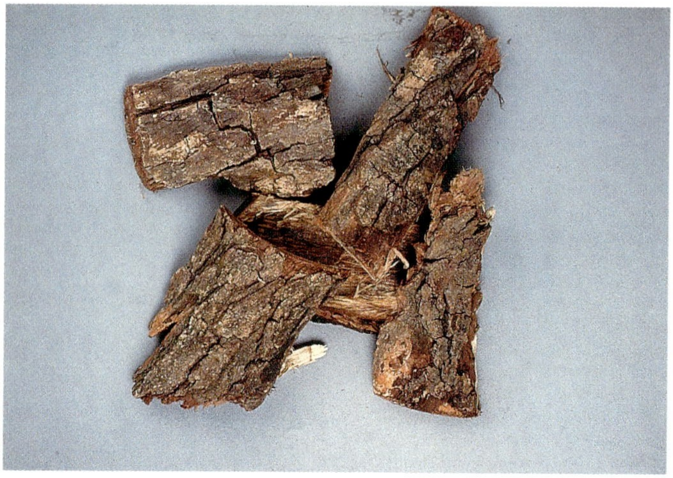

Plate 10 Azadirachta indica. (a) Fresh. (b) Dried.

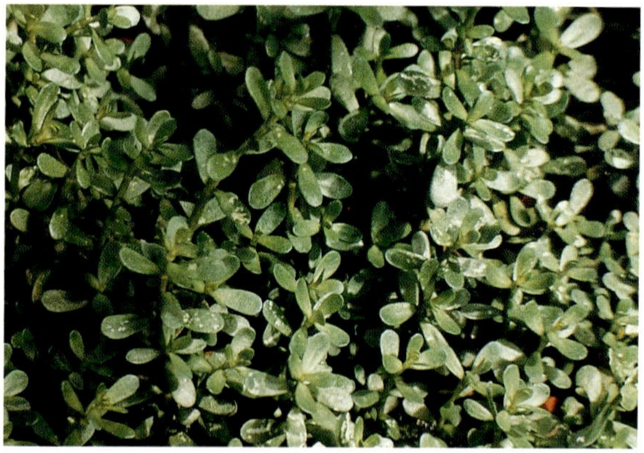
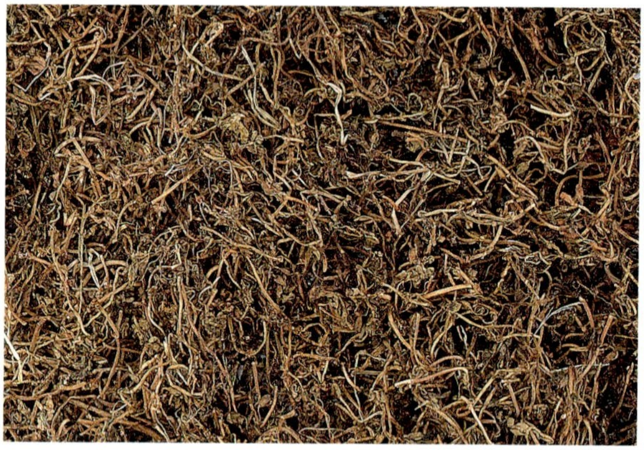

Plate 11 Bacopa monniera. (a) Fresh. (b) Dried.

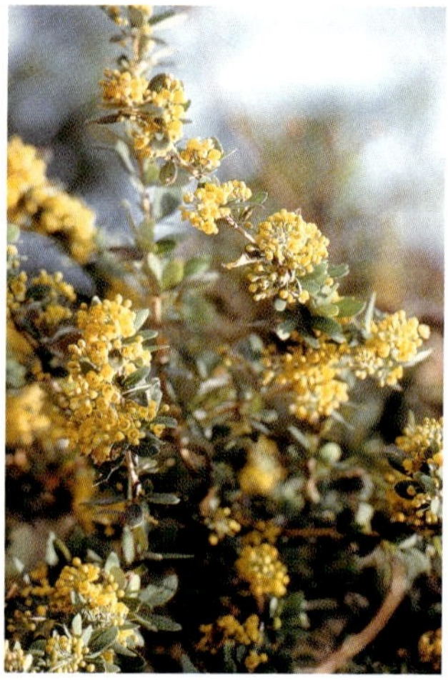
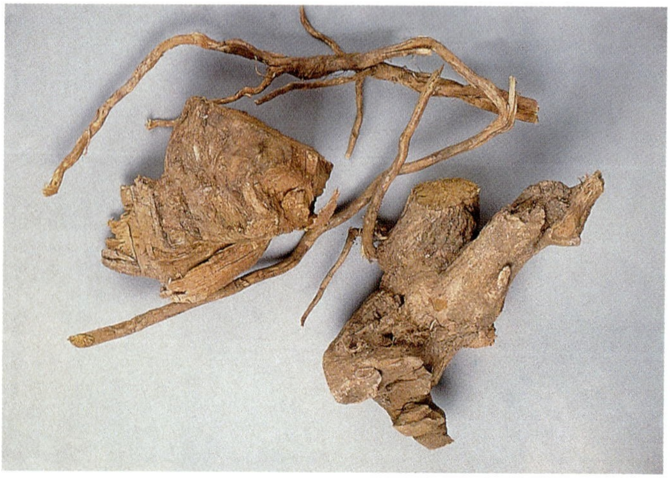

Plate 12 Berberis aristata. (a) Fresh. (b) Dried.

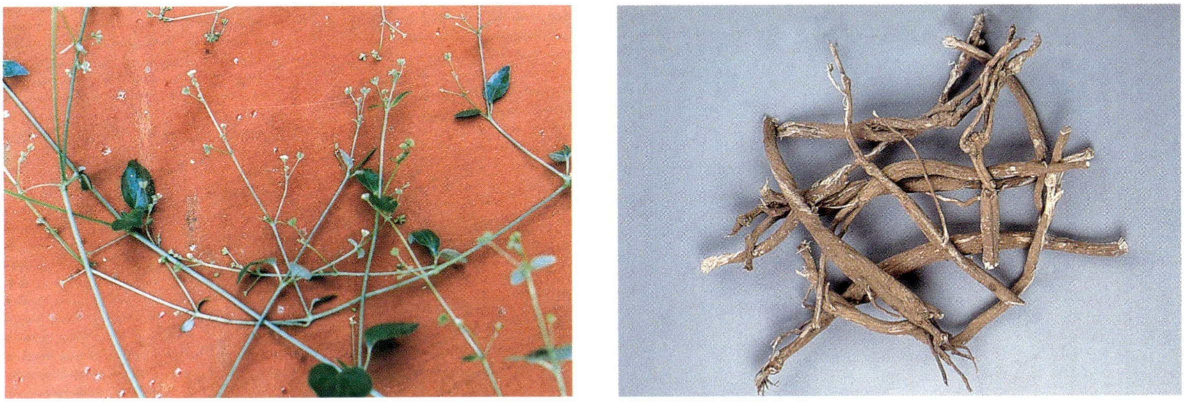

Plate 13 Boerhaavia diffusa. (a) Fresh. (b) Dried.

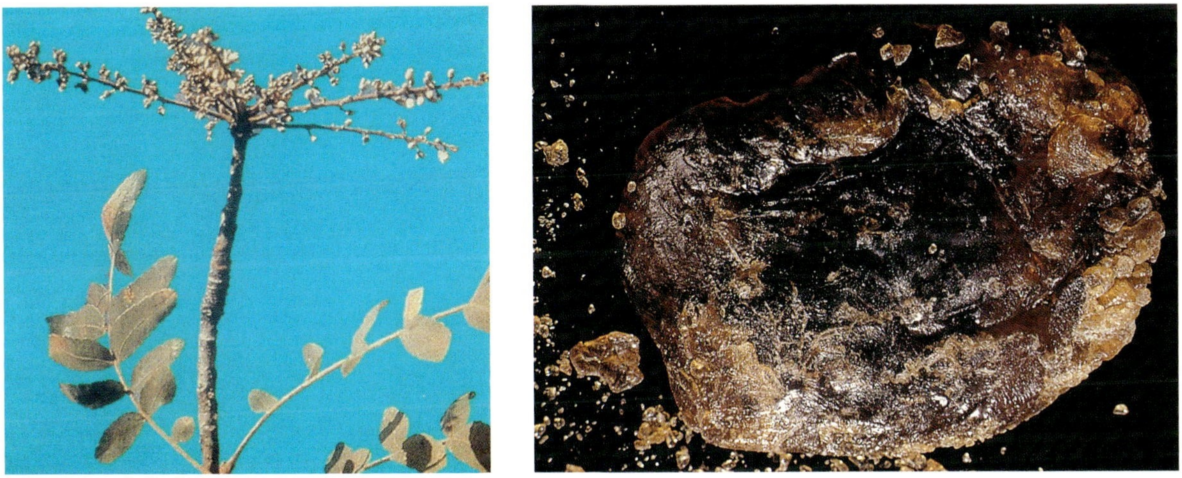

Plate 14 Boswellia serrata. (a) Fresh. (b) Dried.

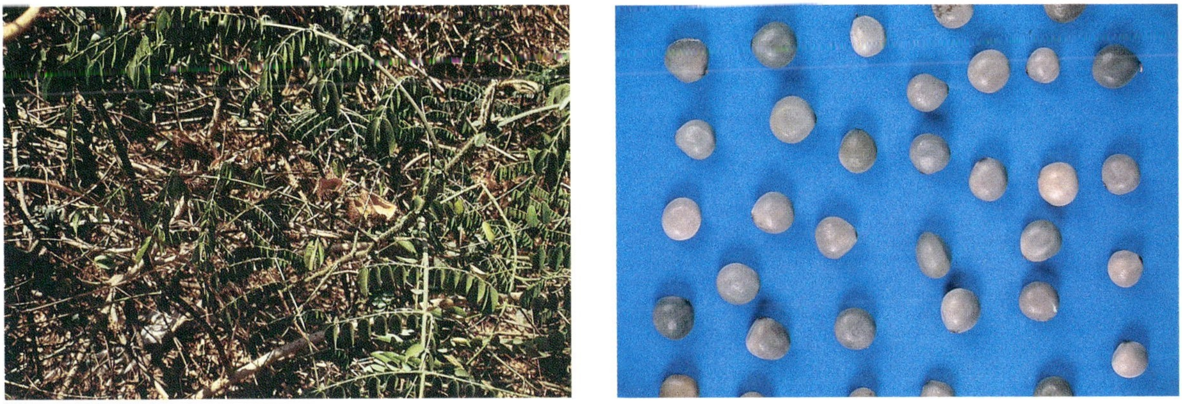

Plate 15 Caesalpinia bonducella. (a) Fresh. (b) Dried.

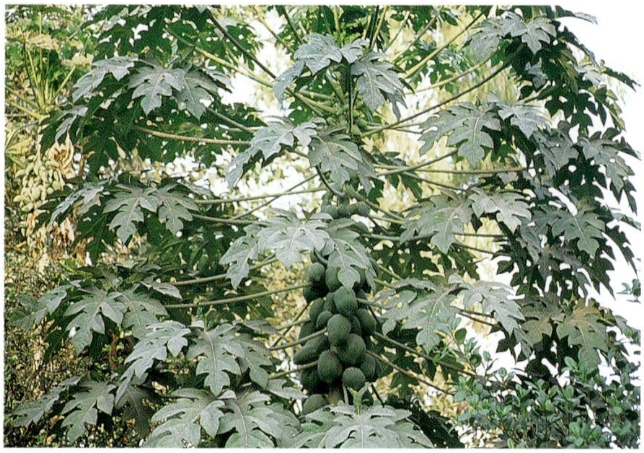
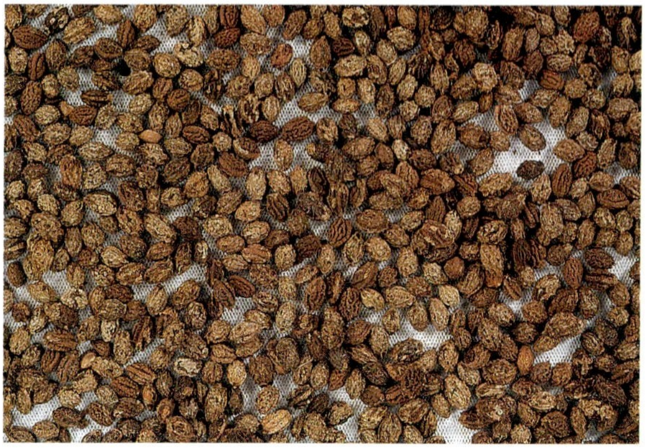

Plate 16 Carica papaya. (a) Fresh. (b) Dried.

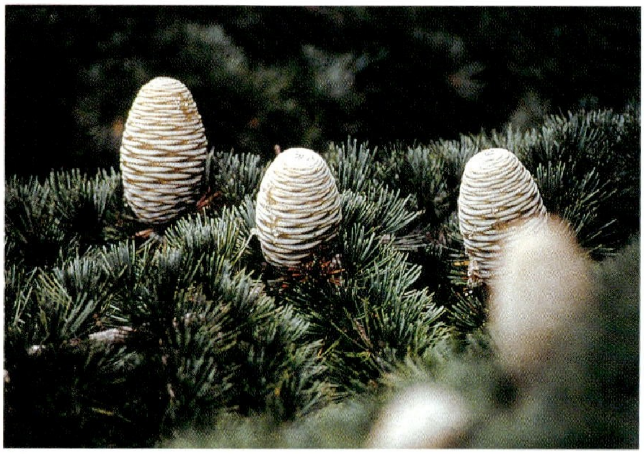
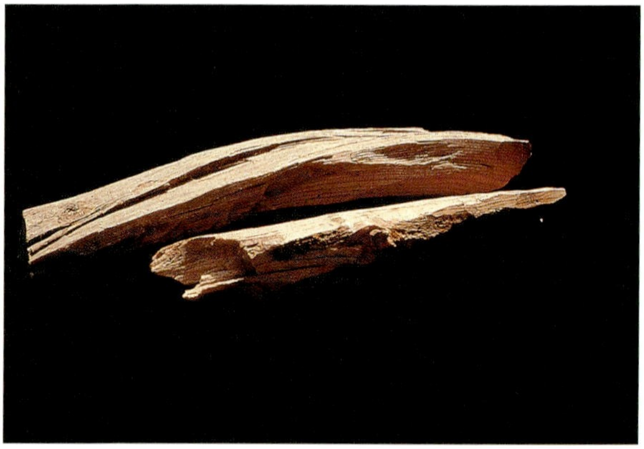

Plate 17 Cedrus deodara. (a) Fresh. (b) Dried.

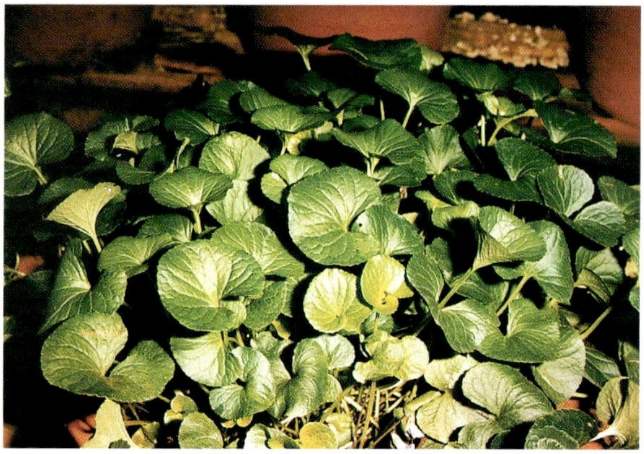
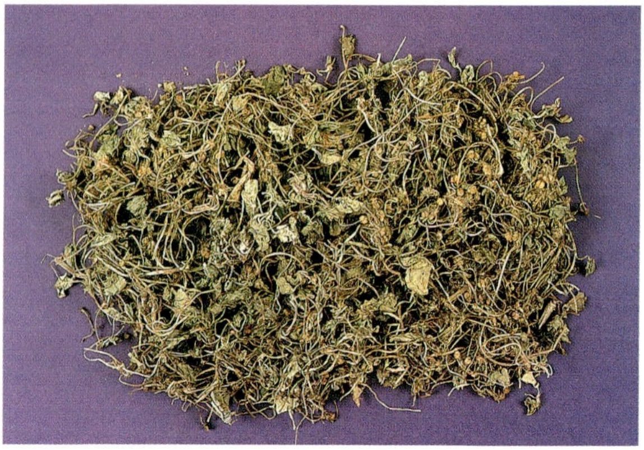

Plate 18 Centella asiatica. (a) Fresh. (b) Dried.

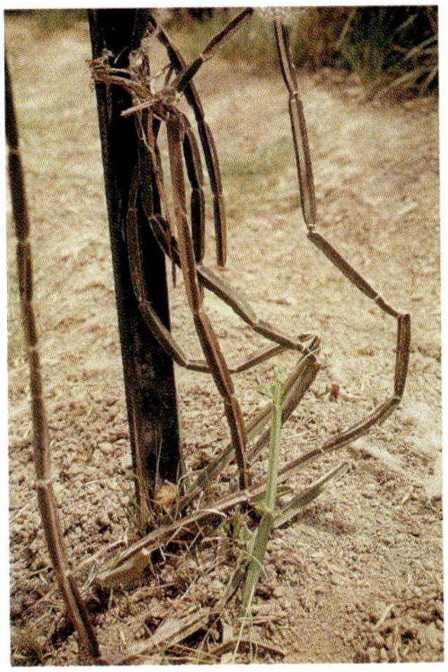
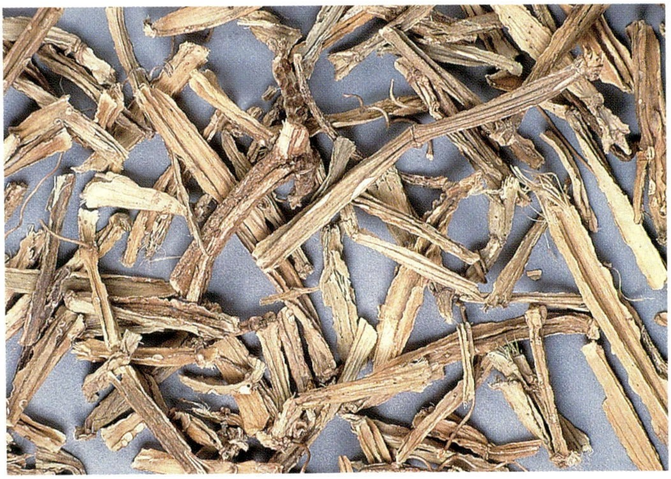

Plate 19 Cissus quadrangularis. (a) Fresh. (b) Dried.

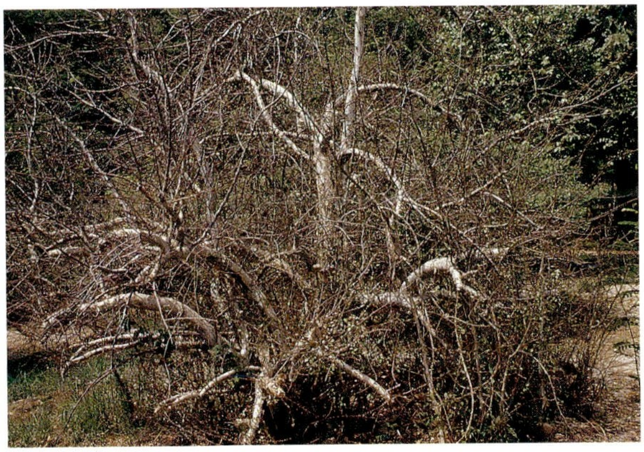
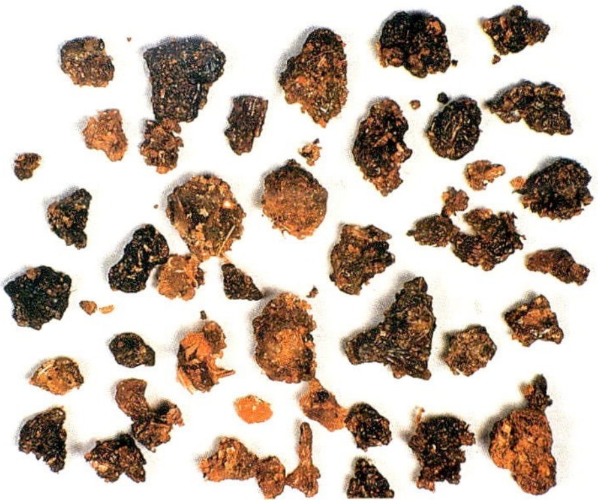

Plate 20 Commiphora mukul. (a) Fresh. (b) Dried.

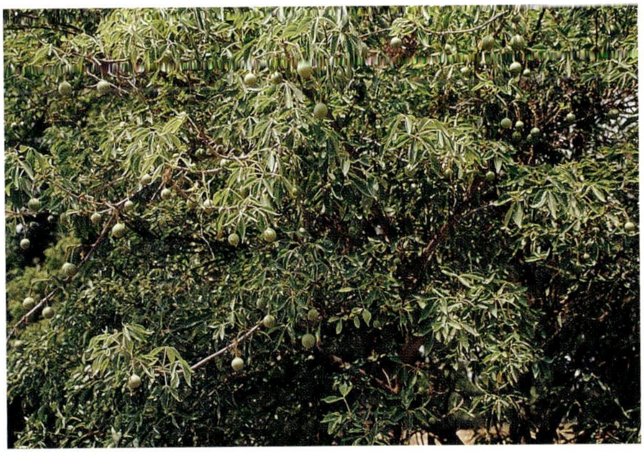
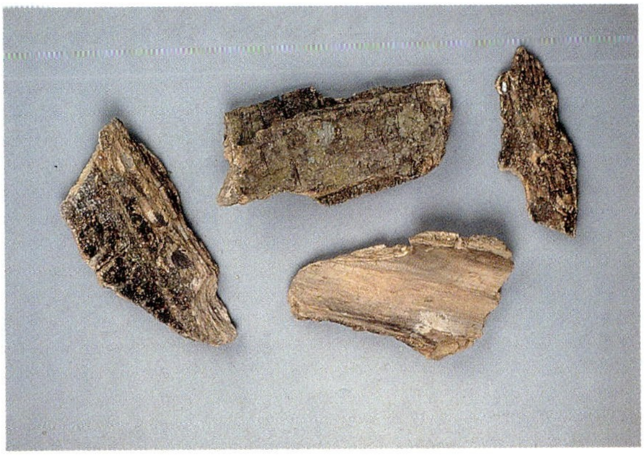

Plate 21 Crataeva nurvala. (a) Fresh. (b) Dried.

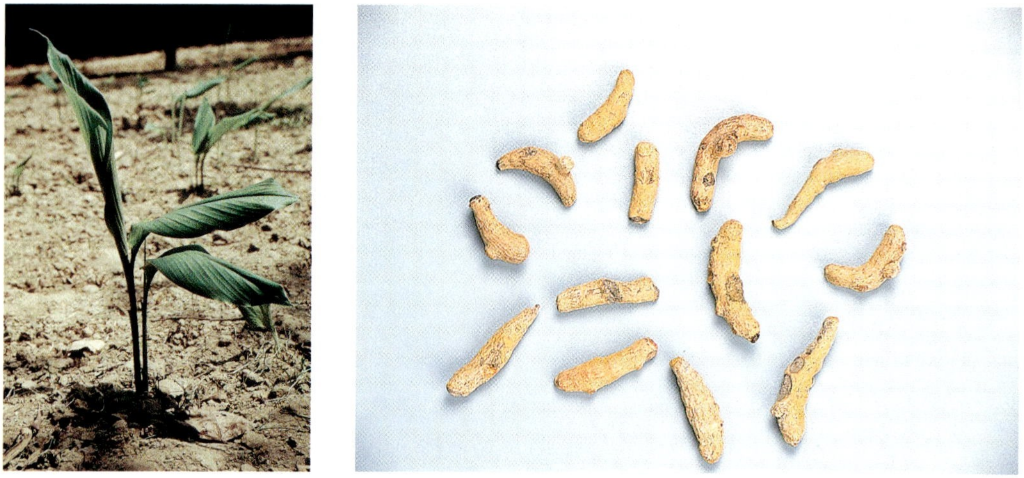

Plate 22 Curcuma longa. (a) Fresh. (b) Dried.

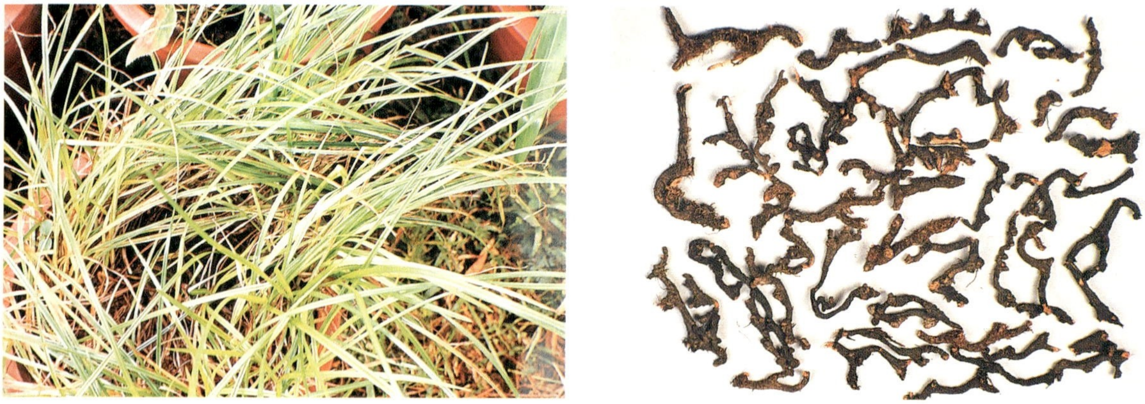

Plate 23 Cyperus rotundus. (a) Fresh. (b) Dried.

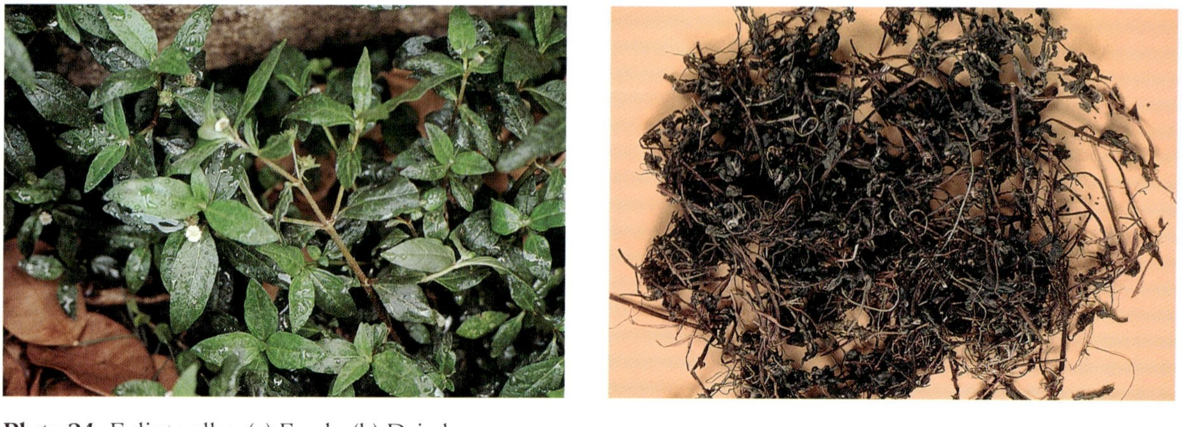

Plate 24 Eclipta alba. (a) Fresh. (b) Dried.

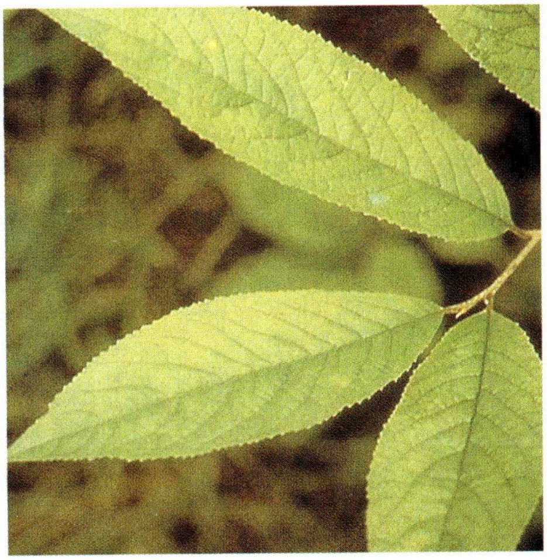

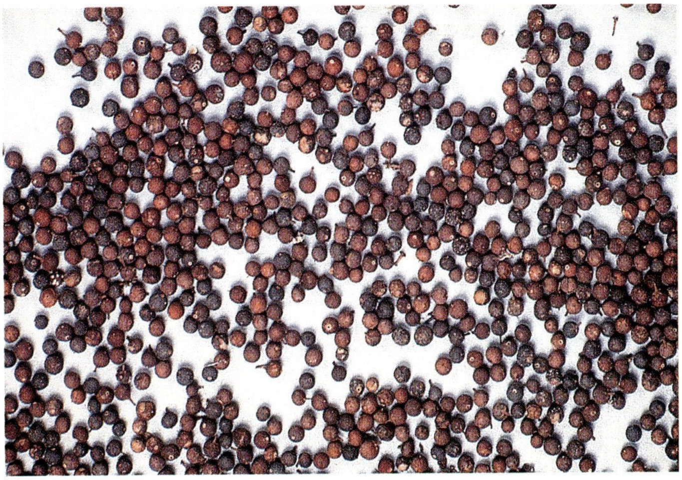

Plate 25 Embelia ribes. (a) Fresh. (b) Dried.

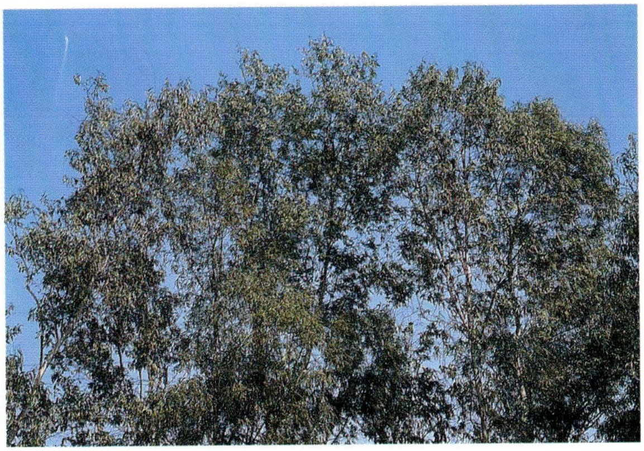

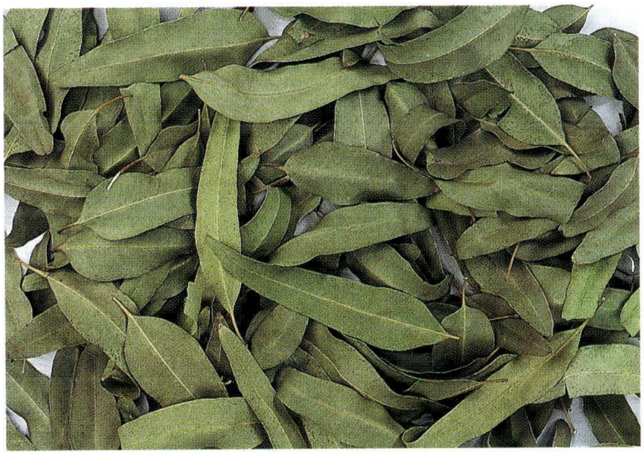

Plate 26 Eucalyptus globulus. (a) Fresh. (b) Dried.

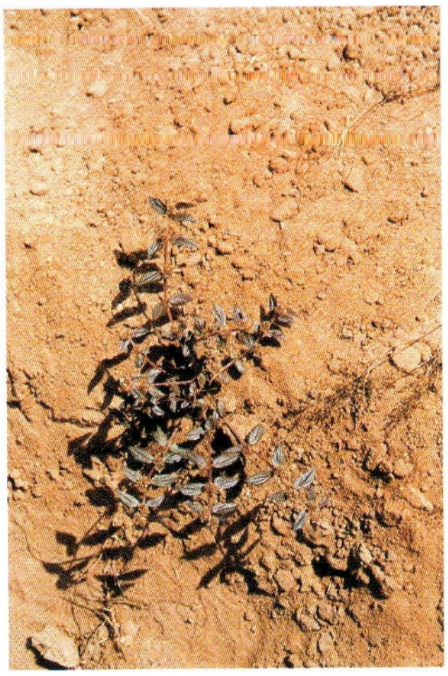

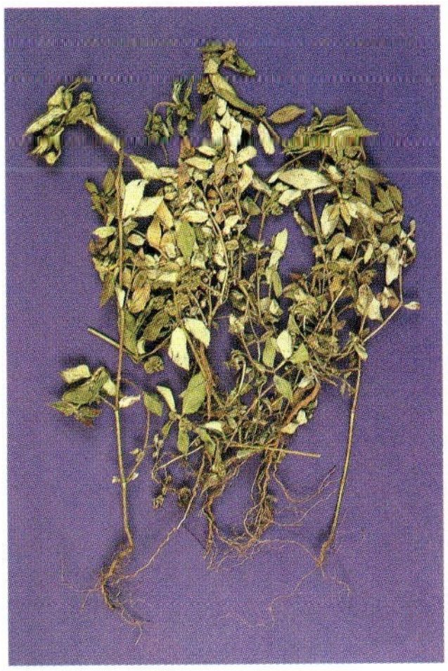

Plate 27 Euphorbia hirta. (a) Fresh. (b) Dried.

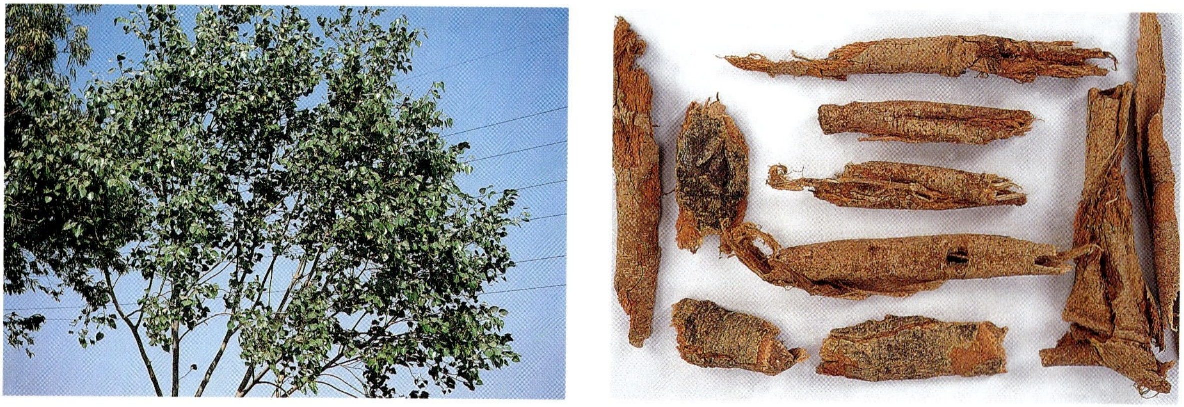

Plate 28 Ficus religiosa. (a) Fresh. (b) Dried.

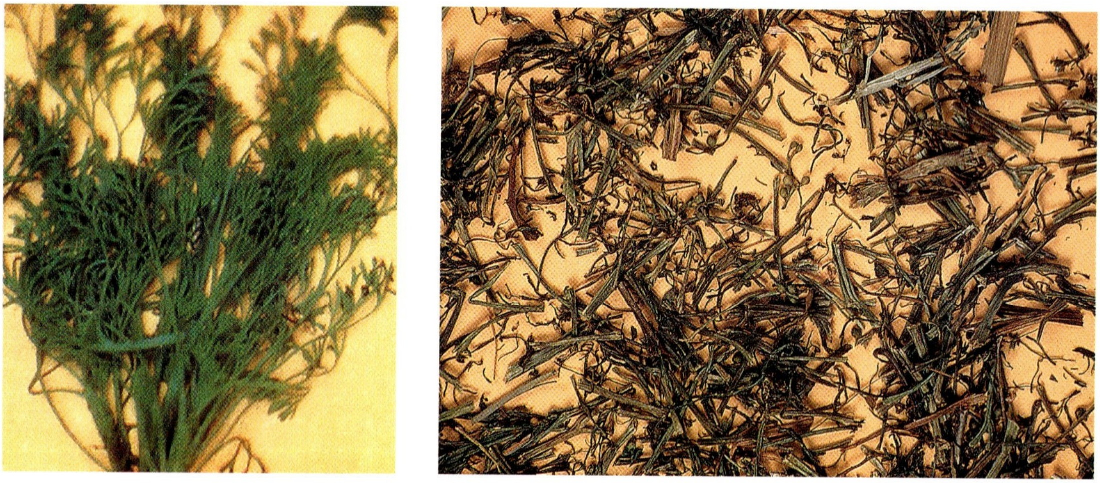

Plate 29 Fumaria indica. (a) Fresh. (b) Dried.

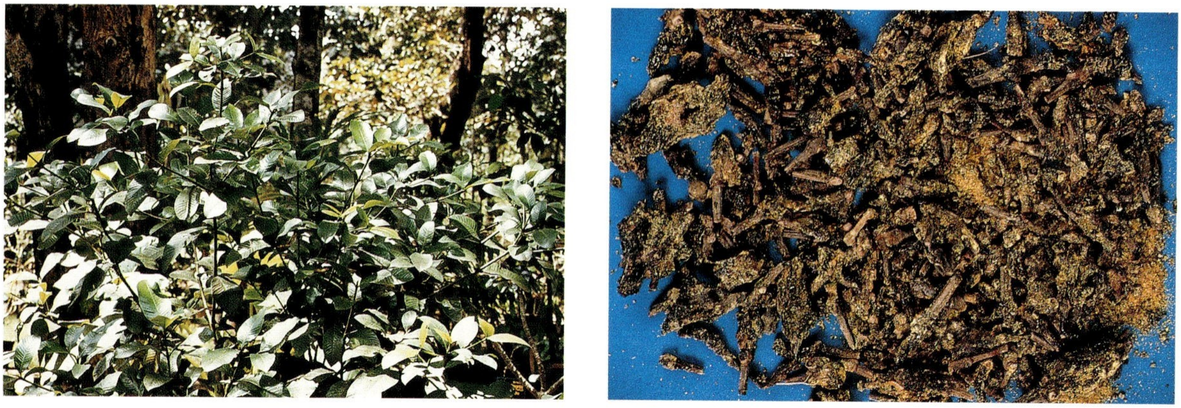

Plate 30 Gardenia gummifera. (a) Fresh. (b) Dried.

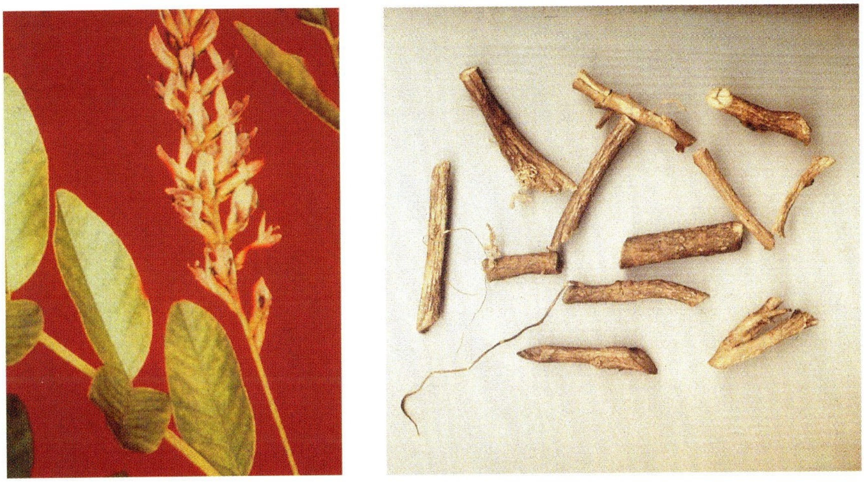

Plate 31 Glycyrrhiza glabra. (a) Fresh. (b) Dried.

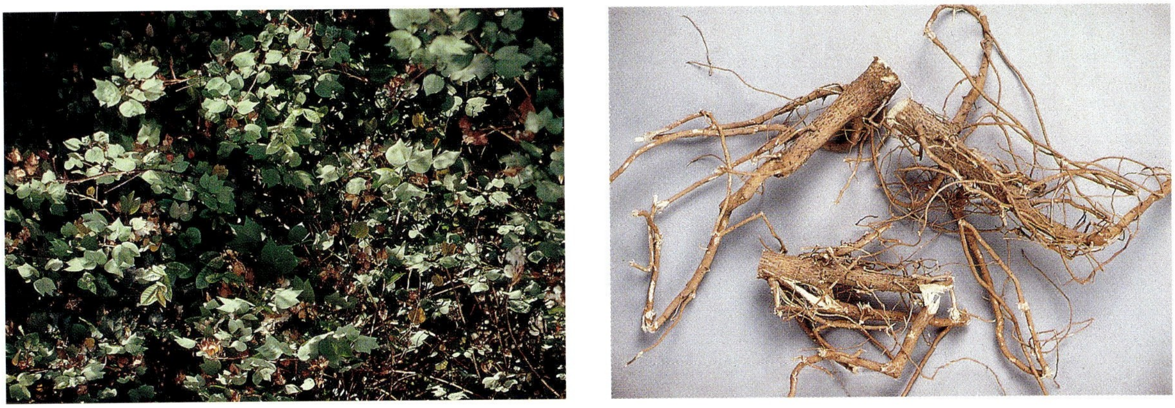

Plate 32 Gossypium herbaceum. (a) Fresh. (b) Dried.

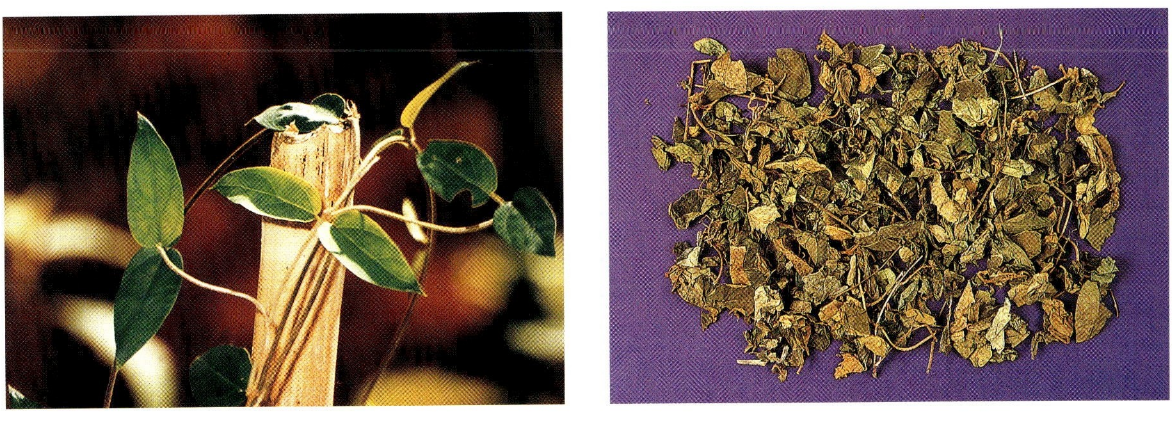

Plate 33 Gymnema sylvestre. (a) Fresh. (b) Dried.

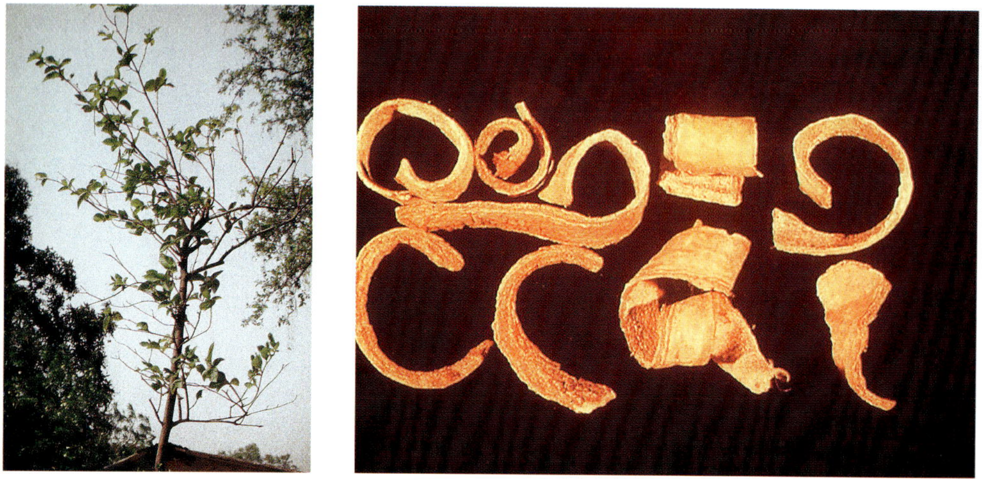

Plate 34 Holarrhena antidysenterica. (a) Fresh. (b) Dried.

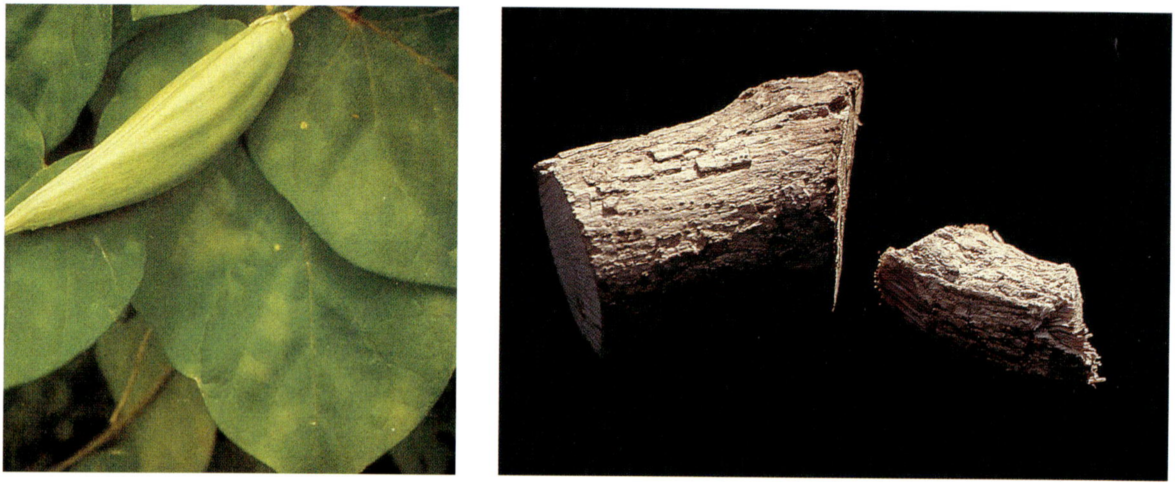

Plate 35 Leptadenia reticulata. (a) Fresh. (b) Dried.

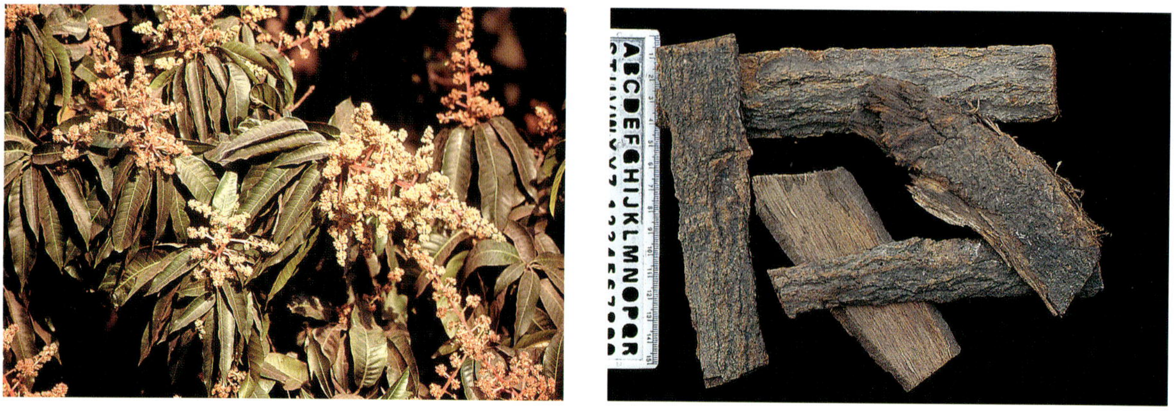

Plate 36 Mangifera indica. (a) Fresh. (b) Dried.

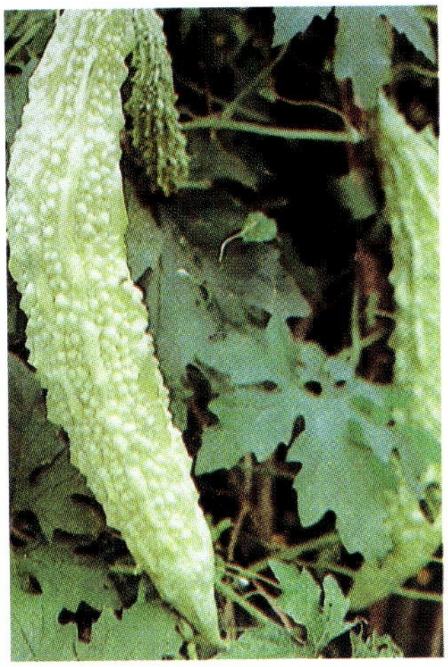
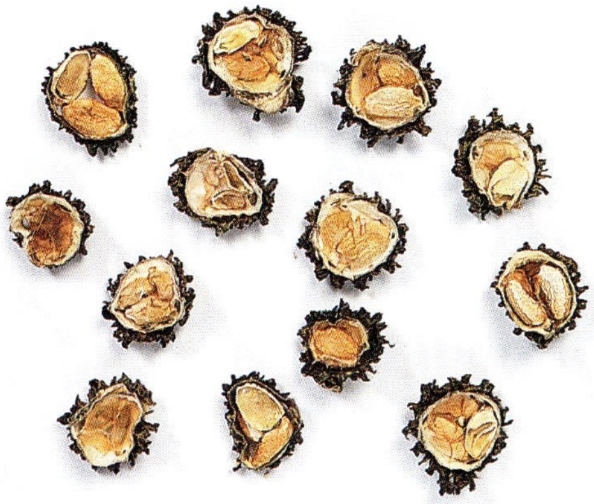

Plate 37 Momordica charantia. (a) Fresh. (b) Dried.

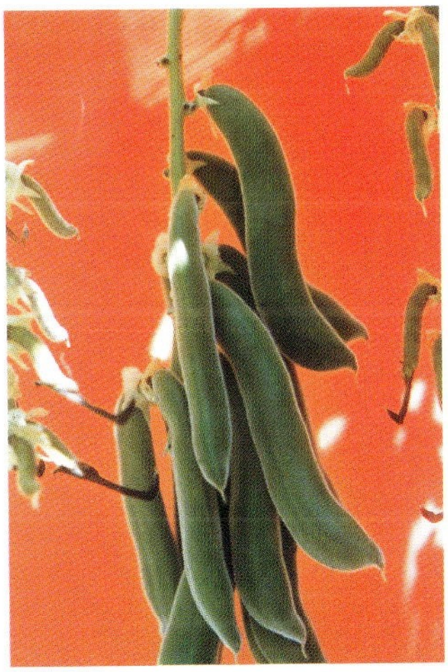
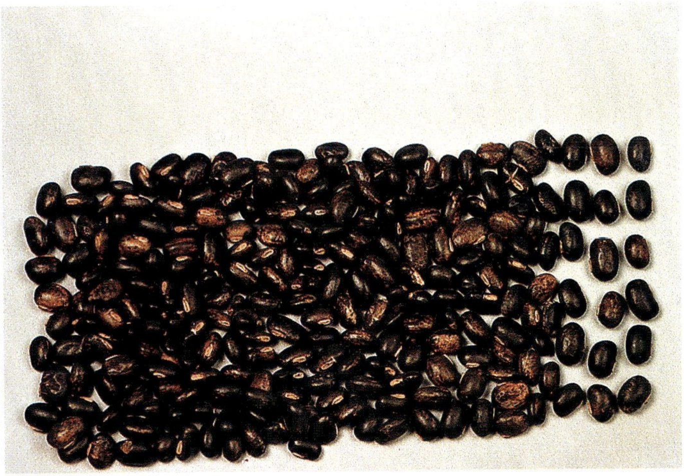

Plate 38 Mucuna pruriens. (a) Fresh. (b) Dried.

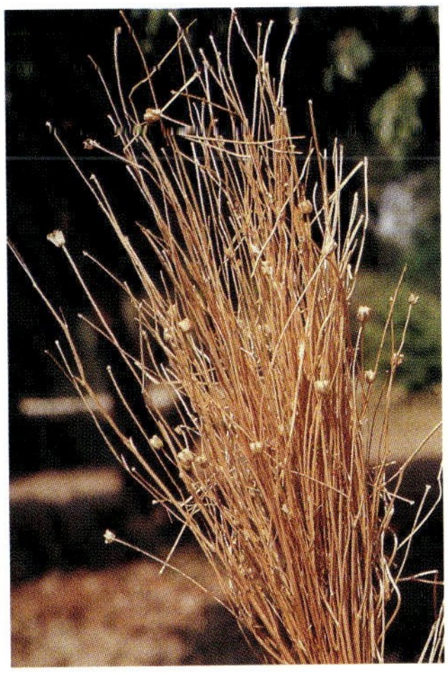
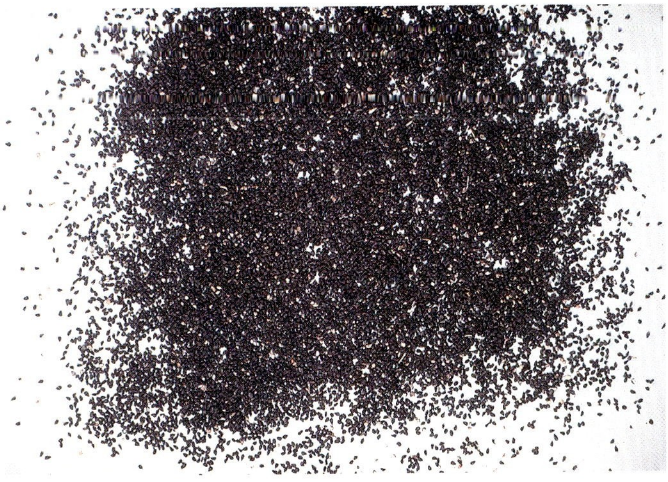

Plate 39 Nigella sativa. (a) Fresh. (b) Dried.

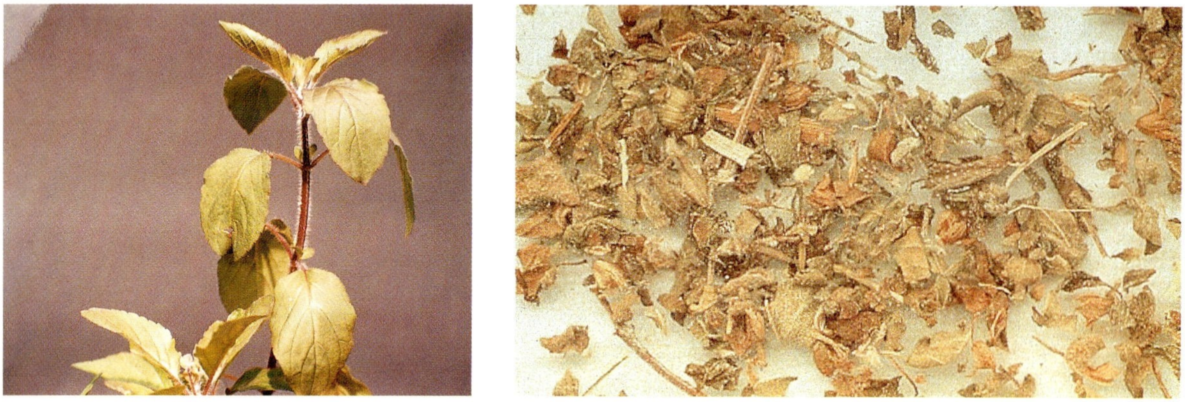

Plate 40 Ocimum sanctum. (a) Fresh. (b) Dried.

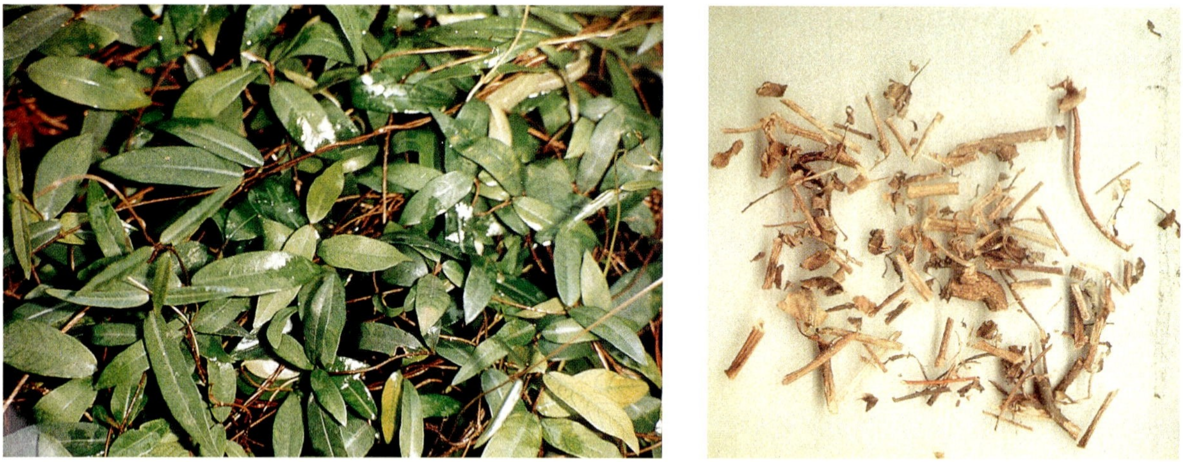

Plate 41 Paederia foetida. (a) Fresh. (b) Dried.

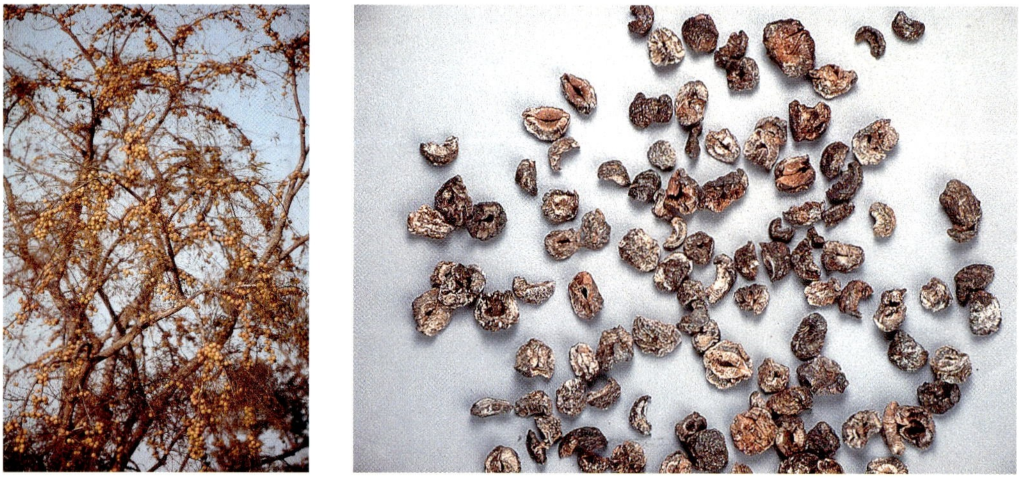

Plate 42 Phyllanthus emblica. (a) Fresh. (b) Dried.

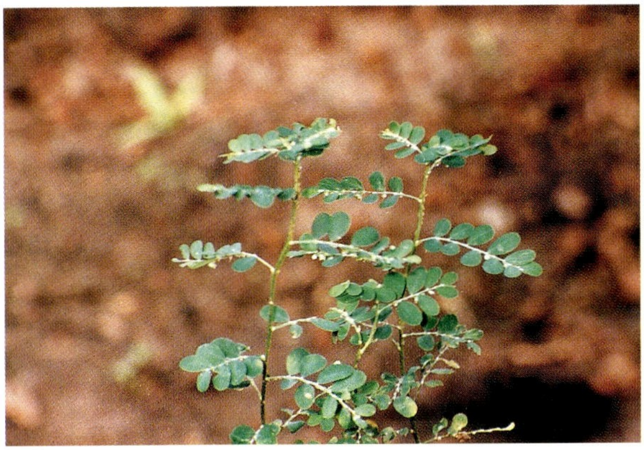
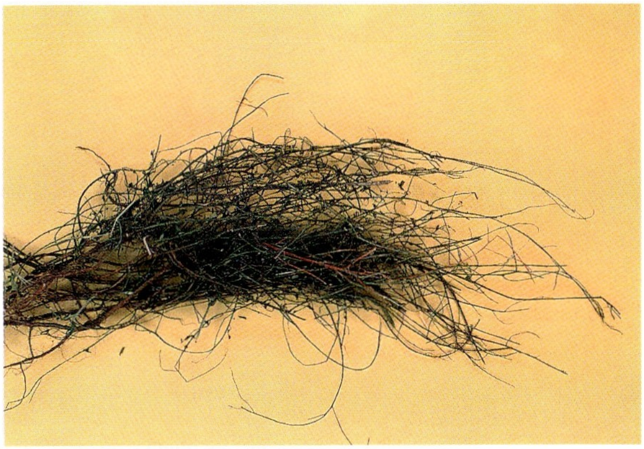

Plate 43 Phyllanthus niruri. (a) Fresh. (b) Dried.

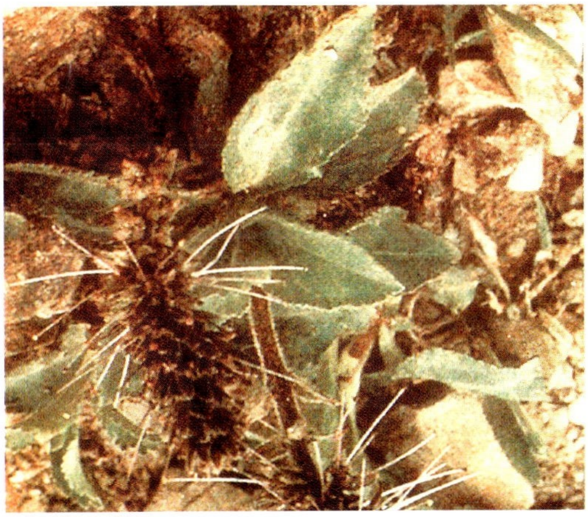
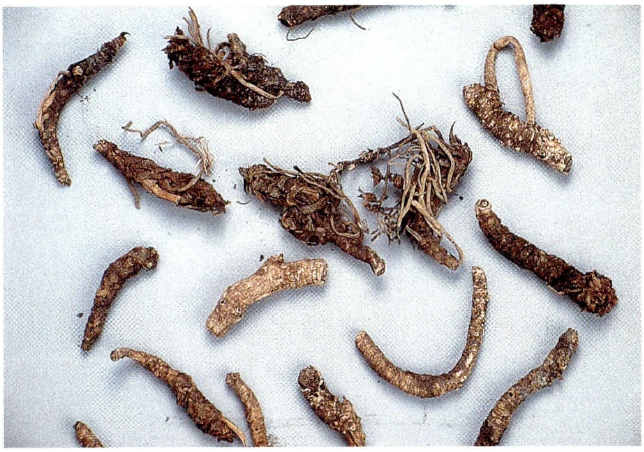

Plate 44 Picrorrhiza kurroa. (a) Fresh. (b) Dried.

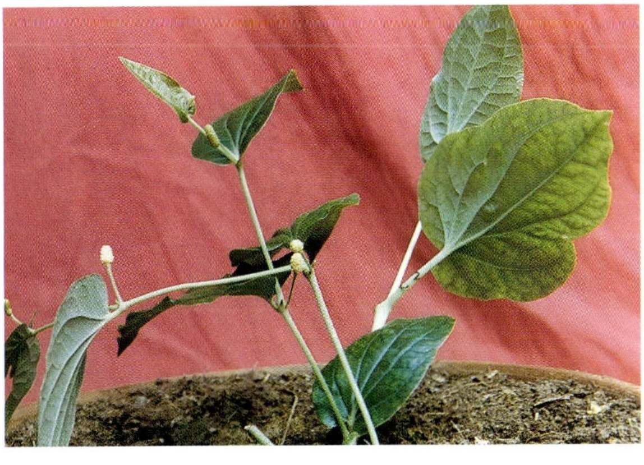
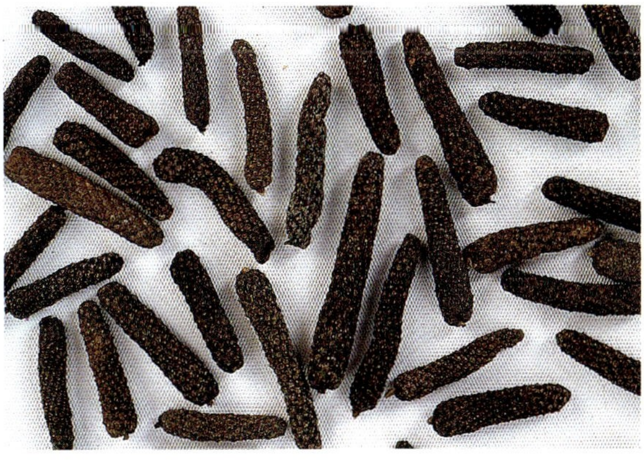

Plate 45 Piper longum. (a) Fresh. (b) Dried.

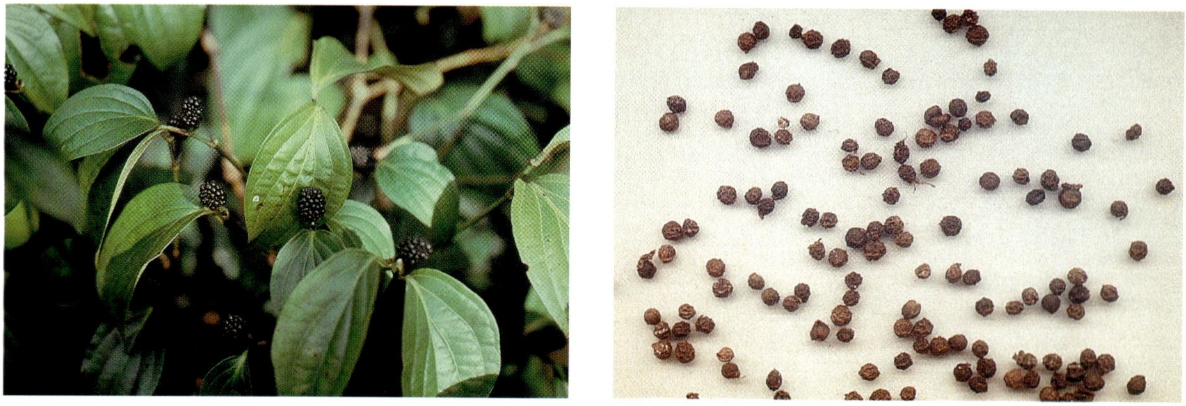

Plate 46 Piper nigrum. (a) Fresh. (b) Dried.

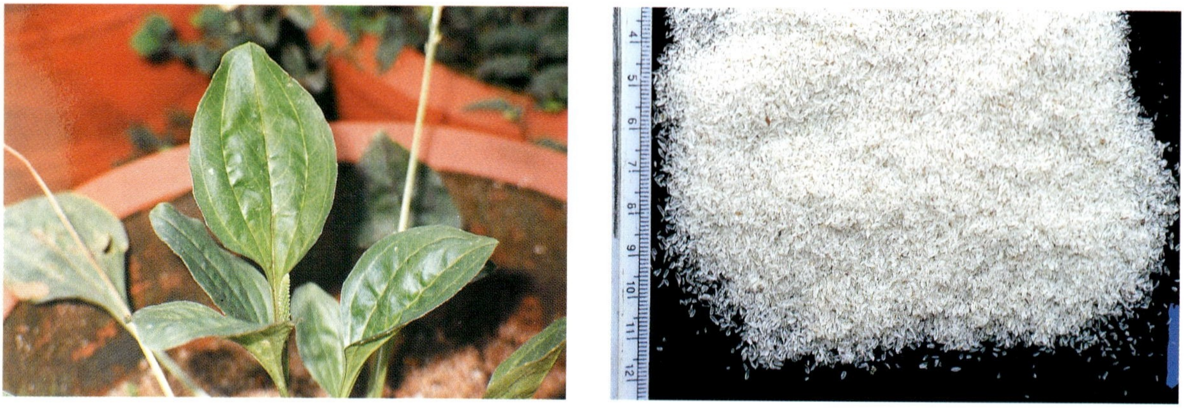

Plate 47 Plantago ovata. (a) Fresh. (b) Dried.

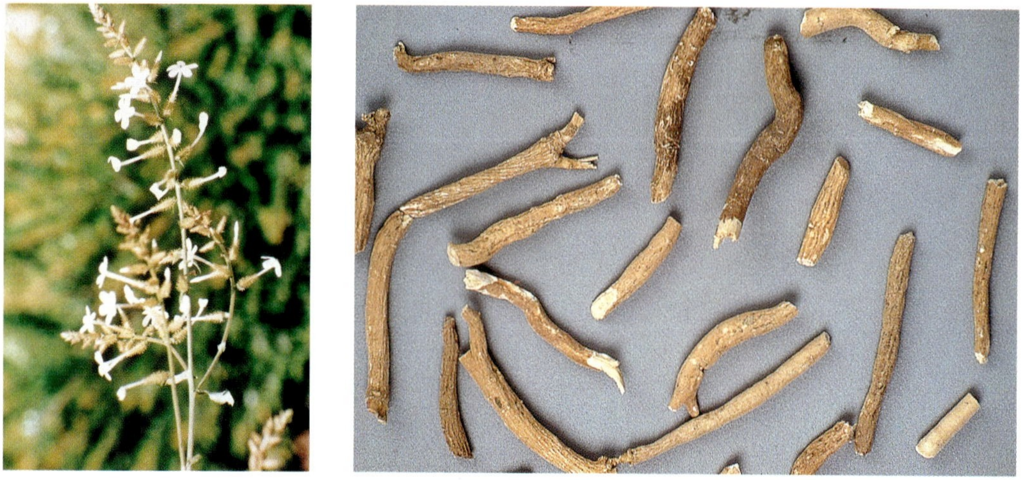

Plate 48 Plumbago zeylanica. (a) Fresh. (b) Dried.

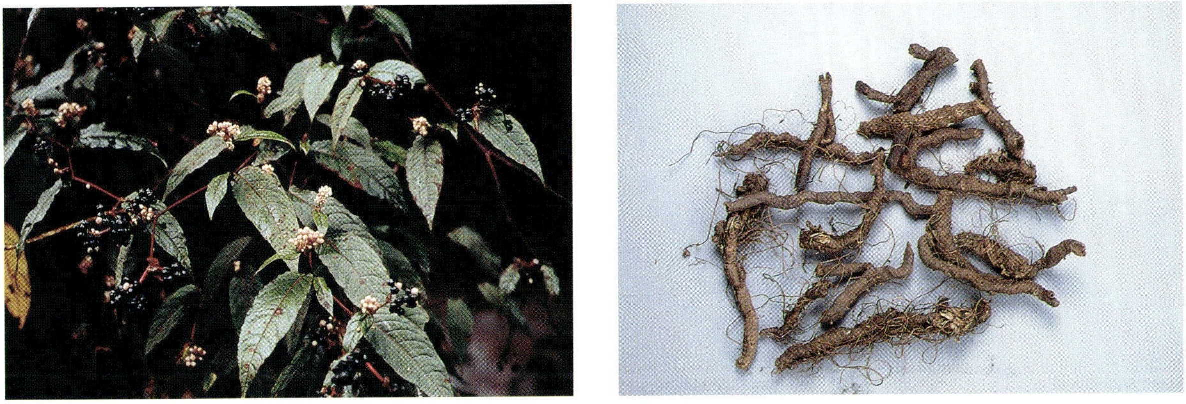

Plate 49 Polygonum aviculare. (a) Fresh. (b) Dried.

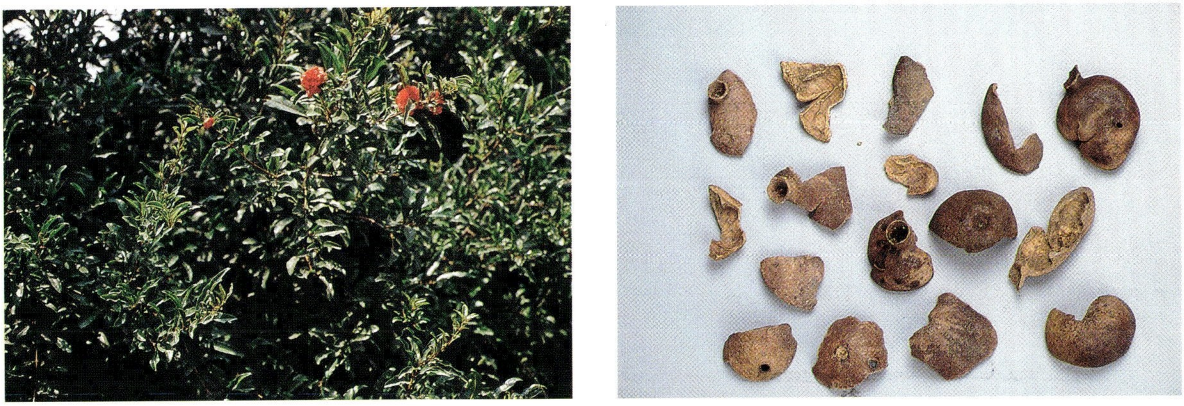

Plate 50 Punica granatum. (a) Fresh. (b) Dried.

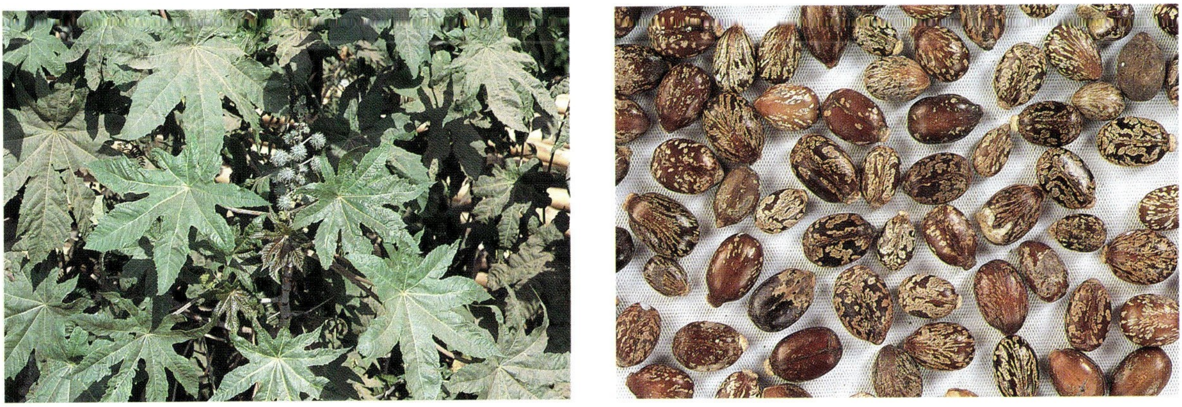

Plate 51 Ricinus communis. (a) Fresh. (b) Dried.

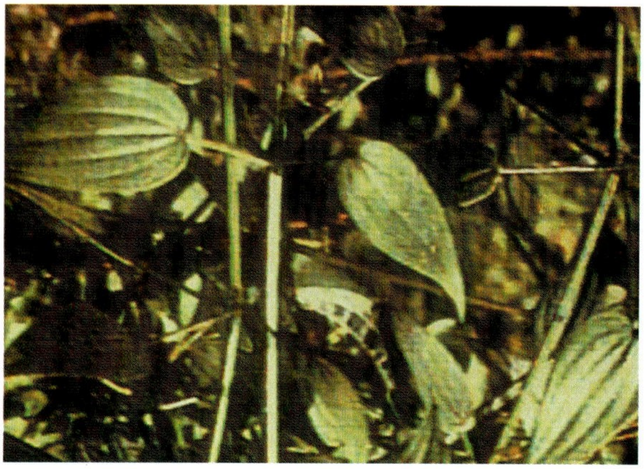
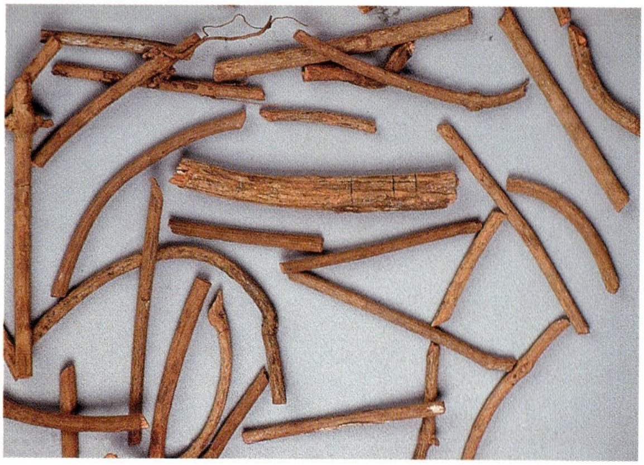

Plate 52 Rubia cordifolia. (a) Fresh. (b) Dried.

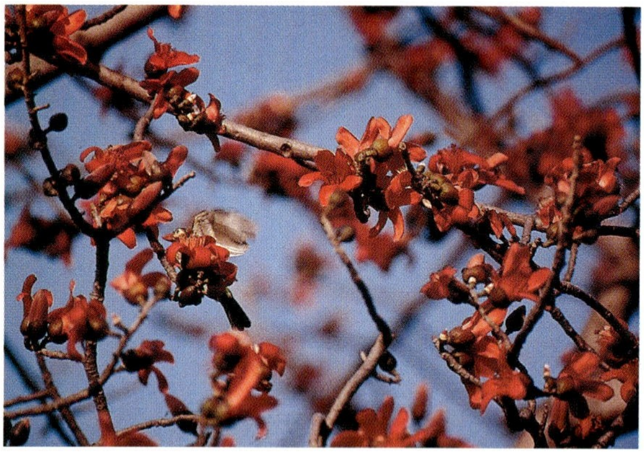
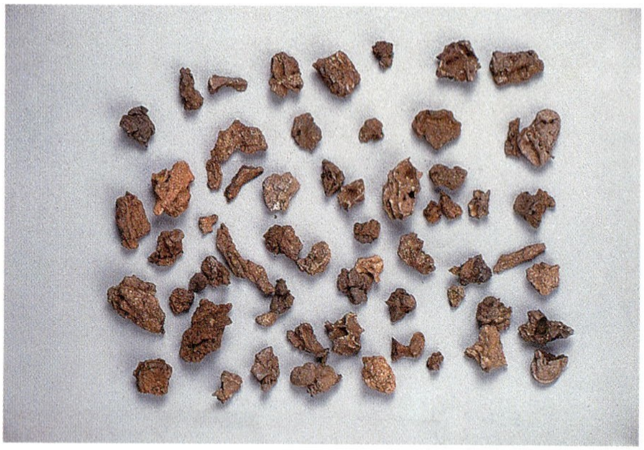

Plate 53 Salmalia malabarica. (a) Fresh. (b) Dried.

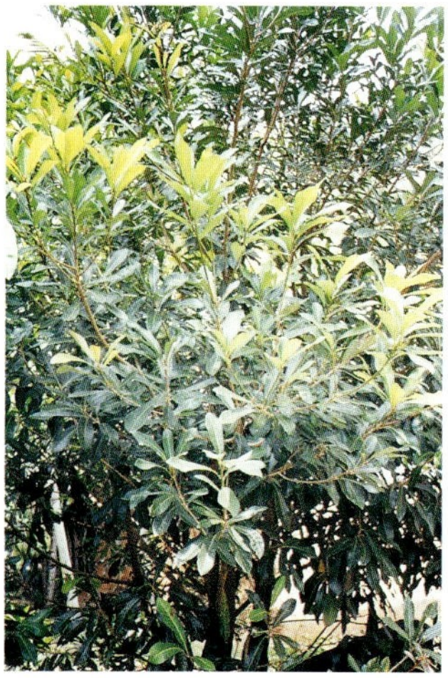
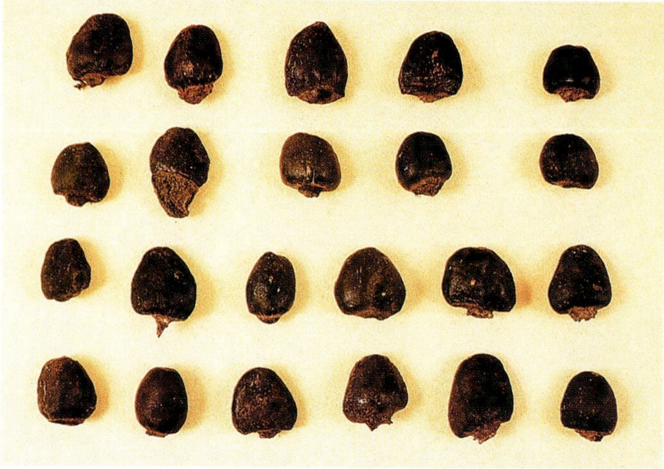

Plate 54 Semecarpus anacardium. (a) Fresh. (b) Dried.

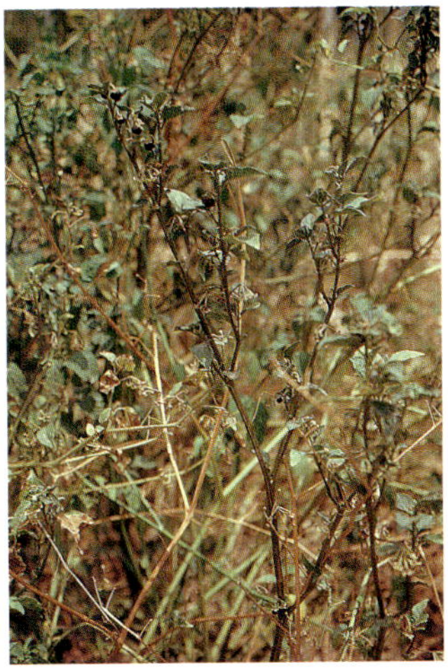
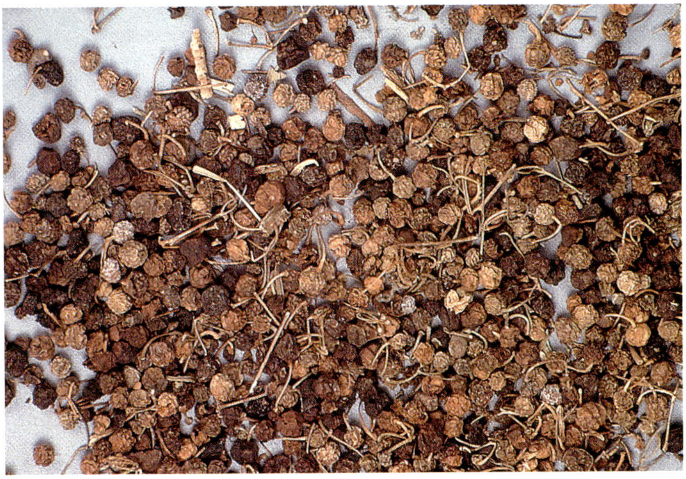

Plate 55 Solanum nigrum. (a) Fresh. (b) Dried.

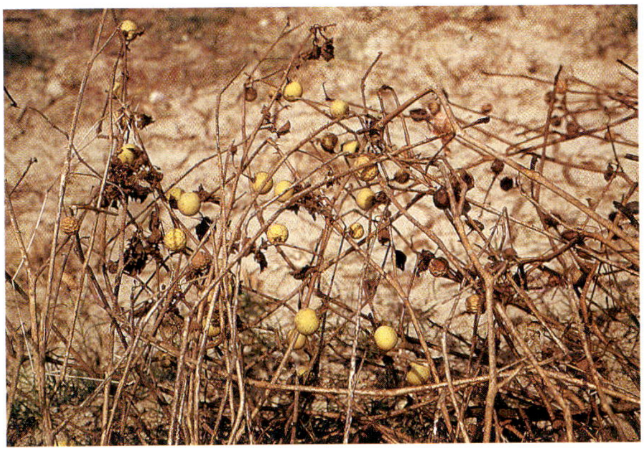
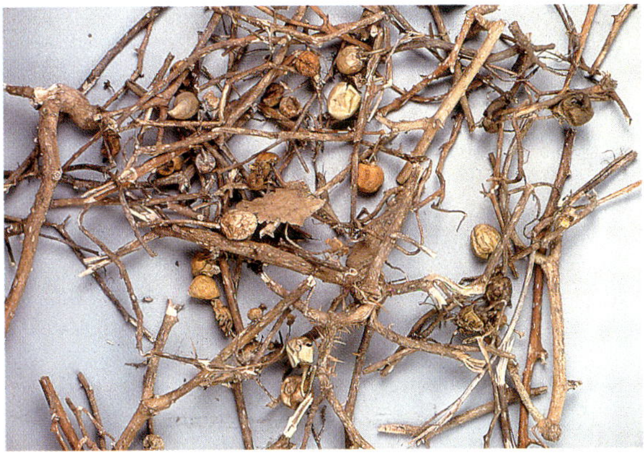

Plate 56 Solanum xanthocarpum. (a) Fresh. (b) Dried.

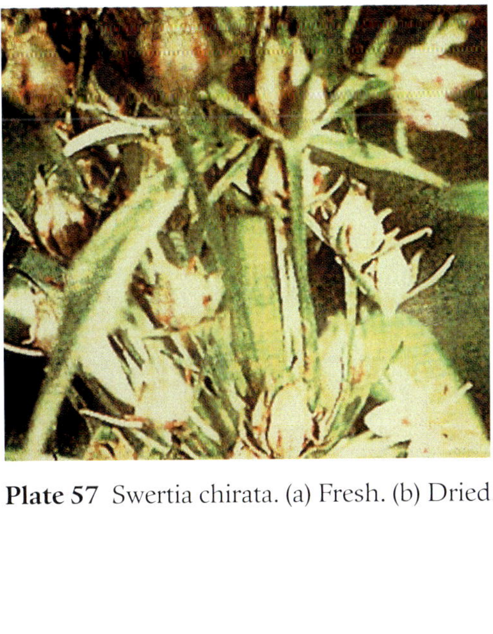
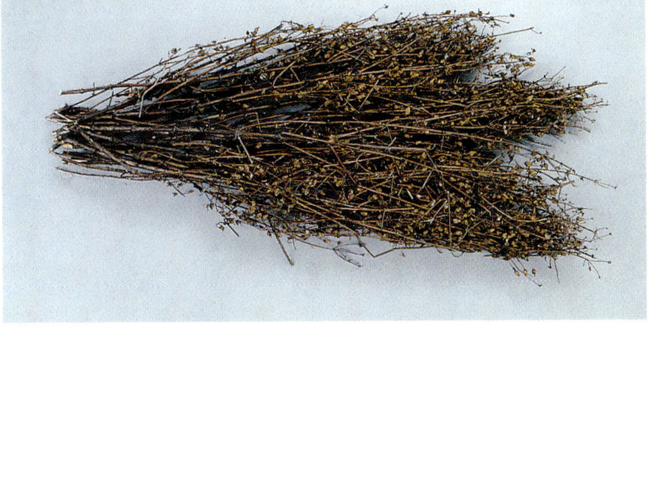

Plate 57 Swertia chirata. (a) Fresh. (b) Dried.

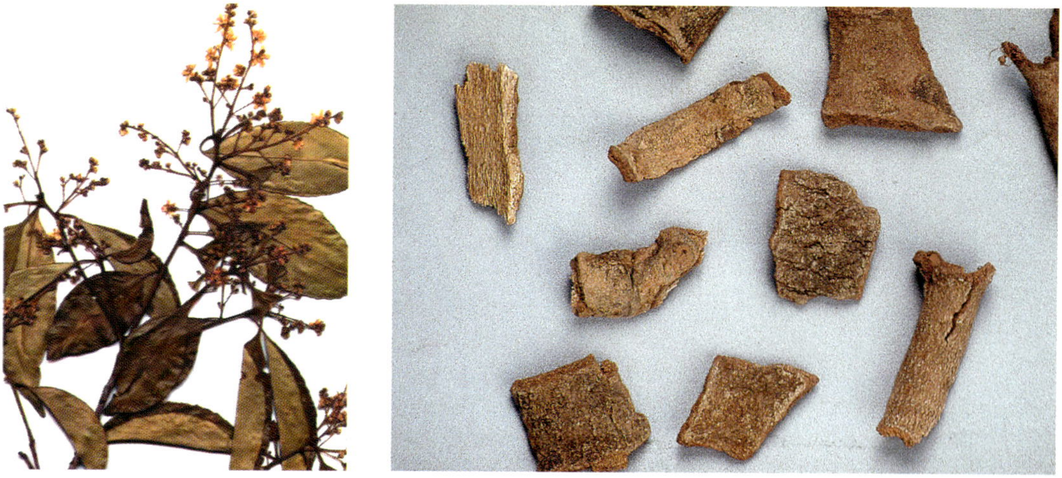

Plate 58 Symplocos racemosa. (a) Fresh. (b) Dried.

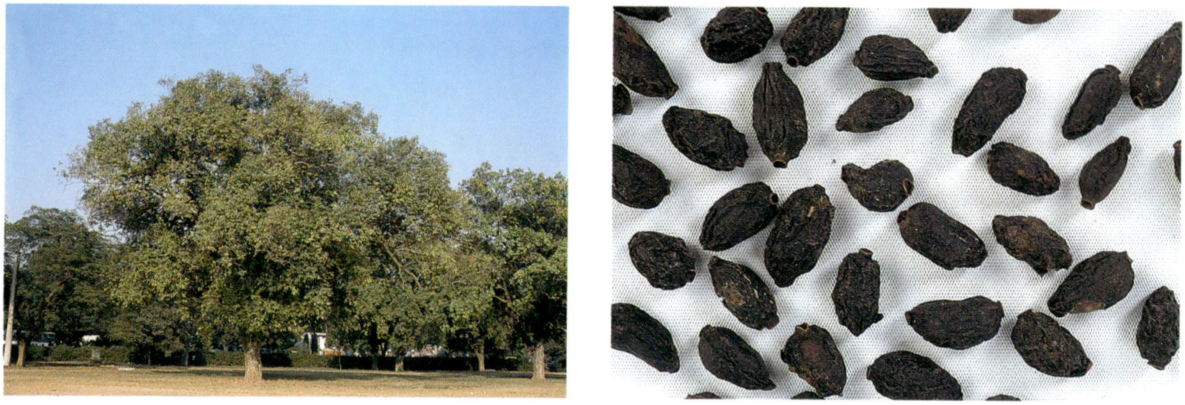

Plate 59 Syzygium cumini. (a) Fresh. (b) Dried.

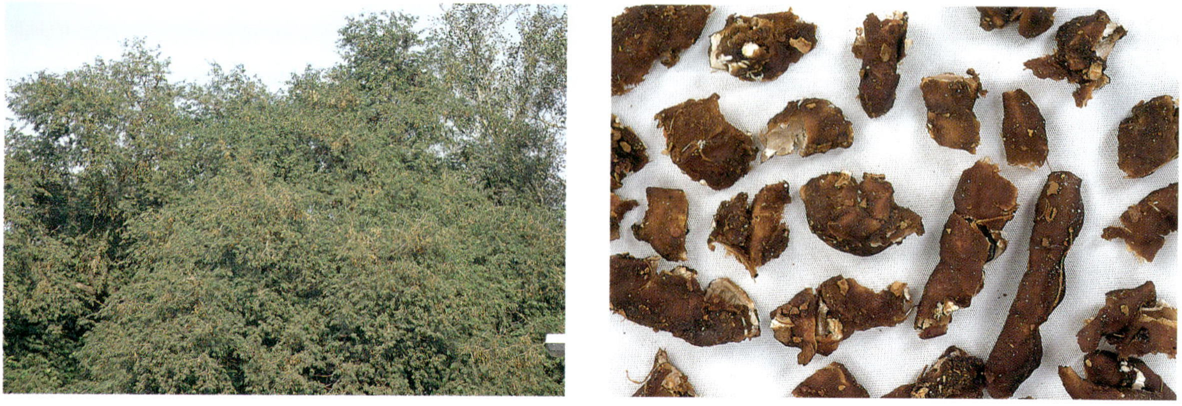

Plate 60 Tamarindus indica. (a) Fresh. (b) Dried.

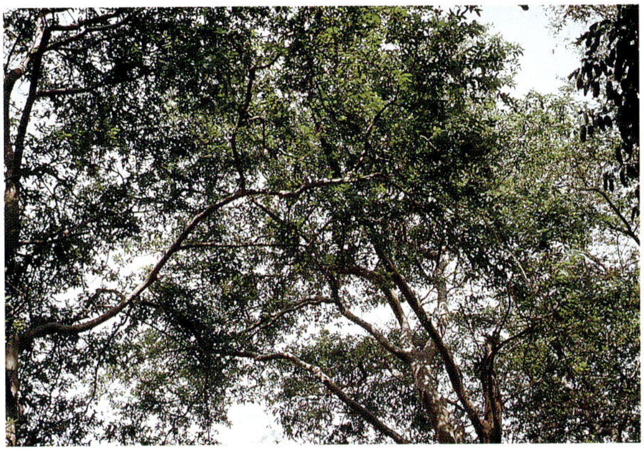

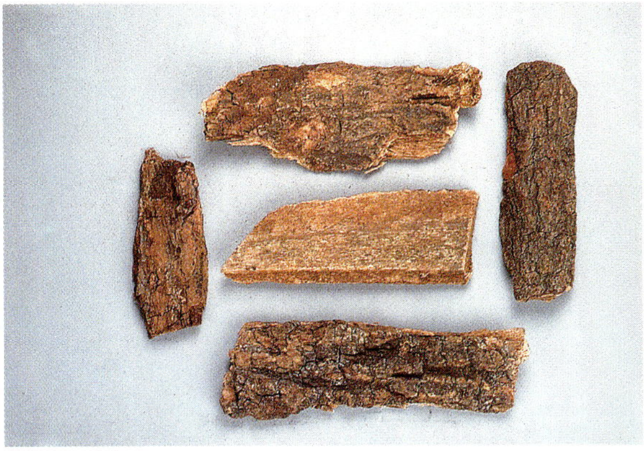

Plate 61 Terminalia arjuna. (a) Fresh. (b) Dried.

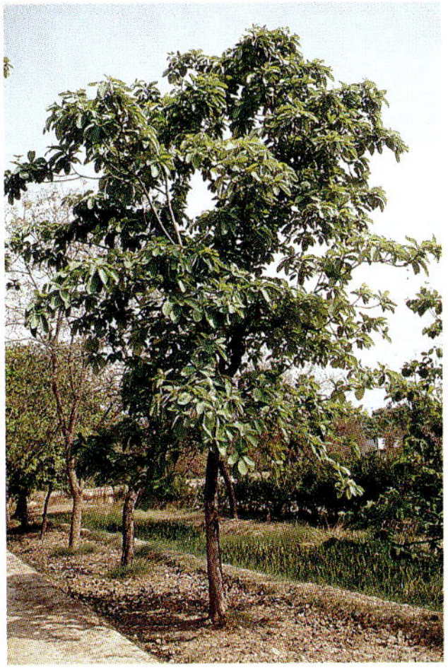

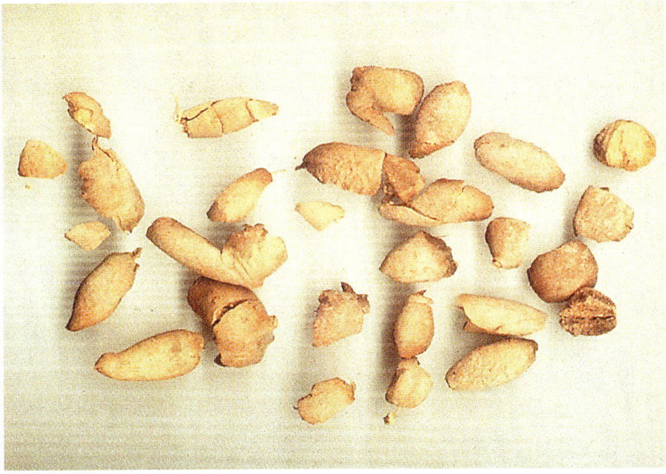

Plate 62 Terminalia belerica. (a) Fresh. (b) Dried.

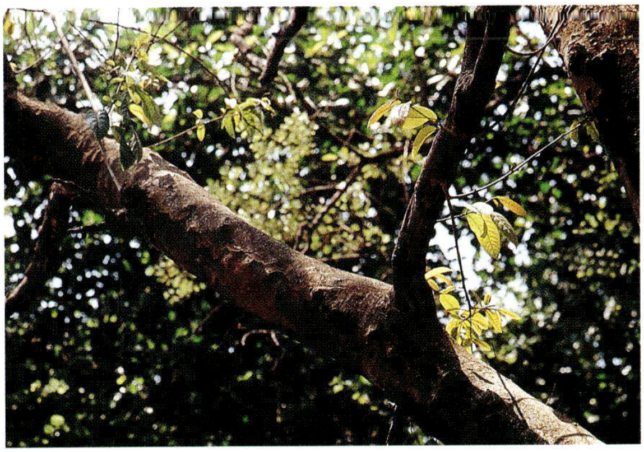

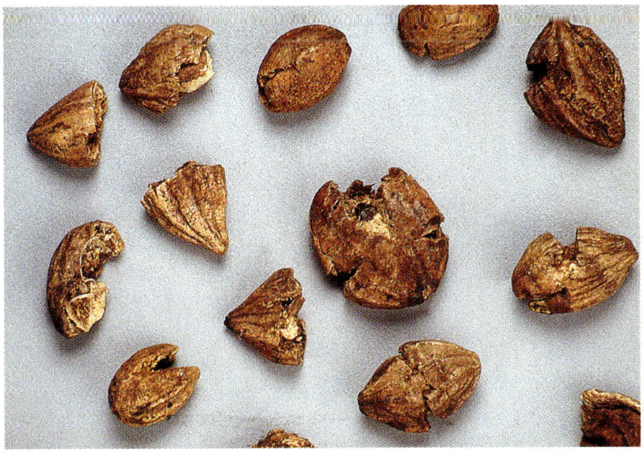

Plate 63 Terminalia chebula. (a) Fresh. (b) Dried.

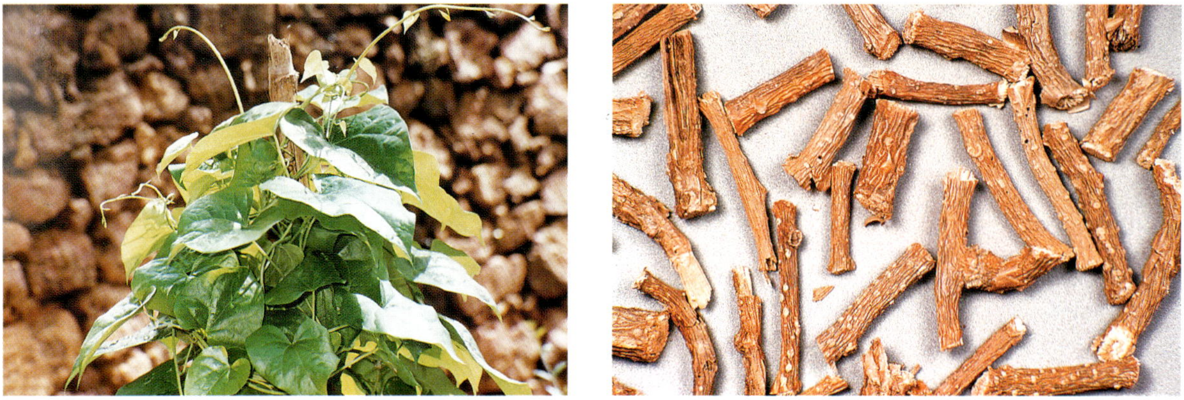

Plate 64 Tinospora cordifolia. (a) Fresh. (b) Dried.

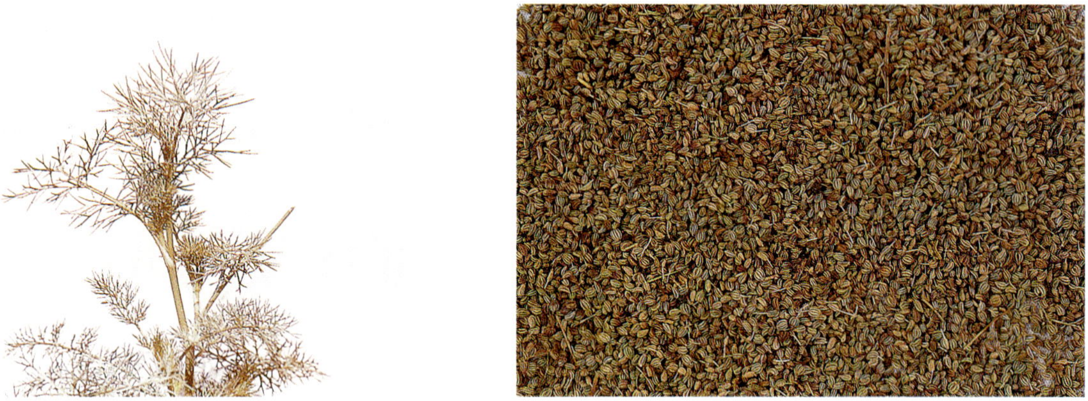

Plate 65 Trachyspermum ammi. (a) Fresh. (b) Dried.

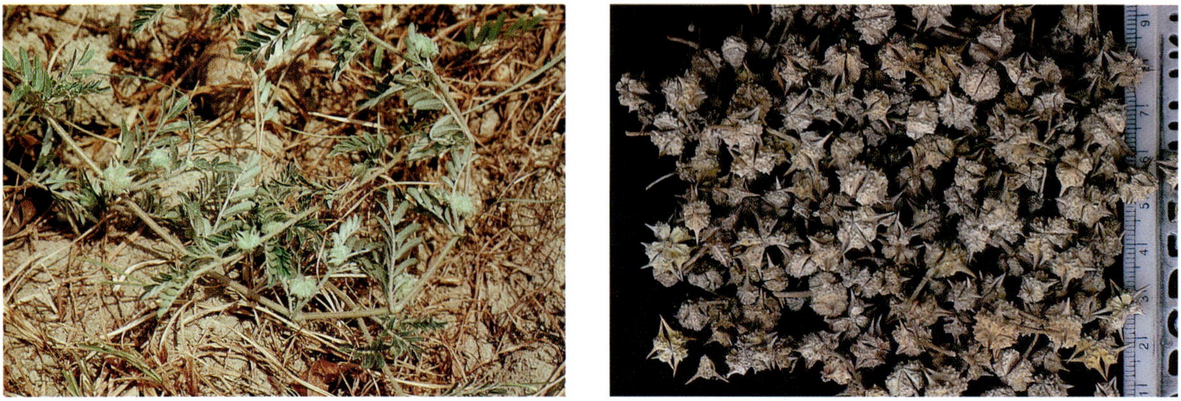

Plate 66 Tribulus terrestris. (a) Fresh. (b) Dried.

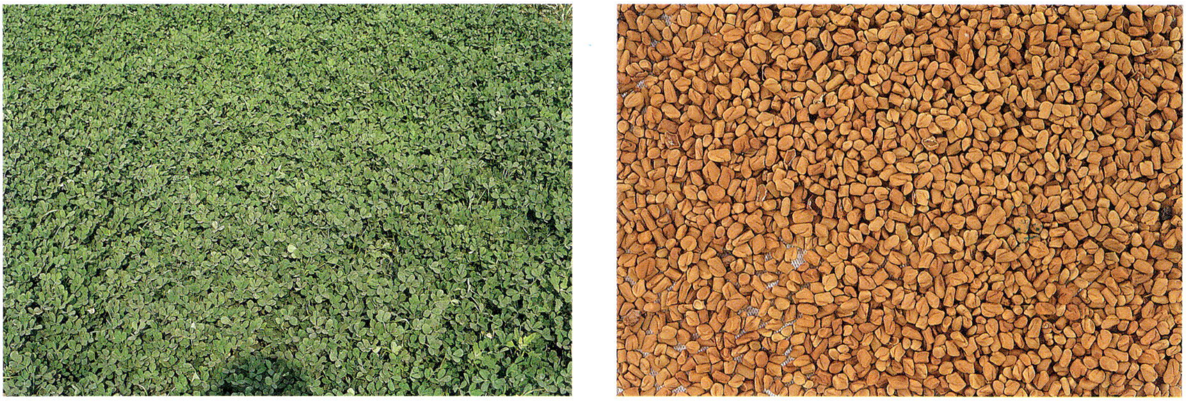

Plate 67 Trigonella foenum-graecum. (a) Fresh. (b) Dried.

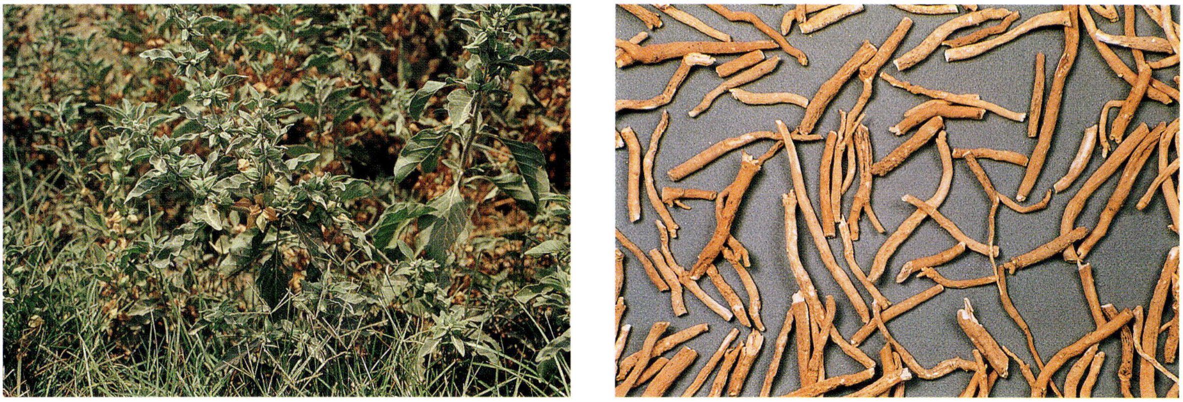

Plate 68 Withania somnifera. (a) Fresh. (b) Dried.

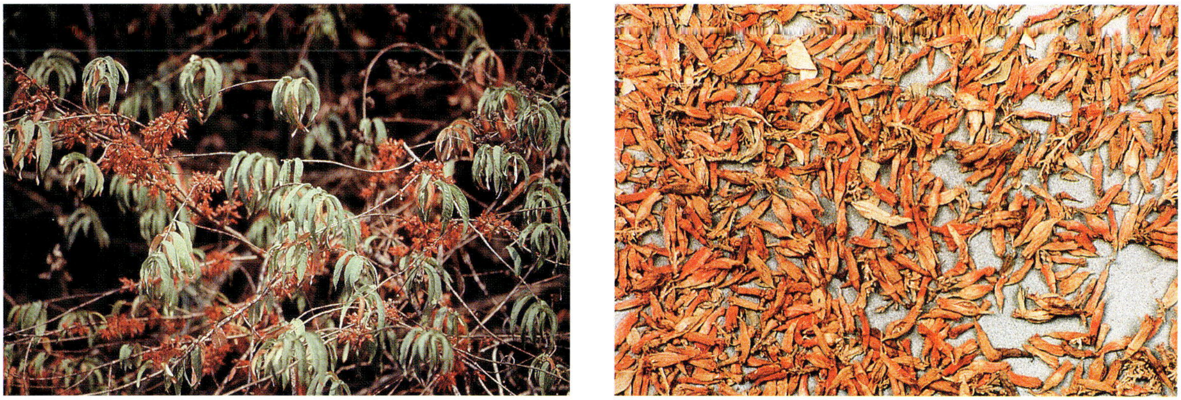

Plate 69 Woodfordia fruticosa. (a) Fresh. (b) Dried.

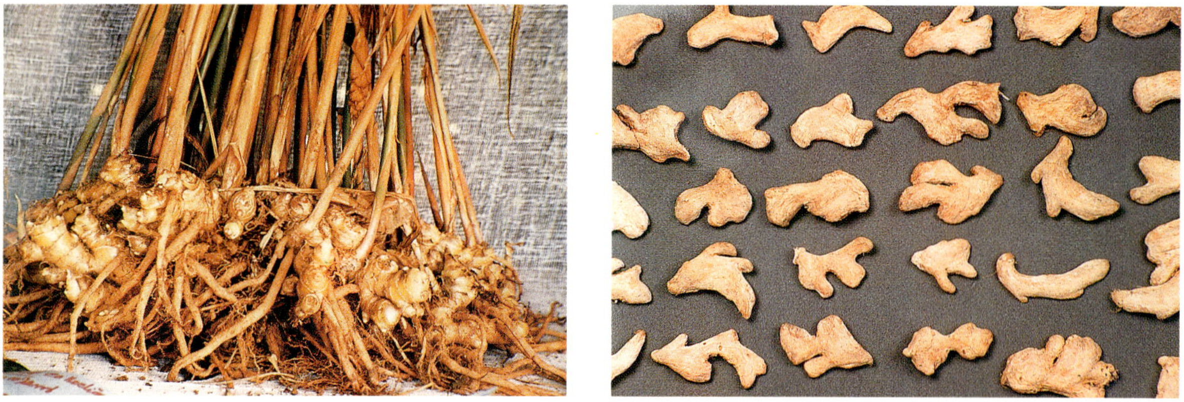

Plate 70 Zingiber officinale. (a) Fresh. (b) Dried.

Introduction: the principles of Ayurveda

Cosmic energy, consciousness and the five elements

Ayurveda encompasses philosophy, science and religion and is a system of knowledge applied to daily life. Man and the universe are interrelated in that cosmic energy manifests in all living and non-living things. In the very beginning, cosmic energy generated consciousness, which manifested as the five elements known as *Ether* (Space), *Air, Fire, Water* and *Earth*.These basic elements exist in all matter. Vasant Lad (see Further Reading) illustrates this using water as an example. The solid state, ice, is an expression of the Earth element; heat (Fire) converts it to a liquid (Water element) and eventually to a gas (Air) which dissipates into the Ether. Therefore all have been manifest in one substance. Since cosmic energy originally gave rise to the five elements, thus energy and matter are one. These ideas predate those of Einstein by several thousand years!

The three humours or *tridosha*

The five basic elements further manifest in the human body as three basic principles or humours known as *tridosha*. The three humours are known as *vata*, *pitta* and *kapha* (individually called *doshas*) and govern all biological, psychological and physiopathological functions of the body, mind and consciousness. The concept of *tridosha* is unique to Ayurveda although the idea of a balance of forces being responsible for health is common to many holistic therapies. The primary requirement to treat a disease is to understand these three humours and their relationships. A slight similarity can be drawn with the Greek system of medicine where the Humour theory holds that the body consists of four fluids, (phlegm, blood, yellow bile and black bile) and disease occurs when these are out of balance. Similarly, when the *tridosha* work in harmony and function in a balanced manner the result is good nourishment and feelings of well-being in an individual. However, in cases of imbalance and disharmony within or between them, the result is disease or poor health.

The *tridosha* monitor the creation, maintenance and destruction of bodily tissue and the elimination of waste products from the body. They are also responsible for psychological phenomena, including emotions such as fear, anger and greed, and also for the more complicated human emotions such as understanding, compassion and love. Hence, the *tridosha* are the foundation of the psychosomatic existence of man.

The three forces, *vata*, *pitta* and *kapha* constitute the 'tripod' of life. They have been redefined by modern scientists as the equilibrium, balance and coordination of the three vital body forces: the central nervous system corresponds to *vata*, the endocrine system to *pitta*, and the immune axis to *kapha*, operating with positive and negative feedback mechanisms. The balance of *vata*, *pitta* and *kapha* is neither geometric nor arithmetic; rather, it is a biological equilibrium.

Vata, derived from Air and Ether, is a

principle of movement. It may be characterised as a form of subtle energy that governs biological movement and thus comprises all phenomena of the central and sympathetic nervous system. It also engenders all subtle changes in the metabolism. *Vata* governs breathing, blinking of the eyelids, movement in muscles and tissues, pulsation of the heart, all expansion and contraction of the body, the movement of cytoplasm, cell membranes and single impulses in nerve cells.

Pitta derives from Fire and Water and signifies bodily heat. It is the manifestation of energy in living organisms. It helps in the regulation of thermogenesis or heat production, metabolism regarding the process of digestion and assimilation, the formation of blood and tissue, activities of the endocrine glands, secretions and excretions. It controls body temperature, skin coloration, lustre of the eyes, intelligence and understanding.

Kapha derives from Water and Earth. It binds the tissues, providing the material for physical structure, and is responsible for biological strength and natural resistance, controlling regulatory functions and the formation of preservative fluids such as mucus and synovial fluid, giving structural integrity and fulfilling a protective role. *Kapha* lubricates joints, provides moisture to skin, helps to heal wounds, fills spaces in the body, gives biological strength, vigour and stability, supports memory retention, gives energy to the heart and lungs and maintains immunity.

Together, the *tridosha* govern all metabolic activities: anabolism (*kapha*), catabolism (*vata*) and metabolism (*pitta*). Excess *pitta* disturbs metabolism, excess *kapha* increases the rate of anabolism and excess *vata* increases catabolism. When anabolism is greater than catabolism there is an increased rate of growth and repair of organs and tissues, so when *vata* is out of balance, the metabolism will be disturbed, resulting in excess catabolism and creating emaciation. In Ayurveda, a state of health exists when the digestive Fire (*agni*) is in a balanced condition, the *tridosha* are in equilibrium and the three waste products (urine, faeces and sweat) are produced at normal levels. The senses are then functioning normally and the body, mind and consciousness are harmoniously working as one. When the balance of any of these systems is disturbed the disease process begins (see Table 1).

The human constitution or *Prakruti*

The constitution includes physical, mental and personality traits and is determined by the balance of the *tridosha* at the time of conception. As such, it depends on the parents, the time of day and year and external factors and could therefore be considered to incorporate genetics, astrology and the environment. People are divided into *vata*, *pitta* and *kapha* groups based on their constitutions, although it is common for a person to possess characteristics of more than one *dosha*.

People of *vata* constitution are generally physically underdeveloped with cold, dry or cracked skin and poor circulation. They may be very tall or short, with a thin frame and poor muscle development. *Vata* people crave sweet, sour and salty tastes, like hot drinks, sleep less than other types and are easily fatigued. Psychologically they are creative and alert, with a quick understanding but short memory and a tendency to suffer from anxiety.

People with *pitta* constitution are of medium height with moderate muscle development. Their skin is warm and soft and the complexion fair. Physiologically, *pitta* people have a good appetite and digestion, a natural craving for sweet, bitter and astringent tastes and enjoy cold drinks. They are natural leaders and are intelligent and sharp.

Kapha people have well-developed bodies but a tendency to put on weight, their skin is lustrous and oily and the hair thick and dark. They crave pungent, bitter or astringent foods and have regular appetites. Psychologically they tend to be calm and tolerant.

The 20 attributes or *Gunas*

Ayurveda also encompasses a subtle science of attributes or qualities called *gunas*. The great Ayurvedic physician Caraka found that all organic and inorganic substances, as well as all thoughts and actions, have definite attributes. The attributes contain potential energy while the actions express kinetic energy. These are closely related since the potential energy of the attributes eventually becomes action or kinetic energy. According to Ayurveda, there are 20 basic attributes, with the following properties.

Guru: heavy	**Laghu**: light
Manda: slow	**Tikshna**: sharp
Shita: cold	**Ushna**: hot
Snigdha: oily	**Ruksha**: dry
Slakshna: slimy	**Khara**: rough
Sandra: dense	**Drava**: liquid
Mrudu: soft	**Kathina**: hard
Sthira: static	**Chala**: mobile
Sukshma: subtle	**Sthula**: gross
Avila: cloudy	**Vishada**: clear

Vata, *pitta* and *kapha* each have their own attributes and substances having similar attributes will tend to aggravate the related bodily humour by the concept of 'like increases like'. On the mental and astral planes, there are also three attributes (also called *gunas*), which correspond to the three humours that make up the physical constitutions. In the Ayurvedic system of medicine, these three attributes provide the basis for distinctions in human temperament and individual differences and psychological and moral dispositions. The three basic attributes are *satva*, *rajas* and *tamas*. *Satva* expresses essence, understanding, purity, clarity, compassion and love. *Rajas* implies movement, aggressiveness and extroversion. The *rajas* mind operates on a sensual level. *Tamas* manifests in ignorance, inertia, heaviness and dullness.

The seven tissues or *Dhatus*

The human body consists of seven basic tissues (constructing elements) or *dhatus*. When there is an imbalance of *vata*, *pitta* and *kapha*, they are directly affected. The health of the *dhatus* can be maintained by taking steps to keep the *tridosha* in balance through a proper diet, exercise and rejuvenation programme. The *dhatus* correspond to the following tissues.

Rasa: plasma

Rakta: blood

Mamsa: muscle

Meda: adipose tissue
Asthi: bone
Majja: bone marrow and nerve tissue
Shukra and Artav: semen and reproductive tissue

Treatment of disease

The concepts governing the pharmacology, therapeutics and food preparation in Ayurveda are based on the action and reaction of the attributes to and upon one another. Through understanding these attributes, balance of the *tridosha* may be maintained. Diseases and disorders ascribed to *vata*, *pitta* and *kapha* are treated with the aid of food and medicines which are characteristic of but opposite to the attributes. *Vata* disorders are therefore corrected with the aid of sweet, sour, saline and warm substances (*madhur*, *amla* and *lavana*). The excitement (or aggravation) of *pitta* is controlled by sweet, bitter, astringent and cooling herbs (*madhur*, *katu* and *kashaya*) and *kapha* disorders are corrected with pungent, bitter, astringent and dry herbs (*tikta*, *katu* and *kashaya*). All of these are essential for the proper functioning of the organism and are obtained through food and medicinal herbs. Correcting the deviation from the natural proportion of the *tridosha* treats the disease by restoring the balance of the three humours and thus the state of health. The use of herbs in achieving this objective is of fundamental importance (see Table 2).

Preparation of medicines

Medicines made from plants are administered in various forms.

- **Juices**: the juice is cold pressed from plants.
- **Powders**: completely dried plants are powdered.
- **Cold infusions** (*sita kasaya*): the herb is steeped in water overnight, then filtered.
- **Hot infusions** (*phanta*): the herbs are steeped in hot water for a few minutes and strained.
- **Decoctions** (*kvatha*): the herb is boiled in water and the volume reduced.
- **Pastes** (*kalka*): the herb is ground to a paste or poultice.
- **Milk preparations** (*ksira paka*): fresh pulp or paste obtained from plant materials converted into a semisolid dosage form (with a consistency of a jam or jelly) using sugar syrup. The product is then topped with a powder of flavouring herbs.
- **Linctuses or jams** (*avaleha*): the plant or extract is preserved in syrup.
- **Medicated oils or ghee** (*sneha*): the extract or paste is added to the oily base and heated gently to extract the constituents.
- **Alcoholic tinctures** (*arava* or *arista*): the water extract of herbal composition is obtained by cold infusion or by decoction. Jaggery (unrefined cane sugar) is added as a nutrient for fermentation. Dried flowers of forest-flame bush (*woodfordia fruticosa*, qv) are added. Since these flowers contain yeast, fermentation is carried out naturally and alcohol is produced within the formulation.
- **Pills or tablets** (*vati* or *gutika*): soft or dry extracts are compressed into pills or tablets.
- **Scale preparations** (*parpati*): molten metals are poured onto leaves so that a flake is formed.
- **Sublimates** (*kupipakva rasayana*): medicines are prepared by sublimation (heating a substance so that it vaporises).

- **Calcined preparations** (*bhasma*): the plant or metal is converted into ash. Minerals, or the horns or shells of animals, are purified to remove impurities and treated by triturating and macerating in herbal extracts. The dough so obtained is calcined to obtain the ashes.
- **Powdered gems** (*pisti*): selected minerals, shells or gems are treated by triturating and mecarating in juices of plants, followed by drying, to obtain a micro-fine powder.
- **Distillates** (*arka*): preparations made by distillation.

Table 1 Relationship between the elements in the *tridosha* and the human body

Functional/structural component of human body	Specific role in human physiology	Dominant elemental composition
Vata	The somatic driving force	*Vayu* (Air) +*Akas'a* (Space)
Pitta	The energy regulator	*Tejas* (Fire) + *Jala* (Water)
Kapha	Somatic integrity	*Prithwi* (Earth) + *Jala* (Water)
Rakta	The cellular fraction of blood and blood forming organs	*Tejas* (Fire) + *Prithwi* (Earth)
Medo	The adipose tissue	*Prithwi* (Earth) + *Jala* (Water)

Table 2 Examples of elemental compositions as interpreted by Ayurveda, their effect on the *tridosha* and therapeutic application

Name of the plant (botanical name)	Taste	Physico-chemical property	Elemental composition	Effect on humour (*dosha*)	Therapeutic application
Neem (*Azadirachta indica*)	Bitter	Light	Air (*Vayu*) + Fire (*Tejas*)	Balances *kapha* and *pitta*	Useful in diabetes
Shatavari (*Asparagus racemosus*)	Sweet	Heavy	Earth (*Prithwi*) + Water (*Jala*)	Balances *vata* and *pitta*, promotes *kapha*	Improves lactation
Pippali (*Piper longum*)	Pungent	Light	Fire (*Tejas*) + Water (*Jala*)	Balances *kapha* and promotes *pitta*	Improves digestion and metabolism

Further reading

Bharatiya Vidya Bhavan's Swami Prakashanandra Ayurveda Research Centre 1992 Selected medicinal plants of India. Chemexcil, Mumbai

Lad V 1985 Ayurveda: the science of self-healing. A practical guide. Lotus Press, Wilmot, Wisconsin

Sairam TV 1999–2000 Home remedies, vol I, II and III. Penguin (India), New Delhi

Sharma PV 1995 Introduction to Dravyaguna (Indian pharmacology). Chaukhambha Orientalia, Varanasi, India

Dash B, Kashyap L 1994 Materia medica of Ayurveda. Concept Publishing Company, New Delhi, India

Sharma PC, Yelne MB, Dennis TJ 2000 Database on medicinal plants used in Ayurveda. Central Council of Research in Ayurveda and Siddha, New Delhi, India

Abrus precatorius L. Fabaceae (Leguminosae)

English: Jequirity, crab's eye, Indian liquorice

Hindi: *Rati*

Sanskrit: *Gunja*

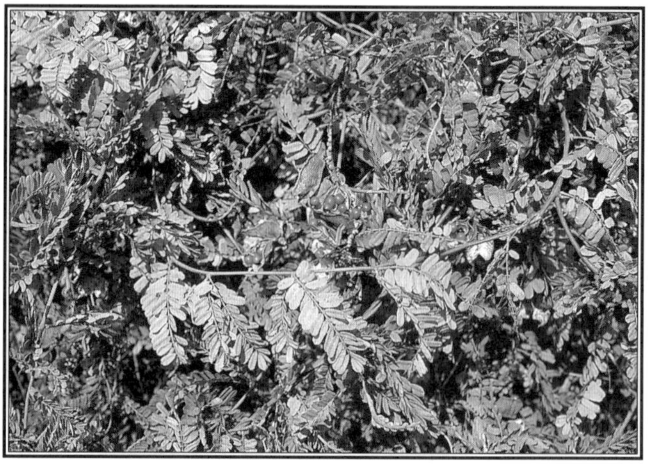

The plant has been used in Hindu medicine from very early times, as well as in China and other ancient cultures. The seeds were formerly used in India to weigh gemstones (they are very uniform in size, a single seed equal to 1.75 g or 1 carat) and in fact the Koh-i-Noor diamond was first weighed by this means. In parts of South America and the Caribbean, necklaces of the seeds were traditionally made for infants to wear as a protection against illness. They are very attractive and hence are popular as jewellery, in rosaries and in noisy toys such as rattles, although this should be avoided because of their toxicity if ingested.

Habitat

A slender vine growing wild in thickets, farms and secondary clearings, generally supported by other plants or a fence. It is native to India, from the Himalayas down to southern India and Sri Lanka, but now grows in all tropical regions throughout the world, most commonly in Florida and Hawaii, Africa, South America and the West Indies.

Botanical description

A twining, climbing shrub, with greenish yellow branches (Plate 1). Leaves 5–17 compound, leaflets obovate or oblong; flowers in crowded racemes, subsessile, pale purple to yellowish. The seeds are slightly smaller than ordinary peas; ovoid scarlet with a black spot round the hilum, or black with a white spot, or uniformly black or white, and glossy. The stout rectangular, bulging, brownish pods ripen by the end of the cold season and curl back on opening to reveal the pendulous red and black seeds, 4–6 in a pod. The root is woody, tortuous and much branched, with a sweet taste, rather like liquorice.

Parts used

Roots, leaves and seeds.

Traditional and modern use

In Ayurveda the plant is considered beneficial for the hair and the seed extract is used externally in the treatment of ulcers and skin affections. The seeds are poisonous and should only be given to patients after proper processing (e.g. 'Shodhan'), as the toxic protein abrin is then denatured.[1] In India a hot water extract of the leaves and roots or seeds is applied topically for eye diseases and taken orally as an emmenagogue.[2,3] The inhabitants of the Andaman Islands eat the boiled seeds.[4] In tropical Africa, a decoction of the root is taken orally as an antiemetic and for treatment of bilharzia, tapeworm infestation, gonorrhoea, asthma, in chest pain and as an aphrodisiac, and the roots are chewed for snakebite.[5] Seeds are taken orally by several Central African tribes for intestinal worms and as an oral contraceptive. A single dose (200 mg) is said to be effective for 13 menstrual cycles.[6] The water extract of the dried leaves and root is taken orally as a nerve tonic in Brazil and powdered leaves are applied to cuts and swellings.[7]

Ethnoveterinary usage

The leaf is used to treat fowl pox in poultry.[8]

Major chemical constituents

Isoflavonoids and quinones

Abruquinones A,B,C,D,E, F and G[2,9,10,11] are present in the root and abrusalactone A, abrusgenic acid and methyl abrusgenate[12] in the aerial parts.

Triterpenoids and saponins

Glycyrrhizin and oleanolic acid are found in the root[13] and abrusosides A, B, C, D and E in the aerial parts.[14–16] Abrus-saponins I and II, abrisapogenol, β-amyrin, squalene, abricin, abridin, cycloartenol, campesterol, cholesterol and β-sitosterol have all been found in the seeds.[17–19]

Proteins

Abrins I, II and III, *Abrus precatorius* agglutinin (APA) I and APA II[20] are present in the seeds.

Alkaloids and nitrogen compounds

Precatorine, trigonelline, choline and abrine are present in the seeds.[21]

Flavonoids and anthocyanins

Abrectorin, dimethoxycentaureidin-7-O-rutinoside, precatorins I, II and III, and xyloglucosyl-delophinidin and p-coumaroyl-galloyl-glucosyl-delphinidin have been isolated from the seeds.[22–24]

Carbohydrates

Galactose, arabinose, and xylose[25] are present in the aerial parts.

Medicinal and pharmacological activities

Antitumour activity: Agglutinin protein purified from the seeds of *Abrus precatorius* showed high antitumour activity.[26] Injection of 1 ng of abrin A into mice bearing Meth-A tumour inhibited the tumour growth by 90%, with abrin A having a higher affinity constant for sarcoma cells than abrin B. Binding inhibition studies with sugars suggested that abrins A and B have different binding sites, although both abrins inhibited sarcoma 180 in mice. Abrin A was more toxic than abrin B. Phytoagglutinins had agglutinating activity in murine ascites cells and inhibited the growth of Yoshida sarcoma cells.[27]

Immunomodulating activity: The abrins have been used in the formulation of antigenic injections with the ability to increase both cellular and humoral immune responses but without causing necrosis and swelling at the injection site. Thus, a mixture of 15 ng abrin and 1 μg bovine serum albumin (BSA), when administered by injection, provided a stronger immune response to the antigen than when abrin and BSA were administered separately. The activity of abrin to increase the humoral immunity was strongest at the 10 ng dose. Abrin also enhanced antitumour immunity.[28]

Antifertility activity, males: An alcoholic extract of the seed produced a lowering of sperm motility, but no effect on concentration, after 60 days of feeding to male rats. Scanning electron microscopic studies on sperm morphology revealed decapitation, acrosomal damage and formation of bulges on the mid-piece region. Biochemical studies on epididymal spermatozoa indicated alterations in energy and/or oxidative metabolism, as evidenced by a fall in succinate dehydrogenase and ATPase levels. The average number of implantation sites in females, after mating with the treated male rats, also markedly declined. However, a significant increase in serum testosterone levels was noted, suggesting that the decrease in fertility rate in treated animals was due to reduced sperm motility, metabolism and altered morphology in the epididymis rather than changes in hormone levels.[29] Dose-dependent degenerative changes in testicular weight, sperm count, later stages of spermatogenesis and Leydig cells were observed in the testis of rats given the steroidal fraction of the seeds. This may be a result of a decrease in the activity of enzymes such as hydroxysteroid dehydrogenases, glucose-6-phosphate and sorbitol dehydrogenases and leucine aminopeptidase or an indirect influence at the pituitary level.[30] In another study, oral administration of a 50% ethanol extract of the seeds (250 mg/kg) in albino rats for 30 and 60 days induced an absolute infertility in males, which was reversible. Suppression of sperm motility in the cauda epididymis was the most pronounced effect of the treatment. Histological and other observations on the testes and para reproductive tissues appeared normal, while the protein, sialic acid, acid phosphatase and succinic dehydrogenase levels were significantly depleted.[31]

Methanol extracts of the seeds showed an inhibitory effect on the motility of washed human spermatozoa, which was essentially irreversible. At the highest concentration tested (20 mg/ml), the onset of the antimotility action was almost immediate and the functional integrity of the plasma membrane and viability impaired. In contrast, with a lower concentration (5 mg/ml), such effects were not evident. It was concluded that at the lower concentrations, the antimotility action may have resulted from a rise in intracellular calcium (not via influx), a decline in cAMP content and/or enhanced generation of reactive oxygen species.[32]

Antifertility activity, females: A partially purified fraction, injected precoitum or immediately postcoitum to female rats, induced 100% sterility, but was ineffective when injected 2–5 days postcoitum. Isolated abridin induced 100% sterility in rats when injected one day pre- or postcoitum.[33] The alcoholic extract of the seeds of *A. precatorius* when injected for 10–12 days disturbed the oestrus cycle of the rat and induced sterility when injected for five consecutive days prior to mating. Similar activity was recorded in the unsaponifiable fraction of the extract. This altered the cyclic rhythm of the animals, lowered plasma oestradiol and progesterone levels and decreased ovarian weight, possibly by altering ovarian steroid metabolism. The petroleum ether and alcoholic extracts of the roots, given 1–5 days postcoitus, completely prevented nidation and the alcoholic extract also showed anti-oestrogenic activity when given simultaneously with 0.05 μg oestradiol. The oral LD_{50} of the alcohol extract was 2 g/kg.[34]

Abortifacient activity: An aqueous suspension of the seeds induced abortion in 51% of rats, when orally administered postcoitally at the daily dose of 125 mg/kg from day 0 to day 10. The activity was reduced when the same dose was administered from day 6 to day 15.[35]

Antiplatelet activity: The isoflavoquinones and abruquinones A, B and D significantly inhibited platelet aggregation. The IC_{50} values of abruquinones A and B for the inhibition of the platelet aggregation induced by arachidonic acid and collagen were less than 5 μg/ml, and that of abruquinone D was less than 10 μg/ml for aggregation induced by arachidonic acid.[36]

Antiinflammatory and antiallergic activity: Abruquinones A, B, D and F showed strong antiinflammatory and antiallergic effects. The IC_{50} for the inhibition of superoxide formation was less than 0.3 μg/ml for the inhibition of the release of both β-glucuronidase and lysozyme from rat neutrophils and less than 1 μg/ml for the release of β-glucuronidase and histamine from mast cells.[36] Saponins isolated from the aerial parts, and their acetates, exhibited antiinflammatory activity in the croton oil ear model.[37] Polymyxin B-induced hind paw oedema was suppressed by abruquinone A, in normal as well in adrenalectomised mice. Unlike dexamethasone, abruquinone A did not increase the liver glycogen content in fasting adrenalectomised mice. It reduced the volume of exuded plasma in neurogenic inflammation and passive cutaneous anaphylactic reaction. Histamine, serotonin, bradykinin and substance P-induced plasma extravasation in ear oedema was also suppressed, to a greater extent than with diphenhydramine and methysergide. These and other results suggested that the antiinflammatory effect of abruquinone A is mediated partly via the suppression of the release of chemical mediators from mast cells and partly via the prevention of vascular permeability changes caused by mediators.[38]

Molluscicidal activity: In vivo and in vitro sublethal exposure to abrin and glycyrrhizin inhibited acetylcholinesterase, lactic dehydrogenase and acid and alkali phosphatase activity in the nervous tissue of *Lymnaea acuminata*. Succinic dehydrogenase activity was increased during the in vivo treatment although in vitro exposure had no significant effect. Abrin and glycyrrhizin also significantly decreased levels of protein, free amino acid, DNA and RNA and abrin caused a reduction in phospholipid levels with a simultaneous increase in the rate of lipid peroxidation in the treated snails.[39]

Insecticidal activity: Abrine produced a dose-dependent depletion of sugars and protein content in mealy bugs and also in lipids at higher concentrations, suggesting that abrine could have a useful effect on reducing the population of this insect.[40]

Use as a sweetening agent: Abrusosides A, B,

C and D have been suggested as sugar substitutes in foods and pharmaceuticals. Preliminary safety studies indicate a lack of acute toxicity in mice and mutagenicity. In sensory tests the abrusosides were 30–100 times sweeter than 2% sucrose. Abrusoside D had a lingering sweetness lasting 30 minutes.[41]

Antibacterial activity: The ethanol (95%) extract was active against *Escherichia coli* and *Staphylococcus aureus*.[42]

Antidiarrhoeal activity: A fraction obtained from the dried seeds was active against castor oil-induced diarrhoea in rats.[43]

Safety profile

Fatal poisoning in children has been reported after the thorough chewing of one seed.[44] They are highly toxic and cause severe stomach cramping accompanied by nausea, severe diarrhoea, cold sweats, tachycardia, coma and circulatory collapse. The LD_{50} of abrin (IP) in mice was found to be 8.34 mg/kg. Prolonged administration of abrin in mice produced initial anaemia, which normalised at the end of the experiment, and an increase in white blood cell count. Intraperitoneal injection of abrin to pregnant rats produced both maternal and fetal changes, whereas abrin given orally produced significant fetal effects only.[45] The ethanol-water (1:1) extract of the aerial parts was much less toxic (when administered to mice the LD_{50} was > 1 g/kg body weight[46]) and the ethanol (95%) extract of the dried leaves, administered to chickens, produced an LD_{50} of 12 mg/kg body weight.[47]

Dosage

Leaf decoction: 56–112 ml

Root powder: 0.5–1 g

Ayurvedic properties

Rasa: *Tikta* (bitter)

Guna: *Laghu* (light), *ruksha* (dry), *tikshna* (sharp)

Veerya: *Ushna* (hot)

Vipaaka: *Katu* (pungent)

Dosha: Pacifies *vata* and *pitta*

Further reading

Bown D 1995 Encyclopaedia of herbs and their uses. Dorling Kindersley, London

Chevallier A 1996 The encyclopedia of medicinal plants. Dorling Kindersley, London

Kapoor LD 1990 Handbook of Ayurvedic medicinal plants. CRC Press, Boca Raton

Ross I 2000 Medicinal plants of the world, vol 2. Humana Press, Totowa, New Jersey

Sairam TV 2000 Home remedies, vol III. Penguin India, New Delhi

References

1 Gautam DN, Singh PN, Mehrotra S 1999 Comparative study of processed (Shodhit) and unprocessed seeds of Gunja-*Abrus precatorius* L. Natural Product Science 5(3):127

2 Jain SP, Verma DM 1981 Medicinal plants in the folk-lore of Northern circle Dehradun, UP India. National Academy of Science Letters (India) 4(7):269

3 Malhi BS, Trivedi VP 1972 Vegetable antifertility drugs of India. Quarterly Journal of Crude Drug Research 12:19

4 Rajaram N, Janardhanan K 1992 The chemical composition and nutritional potential of the tribal pulse, *Abrus precatorius* L. Plants and Foods in Human Nutrition 42(4):285

5 Hedberg I, Hedberg O, Madati PJ, Mshigeni KE, Mshiu EN, Samuelsson G 1983 Inventory of plants used in traditional medicine in Tanzania. Part-III. Plants of the families Papilionaceae-Vitaceae. Journal of Ethnopharmacology 9(2/3):237

6 Watt JM, Breyer-Brandwijk MG 1962 The medicinal and poisonous plants of Southern and Eastern Africa, 2nd edn. E.S. Livingstone, London

7 Elisabetsky E, Figueiro W, Oliveria G 1992 Traditional Amazonian nerve tonics as antidepressant agents. *Chaunochiton kappleri.* A case study. Journal of Herbs, Spices and Medicinal Plants 1(1/2):125

8 International Institute of Rural Reconstruction, 1994 Ethnoveterinary medicine in Asia: an information kit on traditional animal health care practices. IIRR Silang, Philippines

9 Song C-Q, Hu Z-B 1998 Abruquinones A,B,C,D, E, F and G from the root of *Abrus precatorius*. Zhiwu Xue Bao 40(8):734

10 Ross IA 2000 Medicinal plants of the world: chemical constituents, traditional and modern medicinal uses, vol 1. Humana Press, Totowa, New Jersey

11 Saxena VK, Sharma DN 1999 A new isoflavone from the roots of *Abrus precatorius.* Fitoterapia 70(3):328

12 Chinag TC, Chang HM 1983 New oleanane type triterpenes from *Abrus precatorius* and X-ray crystal structure of abrusgenic acid-methanol 1:1 solvate. Planta Medica 49(3):165

13 Chang HM, Chiang TC, Mak TC 1982 Isolation and structure elucidation of abrusalactone-A, a new oleanane type terpene from the roots and vines of *Abrus precatorius*. Journal of the Chemical Society, Chemical Communications 20:1197

14 Akinloye BA, Adalumo LA 1981 *Abrus precatorius* leaves – a source of glycyrrhizin. Nigerian Journal of Pharmacy 12(2):405

15 Kennelly EJ, Cai L, Kim N-C, Kinghorn AD 1996 Potential sweetening agents of plant origin. Part 31. Abrusoside E, a further sweet-tasting cycloartane glycoside from the leaves of *Abrus precatorius.* Phytochemistry 41(5):1381

16 Choi YH, Hussain RA, Pezzuto JM, Kinghorn AD, Morton JF 1989 Abrusosides A-D, four novel sweet-tasting triterpene glycosides from the leaves of *Abrus precatorius*. Journal of Natural Products 52(5):1118

17 Kinjo J, Matsumoto K, Inoue M, Takeshita T, Nohara T 1991 Studies on leguminous plants. Part XIX. A new sapogenol and other constituents in abri semen, the seeds of *Abrus precatorius* L. Chemical and Pharmaceutical Bulletin 39(1):116

18 Siddiqui S, Siddiqui B, Naim Z 1978 Studies of the steroidal constituents of the seeds of *Abrus precatorius* Linn. (Scarlet variety). Pakistan Journal of Scientific and Industrial Research 21(5–6):158

19 Begum S 1993 Chemical investigation of white seeded variety of *Abrus precatorius* Linn. Pakistan Journal of Scientific and Industrial Research 35(7–8):270

20 Hegde R, Maiti TK, Podder SK 1991 Purification and characterization of three toxins and two agglutinins from *Abrus precatorius* seed by using lactamyl-sepharose affinity chromatography. Analytical Biochemistry 194(1):101

21 Ghosal S, Dutta SK 1971 Alkaloids of *Abrus precatorius*. Phytochemistry 10(1):195

22 Bharadwaj DK, Bisht MS, Mehta CK 1980 Flavonoids from *Abrus precatorius.* Phytochemistry 19:2040

23 Karawya MS, El-Gengaihi S, Wassel G, Ibrahim NA 1981 Anthocyanins from seeds of *Abrus precatorius.* Fitoterapia 52(4):175

24 Ma C, Nakamura N, Hattori M 1998 Saponins and C-glycosyl flavones from the seeds of *Abrus precatorius*. Chemical and Pharmaceutical Bulletin 46(6):982

25 Karawya MS, El-Gengaihi S, Wassel G, Ibrahim NA 1981 Carbohydrates of *Abrus precatorius*. Fitoterapia 52(4):179

26 Panneerselvam K, Lin SC, Liu CL, Liaw YC, Lin JY, Lu TH 2000 Crystallization of agglutinin from the seeds of *Abrus precatorius.* Acta Crystallography D: Biological Crystallography 56:898

27 Tomita M, Kurokawa T, Onozaki K, Osawa T, Sakurai Y, Ukita T 1972 Surface structure of

murine ascites tumors. II. Difference in cytotoxicity of various phytoagglutinins toward Yoshida sarcoma cells in vitro. International Journal of Cancer 10(3):602

28 Shionoya H, Arai H, Koyanagi N, Takeuchi H 1980 An immunopotentiator comprising abrin, an injectable preparation and a method of treating microbial infections or cancer. Eisai Co. Ltd., Japan. European Patent EP 28814

29 Rao MV 1987 Antifertility effects of alcoholic seed extract of *Abrus precatorius* Linn. in male albino rats. Acta Europea Fertilitas 18(3):217

30 Sinha S, Mathur RS 1990 Effect of steroidal fraction of seeds of *Abrus precatorius* Linn. on rat testis. Indian Journal of Experimental Biology 28(8):752

31 Sinha R 1990 Post-testicular anti-fertility effects of *Abrus precatorius* seed extract in albino rats. Journal of Ethnopharmacology 28(2):173

32 Ratnasooriya WD, Amarasekera AS, Perera NS, Premakumara GA 1991 Sperm antimotility properties of seed extract of *Abrus precatorius*. Journal of Ethnopharmacology 33(1–2):85

33 Zia-Ul-Haque A, Qazi MH, Hamdard ME 1983 Studies on the antifertility properties of active components isolated from the seeds of *Abrus precatorius* Linn. II. Pakistan Journal of Zoology 15(2):141

34 Agarwal SS, Ghatak N, Arora RB, Bhardwaj MM 1970 Antifertility activity of the root of *Abrus precatorius*. Pharmacological Research Communications 2(2):159

35 Sethi N, Nath D, Singh RK 1990 Teratological aspects of *Abrus precatorius* seeds in rats. Fitoterapia 61(1):61

36 Chukuo S, Chen SC, Chen LH, Wu JB, Teng CM 1995 Potent antiplatelet, antiinflammatory and antiallergic isoflavanquinones from the roots of *Abrus precatorius*. Planta Medica 61(4):307

37 Anam EM 2001 Antiinflammatory activity of compounds isolated from the aerial parts of *Abrus precatorius* (Fabaceae). Phytomedicine 8(1):24

38 Wang J-P, Hsu M-F, Chang L-C, Kuo J-S, Kuo S-C 1995 Inhibition of plasma extravasation by abruquinone A, a natural isoflavanquinone isolated from *Abrus precatorius*. European Journal of Pharmacology 273(1/2):73

39 Singh S, Singh DK 1999 Effect of molluscicidal components of *Abrus precatorius, Argemone mexicana* and *Nerium indicum* on certain biochemical parameters of *Lymnaea acuminata*. Phytotherapy Research 13(3):210

40 Anitha B, Arivalagan M, Sundari MS, Durairaj G 1999 Effect of the alkaloid abrine, isolated from *Abrus precatorius* seeds, on mealy bug, *Maconellicoccus hirsutus*. Indian Journal of Experimental Biology 37(4):415

41 Kinghorn AD, Choi YH 1993 Purification of abrusosides from *Abrus a*nd their use as sweeteners. US Patent 5198427

42 Desai VB, Sirsi M 1966 Antimicrobial activity of *Abrus precatorius*. Indian Journal of Pharmacy 28:164

43 Nwodo OFC, Alumanah EO 1991 Studies on *Abrus precatorius* seeds. II. Anti-diarrhoeal activity. Journal of Ethnopharmacology 31(3):395

44 Lampe KF 1985 American Medical Association handbook of poisonous and injurious plants. Chicago Review Press, Chicago

45 El-Shabrawy OA, El-Gengaihi S, Ali Ibrahim N 1988 Toxicity and teratogenicity of abrin. Egyptian Journal of Veterinary Science 24(2):135–142

46 Dhawan BN, Patnaik GK, Rastogi PR, Singh KK, Tandon JS 1977 Screening of Indian plants for biological activity. Part VI. Indian Journal of Experimental Biology 15:208–219

47 Wambebe C, Amosun SL 1984 Some neuromuscular effects of the crude extracts of the leaves of *Abrus precatorius*. Journal of Ethnopharmacology 11(1):49

Acacia catechu L.f. (Willd.) (Leguminosae)

English: Black catechu, cutch tree, terra japonica

Hindi: *Khair*

Sanskrit: *Khadira*

Known previously as *cacho* or *kat*, this tree formed an important export product from India to China, Arabia and Persia in the 16th century. It was used for tanning and dyeing and the original khaki was dyed and shrunk with it. Japan introduced it to Europe in the 17th century and from there, it was included in the *London Pharmacopoeia* of 1721.

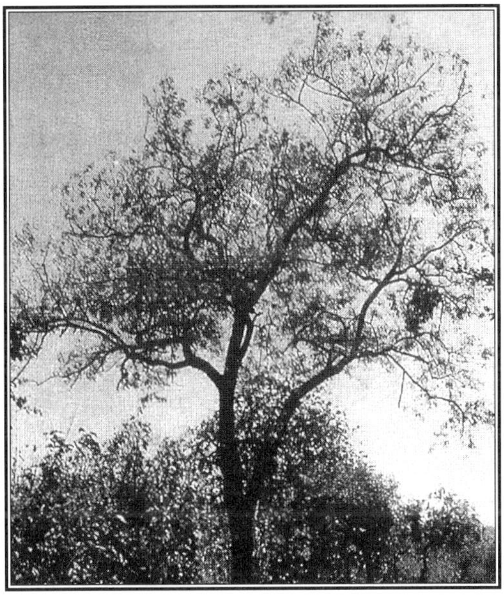

Habitat

A common tree found throughout India and on the eastern slopes of the Western Ghats and the sub-Himalayan tract up to a height of 1500 m. It is also cultivated elsewhere.

Botanical description

A deciduous tree with short hooked spines, reaching 9–12 m in height (Plate 2). The leaves are bipinnately compound with 30–50 pairs of leaflets, a feather-like appearance and a pair of recurved thorns at the base of the rachis. The greyish-brown bark exfoliates in long narrow strips. The flowers are pale yellow, in cylindrical spikes, and the fruit consists of flattened, glabrous and oblong pods with a triangular 'beak' at the apex. The sapwood is yellowish-white but the heartwood is red. The gummy extract of the wood, known as black catechu (to differentiate it from pale catechu or gambir, from *Uncaria gambier*), cutch or kat, is dark brown and brittle and is made from the dried aqueous extract prepared from the heartwood by boiling with water. The extract is concentrated and cooled in moulds; the dried mass formed is then broken into irregular, shiny pieces.

Parts used

Heartwood extract, gum, flowering tops, leaves, young shoots, bark and fruits.

Traditional and modern use

The extract from the heartwood is used as an anodyne, astringent, bactericide, refrigerant, detergent, stimulant, styptic, masticatory, expectorant and antiphlogistic. It is also used in asthma, cough, bronchitis, colic, diarrhoea, dysentery, boils, in skin afflictions and sores and for stomatitis. The bark is used as an anthelmintic, antipyretic, antiinflammatory, in bronchitis, ulcers, psoriasis, anaemia and gum troubles and has been used internally to treat leprosy.[1]

Ethnoveterinary usage

The sap is used for the treatment of wounds and diarrhoea in ruminants.[2] Black catechu and extracts of the bark are used in veterinary folk medicine for broken horn.

Major chemical constituents

Tannins and flavonoids

The outermost bark, inner bark and sapwood contain similar constituents to the extract:[3] 20–35% of catechutannic acid, 2–10% of acacatechin, quercetin and catechu-red.[4] The heartwood contains kaempferol, dihydrokaempferol, taxifolin, isorhamnetin, (+)-afzelchin, a dimeric procyanidin, quercetin, (–)-epicatechin,[5] (–)-catechin, fisetin, quercetagetin and (+)-cyanidanol.[6]

Medicinal and pharmacological activities

Hepatoprotective activity: Cyanidanol, isolated from the heartwood, showed hepatoprotective activity. An ethyl acetate extract in male rats decreased CCl_4-induced elevated enzyme levels in acute and chronic models of liver damage. The results indicated some form of repair of the structural integrity of the hepatocyte cell membrane or regeneration of damaged liver cells. Decreased levels of serum bilirubin after treatment with the extract in both acute and chronic liver damage indicated the efficacy of the extract in restoring normal functional status of the liver and the protective action of the extract was further substantiated by histopathological observations.[7]

Antiinflammatory activity: Cyanidanol demonstrated antiinflammatory activities.[7]

Antifungal activity: The plant extract showed an inhibitory action on the growth of fungi such as *Piricularia oryzae* and *Colletotrichum falcatum*.[8]

Effect on leukaemia: A semi-purified saline extract of the seeds of *Acacia catechu* was tested for agglutinating activity against whole leucocytes and mononuclear cells from patients with chronic myeloid leukaemia, acute myeloblastic leukaemia, acute lymphoblastic leukaemia, various lymphoproliferative or haematological disorders and on normal healthy subjects. The seed extract agglutinated white blood cells from patients with different types of leukaemia; however, it did not react with the peripheral blood cells of normal individuals. It has been suggested that the seed extract may yield leukaemia-specific lectins.[9]

Hypoglycaemic activity: The seed extract exhibited hypoglycaemic action in albino rats.[9]

Safety profile

Side effects are uncommon in normal doses and the drug has been used for centuries without major problems.

Dosage

Powdered bark: 1.5–4.5 g

Extract of heartwood: 0.5–1.8 g

Ayurvedic properties

Rasa: *Tikta* (bitter), *kashaya* (astringent)

Guna: *Laghu* (light), *ruksha* (dry)

Vipaka: *Katu* (pungent)

Veerya: *Shita* (cold)

Dosha: Balances *kapha* and *pitta*

Further reading

Bharatiya Vidya Bhavan's Swami Prakashanandra Ayurveda Research Centre 1992 Selected medicinal plants of India. Chemexcil, Mumbai

British Pharmacopoeia 1998 Pharmaceutical Press, London

Council of Scientific and Industrial Research 1985 The wealth of India. PID, CSIR, New Delhi

Ministry of Health and Family Welfare 1966 The Indian pharmacopoeia. Government of India, New Delhi

Ministry of Health and Family Welfare 1989 Ayurvedic pharmacopoeia of India, vol 1. Government of India, New Delhi

References

1 Council of Scientific and Industrial Research 1985 The wealth of India. A dictionary of Indian raw materials and industrial products. PID, CSIR, New Delhi, pp 21–30

2 International Institute of Rural Reconstruction 1994 Ethnoveterinary medicine in Asia. An information kit on traditional animal health care practices. Part I: General information. IIRR, Silang, Philippines

3 Ali MS, Hye MA, Mondal MIH, Rahman MA 1991, Extraction of catechu from different layers of the stem of *Acacia catechu* tree. Bangladesh Journal of Science and Industrial Research 26(1–4):171

4 British Herbal Medicine Association, 1983 British herbal pharmacopoeia. BHMA, Keighley, UK

5 Deshpande VH, Pati AD 1981 Flavonoids of *Acacia catechu* heartwood. Indian Journal of Chemistry 20 B:628

6 Rege NN, Dahanukar S, Karandikar SM 1984 Hepatoprotective effect of cyanidanol (+) against carbon tetrachloride induced liver damage. Indian Drugs 21:556

7 Jayasekhar P, Mohanan PV, Rathinam K 1997 Hepatoprotective activity of ethyl acetate extract of *Acacia catechu*. Indian Journal of Pharmacology 29:426

8 Council of Scientific and Industrial Research 1985 The wealth of India. A dictionary of Indian raw materials and industrial products. PID, CSIR, New Delhi, pp 1, 24

9 Agrawal S, Agrawal SS 1990 Preliminary observations on leukaemia specific agglutinins from seeds. Indian Journal of Medical Research 92:38–42

Acorus calamus L. (Araceae)(syn. *Acorus aromaticus* Gilib.)

English: Sweet flag, myrtle flag, sweet sedge

Hindi: *Vacha*

Sanskrit: *Vacha, ugragandha*

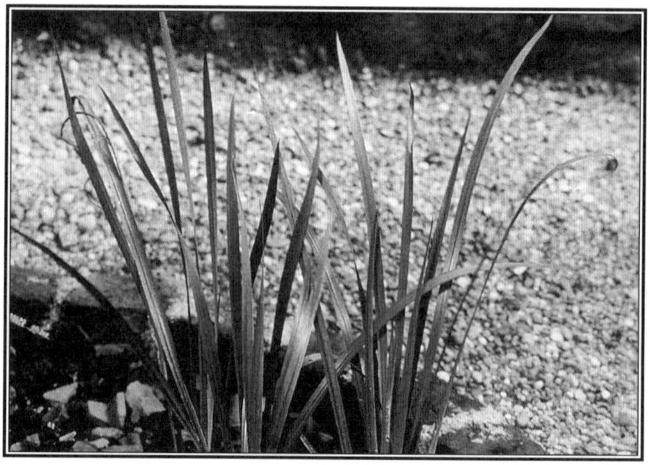

Sweet flag has long been known for its medicinal value. It originated in Europe but has been extensively used in Ayurveda, particularly to enhance memory. *Vacha* powder mixed with ghee is given ritually in India to newborn babies on the seventh day to improve the intellect and speech development. In China it is used in a similar way, to improve speech and aid recovery from stroke. The powder is sometimes blown into the nose of a patient in a coma to help regain consciousness. There are several polypoid varieties to be found, some of which do not contain the toxic constituent β-asarone, and these are preferable for medicinal use.[1]

Habitat

A semi-aquatic plant growing in damp, marshy places throughout the world.

Botanical description

A perennial, aromatic herb with creeping rhizomes (Plate 3). The leaves are long, slender, sword-shaped and simple, arising alternately from the horizontal rhizomes. These are longitudinally fissured with nodes, somewhat vertically compressed and spongy internally. Flowers small, fragrant, pale green in a spadix; fruits are a three-celled fleshy capsule.

Parts used

Rhizomes, rootstock.

Traditional and modern use

The rhizome is used in many different disorders, mainly as a nerve stimulant, to enhance memory and as an aromatic digestive. It is considered to be thermogenic, rejuvenative and sedative.[2] Other uses for the plant include as a diuretic, expectorant, decongestant, antiinflammatory, aphrodisiac, anticonvulsant and antibacterial. It has also been used in the treatment of epilepsy, chronic diarrhoea, dysentery, bronchial catarrh, intermittent fever and certain tumours. Ayurveda recommends the use of *vacha* in the kidney and liver diseases, rheumatism and eczema. A poultice made of *vacha* is applied to paralysed limbs.[3]

Ethnoveterinary usage

It is used in birds to get rid of lice; dusting the birds with dry powdered rhizomes kills lice within 12 hours. An infusion of the rhizome is used to wash newborn calves as a protection against vermin. It is also helpful in killing houseflies, repelling ticks and treating eye diseases in ruminants.[4,5]

Major chemical constituents

Essential oil

β-Asarone (isoasarone) is usually the major constituent but is present in highly variable proportions and occasionally absent. α-Asarone, elemicine, cis-isoelemicine, cis and trans isoeugenol and their methyl ethers, camphene, P-cymene, β-gurjunene, α-selinene, β-cadinene, camphor, terpinen-4-ol, α-terpineol and α-calacorene, acorone, acorenone, acoragermacrone, 2-deca-4,7-dienol, shyobunones, isoshyobunones, calamusenone, linalool and pre-isocalamendiol are also present.[1,6,7,8]

Others

Acoradin, galangin, 2,4,5-trimethoxy benzaldehyde, 2,5-dimethoxybenzoquinone, calamendiol, spathulenol and sitosterol have been isolated from *Acorus calamus*.[1,5,6]

Medicinal and pharmacological activities

Antiulcer and cytoprotective activity: The ethanolic extract of the rhizome was studied in rats, for protection of the gastroduodenal mucosa against injuries caused by indomethacin, reserpine and cysteamine, and also in a pyloric ligation model. The extract produced a marked reduction in the volume and acidity of basal gastric secretions and ulcer index and helped to protect against chemically induced lesions.[9]

Antispasmodic activity: Experiments on the ileum, uterus, bronchial muscles, tracheal chain and blood vasculature showed the relaxant and antispasmodic activity of β-asarone and the essential oil of the rhizome.[10,11] The rhizome is useful in the treatment of diarrhoea and dysentery, combined with ginger for relief in flatulent colic.[12]

Analgesic activity: The essential oil and alcoholic extract of the rhizome were shown to possess analgesic properties and also mild hypotensive and sedative action.[13]

Antiinflammatory activity: An extract of the rhizome was studied in acute, chronic and immunological models of inflammation, including carrageenan-induced rat paw oedema, and compared with the activity of hydrocortisone. The extract showed significant antiinflammatory activity with a reduction of up to 44%. The essential oil is also an effective antiinflammatory agent and a coconut oil extract of the rhizome produced a 45% inhibition of carrageenan-induced rat paw oedema and 61% inhibition using the granuloma pouch method.[14,15,16]

Anticonvulsant activity: A polyherbal compound containing rhizome of *Acorus calamus* as one of the ingredients has been reported clinically to reduce epileptic attacks in patients by up to 50%. Treatment continued for 6 months resulted in cure in 66 out of 88 patients and no repeat episodes were reported after 2 years of the treatment. The isolated constituents of the rhizomes, asarone and β-asarone, showed anticonvulsant activity in experimental models. There was a decrease in sociability scores with a reduction in anticholinergic action. Experiment on animal models also revealed the depressant action of the essential oils and the crude alcoholic and aqueous extracts of the rhizomes.[17,18]

Antibacterial activity: Growth of cultured Gram-positive and Gram-negative organisms was inhibited significantly by an extract of the rhizome. A consistent and gradual decrease in replication of standard cultures of *Staphylococcus aureus*, *Escherichia coli* and *Shigella flexneri* was observed after treatment with the essential oil.[12,19]

Safety profile

No health hazards or side effects are known with the administration of designated therapeutic dose, although β-asarone is known to be carcinogenic in animals.[1] It also induces vomiting in large doses.

Dosage

Rhizome: 60–120 mg

(To induce vomiting: 1–2 g)

Ayurvedic properties

Rasa: *Katu* (pungent), *tikta* (bitter)

Guna: *Laghu* (light), *tikshna* (sharp)

Veerya: *Ushna* (hot)

Vipaka: *Katu* (pungent)

Dosha: Pacifies *kapha* and *vata*

Further reading

Council of Scientific and Industrial Research 1985 The wealth of India. PID, CSIR, New Delhi

Kapoor LD 1990 Handbook of Ayurvedic medicinal plants. CRC Press, Boca Raton

Rastogi RP, Mehrotra BN 1993 Compendium of Indian medicinal plants, vol 3. PID, New Delhi

Shastri B 1988 Bhavprakash. Chaukhamba Sanskrit Sansthan Publications, Varanasi

References

1 Williamson EM, Evans FJ 1988 Potter's new cyclopedia of botanical drugs and preparations. CW Daniels, Saffron Walden

2 Tyler VE 1986 Recent advances in herbal medicines. Pharmacology International 7:203

3 Motley TJ 1994 The ethnobotany of sweet flag, *Acorus calamus* (Araceae). Economic Botany 48(4):397

4 Matzigkeit U 1990 Natural veterinary medicine. Ectoparasites in the tropics. AGRECOL, Langerbruck, Switzerland

5 International Institute of Rural Reconstruction 1994 Ethnoveterinary medicine in Asia. An information kit on traditional animal health care practices. IIRR, Silang, Philippines, vol 1, p58

6 Mazza G 1985 Gas chromatographic and mass spectrometric studies of the constituents of the rhizome of *Acorus calamus*. II. The volatile constituents of the essential oil. Journal of Chromatography 328:179

7 Harborne JB, Baxter H 1993 Phytochemical dictionary. Taylor and Francis, London

8 Keller K, Stahl E 1983 Extraction of thermolabile compounds with supercritical gasses. Part 12, Extraction of beta-asarone from calamus rhizomes. Planta Medica 47:75

9 Rafatullah S, Tariq M, Mossa JS, Al-Yahaya MA, Al-Said MS, Ageel AM 1994 Anti-secretagogue, anti-ulcer and cytoprotective properties of *Acorus calamus* in rats. Fitoterapia 65:19

10 Das PK, Malhotra CL, Dhalla NS 1962 Spasmolytic activity of asarone and essential oil of *Acorus calamus* Linn. Archives of Internal Pharmacodynamics 135:167

11 Maj M, Malec D, Laastowski Z 1966 Pharmacological properties of native *calamus* (*Acorus calamus* L). 3. Spasmolytic effect of ethereal oil. Acta Poloniae Pharmaceutica 23(5):477

12 Dey D, Das MN 1988 Pharmacognosy of antidysenteric drugs of Indian medicine. Acta Botanica Indica 16:216

13 Menon MK, Dandiya PC 1967 The mechanism of the tranquilizing action of asarone from *Acorus calamus* Linn. Journal of Pharmacology 19(3):170

14 Vohora SB, Shah AS, Sharma K, Naqvi SAH, Dandiya PC 1989 Anti-bacterial, anti-pyretic, analgesic and anti-inflammatory studies on *Acorus calamus* Linn. Annals of the National Academy of Medical Science 25(1):13

15 Varde AB, Ainapure SS, Naik SR, Amladi SR 1988 Anti-inflammatory activity of coconut oil extract of *Acorus calamus*, *Ocimum sanctum* and *Ocimum bascilicum* in rats. Indian Drugs 25(6):226

16 Siddiqui MTA, Asif M 1991 Anti-inflammatory activity of *Acorus calamus* Linn. Proceedings of a Symposium on Herbal Drugs. New Delhi

17 Narayan J, Pandit BSV, Rangesh PRMD 1987 Clinical experience of a compound Ayurvedic preparation on *apasmara* (epilepsy). Ayurveda Vignyana 9(5):7

18 Martis G, Rao A, Karanth KS 1991 Neuropharmacological activity of *Acorus calamus*. Fitoterapia 62(4):331

19 Syed M, Riaz M, Chaudhari FM 1991 The antibacterial activity of the essential oils of the Pakistani *Acorus calamus*, *Callistemon lanceolatus* and *Laurus nobilis*. Pakistan Journal of Science and Industrial Research 34(11):456

Adhatoda vasica L. Nees (Acanthaceae) syn. *A. zeylanica* Medik, *Justicia adhatoda* L.

English: Malabar nut

Hindi: *Adosa*

Sanskrit: *Vasaka*

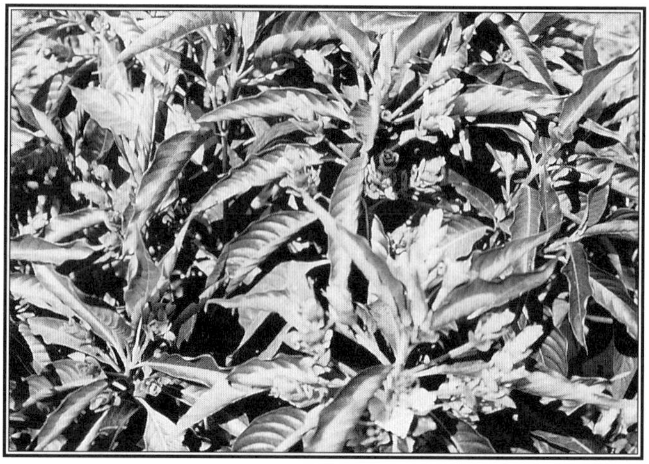

Vasaka has been used in Indian medicine for over 2000 years. The leaf buds are chewed, sometimes with ginger, by sadhus. This helps to clear the respiratory passages during their yogic breathing exercises.

Habitat

The plant grows throughout the Indian peninsula up to an altitude of 1300 m, on wastelands in a variety of habitats and types of soil. It is sometimes cultivated as a hedge plant and the twigs and leaves used as 'green manure'. It is also found in Sri Lanka and Malaysia.

Botanical description

Vasaka is a small, evergreen, perennial shrub, reaching 1–2.5 m high with opposite, ascending branches (Plate 4). The leaves are simple, opposite, lanceolate and leathery, 7–19 cm long and 4–7 cm wide, pubescent, and light green in colour above, darker on the lower surface. The flowers are large, dense, terminal spikes with large bracts. The corolla is white, the lower lip often streaked with pink or purple, and the capsule small, clavate and longitudinally channelled, containing four globular seeds.

Parts used

Leaves, roots, flowers and bark.

Traditional and modern use

Adhatoda vasica has been most commonly used for the treatment of respiratory complaints and diseases such as coughs, colds and asthma.[1] The leaves are boiled and taken orally for fevers and warmed leaves are applied externally for rheumatic pains and dislocation of joints. The powder, boiled in sesame oil, is used as a local application for ear infection and to stop bleeding. In Nepal, a dried water extract of leaves is used to relieve stomach acidity and in Bihar and other parts of India, a decoction of the leaves is used to facilitate childbirth or induce abortion. A paste of the leaves is sometimes applied to the abdomen to treat urinary disorders.[2,3] The leaves and flowers are cooked as a vegetable by the Khasi tribe in India.[4] It has been used by European herbal practitioners as an antispasmodic, expectorant and febrifuge.

Ethnoveterinary usage

The leaves and rhizome are used in coughs and colds in ruminants and generally in treating diseases such as abscesses, anthrax, throat diseases, asthma, tuberculosis, jaundice, scabies, urticaria, rheumatism, pneumonia, haematuria and contagious abortion.[5]

Major chemical constituents

Alkaloids

Vasicine (= peganine), a quinazoline alkaloid, is the major alkaloid present in all parts of the plant. The leaves also contain vasicinone, 7-methoxyvasicinone, vasicinol, adhatodine, adhatonine, adhavasinone, anisotine, 3-hydroxyanisotine, desmethoxyaniflorine, vasicoline and vasicolinone.[6–9] The root contains vasicinol, vasicinolone, vasicinone, adhatonine[10,11] and vasicol.[12]

Phytosterols and triterpenes

Daucosterol, α-amyrin and epitaraxerol are present.[8,13]

Flavonoids

Apigenin, astragalin, kaempferol, quercetin, vitexin, isovitexin, violanthin, 2''-O-xylosylvitexin, rhamnosylvitexin, 2'-hydroxy-4-glucosyloxychalcone are present in the leaf and flower.[14,15]

Essential oil

The flower volatile oil contains a ketone identified as 4-heptanone as the major compound, together with at least 36 other components including 3-methylheptanone.[14]

Fatty acids and hydrocarbons

The leaf oil is a complex mixture of over 50 compounds, the major component being decane, together with the hydroxyalkanes 37-hydroxyhexatetracont-1-en-15-one and 29-methyltriacontan-1-ol and linolenic, arachidonic, linoleic, palmitic and oleic acids.[16,17]

Medicinal and pharmacological activities

Bronchodilatory and antiasthmatic activity: Vasicine showed bronchodilatory activity both in vitro and in vivo, the activity being comparable to that of theophylline.[18] Vasicinone, however, showed bronchodilatory activity in vitro but bronchoconstriction in vivo. The two alkaloids in combination had a more potent bronchodilatory activity and the combination of vasicinone with aminophylline also had an additive effect.[19] *Adhatoda vasica* reduced ovalbumin and PAF-induced allergic reactions. A fraction containing the minor alkaloid vascinol and about 20% vasicine inhibited ovalbumin-induced allergic reactions by about 37% at a concentration of 5 mg.[20]

Antibacterial activity: A methanolic extract of the leaves was investigated for antibacterial activity using the paper disc and dilution methods. The in vitro screening showed a strong activity of the alkaloid fraction against *Pseudomonas aeruginosa* (MIC=164 μg/ml). Significant antibacterial activity against the Gram-positive bacteria *Streptococcus faecalis*, *Staphylococcus aureus*, *Staph epidermidis* and the Gram-negative *E. coli* was also noted.[21] In another study the plant was tested for inhibition of bacterial population of untreated water (in vitro). At pH 7, growth of the bacterial population was inhibited by 82% and at pH 6.5, various coliforms were also inhibited, suggesting a possible use for the plant in the improvement of drinking water.[22]

Antitubercular activity: Bromhexine and ambroxol are semi-synthetic derivatives of vasicine, an alkaloid from *Adhatoda vasica*, and are widely used as mucolytics. They also have a pH-dependent growth inhibitory effect on *Mycobacterium tuberculosis*. This, combined with indirect effects including enhancement of lysozyme levels in bronchial secretions and levels of rifampicin in lung tissue and sputum, suggests a useful adjunctive role in the therapy of tuberculosis.[23]

Cholagogue activity: In acute experiments on cats and chronic experiments using dogs, peganine (vasicine) at an IV dose of 5 mg/kg had a cholagogue action. In dogs, the amount of excreted bile increased by 40–100%, with a tendency towards dilution of the bile and an increase in bilirubin excretion.[24]

Antidyspepsia activity: A syrup of *Adhatoda vasica* improved symptoms of dyspepsia.[25]

Insecticidal activity: *Adhatoda vasica* leaves were found to control insect pests in oil seeds, in both laboratory and warehouse conditions.[26] In another study, vasicinol produced antifertility effects in *Dysdercus koenigii* and *Tribolium castaneum*, due to blocking of the oviduct. Feeding deterrence was observed against *Aulacophora foveicollis* and *Epilachna vijintioctopunctata* at 0.05% and 0.01% levels.[27] The essential oil showed insecticidal activity against granary pests, e.g. *Sitophilus oryzae, Rhizopertha dominica* and *Bruchus chinensis*, and also juvenile hormone-mimicking activity in *Dysdercus koenigii*. It exhibited repellent activity against *S. oryzae* and *B. chinensis*.[28]

Abortifacient and uterotonic activity: Vasicine showed an abortifacient effect in guinea pigs (although not in rats), depending on the stage of pregnancy. The effect was more marked under the priming influence of oestrogens, indicating that the action of the vasicine was probably mediated via the release of prostaglandins.[29] Vasicine also has a uterotonic activity in various other species, including humans, again influenced by the degree of priming of the uterus by oestrogens. It initiated rhythmic contractions of human myometrial strips from both non-pregnant and pregnant uteri and the effect was comparable with that of oxytocin.[30]

Wound-healing activity: In a small study, 12–18-month-old male buffalo calves were randomly divided into four groups of three animals each. Six wounds were created on either side of the vertebral column in each animal. The wounds were treated with powdered plant, alcoholic and chloroform extracts of *Adhatoda vasica*. An increase in rate of healing, breaking strength, tensile strength, absorption and extensibility was observed and collagen, elastin, hydroxyproline, hexosamine and zinc in biopsy specimens significantly increased from the third to the 30th day in the treated groups. The alcoholic extract was the most effective.[31]

Safety profile

Large doses cause diarrhoea and vomiting and because of the uterotonic activity it should not be used during pregnancy. The

LD_{50} for vasicine in mice via different routes are: 290 (PO), 125 (IP), 200 (SC) and 79 (IV) mg/kg body weight.[1]

Dosage

Liquid extract: 2–5 ml

Leaf juice: 10–20 ml

Flower juice: 10–20 ml

Root decoction: 40–80 ml

Ayurvedic properties

Guna: *Laghu* (light), *ruksha* (dry)

Rasa: *Tikta* (bitter), *kashaya* (astringent)

Veerya: *Shita* (cold)

Vipaka: *Katu* (pungent)

Dosha: Pacifies *kapha* and *pitta*

Further reading

Kirtikar KR, Basu BD, An LCS 1975 Indian medicinal plants, vol 3. Bishen Singh Mahendra Pal Singh, Dehradun

Ministry of Health and Family Welfare 1966 Indian pharmacopoeia. Government of India, New Delhi

Ministry of Health and Family Welfare 1989 Ayurvedic pharmacopoeia, part I, vol I. Government of India, New Delhi

Council of Scientific and Industrial Research 1985 The wealth of India. PID, CSIR, New Delhi

Nadkarni AK 1976 Indian materia medica, vol 1. Popular Prakashan Pvt Ltd, Bombay

Sairam TV 1999 Home remedies, vol II. Penguin India, New Delhi

References

1 Claeson UP, Malmfors T, Wikman G, Bruhn JG 2000 *Adhatoda vasica*: a critical review of ethnopharmacological and toxicological data. Journal of Ethnopharmacology 72:1

2 Jain SP, Singh SC, Puri HS 1994 Medicinal plants of Neterhat, Bihar, India. International Journal of Pharmacognosy 32: 44

3 Siddiqui MB, Husain W 1994 Medicinal plants of wider use in India with special reference to Sitapur district (Uttar Pradesh). Fitoterapia 65:3

4 Maikhuri RK, Gangwar AK 1965 Ethnobiological notes on the Khasi and Garo tribes of Meghalaya, Northeast India. Economic Botany 47:345

5 Jha MK 1992 The folk veterinary system of Bihar – a research survey. NDDB, Anand, Gujrat

6 Lahiri PK, Pradhan SN 1964 Pharmacological investigation of vasicinol, an alkaloid from *Adhatoda vasica* Nees. Indian Journal of Experimental Biology 2:219

7 Willaman JJ, Li HL 1970 Alkaloid-bearing plants 1957–1968. Lloydia 33S :1

8 Thappa RK, Agarwal SG, Dhar KL, Gupta VK, Goswami KN 1996 Two pyrroloquinazolines from *Adhatoda vasica*. Phytochemistry 42(5):1485

9 Abd El-Megeed Hashem F, Ahmed El-sawi S 1998 Isoquinoline and quinazoline alkaloids of *Adhatoda vasica*. Pharmacy and Pharmacology Letters 8(4):167

10 Jain MP, Koul SK, Dhar KL Atal CK 1980 Novel nor-harmal alkaloid from *Adhatoda vasica*. Phytochemistry 19:1880

11 Jain MP, Sharma VK, 1982 Phytochemical investigation of roots of *Adhatoda vasica*. Planta Medica 46:250

12 Dhar KL, Jain MP, Koul SK, Atal CK 1981 Vasicol, a new alkaloid from *Adhatoda vasica*. Phytochemistry 20(2):319

13 Rahman AU, Sultana N, Akhter F, Nighat F, Choudhary MI 1997 Phytochemical studies on *Adhatoda vasica*. Pakistan Natural Product Letters 10(4):249

14 Bhartiya HP, Gupta PC 1982 A chalcone glycoside from the flowers of *Adhatoda vasica*. Phytochemistry 21(1):247

15 Ahmed El-Sawi S, Abd El-Megeed Hashem F, Ali AM 1999 Flavonoids and antimicrobial volatiles from *Adhatoda vasica* NEES. Pharmacy and Pharmacology Letters 9(2):52

16 Singh RS, Misra TN, Pandey HS, Singh BP 1991 Aliphatic hydroxyketones from *Adhatoda vasica*. Phytochemistry 30(11):3799

17 Singh RS, Misra TN, Pandey HS, Singh BP 1992 A new aliphatic alcohol from *Adhatoda vasica*. Fitoterapia 63(3):262

18 Gupta OP, Anand KK, Ghatak BJ, Atal CK 1977 Pharmacological investigations of vasicine and vasicinone – the alkaloids of *Adhatoda vasica*. Indian Journal of Medical Research 66(4):680

19 Bhalla HL, Nimbkar AY 1982 Preformulation studies III. Vasicinone, a bronchodilatory alkaloid from *Adhatoda vasica* Nees (absorption, potency and toxicity studies). Drug Dev. Indian. Pharm 8(6):833

20 Mullar A, Antus S, Bittinger M et al 1993 Chemistry and pharmacology of the antiasthmatic plants, *Galpinia glauca, Adhatoda vasica, Picrorrizha kurroa.* Planta Medica 59S:A586

21 Brantner AH, Chakraborty A 1998 *In vitro* antibacterial activity of alkaloids isolated from *Adhatoda vasica* NEES. Pharmacy and Pharmacology Letters 8(3):137

22 Kumar S, Gopal K 1999 Screening of plant species for inhibition of bacterial population of raw water. Journal of Environmental Science and Health A34(4):975

23 Grange JM, Snell NJC 1996 Activity of bromhexine and ambroxol, semi-synthetic derivatives of vasicine from the Indian shrub *Adhatoda vasica*, against *Mycobacterium tuberculosis in vitro*. Journal of Ethnopharmacology 50(1):49

24 Rabinovich MI, Leskov AI, Gladkikh AS 1966 Cholegogic properties of peganine. Vrachei: 181

25 Chaturvedi GN, Rai NP, Dhani R, Tiwari SK, 1983 Clinical trial of *Adhatoda vasica* syrup (vasa) in the patients of non-ulcer dyspepsia (Amlapitta). Ancient Science of Life 3(1):19

26 Srivastava AS, Saxena HP, Singh DR 1965 *Adhatoda vasica*, a promising insecticide against pests of storage. Lab. Dev 3(2):138

27 Saxena BP, Tikku K, Atal CK 1986 Insect antifertility and antifeedant alleochemics in *Adhatoda vasica*. Insect Sci. Appl. 7(4):489

28 Kokate CK, D'Cruz JL, Kumar RA, Apte SS 1985 Anti-insect and juvenoidal activity of phytochemicals derived from *Adhatoda vasica* Nees. Indian Journal of Natural Products 1(1–2):7

29 Gupta OP, Anand KK, Ghatak BJ, Ray, Atal CK 1978 Vasicine, alkaloid of *Adhatoda vasica*, a promising uterotonic abortifacient. Indian Journal of Experimental Biology 16(10):1075

30 Atal CK 1980 The chemistry and pharmacology of vasicine, a new oxytocic and abortifacient. Regional Research Laboratory, CSIR, Jammu-Tawi, India

31 Bhargava MK, Singh H, Kumar A 1988 Evaluation of *Adhatoda vasica* as a wound healing agent in buffaloes. Clinical, mechanical and biochemical studies. Indian Veterinary Journal 65(1):33

Aegle marmelos L. Corr. ex Roxb. (Rutaceae)

English: Bengal quince

Hindi: *Bael, bel, beli*

Sanskrit: *Bilva*

Bael is considered to be an auspicious tree by the Hindus and has been called '*shivadruma*' (the tree of Shiva). It is often planted near temples and the leaves and wood of the plant have been used for worshipping Lord Shiva and Parvati since time immemorial. All parts, but especially the fruits, are commonly used in traditional medicine and the drug has been described as a *rasayana*.

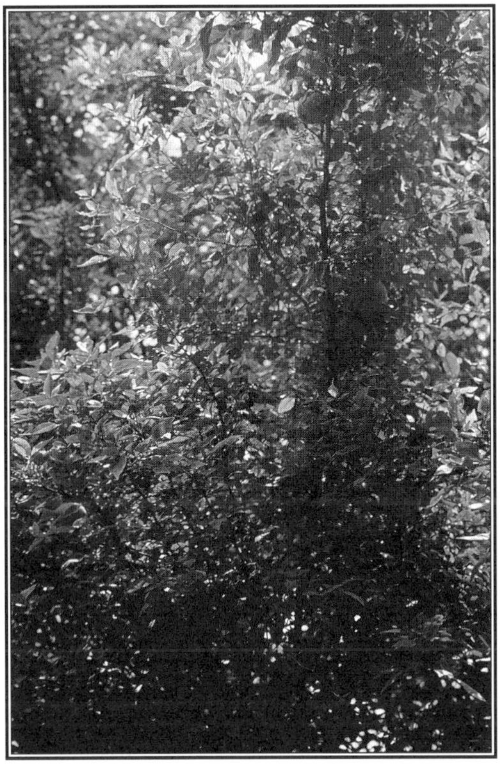

Habitat

It is commonly found in the sub-Himalayan tract up to an altitude of 1200 m, in the dry deciduous forests of central and southern India, the Andaman islands, Myanmar, south-east Asia and Baluchistan.

Botanical description

A medium-sized, deciduous tree, up to 7.5 m in height; the branches are armed with sharp spines about 2.5 mm long (Plate 5). Leaves glabrous, attenuate and trifoliate; flowers large, greenish-white and sweet scented, with numerous seeds, oblong, compressed, embedded in sacs and covered with thick orange-coloured sweet pulp. The ripe fruits are large and subspherical, greenish-white with a tough, woody outer coat. The roots are woody, fairly large and often curved. The bark is corky and light grey in colour.

Parts used

Fruit, pulp, unripe fruit, ripe fruit, rind of ripe fruit, bark, root and root bark.

Traditional and modern use

The ripe bael fruit is usually eaten fresh. The pulp is often combined with sugar and tamarind to prepare a refreshing drink in Indian homes, as well as squash, jam and nectar. The green fruits have digestive, stomachic and astringent properties and are used to make the preparation *murabbas*. Ripe fruits are used in chronic diarrhoea and dysentery and act as a tonic for the heart and brain. They are also useful in adjuvant treatment of bacillary dysentery, assisting the healing of the ulcerated mucosa of the intestines. The roots, in the form of a decoction, are used to treat melancholia, intermittent fevers and heart palpitations and also form a component of a popular Ayurvedic medicine *dashmool*. The bitter-tasting leaves are used as a febrifuge and a poultice made of them is used for ophthalmic disorders and ulcers. Fresh leaves have been used to treat weakness of the heart, dropsy and beri-beri. Bengal quince has also been used for stomach ache, snakebite, cholera, convulsions, dyspepsia, malaria, nausea, spasms, thirst, tumours, sores, itches and proctitis and as an abortifacient. It also finds use as an anodyne, astringent, dentifrice, digestive, piscicide, refrigerant, restorative and laxative.

Ethnoveterinary usage

Bark, flower, fruit, leaf, root and stem are all used in the treatment of diarrhoea and dehydration of ruminants.[1] The fruit pulp (both ripe and unripe), leaves, roots and bark (also the 'powdery mildew' on the bark) are used in folk veterinary medicine to treat wounds, burns, poisoning and disorders of the digestive systems including dysentery, enteritis and intestinal lesions, tympanitis and for flat and thread worms. It also finds use in ailments of the reproductive system such as miscarriage, retention of the placenta, repeated oestrus in cows and buffaloes, vaginal haemorrhage, orchiditis, and in addition, milk fever, tachycardia, bradycardia, swelling of the throat, haemorrhagic septicaemia, pneumonia, polyurea, lumbar fracture and others.

Major chemical constituents

Alkaloids

The leaves contain alkaloids including aegelenine and aegeline. The roots and aerial parts contain skimmianine.[2]

Anthraquinones

7,8-Dimethoxy-1-hydroxy-2-methyl anthraquinone and 6-hydroxy-1-methoxy-3-methyl anthraquinone.[3]

Coumarins

The fruit contains marmelosin, allo-imperatorin, marmelide and psoralen and the roots umbelliferone, psoralen, xanthotoxin, dimethoxy coumarin, scopoletin.[4] The heartwood yields α-xanthotoxol-8-O-β-D-glucoside and the seeds contain luvangetin.[5]

Tannins

The fruit contains tannic acid. The tannin content of the fruit and rind is 7–9% and 18–22% respectively. The leaves also contain condensed tannins.[3]

Triterpenes

The roots contain β-sitosterol and lupeol.[3]

Medicinal and pharmacological activities

Antiulcer activity: Luvangetin, at a dosage of 25 mg/kg by oral administration, showed significant protection against pylorus-ligated and aspirin-induced gastric ulcers in rats and cold restraint stress-induced gastric ulcers in rats and guinea pigs. The mechanism of action appeared to be due to mucosal defensive factors.[5]

Antimicrobial activity: The essential oil isolated from the leaves was evaluated in a spore germination assay and variable efficacy observed against different fungal isolates. Complete inhibition of germination of all fungal spores was observed at 500 ppm, except for the most resistant, *Fusarium udum*, which was inhibited 80% at 400 ppm.[6] It also inhibited the growth of 21 bacteria including Gram-positive (cocci and rods), Gram-negative (rods) and 12 fungi including three yeast-like and nine filamentous.[7] The seed oil was also antibacterial and an ethanolic extract of the roots showed appreciable activity against *Vibrio cholerae, Salmonella typhimurium, Klebsiella pneumoniae, Candida albicans, Aspergillus fumigatus* and *Trichophyton mentagrophytes*. An ethanolic extract was effective against *Curvularia lanata, Aspergillus niger* and *Rhizopus nodulens*.[8]

Hypoglycaemic activity: The aqueous extract of the leaves exhibited significant hypoglycaemic activity in both normoglycaemic and streptozotocin-diabetic rats, assessed as a stimulation of the surviving cells to release more insulin and substantiated by elevated levels of plasma insulin. The extract was found to be as effective as insulin in restoring blood glucose levels and body weight to normal.[9] In streptozotocin-induced diabetic rats, histopathological changes in the acinar cells and hepatocytes, liver fibrosis and decrease in glycogen content and changes in kidney glomeruli were restored to near normal. The extract also appeared to help in the regeneration of the damaged pancreas.[10] In an alloxan-induced animal model, the oral administration of a leaf extract (1 g/kg) prior to the experiment resulted in a significant increase in glucose tolerance. Administration to diabetic rats resulted in the decrease of liver glycogen, blood urea and a reduction of elevated serum cholesterol levels, once again exhibiting a similar action to that of insulin.[11]

Antidiarrhoeal activity, Irritable Bowel Syndrome: An Ayurvedic preparation consisting of *Aegle marmelos* (3 g) and *Bacopa monnieri* (1 g) was compared with a standard therapy (clidinium bromide with chlordiazepoxide and ispaghula) and a matching placebo, in a randomised trial for 6 weeks. In 57 patients (33.7%) improvement was seen with the Ayurvedic preparation, in 60 patients (35.5%) an effect was observed with the standard therapy and in 52 patients (30.8%) an effect was observed with the placebo. The Ayurvedic preparation was the most useful in the diarrhoea-predominant form as compared to the placebo. Long-term therapy (longer than 6 months) showed that neither was better than placebo in limiting relapse.[12]

Antiinflammatory activity: An aqueous extract of the root (5 mg/kg) exhibited significant antiinflammatory activity against both acute and chronic inflammation.[13] The acute experimental model was carrageenan-induced rat paw oedema and a 'dead space' wound model was used to monitor chronic inflammation. Marmin also showed an antiinflammatory effect in carrageenan-induced paw oedema in rats.[14]

Effects on the cardiovascular system: A methanolic extract of root bark (100 μg/ml) inhibited the spontaneous beating rate of cultured mouse myocardial cells by approximately 50%. Aurapten, a pure compound isolated from the same, was found to be the most potent with IC_{50} of 0.6 μg/ml.[15]

Immunomodulatory activity: A C-glucosylated propelargonidin from the aqueous extract of the unripe fruit of *A. marmelos* exhibited a moderate inhibition of the classic pathway of complement activation and of luminal-enhanced chemiluminescence by zymosan-activated polymorphonuclear leucocytes. It had no effect on the alternative pathway of complement activation.[16]

Safety profile

The fruits are generally regarded as safe, although feeding large amounts to rats produced hepatic lesions, including vein abnormalities.[17] The maximum tolerated dose of the 50% ethanolic extract of roots was 1000 mg/kg in adult albino mice.[18]

Dosage

Fruit Powder: 2–12 g

Infusion: 12–20 ml

Decoction: 28–56 ml

Ayurvedic properties

Rasa: *Tikta* (bitter), *kashaya* (astringent)

Guna: *Laghu* (light), *ruksha* (dry)

Vipaka: *Katu* (pungent)

Veerya: *Ushna* (hot)

Dosha: Pacifies *kapha* and *vata* and promotes *pitta*

Further reading

Bharatiya Vidya Bhavan's Swami Prakashanandra Ayurveda Research Centre 1992 Selected medicinal plants of India. Chemexcil, Mumbai

Kapoor LD1990 Handbook of Ayurvedic medicinal plants. CRC Press, Boca Raton

Pandey GS (ed) 1998 Ayurvedic pharmacopoeia. Chaukhambha Bharati Academy, Gokul Bhawan, Varanasi

Sairam TV 1999 Home remedies, vol I. Penguin India, New Delhi

References

1 International Institute of Rural Reconstruction, 1994 Ethnoveterinary medicine in Asia. An information kit on traditional animal health care practices, Part I, General Information. IIRR Silang, Philippines

2 Bhavan B 1992 *Aegle marmelos*. In: Bharatiya Vidya Bhavan Selected medicinal plants of India. Chemexcil, Mumbai

3 Srivastava SD, Srivastava S, Srivastava SK 1996 New anthraquinones from heartwood of *Aegle marmelos*. Fitoterapia 67:83

4 Barthakur NN, Arnold NP 1989 Central organic and inorganic constituents in bael (*Aegle marmelos* Correa) fruit. Tropical Agriculture 66(1):65

5 Goel RK, Maiti RN, Manickam M, Ray AB 1997 Antiulcer activity of naturally occurring pyrano-coumarin and isocoumarins and their effect on prostanoid synthesis using human colonic mucosa. Indian Journal of Experimental Biology 35(10):1080

6 Rana BK, Singh UP, Taneja V 1997 Antifungal activity and kinetics of inhibition by essential oil isolated from leaves of *Aegle marmelos*. Journal of Ethnopharmacology 57(1):29

7 Patnaik S, Subramanyam VR, Kole C 1996 Antibacterial and antifungal activity of ten essential oils *in vitro*. Microbios 86(349):237

8 Rusia K, Srivastava SK 1988 Antimicrobial activity of some Indian medicinal plants. Indian Journal of Pharmaceutical Sciences 50(1):57

9 Seema PV, Sudha B, Padayatti PS, Abraham A, Raghu KG, Paulose CS 1996 Kinetic studies of

purified malate dehydrogenase in liver of streptozotocin-diabetic rats and the effect of leaf extract of *Aegle marmelos* (L.) Correa ex Roxb. Indian Journal of Experimental Biology 34(6):600

10 Das AV, Padayatti PS, Paulose CS 1996 Effect of leaf extract of *Aegle marmelos* (L.) Correa ex Roxb. on histological and ultrastructural changes in tissues of streptozotocin induced diabetic rats. Indian Journal of Experimental Biology 34(4):341

11 Ponnachan PT, Paulose CS, Panikkar KR 1993 Effect of leaf extract of *Aegle marmelos* in diabetic rats. Indian Journal of Experimental Biology 31(4):345

12 Yadav SK, Jain AK, Tripathi SN, Gupta JP 1989 Irritable bowel syndrome: therapeutic evaluation of indigenous drugs. Indian Journal of Medical Research 90:496

13 Udupa SL, Udupa AL, Kulkarni DR 1994 Studies on the antiinflammatory and wound healing properties of *Moringa oleifera* and *Aegle marmelos*. Fitoterapia 65(2):119

14 Pitre S, Srivastava SK 1987 Pharmacological, microbiological and phytochemical studies on roots of *Aegle marmelos*. Fitoterapia 58(3):194

15 Kakiuchi N, Senaratne LR, Huang SL et al 1991 Effects of constituents of Beli (*Aegle marmelos*) on spontaneous beating and calcium paradox of myocardial cells. Planta Medica 57(1):43

16 Abeysekera AM, De Silva KTD, Samarsinghe S, Seneviratne PAK, Van Den Berg AJJ, Labadie RP 1996 An immunomodulatory C-glucosylated propelargonidin from the unripe fruit of *Aegle marmelos*. Fitoterapia 67(4):367

17 Arseculeratne SN, Gunatilaka AA, Panabokke RG 1985 Studies of medicinal plants of Sri Lanka. Part 14: Toxicity of some traditional medicinal herbs. Journal of Ethnopharmacology 13(3):323

18 Dhar ML, Dhar MM, Dhawan BN, Mehrotra BN, Ray C 1968 Screening of Indian plants for biological activity: Part I. Indian Journal of Experimental Biology 6:232

Allium sativum L. (Liliaceae)

English: Garlic

Hindi: *Lasan*

Sanskrit: *Lasuna, rasonam*

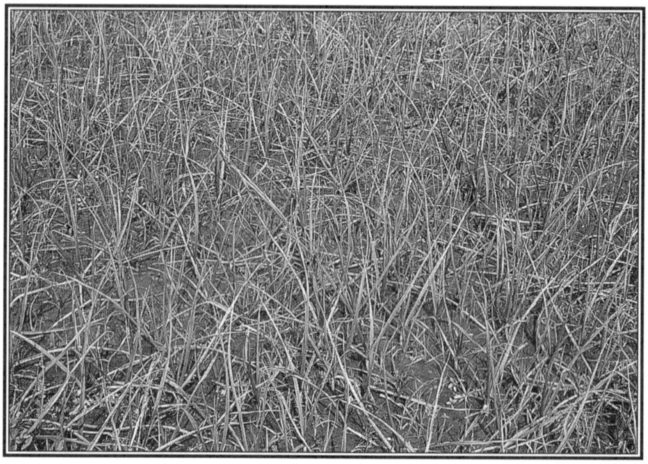

The first mention of garlic appears in a Sumerian recipe written in about 3000 BC. The Assyrians also used garlic as a food, brewed as a tea or mixed with wine for a variety of medicinal purposes and to strengthen the system and ward off diseases. In ancient India, there are records in the Sanskrit language documenting the use of garlic remedies about 5000 years ago and the Ebers papyrus written in 1550 BC appears to contain the first mention of garlic in Egyptian medicine. This codex gives 22 uses for garlic, including treatments for heart problems, tumours, headaches, worms and bites. The Holy Bible also mentions garlic as a common food in Egypt.

Athletes in the early Olympic games used to eat garlic before competitions to gain strength and Greek soldiers ate it before battle. It was used as a battlefield medicine to prevent infection in wounds. Hippocrates himself recommended garlic for infections, cancer, leprosy and digestive problems. Galen, the greatest physician of Roman history, referred to garlic as *theriaca rusticorum*, 'peasant's heal all', a name which eventually reached England in the Middle Ages as 'poor man's theriacle', and it was known in Arabia as *theriaka-al-fuqara* (theriac of the poor).

It has been suggested that the wild ancestor of garlic was a flowering form producing seeds on aerial 'bulbils'. Under different soil and climate conditions, and different methods of cultivation in the ancient centres of civilisation, other varieties arose.

Habitat

A hardy perennial, native to Central Asia and cultivated worldwide, garlic requires a fertile soil and a warm, sunny climate. The culture is annual or biannual.[1] It is grown by dividing the bulb and is harvested late the following summer.

Botanical description

A perennial, erect, bulbous herb, 30–60 cm tall (Plate 6), strong smelling especially when crushed. The underground portion consists of a compound bulb giving rise above ground to a number of narrow, keeled, grass-like leaves. The leaf blade is linear, flat, solid, 1.0–2.5 cm wide, 30–60 cm long, and has an acute apex. The leaf sheaths form a pseudo-stem. The inflorescence is umbellate; the scape coiled at first and subtended by a membranous, long-beaked spathe, splitting on one side and remaining attached to the umbel. Small bulbils are produced in the inflorescences. The flowers are variable in number and sometimes absent, seldom open and may wither in the bud. They occur on slender pedicles, consisting of a perianth of six segments, about 4–6 mm long and pinkish. There are six stamens with the anthers exserted and a superior, three-locular ovary. Seeds are rarely produced.

Parts used

Bulb.

Traditional and modern use

Ayurveda uses garlic as a tonic, to build the health in general rather than treat a particular disease, although it recognises garlic's effects on the digestive, respiratory, nervous, reproductive and circulatory systems. In Unani medicine garlic is used to treat dysentery, intestinal infection, colic in children, arthritis and food poisoning. In south-west America it is used as a cough remedy, and the Appalachians used garlic for treating pneumonia and chest colds. It is also recommended for earaches and deafness. In Thailand it is eaten to avoid diarrhoea from parasites and a decoction of fresh bulb is taken orally as an antiinflammatory. The crushed bulb is also used as a poultice on inflamed joints.[2] In France it is used to treat allergies, arteriosclerosis, arthritis, asthma, urinary incontinence, bronchial diseases, acne, emphysema, hypertension and liver diseases. A hot water extract of fresh bulb has been taken in Yugoslavia for treating diabetes.[3] In the West Indies extracts of the bulb are taken for hypertension and rubbed on the abdomen to facilitate parturition and in Africa it is used as an antibacterial for sore throats, infected wounds and boils. The essential oil is occasionally used as an antispasmodic, antimicrobial, diuretic, antiasthmatic and emmenagogue.

Ethnoveterinary usage

The bulb is used in fungal infections and swelling of the tongue, oral blisters and wounds, rheumatism, contagious abortion, tetanus, milky diarrhoea, abdominal pain, asthma, polyuria, sores, compound fracture, epilepsy and swelling of the kidney.[4]

Major chemical constituents

Sulphur compounds

Allicin, mercaptan, allyl methyl thiosulphinate, allyl methyl trisulphide, allyl propyl disulphide, diallyl disulphide, diallyl heptasulphide, diallyl hexasulphide, diallyl pentasulphide, diallyl sulphide, diallyl tetrasulphide, diallyl trisulphide, dimethyl disulphide, methyl allyl thiosulphinate, S-allyl cysteine sulphoxide, and others.[1,3,8]

Glycosides

Sativoside-B1, proto-desgalactotigonin.[5]

Aminoacids

Alanine, arginine, aspartic acid, asparagine, histidine, leucine, methionine, phenyl alanine, proline, serine, threonine, tryptophan, valine.[6]

Monoterpenoids

Citral, geraniol, linalool, α- and β-phellandrene, and others.[7]

Minerals

Calcium, phosphorus, iron, iodine, cobalt, copper, sodium, potassium, selenium and zinc.[3,7]

Vitamins

β-Carotene, biotin, niacin, riboflavin, ascorbic acid, thiamin, folic acid and others.[8]

Flavones and flavonols

Kaempferol, quercetin, rutin.[1,3,7]

Peptides

γ-L-glutamyl-S-methyl-L-cysteine sulphoxide, γ-L-glutamyl-S-methyl-L-cysteine, γ-L-glutamyl-S-allyl-L-cysteine, γ-L-glutamyl-L-phenylalanine, γ-L-glutamyl-S-propylcysteine, γ-L-glutamyl-S-(2-carboxy-propyl)-cysteinyl-gly cine.[9]

Medicinal and pharmacological activities

Immunomodulatory activity: Aged garlic extracts (AGE) have shown immunomodulatory activity in various experimental models. In the immunoglobulin (Ig)E-mediated allergic mouse model, AGE significantly decreased the antigen-specific ear swelling induced by picryl chloride ointment to the ear and intravenous administration of anti-trinitrophenyl antibody. In the transplanted carcinoma cell model, AGE significantly inhibited the growth of sarcoma-180 (allogenic) and LL/2 lung carcinoma (syngenic) cells transplanted into mice and increased natural killer (NK) activities of spleen cells observed in the sarcoma-180 bearing mice. In a psychological stress model, AGE significantly prevented the decrease in spleen weight and restored the reduction of anti-SRBC haemolytic plaque-forming cells caused by electrical stress. These studies suggest that AGE may be an immune modifier, maintaining the homeostasis of immune functions.[10]

Diallyl sulphide (DAS) showed chemopreventive effects at several organ sites in rodents after administration of chemical carcinogens, possibly by inhibiting carcinogen activation via cytochrome P450-mediated oxidative metabolism. It also exerted a protective effect on N-nitrosodimethylamine (NDMA)-induced immunosuppression of humoral and cellular responses in BALB/c mice. This effect may, at least in part, be due to its ability to block bioactivation of NDMA by the inhibition of cytochrome P450 2E1.[11]

Antiageing activity: The Hayflick system of cellular ageing in culture method was adopted to evaluate garlic for its effects on long-term growth characteristics, morphology and macromolecular synthesis of human skin fibroblasts. The rejuvenating effects were demonstrated after the addition of garlic extract into a normal cell culture medium, which supported serial subculturing for over 55 population doublings in 475 days. This suggests antiageing and other beneficial effects on human fibroblasts, in terms of the maximum proliferative capacity and morphological characteristics.[12]

Hypolipidaemic activity: Rats fed with a sucrose-rich high-fat diet had a higher level of triglycerides and cholesterol in the serum, liver and kidneys. When the animals were given ethanol (instead of water) to drink, triglycerides and cholesterol levels in the liver and kidneys significantly increased although serum levels did not change significantly. However, when the sucrose-rich high-fat diet fed rats were given garlic extracts, these lipid levels were significantly reduced to almost the same extent in both cases.[13] An ethanol and high-fat, high-cholesterol diet fed to rats markedly increased the total lipids in the liver and cholesterol and triglyceride levels in the serum, liver and kidneys. When ethanol was mixed with garlic oil (0.5%) and fed to these animals, lipid levels were significantly reduced to near those seen in untreated control rats. Garlic oil may enhance the catabolism of dietary cholesterol and fatty acids.[14] In an experiment using female kid goats, the concentration of serum lipids and cholesterol in animals fed with cholesterol was increased but was lower in those fed with garlic. The involvement of fatty streaks and spots in the aorta was maximal in kids fed cholesterol alone but minimal in those fed with both cholesterol and garlic, indicating that garlic produced both hypocholesterolaemic and antiatherosclerotic effects in the goat.[15]

Hepatoprotective acitvity:
S-Allylmercaptocysteine (SAMC), a water-soluble organosulphur compound, was shown to protect mice against acetaminophen (APAP)-induced liver injury at a dose of 100 mg/kg (PO). When given 2 and 24 hours before APAP administration (500 mg/kg, PO) it suppressed the plasma alanine aminotransferase activity significantly. The mode of action was suggested to be the inhibition of cytochrome P450 2E1 activity. Pretreatment with SAMC also suppressed the increase in hepatic lipid peroxidation and the decrease in hepatic reduced coenzyme Q9 (CoQ9H2) levels, indicating another mechanism of action of SAMC may be its antioxidant activity.[16]

Spermatogenic activity: A water extract of garlic was administered to male mice in drinking water (100 mg/kg/day) for 3 months. A significant increase in the weight of the seminal vesicles and epididymides, as compared to controls, was observed and the sperm count was significantly elevated.[17]

Antibacterial activity: Garlic has long been recognised as a natural antibiotic and recent publications indicate that the extract has broad-spectrum antimicrobial activity against bacteria and fungi. Many of these are medically significant and garlic shows promise as a broad-spectrum therapeutic agent.[18] Louis Pasteur was the first to describe its antibacterial effects. Garlic exhibits activity against both Gram-positive and Gram-negative bacteria and is effective against those strains that have become resistant to antibiotics. Resistance to garlic itself has not been seen. The raw juice was found to be effective against many common pathogenic bacteria-intestinal bacteria, which are responsible for diarrhoea in humans and animals. The combination of garlic with antibiotics leads to partial or total synergism. *Helicobacter pylori*, a bacterium implicated in the aetiology of stomach cancer and ulcers, is inhibited by garlic in vitro and the incidence of stomach cancer is lower in populations with a high intake of Allium vegetables.[19] A study carried out to evaluate the antibacterial properties of garlic before and after heat treatment used test microorganisms including *Escherichia coli, Salmonella typhimurium, Vibrio parahaemolyticus, Pseudomonas aeruginosa, Proteus vulgaris,*

Staphylococcus aureus, Mycobacterium phlei, Streptococcus faecalis, Bacillus cereus and *Micrococcus luteus*. Raw garlic bulb inhibited all of the test strains except the antibacterial activity within 20 minutes of heat treatment at 100°C.[20] Allicin, one of the active principles of freshly crushed garlic, has a variety of antimicrobial activities. In the pure form it was found to exhibit antibacterial activity against a wide range of Gram-negative and Gram-positive bacteria, including multidrug-resistant enterotoxicogenic strains of *E. coli*. It had antiviral and antifungal activity, particularly against *Candida albicans*, and antiparasitic activity against *Entamoeba histolytica* and *Giardia lamblia*. These effects are thought to be mediated through reaction with the thiol groups of various enzymes, including alcohol dehydrogenase, thioredoxin reductase and RNA polymerase. These can affect essential metabolism of cysteine proteinase activity involved in the virulence of *E. histolytica*.[21]

Antidermatophytic activity: The aqueous extract of garlic demonstrated activity against 88 clinical isolates of dermatophytes using an agar dilution technique. The isolates included *Microsporum canis* (50), *M. audouinii* (5), *Trichophyton rubrum* (6), *T. mentagrophytes* (5), *T. violaceum* (12), *T. simii* (5), *T. verrucosum* (1), *T. erinacei* (1) and *Epidermophyton floccosum* (2).[22]

Antiviral activity: The in vitro antiviral activity of garlic extract (GE) on human cytomegalovirus (HCMV) was shown using tissue culture, plaque reduction and early antigen assay. A dose-dependent inhibitory effect was evident when applied simultaneously with HCMV and the effect was stronger when the monolayers were pretreated with GE. In addition, the antiviral effect persisted in infected cells long after the garlic was removed from the culture medium and was strongest when applied continuously. It was therefore suggested that clinical use of GE against HCMV infection should be long term and the prophylactic use of GE is recommended for immunocompromised patients.[23]

Anticancer activity: Epidemiological and laboratory studies provide insight into the anticarcinogenic potential of garlic and its constituent compounds. Both water- and lipid-soluble allyl sulphur compounds are effective in blocking many chemically induced tumours, thought to be partly related to inhibition of nitrosamine formation and metabolism. However, blocking the initiation and promotion phases of various carcinogens, including polycyclic hydrocarbons, provides evidence that garlic and its constituents can affect several phase I and II enzymes. The ability to prevent experimentally induced tumours in a variety of sites, including the skin, mammary glands and colon, suggests a general mechanism of action. Changes in DNA repair and in immunocompetence may also account for some of this protection. Some allyl sulphur compounds can effectively retard tumour proliferation and induce apoptosis and changes in cellular thiol and phosphorylation stains may account for some of these properties.[24] There is further evidence that organosulphur compounds, including diallyl sulphides, can inhibit the induction and growth of cancer and epidemiological studies have suggested that consumption of garlic can decrease cancer incidence.[25] The effect of pretreatment with DAS on experimentally induced nuclear aberrations (NA) and ornithine decarboxylase (ODC) activity in rat glandular stomach mucosa was studied and a significant and dose-dependent inhibition was found for both, supporting the epidemiological evidence for the chemopreventive effect of garlic on gastric ulcer.[26] A 50% aqueous extract of garlic significantly inhibited precancerous lesions of the oesophagus induced by N-methyl-N-amyl-nitrosamine, and increased the percentage of peripheral T-lymphocytes in rats. The results suggested a preventive action against carcinoma of the oesophagus, which could be attributed to increasing the immunity.[27] Administration of garlic (250 mg/kg PO, three times a week) effectively suppressed 4-nitroquinoline 1-oxide (4NQO)-induced tongue carcinogenesis in the rat, as revealed by an absence of carcinomas in the initiation phase and their reduced incidence in the postinitiation phase. These results suggest that garlic may exert its chemopreventive effects by modulating lipid peroxidation and enhancing the levels of reduced glutathione (GSH), glutathione peroxidase (GPx) and glutathione S-transferase (GST).[28] Diallyl sulphide (DAS), at doses above 50 mg/kg administered 1hour before 1,2-dimethylhydrazine (DMH) in male rats partially reduced the numbers of γ-glutamyl transpeptidase and glutathione-S-transferase-P positive foci. In comparison, all doses of DAS (25–100 mg/kg) completely prevented liver necrosis by DMH (200 mg/kg), suggesting that low doses of DAS, which reduce DMH binding, appear more likely to inhibit hepatocarcinogenicity by reducing the promoting influences of postnecrotic regeneration rather than preventing initiation.[29] The antitumour activity of pure garlic oil against tumours of the cervix has also been demonstrated, in that treatment before and after insertion of a 3-methylcholanthranene thread in the uterus of rats led to a reduction of 22% in cervical weight compared to the control.[30] Phorbol myristate acetate-induced tumour promotion was also inhibited by garlic oil in a dose-dependent manner.[31]

Antimutagenic activity: The acetone extract of garlic was tested in the Ames test against a variety of known mutagens and significant activity found, providing further evidence for the chemoprevention of cancer.[32] An aqueous extract prepared from garlic bulbs also markedly suppressed both *E. coli* WP2 trp- and *E. coli* WP2 trp- uvrA-induced mutagenesis by 4-nitroquinoline 1-oxide (4NQO), but not that induced by UV. It may be inactivating the electrophilic group(s) of 4NQO or inhibiting metabolic activation.[33]

Antioxidant effects: Garlic is claimed to be effective against those diseases in which the pathophysiology of oxygen free radicals (OFRs) has been implicated, due to its ability to scavenge OFRs. Allicin produced concentration-dependent decreases in 2,3 and 2,5-dihydroxybenzoic acid (DHBA) generated by photolysis of hydrogen peroxide, by scavenging hydroxyl radicals, but not the formed hydroxyl adduct products. It also prevented lipid peroxidation in liver homogenates in a concentration-dependent manner. The results suggest that allicin has antioxidant activity.[34] The effect of AGE on oxidant injury in bovine pulmonary artery endothelial cells was shown after overnight preincubation. AGE (1–4 mg/ml) pretreatment significantly prevented the loss of cell viability induced by hydrogen peroxide. Both AGE and s-allyl cysteine (SAC) exhibited dose-dependent inhibition of lactate dehydrogenase (LDH) release and lipid peroxidation (TBA-RS) production induced by hydrogen peroxide leading to the protection of vascular endothelial cells.[35] Similar results were obtained on lipid peroxidation in mice liver homogenate, shown by a decrease in hyaluronic acid depolymerisation induced by oxygen and an inhibition of adenosine deaminase activity.[36]

Antiatherosclerotic activity: Garlic extract protected endothelial cells from oxidised LDL-induced injury in endothelial cells (EC), by preventing intracellular glutathione depletion and by minimising release of peroxides from endothelial cells and macrophages. This indicates a role in the prevention of atherosclerosis.[36]

Diuretic activity: Intravenous administration of purified fractions of garlic to anaesthetised rabbits elicited a dose-dependent diuretic and natriuretic response. A gradual decrease in heart rate but not arterial blood pressure was observed. The electrocardiogram was not affected.[37]

Antiplatelet activity: In a randomised, double-blind study of normal healthy individuals, the effect of AGE was evaluated in doses between 2.4 and 7.2 g/day vs equal amounts of placebo. Adherence of platelets was inhibited by AGE in a dose-dependent manner when collagen was the adhesive surface. Adhesion to von Willebrand factor was reduced at 7.2 g/day AGE but adherence to fibrinogen was inhibited at all levels of supplementation. Thus, AGE appears to exert selective inhibition of platelet aggregation and adhesion, which are considered to be important in the development of cardiovascular events such as myocardial infarction and ischaemic stroke.[38] Adenosine and guanosine, isolated from *Allium sativum*, showed a significant inhibitory activity against both primary and secondary aggregation of human platelets induced by 2 μM ADP.[39] The effects of aqueous extracts of raw and boiled garlic were studied in vitro on collagen-induced rabbit and human platelet aggregation. Boiled garlic was less effective than raw garlic.[40]

Antihypertensive activity: Garlic juice inhibited contractions of isolated rabbit and guinea pig aortic rings induced by norepinephrine and contractions of tracheal smooth muscles induced by acetylcholine and histamine. Furthermore, garlic juice inhibited the spontaneous movements of rabbit jejunum and guinea pig ileum and reduced the force of contraction of isolated rabbit heart in a concentration-dependent manner. These data suggest that the hypotensive action of garlic juice may be due, at least in part, to a direct relaxant effect on smooth muscles.[41] An aqueous ethanol extract of garlic administered to conscious unrestrained rats showed antihypertensive activity.[42]

Larvicidal activity: The crude extract was effective against *Aedes fluviatilis* at 1 ppm concentrations.[43]

Anthelmintic activity: Minced garlic at a concentration of 200 mg/l showed 100% anthelmintic activity in carp infested with Capillaria spp. The hexane extract in equivalent amounts showed a 75% effectiveness while the aqueous extract showed no anthelmintic effect. Ammonium potassium tartrate (1.5 mg/ml) used as a comparison gave 86% anthelmintic effectiveness.[44]

Safety profile

The level of safety is reflected by its worldwide use as a food. Ingestion of fresh garlic bulbs, extracts or the oil may occasionally cause heartburn, nausea, vomiting and diarrhoea. LD_{50} measurements in animals were too high to be relevant.

Dosage

Fresh garlic: 2–5 g
Dried powder: 0.4–1.2 g
Oil: 2–5 mg
Solid Extract: 300–1000 mg[45]

Ayurvedic properties

Rasa: *Tikta* (bitter), *kashaya* (astringent)
Guna: *Snigdha* (unctuous), *tikshna* (sharp)
Veerya: *Ushna* (hot)
Vipaka: *Katu* (pungent)
Dosha: Pacifies *vata* and *kapha*

Further Reading

Chevallier A 1996 The encyclopedia of medicinal plants. Dorling Kindersley, London

Council of Scientific and Industrial Research 1985 The wealth of India. PID, CSIR, New Delhi

Ministry of Health and Family Welfare 1989 Ayurvedic pharmacopoeia of India, vol 1. Government of India, New Delhi

References

1 Sendi A 1995 *Allium sativum* and *Allium ursinum*: Part 1 Chemistry, analysis, history, botany. Phytomedicine 4:323

2 Panthong A, Kanjanapothi D, Taylor WC 1986 Ethnobotanical review of medicinal plants from Thai traditional books, Part-I, Plants with antiinflammatory, anti-asthmatic and antihypertensive properties. Journal of Ethnopharmacology 18(3):213

3 Ross IA 1999 Medicinal plants of the world, vol 1. Humana Press, Totowa, New Jersey

4 Jha MK 1992 The folk veterinary system of Bihar – a research survey. NDDB, Anand, Gujrat

5 Matsuura H, Ushiroguchi T, Itakura Y, Fuwa T 1989 Further studies on steroidal glycosides from bulbs, roots and leaves of *Allium sativum* L. Chemical and Pharmaceutical Bulletin 37(10):2741

6 Atal CK, Sethi JK 1961 Occurrence of amino acids and allicin in Indian *Allium* (garlic). Current Science 30:308

7 Leung AY, Foster S 1996 Encyclopedia of common natural ingredients used in food, drugs and cosmetics, 2nd edn. Wiley-Interscience, New York

8 Ross I 1999 Medicinal plants of the world, vol 1. Humana Press, Totowa, New Jersey

9 Suzuki T, Sugii M, Kakimoto T 1961 New γ-glutamyl peptides in garlic. Chemical and Pharmaceutical Bulletin 9:77

10 Kyo E, Uda N, Kasuga S, Itakura Y 2001 Immunomodulatory effects of aged garlic extract. Journal of Nutrition 131:1075S

11 Jeong HG, Lee YW 1998 Protective effects of diallyl sulfide on N-nitrosodimethylamine-induced immunosuppression in mice. Cancer Letters 134(1):73

12 Svendsen L, Rattan SI, Clark BF 1994 Testing garlic for possible anti-ageing effects on long-term growth characteristics, morphology and macromolecular synthesis of human fibroblasts in culture. Journal of Ethnopharmacology 43(2):125

13 Ikpeazu OV, Agusti KT, Joseph PK 1987 Hypolipidemic effect of garlic extracts mixed with 3% ethanol in rats fed sucrose-high fat diet. Indian Journal of Biochemical Biophysics 24(4):252

14 Shoetan A, Agusti KT, Joseph PK 1984 Hypolipidemic effects of garlic oil in rats fed ethanol and a high lipid diet. Experientia 40(3):261–263

15 Kaul PL, Prasad MC 1990 Hypocholesterolemic and antiatherosclerotic effects of garlic (*Allium*

sativum L.) in goats – an experimental study. Indian Veterinary Journal 67(12):1112

16 Sumioka I, Matsura T, Kasuga S, Itakura Y, Yamada K 1998 Mechanisms of protection by S-allylmercaptocysteine against acetaminophen-induced liver injury in mice. Japanese Journal of Pharmacology 78(2):199

17 Al-Bekairi AM, Shah AH, Qureshi S 1990 Effect of *Allium sativum* on epididymal spermatozoa, estradiol-treated mice and general toxicity. Journal of Ethnopharmacology 29(2):117

18 Adetumbi MA, Lau BH 1983 *Allium sativum* (garlic) – a natural antibiotic. Medical Hypotheses 12(3):227

19 Sivam GP 2001 Protection against *Helicobacter pylori* and other bacterial infections by garlic. Journal of Nutrition 131:1106S

20 Chen HC, Chang MD, Chang TJ 1985 Antibacterial properties of some spice plants before and after heat treatment. Zhong Min Guo Wei Sheng Wu Ji Mian Yi Xue Za Zhi 18(3):190

21 Ankri S, Mirelman D 1999 Antimicrobial properties of allicin from garlic. Microbes and Infection 1(2):125

22 Venugopal PV, Venugopal TV 1995 Antidermatophytic activity of garlic (*Allium sativum*) in vitro. International Journal of Dermatology 34(4):278

23 Guo NL, Lu DP, Woods GL et al 1993 Demonstration of the anti-viral activity of garlic extract against human cytomegalovirus *in vitro*. Chinese Medical Journal 106(2):93

24 Milner JA 2001 A historical perspective on garlic and cancer. Journal of Nutrition 131:1027S

25 Lea MA 1996 Organosulfur compounds and cancer. Advances in Experimental Medicine and Biology 401:147

26 Hu PJ 1990 Protective effect of diallyl sulfide, a natural extract of garlic, on MNNG-induced damage of rat glandular stomach mucosa. Zhong Zhong Liu Za Zhi 12(6):429

27 Cao ZL 1991 The effect of Bulbus allii on precancerous lesions of the esophagus due to N-methyl-N-amylnitrosamine in rats. Zhong. Yu Fang Yi Xue Za Zhi 25(4):208

28 Balasenthil S, Ramachandran CR, Nagini S 2001 Prevention of 4-nitroquinoline 1-oxide-induced rat tongue carcinogenesis by garlic. Fitoterapia 72(5):524

29 Hayes MA, Rushmore TH, Goldberg MT 1987 Inhibition of hepatocarcinogenic responses to 1,2-dimethylhydrazine by diallyl sulfide, a component of garlic oil. Carcinogenesis 8(8):1155–1157

30 Rai L, Ahujarai PL 1990 Effect of pure garlic oil (*Allium sativum*) on the protection against 3-methylcholanranthrene-induced uterine and cervical tumorigenesis. Journal of Research and Education in Indian Medicine 9(4):20

31 Belman S 1983 Onion and garlic oils inhibit tumor promotion. Carcinogenesis 4(8):1063

32 Ruan CC 1989 Research on the anti-mutagenic effect of six natural foods. Zhong Yu Fang Yi Xue Za Zhi 23(3):160

33 Zhang YS, Chen XR, Yu YN 1989 Antimutagenic effect of garlic (*Allium sativum* L.) on 4NQO-induced mutagenesis in *Escherichia coli* WP2. Mutation Research 227(4):215

34 Prasad K, Laxdal VA, Yu M, Raney BL 1995 Antioxidant activity of allicin, an active principle in garlic. Molecular and Cellular Biochemistry 148(2):183

35 Yamasaki T, Lau BH 1997 Garlic compounds protect vascular endothelial cells from oxidant injury. Nippon Yakurigaku Zasshi 110 (suppl 1):138P

36 Ide N, Lau BH 2001 Garlic compounds minimize intracellular oxidative stress and inhibit nuclear factor kappa B activation. Journal of Nutrition 131:1020S

37 Pantoja CV, Norris BC, Contreras CM 1996 Diuretic and natriuretic effects of chromatographically purified fraction of garlic (*Allium sativum*). Journal of Ethnopharmacology 52(2):101

38 Steiner M, Li W 2001 Aged garlic extract, a modulator of cardiovascular risk factors: a dose-finding study on the effects of AGE on platelet functions. Journal of Nutrition 131:980S

39 Okuyama T, Fujita K, Shibata S et al 1989 Effects of chinese drugs 'Xiebai' and 'Dasuan' on human

platelet aggregation (*Allium bakeri, A. sativum*). Planta Medica 55(3):242

40 Ali M, Bordia T, Mustafa T 1999 Effect of raw versus boiled aqueous extract of garlic and onion on platelet aggregation. Prostaglandins, Leukotrienes and Essential Fatty Acids 60(1):43

41 Aqel MB, Gharaibah MN, Salhab AS 1991 Direct relaxant effects of garlic juice on smooth and cardiac muscles. Journal of Ethnopharmacology 33(1–2):13

42 Ribeiro RD, Fiuza de Melo MM, De Barros F, Gomes C, Trolin G 1986 Acute antihypertensive effect in conscious rats produced by some medicinal plants used in the state of Sao Paulo. Journal of Ethnopharmacology 15(3):261

43 Consoli RA, Mendes NM, Pereira JP, Santos BD, Lamounier MA 1988 Effect of several extracts derived from plants on the survival of larvae of *Aedes fluviatilis* (Lutz) (Diptera: Culicidae) in the laboratory. Memorias do Instituto Oswaldo Cruz 83(1):87

44 Pena N, Auro A, Sumano H 1988 A comparative trial of garlic, its extract and ammonium-potassium tartrate as anthelmintics in carp. Journal of Ethnopharmacology 24(2–3):199

45 Bradley, PR (ed) 1992 British herbal compendium, vol 1. British Herbal Medicine Association, Bournemouth

Andrographis paniculata (Burm. f) Nees (Acanthaceae) (syn. *Justicia paniculata* Burm. f.)

English: Green chiretta, creat

Hindi: *Kalmegh*

Sanskrit: *Bhunimba*

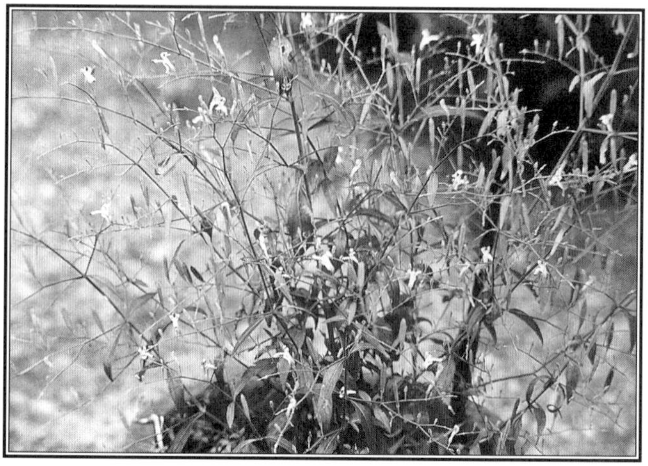

Kalmegh has been used over many centuries as a household remedy specifically for jaundice and fevers, especially the intermittent type. It is a component of over 50% of the multi-ingredient herbal formulations available in India for the treatment of liver ailments and many books on Indian materia medica equate the therapeutic applications of the plant with those of chiretta, *Swertia chirata* (qv).

Habitat

The herb is found on plains and in forests throughout India, especially the south, and in other tropical Asian countries. It grows abundantly in shady and moist places.

Botanical description

An erect, branched, annual herb with dark green stems, growing up to 1 m in height (Plate 7). Leaves glabrous, about 8 cm long and 2.5 cm broad, lanceolate and pinnate. Flowers are small, whitish or pale pink, with brown or purple blotches, in loose spreading axillary and terminal pannicles. Capsules linear or oblong, containing numerous seeds which are subquadrate and yellowish-brown in colour.

Parts used

Whole plant, leaves and roots.

Traditional and modern use

Kalmegh is used mainly for liver disorders and jaundice. A decoction or infusion of leaves is used in general debility and dyspepsia and a tincture of the root as a tonic, stimulant and aperient. The macerated leaves and juice, together with carminative spices such as cardamom, clove and cinnamon, may be made into pills and prescribed for gripe and other stomach ailments in infants. The leaves and roots also find use as an antispasmodic, febrifuge, stomachic, alterative, anthelmintic anodyne, antiseptic, laxative, astringent, and antipyretic and have been used as an adjunct in the treatment of diabetes, malaria, cholera, dysentery, enteritis, gastritis, pneumonia, pyelonephritis and even rabies. It is also a major constituent of *switradilepa*, an

Ayurvedic preparation which is used to treat vitiligo.

Ethnoveterinary usage

The juice of the stem, and the whole plant, are used to treat diarrhoea, Newcastle disease and respiratory problems in poultry.[1] The plant, especially the leaves, has been used to treat dhatoora (*datura*) poisoning, maggots in wounds, worms in the eye and abdomen, liver fluke, glossitis, holes in the hard palate, constipation, tuberculosis, pneumonia, leeches in the nostrils, contagious abortion, retention of placenta, tetanus and scabies.[2]

Major chemical constituents

Diterpenes

Andrographolide is the major component, with neoandrographolide, deoxyandrographolide and various derivatives, andrographiside, andropanoside, andrographin and panicolin also present.[3]

Flavonoids

5-Hydroxy-2′,7,8-trimethoxy flavone, 2′,5-dihydroxy-7,8-dimethoxyflavone, apigenin-4′,7-dimethylether, 5-hydroxy-7,8-dimethoxyflavanone and others.[4] The roots contain apigenin-7-4′-di-O-methyl ether and 5-hydroxy-7,8,2′,3′-tetramethoxy flavone.[5]

Medicinal and pharmacological activities

Antiviral activity: A dry extract of *A. paniculata* was shown to have some efficacy in the initial treatment of common cold and sinusitis, decreasing the symptoms and shortening their duration.[6,7] Dehydroandrographolide succinic acid monoester inhibited the human immunodeficiency virus (HIV) in vitro. The methanolic extract of the leaves also exhibited activity in HIV-1 infected MT-4 cells and suppressed the formation of syncytia in co-cultures of MOLT-4 and MOLT-4/HIV-1 cells.[8,9]

Anthelmintic activity: An alcoholic extract showed in vitro anthelmintic action against human *Ascaris lumbricoides*.[10]

Antidiarrhoeal activity: The alcoholic extract exhibited significant activity against diarrhoea induced by *Escherichia coli* enterotoxins in animal models. Andrographolide and neoandrographolide showed activity similar to that of loperamide against *E. coli* LT and LT/ST enterotoxins and andrographolide was found to be superior against enterotoxin-induced neonatal diarrhoea.[11]

Antimalarial activity: An ethanolic extract, fractions and pure isolated compounds were studied in a 4-day suppressive test against *Plasmodium berghei* NK 65 in *Mastomys natalensis*. The ethanolic extract suppressed the level of parasites in a dose-dependent manner and 15 days' administration of neoandrographolide before infection also suppressed parasitaemia.[12]

Antiplatelet aggregation activity: The crude extract of *Andrographis paniculata* inhibited platelet aggregation, being more potent than ligustrazine and persantin in vitro. Efficient absorption of the extract was assumed since rapid effects were observed in vivo, suggesting a potential use in the treatment of thrombotic diseases.[13] A study carried out on 63 patients with cardiac and cerebral vascular diseases, where the extract was administered and observations made after 3 hours and/or 1 week, found ADP-induced aggregation to be significantly delayed. The release of both dense and α granules from platelets was inhibited and a dilation of the canalicular system observed; the mechanism of action was attributed to a rise in the platelet cAMP level.[14] Similar results were observed with an IV administered flavone extract of the roots, where development of thrombi and myocardial infarction were prevented.[15]

Antipyretic activity: Oral administration of the juice of *Andrographis paniculata* normalised induced pyrexia conditions in experimental rats.[16] This activity was shown to be due in part to the ability of andrographolide to inhibit tumour necrosis factor (TNF)-α- induced intercellular adhesion molecule-1 (ICAM-1) and endothelial-monocyte adhesion.[3]

Antiatherosclerotic activity: *A. paniculata* alleviated atherosclerotic artery stenosis induced by both de-endothelialisation and a high cholesterol diet, as well as lowering the restenosis rate after experimental angioplasty.[17]

Cardiovascular activity: Polar extracts of *A. paniculata* produced a significant fall in the mean arterial blood pressure of anaesthetised rats. The most active n-butanol fraction appeared to act through α–receptors, autonomic ganglion and histaminergic receptors.[18]

Induction of cell differentiation: The methanolic extract of the aerial parts exhibited potent cell differentiation, inducing activity on mouse myeloid leukaemia cells.[19]

Hepatoprotective activity: Significant, dose-dependent protection by andrographolide was observed using an in vitro preparation of isolated rat hepatocytes[20] and both andrographiside and neoandrographolide exhibited a protective action equal to that of silymarin in liver damage induced by carbon tetrachloride or tert-butylhydroperoxide in mice.[21] Andrographolide was also effective in an in vivo system against galactosamine and paracetamol-induced hepatotoxicity in rats.[22] The ethanolic extract of the plant, and andrographolide and neoandrographolide at a dose of 6 mg/kg/day for 2 weeks, protected against hepatic damage induced by *Plasmodium berghei* K-173 in *Mastomys natalensis*. All reduced the levels of serum lipoprotein-X, alkaline phosphatase, GOT, GPT and bilirubin, as well as lipid peroxidation products, and facilitated the recovery of superoxide dismutase and glycogen in the liver.[23] An aqueous extract of *kalmegh* also improved biliary flow in rats, increased liver weight and decreased the duration of action of hexabarbital in hepatotoxicity induced by CCl_4, tetracycline and isoniazide.[24,25] Clinically, a decoction of the plant administered to patients with infectious hepatitis produced significant symptomatic relief, with a marked decrease in serum bilirubin, thymol turbidity, alkaline phosphatase, SGOT, SGPT and serum globulin fraction of protein. Eighty percent of the patients experienced symptomatic relief and 20% showed some improvement.[26]

Hypoglycaemic activity: A water extract prevented hyperglycaemia induced by oral administration of glucose, possibly by preventing the absorption of glucose from the gut.[27]

Hypotensive activity: The aqueous extract exhibited a dose-dependent, hypotensive effect on the systolic blood pressure of spontaneously hypertensive rats, thought to be due to reducing circulating angiotensin-converting enzyme (ACE) as well as reducing free radical levels in the kidneys.[28]

Immunomodulator activity: The ethanolic extract and some isolated compounds induced significant stimulation of antibody and delayed-type hypersensitivity response to sheep RBC in mice. The non-specific immune response was also stimulated.[29]

Filaricidal activity: An aqueous decoction of the leaves killed the microfilaria of *Dipetalonema reconditum* in 40 minutes in vitro and subcutaneous injections in infected dogs reduced the level of microfilariae in blood by more than 85%.[30]

Safety profile

Generally regarded as safe. The LD_{50} of the 50% ethanolic extract of plant is 215 mg/kg IP in adult male albino mice.[31]

Dosage

Infusion or decoction: 20–40 ml tid
Juice of leaves and stem: 1–4 ml tid

Ayurvedic properties

Rasa: *Tikta* (bitter)
Guna: *Laghu* (light), *ruksha* (dry)
Vipaka: *Katu* (pungent)
Veerya: *Ushna* (hot)
Dosha: Pacifies *kapha* and *pitta*

Further reading

Bharatiya Vidya Bhavan's Swami Prakashanandra Ayurveda Research Centre 1992 Selected medicinal plants of India. Chemexcil, Mumbai

Japan Pharmaceutical Traders Association 1973 Japanese drug directory – sources of crude drugs. JPTA, Tokyo

Kapoor LD 1990 Handbook of Ayurvedic medicinal plants. CRC Press, Boca Raton

References

1 International Institute of Rural Reconstruction 1994 Ethnoveterinary medicine in Asia. An information kit on traditional animal health care practices. Part I, General Information. IIRR, Silang, Philippines

2 Jha MK 1992 Folk veterinary medicine of Bihar – a research project. NDDB, Anand, Gujrat

3 Kapil A, Koul IB, Banerjee SK, Gupta BD 1993 Antihepatotoxic effects of major diterpenoid constituents of *Andrographis paniculata*. Biochemical Pharmacology 46(1):182

4 Abeysekera AM, De Silva KTD, Ratnayake S and Labadie PR 1990 An iridoid glucoside from *Andrographis paniculata*. Fitoterapia 61(5):473

5 Govindachari TR, Pai BR, Srinivasan M, Kalyanaraman PS 1969 Chemical investigation of *Andrographis paniculata*. Indian Journal of Chemistry 7:306

6 Hancke J, Burgos R, Caceres D, Wikman G 1995 A double-blind study with a new monodrug Kan Jang: decrease in symptoms and improvement in the recovery from common colds. Phytotherapy Research 9(8):559

7 Melchior J, Palm S. Wikman G 1996 Controlled clinical study of standardized *Andrographis paniculata* extract in common cold – a pilot trial. Phytomedicine 3(4):315

8 Chang RS, Ding L, Chen GQ, Pan QC, Zhao ZL, Smith KM 1991 Dehydroandrographolide succinic acid monoester as an inhibitor against the human immunodeficiency virus. Proceedings of the Society for Experimental Biology and Medicine 197(1):59–66

9 Otake T, Mori H, Morimoto M et al 1995 Screening of Indonesian plant extracts for anti-human immunodeficiency virus type-1 (HIV-1) activity. Phytotherapy Research 9(1):6

10 Raj RK 1975 Screening of indigenous plants for anthelmintic action against human *Ascaris lumbricoides*: Part II. Indian Journal of Physiology and Pharmacology 19(1):47

11 Gupta S, Choudhry MA, Yadava JNS, Srivastava V, Tandon JS 1990 Antidiarrhoeal activity of diterpenes of *Andrographis paniculata* (Kal-Megh) against *Escherichia coli* enterotoxin in *in vivo* models. International Journal of Crude Drug Research 28(4):273

12 Misra P, Pal NL, Guru PY, Katiyar JC, Srivastava V, Tandon JS 1992 Antimalarial activity of *Andrographis paniculata* (Kalmegh) against *Plasmodium berghei* NK 65 in *Mastomys natalensis*. International Journal of Pharmacognosy 30(4):263

13 Huo T, Jinzhi T 1989 Study on antiplatelet aggregation effect of *Andrographis paniculata*. Chinese Journal of Internal Traditional and Western Medicine 9(9):540

14 Zhang YZ, Tang JZ, Zhang YJ 1994 Study of *Andrographis paniculata* extract on antiplatelet aggregation and release reaction and its mechanism. Chung Kuo Chung Hsi I Chieh Ho Tsa Chih 14(1):28

15 Zhao HY, Fang WY 1991 Combined traditional Chinese and western medicine. Antithrombotic effects of *Andrographis paniculata* Nees in preventing myocardial infarction. Chinese Medical Journal 104(9):770

16 Kanniappan M, Mathuram LN, Natarajan, R 1991 Study of the antipyretic effect of Chiretta (*Andrographis paniculata*). Indian Veterinary Journal 68(4):314

17 Wang DW, Zhao HY 1994 Prevention of atherosclerotic arterial stenosis and restenosis after angioplasty with *Andrographis paniculata* Nees and fish oil. Experimental studies of effects and mechanisms. Chinese Medical Journal 107(6):464

18 Zhang CY, Tan BK 1997 Mechanism of cardiovascular activity of *Andrographis paniculata* in the anaesthetized rat. Journal of Ethnopharmacology 56(2):97

19 Matsuda T, Kuroyanagi M, Sugiyama S, Umehara K, Ueno A, Nishi K 1994 Cell differentiation inducing diterpenes from *Andrographis paniculata* Nees. Chemical and Pharmaceutical Bulletin 42(6):1216

20 Visen PK, Shukla B, Patnaik GK, Dhawan BN 1993 Andrographolide protects rat hepatocytes against paracetamol-induced damage. Journal of Ethnopharmacology 40(2):131

21 Kapil A, Koul IB, Banerjee SK, Gupta BD 1993 Antihepatotoxic effects of major diterpenoid constituents of *Andrographis paniculata*. Biochemical Pharmacology 46(1):182

22 Handa SS and Sharma A 1990 Hepatoprotective activity of andrographolide against galactosamine and paracetamol intoxication in rats. Indian Journal of Medical Research 92:284

23 Chander R, Srivastava V, Tandon JS and Kapoor NK 1995 Antihepatotoxic activity of diterpenes of *Andrographis paniculata* (Kal-megh) against *Plasmodium berghei* induced hepatic damage in *Mastomys natalensis*. International Journal of Pharmacognosy 33(2):135

24 Chaudhuri SK 1978 Influence of *Andrographis paniculata* (Kalmegh) on bile flow and hexabarbitone sleeping in experimental animals. Indian Journal of Experimental Biology 16:830

25 Tripathi GS, Tripathi YB 1991 Choleretic action of andrographolide obtained from *Andrographis paniculata* in rats. Phytotherapy Research 5(4):176

26 Chaturvedi GN, Tomar GS, Tiwari SK and Singh KP 1983 Clinical studies on Kalmegh (*Andrographis paniculata* Nees) in infective hepatitis. Ancient Science of Life II(4):208

27 Borhanuddin M, Shamsuzzoha M, Hussain AH 1994 Hypoglycaemic effects of *Andrographis paniculata* Nees on non-diabetic rabbits. Bangladesh Medical Research Council Bulletin 20(1):24.

28 Zhang CY, Tan BK 1996 Hypotensive activity of aqueous extract of *Andrographis paniculata* in rats. Clinical and Experimental Pharmacology and Physiology 23(8):675

29 Puri A, Saxena R, Saxena RP, Saxena KC, Srivastava V, Tandon JS 1993 Immunostimulant agents from *Andrographis paniculata*. Journal of Natural Products 56(7):995

30 Dutta A, Sukul NC, 1982 Filaricidal properties of a wild herb *Andrographis paniculata*. Journal of Helminthology 56(2):81

31 Aswal BS, Bhakuni DS, Goel AK, Kar K, Mehrotra BN 1984 Screening of Indian plants for biological activity. Indian Journal of Experimental Biology 22:487

Aristolochia indica L. (Aristolochiaceae)

English: Indian birthwort

Hindi: *Isharmul*

Sanskrit: *Sunanda*

The plant is commonly known by the names birthwort and snakeroot, which refer to its use in traditional medicine for postpartum infections and snakebite respectively. These indications may have originated in the medieval Doctrine of Signatures, which believed that the appearance of a plant pointed to its purpose. The flowers of Aristolochia were thought to resemble a curved foetus or a snake. The Hindi name *iswari* suggests that the plant has the property of neutralising snake poison. Unfortunately, aristolochic acid, one of the major constituents, is now known to be too toxic for the plant to be used in human medicine. It is included only for information.

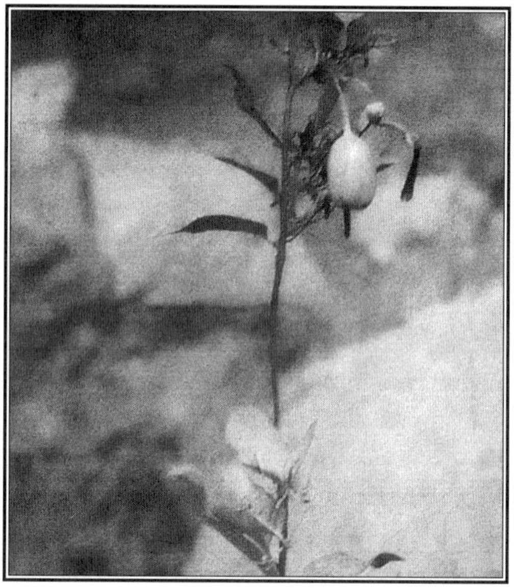

Habitat

The plant is distributed throughout all the provinces of India and in Sri Lanka, Nepal and Bangladesh. It is usually found scrambling over hedges and bushes.

Botanical description

Leaves simple, alternate, short petioled, the blade ovate or somewhat wedge shaped, very variable in shape and size (Plate 8). The young leaves are light purplish. The fruit is a capsule, roundish or oblong and hexagonal, 2.5–4 cm long and slightly less broad, with shallow grooves and six valves, containing many triangular seeds. The young roots are light brown and fairly smooth, whereas the older ones are comparatively rough due to the development of cork, lenticels and the presence of scars of rootlets. The cork layer is somewhat friable. In a freshly cut transverse section of the root the entire bark appears as a narrow, cream-coloured strip, surrounding a wide woody core. The wood has a light yellow colour and appears highly porous, with the pores being sufficiently large to be easily visible with the naked eye; the medullary rays are soft and creamy white in colour; there is no pith in the centre.

Parts used

Roots, rhizomes and leaves.

Traditional and modern use

The plant has been used in skin diseases where there is morbidity of *vata*, *pitta* and *kapha*. It is used as a appetiser, aphrodisiac and anthelmintic. The fresh juice of the leaves is a popular antidote to snake poison. The leaves and bark are used in bowel complaints of children, diarrhoea and in intermittent fevers. In traditional medicine the underground parts of the plant are rubbed with honey and given to treat leprosy; and, macerated with black pepper, it is prescribed in diarrhoea.

Ethnoveterinary usage

The root and stem of the plant are used in aches and pains, rheumatism, anthrax, madness and snakebite.[1]

Major chemical constituents

Phenanthrene derivatives

Aristolochic acid,[2] aristolochic acid-D, aristolochic acid-D methyl ether lactam, aristololactam β-D-glucoside,[3] aristolic acid, aristolic acid methyl ester, methyl aristolochate, aristolamide, aristolinic acid, aristolonitrite.[20]

Quinones

Aristolindiquinone.[4]

Lactones

Aristololide.[5]

Sesquiterpenes

(12S)-7,12-Secoishwaran-12-ol,[6] ishwarol,[7] ishwarone,[8] ishwarane, aristolochene,[9] ishwarene, selina-4(14),11-diene,[10] ledol.[11]

Alkaloid

Aristolochine.[12]

Terpenes

The essential oil of the aerial parts contains mono- and sesquiterpenes including linalool, β-caryophyllene, α-humulene, ishwarone, caryophyllene oxide, ishwarol, ishwarane and aristolochene, and α-terpinolene.[13]

Others

Ceryl alcohol, allantoin, p-coumaric acid,[20] d-camphor,[15] sitosterol and stigmast-4-en-3-one.[14]

Medicinal and pharmacological activities

General antifertility activity: Aristolic acid, from *Aristolochia indica*, disrupted nidation in mice when administered on day 1 of pregnancy. The implantation-inhibiting effect of the compound was assessed with respect to tubal transport of ova into the uterus, hyperpermeability of endometrial capillaries, increase in uterine weight and total protein content, endometrial bed preparation and changes in uterine phosphatase enzymes during days 4–6 of pregnancy. The plant induces impairment of development, with a decrease in uterine weight and total protein content, in treated animals. Aristolic acid interfered with steroidal conditioning of the uterus, rendering it hostile to ovum implantation.[15] An ethanol extract of *A. indica* root was found to decrease fertility in both rats and hamsters when administered postcoitally (on days 1–10 and 1–6 respectively).[16] Methyl aristolate (60 mg/kg, orally) decreased the number of implantation sites when administered on the first two days of pregnancy in mice. When given at doses of 50 mg/kg (but not at

30 mg/kg) consecutively on days 1–4 of pregnancy, the number of implantation sites was also decreased, possibly by disturbing the hormone balance and thereby disrupting implantation.[17] The aqueous alcoholic and petroleum ether extracts of *Aristolochia indica* at 1:20 concentration affected the oestrus cycle adversely, terminating at the dioestrous stage. These extracts also showed a marked reduction in RNA, sialic acid, glycogen of the uterus and vagina, and ascorbic acid of the adrenal glands. An aqueous alcoholic extract (at 0.2 ml) was found to be more effective than the petroleum ether extract.[18]

Antioestrogenic activity: Aristolic acid exhibited antioestrogenic activity as shown by the prevention of oestrogen-induced weight increase and epithelial growth in the mouse uterus. It caused a decrease in alkaline phosphatase activity, glycogen content and mitotic counts in the oestrogen-treated uterus and prevented implantation in the early stages of pregnancy in mice.[19]

Abortifacient activity: In female mice, methyl aristolate produced 100% abortifacient activity at a single oral dose of 60 mg/kg when administered on the sixth or seventh day of pregnancy and 20–25% when given on days 10 or 12, respectively.[20]

Interceptive activity: Fractions isolated from the chloroform extract of *Aristolochia indica* at doses of 35–60 mg/kg demonstrated interceptive activity. Histological studies of the uterus and ovary at the minimum effective dose levels with each fraction revealed no overt changes apart from the presence of degenerated corpora lutea in the ovary of the animals treated, and no teratogenic effects were observed.[21] A sesquiterpene isolated from the roots demonstrated 100% interceptive activity and 91.7% antiimplantation activity in mice at a single oral dose of 100 mg/kg, with no other toxic effects at the dose levels used.[22] P-coumaric acid isolated from *Aristolochia indica* also showed 100% interceptive activity when administered at 50 mg/kg to mice, with a high margin of safety (>1000 mg/kg) and no teratogenic activity.[23]

Antitumour activity: Aristolochic acid was found to have activity against adenocarcinoma 755 in mice.[16]

Immunomodulatory activity: Aristolochic acid has been shown to bind to surface receptors of lymphocytes, altering immune response.[24] An immune-stimulating action was reported in a human study which measured increased phagocytic activity after 3 days of treatment at a dosage of 0.9 mg/day.[25]

Antiinflammatory activity: Aristolochic acid also played a regulatory role in prostaglandin synthesis. It inhibited inflammation by both immunological and non-immunological agents. One mechanism of activity was thought to be as a direct inhibitor of phospholipase A2, decreasing the generation of eicosanoids and platelet-activating factors. Another antiinflammatory mechanism may be the effect on arachidonic acid mobilisation in human neutrophils.[26,27]

Safety profile

The plant is carcinogenic and nephrotoxic.[28] The LD_{50} value of the 50% alcoholic extract of the whole plant, when administered to mice, was 375 mg/kg.[29] Its usage is not recommended.

Dosage

Root powder: 1–3 g

Leaf infusion: 5–10 ml

Ayurvedic properties

Guna: *Laghu* (light), *ruksha* (dry)

Rasa: *Katu* (bitter), *kasaya* (astringent)

Veerya: *Ushna* (hot)

Vipaka: *Katu* (bitter)

Dosha: Balances *kapha* and *vata*

Further reading

Bown D 1995 Encyclopaedia of herbs and their uses. Dorling Kindersley, London

Kapoor LD 1990 Handbook of Ayurvedic medicinal plants. CRC Press, Boca Raton

Nadkarni AK 1976 Indian materia medica. Popular Prakashan PVT Ltd, Bombay

Sivarajan VV, Balachandran I 1994 Ayurvedic drugs and their plant sources. Oxford and IBH Publishing, New Delhi

Thakur RS, Puri HS, Husain A 1989 Major medicinal plants of India. CIMAP, Lucknow

References

1 Jha MK 1992 The folk veterinary system of Bihar – a research survey. NDDB, Anand, Gujrat

2 Kupchan SM, Doskotch RW 1962 Tumor inhibitors I. Aristolochic acid, the active principle of *Aristolochia indica*. Journal of Medicinal and Pharmaceutical Chemistry 5:657

3 Kupchan SM, Merianos JJ 1968 The isolation and structural elucidation of novel derivatives of Aristolochic acid from *Aristolochia indica*. Journal of Organic Chemistry 33(10): 3735

4 Che CT, Cordell GA, Fong HS, Evans C 1983 Studies on *Aristolochia*. Part 2. Aristolindiquinone, a new naphthoquinone from *Aristolochia indica* L. (Aristolochiaceae). Tetrahedron 24(13):1333

5 Achari B, Bandyopadhyay S, Saha CR, Pakrashi SC 1983 A phenanthroid lactone, steroid and lignans from *Aristolochia indica*. Heterocycles 20(5):771

6 Pakrashi SC, Dastidar PP, Ghosh, Chakrabarty S, Achari B 1980 (12S)-7,12-Secoishwaran-12-ol, a new type of sesquiterpene from *Aristolochia indica* Linn. Journal of Organic Chemistry 45(23):4765

7 Govindachari TR, Parthasarathy PC 1971 Ishwarol, a new tetracyclic sesquiterpene alcohol from *Aristolochia indica*. Indian Journal of Chemistry 9(11):1310

8 Fuhrer H, Ganguly AK, Gopinath KW et al 1970 Ishwarone. Tetrahedron 26(10):2371

9 Govindachari TR, Mohamed PA, Parthasarathy PC 1970 Ishwarane and aristolochene, two new sesquiterpene hydrocarbons from *Aristolochia indica*. Tetrahedron 26(2):615

10 Govindachari TR, Parthasarathy PC, Desai HK, Mohamed PA 1973 5βH,7β,10α-selina-4(14),11-diene, a new sesquiterpene hydrocarbon from *Aristolochia indica*. Indian Journal of Chemistry 11(10):971

11 Rao AS, Muthana MS 1955 Preliminary studies on the essential oil from *Aristolochia indica*. Journal of the Indian Institute of Science 37A:266

12 Govindachari TR, Viswanathan N 1967 The identity of aristolochine. Indian Journal of Chemistry 5(12):655

13 Jirovetz L, Buchbauer G, Puschmann C, Fleischhacker W, Shafi PM, Rosamma MK 2000 Analysis of the essential oil of the aerial parts of the medicinal plant *Aristolochia indica* (Aristolochiaceae) from South-India. Science and Pharmacy 68(3):309

14 Pakrashi SC, Ghosh, Dastidar P, Basu S, Achari B 1977 Studies on Indian medicinal plants, part 46. New phenanthrene derivatives from *Aristolochia indica*. Phytochemistry 16(7):1103

15 Ganguly T, Pakrashi A, Pal AK 1986 Disruption of pregnancy in mouse by aristolic acid: I. Plausible explanation in relation to early pregnancy events. Contraception 34(6):625

16 Che CT, Ahmed MS, Kang SS et al 1984 Studies on *Aristolochia* III. Isolation and biological evaluation of constituents of *Aristolochia indica* roots for fertility-regulating activity. Journal of Natural Products 47(2):331

17 Pakrashi A, Shaha C 1979 Effect of methyl aristolate from *Aristolochia indica* Linn. on implantation in mice. IRCS Medical Science Library Compendium 7(2):78

18 Pandey D, Bisht M, Naba Chandra Singh Y 1993 Antifertility and antiestrogenic activity of *Aristolochia indica* Linn. on female Wister rat. Himalayan Journal of Environment and Zoology 7(1):1

19 Pakrashi A, Chakrabarty B 1978 Anti-estrogenic and anti-implantation effect of aristolic acid from *Aristolochia indica* (Linn.). Indian Journal of Experimental Biology 16(12):1283

20 Pakrashi A, Shaha C 1978 Effect of methyl ester of aristolic acid from *Aristolochia indica* Linn. on fertility of female mice. Experientia 34(9):1192

21 Pakrashi A, Chakrabarty B 1977 Biological properties of interceptive agents from *Aristolochia indica* Linn. Indian Journal of Medical Research 66(6):991

22 Pakrashi A, Shaha C 1977 Effect of a sesquiterpene from *Aristolochia indica* Linn. on fertility in female mice. Experientia 33(11):1498

23 Pakrashi A, Pakrasi P 1978 Biological profile of p-coumaric acid isolated from *Aristolochia indica* Linn. Indian Journal of Experimental Biology 16(12):1285

24 Siering H, Muller H 1981 Antagonistic effects of glucorticoids and aristolochic acid on the immunocyte adherence phenomenon. Arzneimittel-Forschung 31(8):1260

25 Kluthe R, Vogt A, Batsford S 1982 Double blind study of the influence of aristolochic acid on granulocyte phagocytic activity. Arzneimittel-Forschung 32:443

26 Moreno JJ 1993 Effect of aristolochic acid on arachidonic acid cascade and *in vivo* models of inflammation. Immunopharmacology 26(1):1

27 Rosenthal MD 1992 The effects of the phospholipase A2 inhibitors aristolochic acid and PGBx on A23187-stimulated mobilization of arachidonate in human neutrophils are overcome by diacylglycerol or phorbol ester. Biochimica et Biophysica Acta 1126(3):319

28 Mcguffin M, Hobbs C, Upton R, Goldberg A (eds) 1997 Botanical safety handbook. CRC Press, Boca Raton

29 Dhawan BN, Patnaik GK, Rastogi RP, Singh KK, Tandon JS 1977 Screening of Indian plants for biological activity: Part VI. Indian Journal of Experimental Biology 15:208

Asparagus racemosus (Willd.) (Liliaceae)

English: Wild asparagus, sparrow-grass

Hindi: *Shatavari, satavari*

Sanskrit: *Shatavari, abhiru*

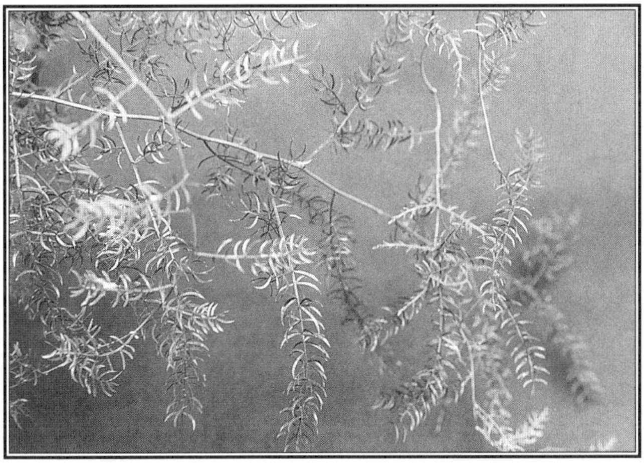

The plant has been used medicinally for centuries and the common name *shatavari* means 'she who possesses a hundred husbands', referring to the rejuvenative effect of the herb on the female reproductive organs. It is characterised in Ayurveda as a powerful *rasayana* and is sometimes used as a vegetable.

Habitat

It grows wild and is cultivated throughout tropical and subtropical parts of India, including the Andamans, and other Asian and African countries.

Botanical description

It is a climber, growing up to 2 m in height and extensively branched (Plate 9). The leaves are reduced to needle-like, suberect, soft spines. The rootstocks are tuberous, bearing numerous fusiform, succulent tuberous roots 30–100 cm long and 1–2 cm thick and the stem is woody, pale grey or brown in colour and armed with strong spines. Flowers are tiny, white in colour, fragrant and profuse, in simple or branched racemes.

Parts used

Root and leaves.

Traditional and modern use

The roots are used mainly to promote milk secretion and as a demulcent, diuretic, aphrodisiac, tonic, alterative, antiseptic and antidiarrhoeal. It is also used to treat debility, especially in women, and infertility, impotence, menopause, stomach ulcers, hyperacidity, dehydration, lung abscess, haematemesis, cough, herpes, leucorrhoea and chronic fevers.

Ethnoveterinary usage

The fresh roots are fed to buffaloes in order to increase the milk yield and to promote lactation after the death of a calf,[1] and also for maggots in wounds, constipation and as a demulcent.

Major chemical constituents

Steroidal glycosides and aglycones

Shatavarins I–IV, β-D-Glc-(1-4)-β-D-Glc-(1-2) α-L-rha(1-2)sarasapogenin,[2] arasosapogenin,[3] sterols and diosgenin have also been isolated from the roots.[4]

Alkaloids

Asparagamine A has been isolated from the roots.[5]

Flavonoids

The ripe fruits yielded quercetin, rutin, hyperoside, cynidin-3-galactoside and cynidin-3-glucorhamnoside. Quercetin-3-glucuronide has been isolated from the leaves.[6]

Medicinal and pharmacological activities

Anticancer activity: An alcoholic extract of the aerial parts of *Asparagus racemosus* exhibited anticancer activity in human epidermal carcinoma of the nasopharynx in tissue culture.[7]

Adaptogenic activity: Aqueous extracts administered orally to experimental animals, in a dose extrapolated from the human dose, protected against a variety of biological, physical and chemical stressors. A model of cisplatin-induced alterations in gastrointestinal motility was used to test the ability of extract to exert a normalising effect, irrespective of direction of pathological change. The extract reversed the effects of cisplatin on gastric emptying and also normalised cisplatin-induced intestinal hypermotility.[8]

Antibacterial activity: A methanolic extract of the roots at 50, 100 and 150 μg/ml showed significant in vitro antibacterial efficacy against *Escherichia coli, Shigella dysenteriae, Shigella sonnei, Shigella flexneri, Vibrio cholerae, Salmonella typhi, Salmonella typhimurium, Pseudomonas putida, Bacillus subtilis* and *Staphylococcus aureus*. Chloramphenicol was used for comparison.[9]

Antitussive activity: The methanolic extract of the root, at a dose of 200 and 400 mg/kg PO, showed significant antitussive activity on sulphur dioxide-induced cough in mice. The cough inhibition of 40% and 58.5%, respectively, was comparable to that of 10–20 mg/kg of codeine phosphate, where the inhibition observed was 36% and 55.4%, respectively.[10]

Antiprotozoal activity: An aqueous solution of the crude alcoholic extract of the roots exhibited an inhibitory effect on the growth of *E. histolytica* in vitro.[11]

Antiulcer activity: Efficacy of *Asparagus racemosus* was evaluated in 32 patients by administering the root powder 12 g/day in four doses, for an average duration of 6 weeks. *Shatavari* was found to relieve most of the symptoms in a majority of patients. The ulcer-healing effect of the drug was attributed to a direct healing effect, possibly by potentiating intrinsic protective factors as it has neither antisecretory activity nor antacid properties, by strengthening mucosal resistance, prolonging the lifespan of mucosal cells, increasing secretion and viscosity of mucus and reducing H^+ ion back diffusion. It has been found to maintain the continuity and thickness of aspirin-treated gastric mucosa with a significant increase in mucosal mucin. As *A. racemosus* heals duodenal ulcers without inhibiting acid secretion, it may have cytoprotective action similar to that of prostaglandins. Other possible mechanisms may be deactivation and binding of pepsin or binding of bile salts.[12]

Galactagogue activity: The roots exhibited a galactagogue action in buffaloes, the milk yield being significantly increased after administration of the drug.[13] In another study the aqueous fraction of the alcoholic extract of the roots at 250 mg/kg, administered intramuscularly, was shown to cause both an increase in the weight of mammary lobulo-alveolar tissue and in the milk yield in oestrogen-primed rats. This activity was attributed to the action of released corticosteroids or an increase in prolactin.[14]

Immunomodulatory activity: *A. racemosus* protected rats against mixed bacterial abdominal sepsis induced by caecal ligation. It also produced polymorphonuclear leucocytosis and prevented cyclophosphamide-induced neutropenia. *A. racemosus* also protected mice against *E. coli*-induced abdominal sepsis via immunomodulation.[15] The effect of *A. racemosus* was studied on the functions of macrophages obtained from mice treated with a carcinogen, ochratoxin A (OTA). The chemotactic activity of murine macrophages was significantly decreased by 17 weeks of treatment with OTA compared with controls. Production of interleukin-1 (IL-1) and tumour necrosis factor (TNF) was also markedly reduced. Treatment with *A. racemosus* significantly inhibited OTA-induced suppression of chemotactic activity and production of IL-1 and TNF-α by macrophages and also induced excess production of TNF-α when compared with controls.[16] This has implications for the treatment of intraabdominal sepsis, which continues to be a major cause of morbidity and mortality following trauma and abdominal surgery for bowel perforations. Treatment of this condition has always been focused on appropriate surgery, supplemented with antibiotics and good nutritional support. An important factor influencing recovery from any infective process is the host's defence mechanisms and the approach of fortifying the cellular immune functions in order to increase resistance against infection. *A. racemosus* exhibits protective effects against myelosuppression induced by single doses of cyclophosphamide. A comparative study was done between *Asparagus racemosus*, glucan and lithium carbonate against the myelosuppressive effects of single and multiple doses of cyclophosphamide in mice. Cyclophosphamide was administered as a single dose of 200 mg/kg subcutaneously to one group of mice, while a second group received three doses of 30 mg/kg of the same compound intraperitoneally. Both the groups received *A. racemosus* and lithium orally, for 15 days before cyclophosphamide. Glucan was given intravenously in three doses before cyclophosphamide in the first group and together with cyclophosphamide in the second group. Peripheral and differential white blood cell counts were done before and after drug treatment and serially after cyclophosphamide injection. All the drugs were found to produce leucocytosis and neutrophilia.[17] When compared to the control group, all four drugs prevented leucopenia produced by cyclophosphamide to varying degrees; it was therefore concluded that *A. racemosus* is an immunostimulant with effects comparable to those of lithium and glucan.

Molluscicidal activity: Aqueous and ethanolic extracts of *Asparagus racemosus* exhibited a high mortality rate (100%) against *Biomphalaria pfeifferi* and *Lymnaea natalensis*. The LC_{50} was found to be 0.1, 5, 5, 10 and 50 mg/ml for *Biomphalaria pfeifferi* and 0.5, 5, 1, 10 and 10 mg/ml for *Lymnaea natalensis*. The activities were attributed to the presence of terpenoids, steroids and saponins in the extracts.[18]

Safety profile

No adverse effects due to the use of the root powder have been reported and the plant is also consumed as food. The maximum tolerated oral dose of the 50% ethanolic extract of the whole plant (excluding roots) was 1000 mg/kg body weight in adult male albino rats.[19]

Dosage

Infusion: 12–20 ml

Decoction: 56–112 ml

Powder: 20–30 g

Ayurvedic properties

Rasa: *Madhur* (sweet), *tikta* (bitter)

Guna: *Guru* (heavy), *snigdha* (unctuous)

Vipaka: *Madhur* (sweet)

Veerya: *Shita* (cold)

Dosha: Pacifies *pitta* and *vata*, promotes *kapha*

Further reading

Bharatiya Vidya Bhavan's Swami Prakashanandra Ayurveda Research Centre 1992 Selected medicinal plants of India. Chemexcil, Mumbai

Nadkarni AK 1976 Indian materia medica. Popular Prakashan PVT Ltd, Bombay

Council of Scientific and Industrial Research 1985 The wealth of India. PID, CSIR, New Delhi

Sairam TV 1999 Home remedies, vol II. Penguin India, New Delhi

References

1 Jha MK 1992 Folk veterinary system of Bihar – a research survey. NDDB, Anand, Gujrat

2 Ravikumar PR, Soman R, Chetty GL 1987 Chemistry of Ayurvedic crude drugs: Part 6-(shatavari-1) Structure of shatavarin -IV. Indian Journal of Chemistry 26B(11):1012

3 Ahmed S, Ahmed S, Jain PC 1991 Chemical examination of *Asparagus racemosus*. Bulletin of Medico Ethnobotanical Research 12(3–4):157

4 Singh J, Tiwari HP 1991 Chemical examination of roots of *Asparagus racemosus*. Journal of the Indian Chemical Society 68(7):427

5 Sekine T, Fukasawa N, Kashiwagi Y, Ruangrungsi N, Murakoshi I 1994 Structure of asparagamine A, a novel polycyclic alkaloid from *Asparagus racemosus*. Chemical and Pharmaceutical Bulletin 42(6):1360

6 Singh J, Tiwari HP 1991 Chemical examination of roots of *Asparagus racemosus*. Journal of the Indian Chemical Society 68(7):427

7 Dhar ML, Dhar MM, Dhawan BN, Mehrotra BN, Ray C 1968 Screening of Indian medicinal plants for biological activity I. Indian Journal of Experimental Biology 6:232

8 Rege NN, Thatte UM, Dahanukar SA 1999 Adaptogenic properties of six rasayana herbs used in Ayurvedic medicine. Phytotherapy Research 13(4):275

9 Mandal SC, Nandy A, Pal M, Saha BP 2000 Evaluation of antibacterial activity of *Asparagus racemosus* Willd. root. Phytotherapy Research 14(2):118

10 Mandal SC, Kumar CKA, Mohana Lakshmi S et al 2000 Antitussive effect of *Asparagus racemosus* root against sulfur dioxide-induced cough in mice. Fitoterapia 71(6):686

11 Roy RN, Chavan SR, Bhagwager S, Dutta NK, Iyer NS 1968 Preliminary pharmacological studies on different extracts of roots of *Asparagus racemosus* (Satawari) Willd. Indian Journal of Pharmacy 30:289

12 Singh KP, Singh RH 1986 Clinical trial on Satavari (*Asparagus racemosus* Willd.) in duodenal ulcer disease. Journal of Research in Ayurveda and Siddha 7(3–4):91

13 Patel AB, Kantikar UK 1969 *Asparagus racemosus* Willd.–form bordi, as a galactagogue, in buffaloes. Indian Veterinary Journal 46(8):718

14 Sabnis PB, Gaitonde BB, Jethmalani M 1968 Effects of alcoholic extract of *Asparagus racemosus* on mammary glands of rats. Indian Journal of Experimental Biology 6:55

15 Thatte U, Chhabria S, Karandikar SM, Dahanukar S 1987 Immunotherapeutic modification of *E.coli* induced abdominal sepsis and mortality in mice by Indian medicinal plants. Indian Drugs 25(3):95

16 Dhuley JN 1997 Effect of some Indian herbs on macrophage functions in ochratoxin A treated mice. Journal of Ethnopharmacology 58(1):15

17 Thatte UM, Dahanukar SA 1988 Comparative study of immunomodulating activity of Indian medicinal plants, lithium carbonate and glucan. Methods and Findings in Experimental and Clinical Pharmacology 10(10):639–644

18 Chifundera K, Baluku B, Mashimango B 1993 Phytochemical screening and molluscicidal potency of some Zairean medicinal plants. Pharmacological Research 28(4):333

19 Dhar ML, Dhar ML, Dhawan BN, Mahrotra BN, Ray C 1968 Screening of Indian plants for biological activity Part I. Indian Journal of Experimental Biology 6:232

Azadirachta indica A. Juss. (Meliaceae)

English: Neem tree, margosa

Hindi: *Neem, nim*

Sanskrit: *Nimba*

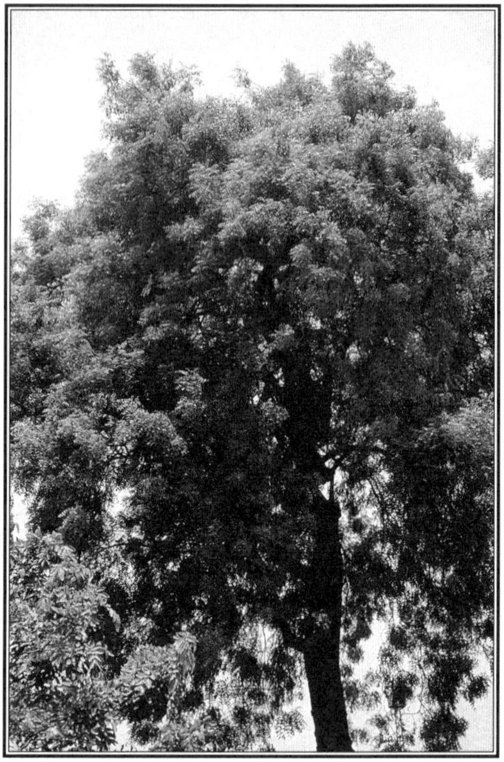

Neem, *Azadirachta indica*, has similar properties to its close relative, *Melia azederach*. It is one of the most important detoxicants in Ayurvedic medicine. The young shoots of neem, known as *datoon*, are used to clean teeth in the villages. It is used as an insecticide, for fumigation and as an air purifier. The word *Azadirachta* is derived from the Persian *azaddhirakt*, meaning 'noble tree'.

Habitat

It is indigenous to the warmer parts of India and south-east Asia and found commonly in the forests of Andhra Pradesh, Tamil Nadu and Karnataka. It is also widespread in West Africa, the Caribbean and South and Central America.

Botanical description

It is a hardy, fast-growing evergreen tree with a straight trunk, long spreading branches and moderately thick, rough, longitudinally fissured bark (Plate 10). Mature trees attain a height of 7–20 m with a spread of 5–10 m. The tree starts producing the yellowish ellipsoidal drupes (fruits) in about 4 years, becomes fully productive in 10 years and may live for more than 200 years. The leaves are compound, imparipinnate, comprising up to 15 leaflets arranged in alternate pairs with terminal leaflets. The leaflets are narrow, lanceolate, up to 6 cm long. The flowers are abundant, sweet-smelling white panicles in the leaf axils.

Parts used

Seeds, seed kernel, leaves, flowers, stem and stem bark.

Traditional and modern use

All parts of the plant are highly regarded in medicine. The stem bark is an astringent and antiperiodic and the root bark and young fruits are used in a similar way and as a bitter tonic. The flowers are used for dyspepsia and the berries are purgative, emollient and anthelmintic. Fresh twigs are often used for cleaning the teeth in pyorrhoea. The seed is stimulant and applied externally in rheumatism and skin diseases. The oil extracted from the leaf and seed is important as an antiseptic, insecticide and applied to boils, ulcers and eczema. It is also applied externally in rheumatism, leprosy and sprains.

Ethnoveterinary usage

In poultry, the bark is used to treat wounds, diarrhoea, ticks and lice. The leaves are used to treat abscesses and applied after castration. They are also effective against bleeding, udder infections, fever, foot rot and lice in ruminants. The seeds are used for ticks in ruminants and the bark, seeds, leaves and roots are used as an insect repellent.[1] All parts of the plant, as well as the gum and oil, are effective against worms, wounds in the mouth, glossitis, *E. coli* bacillosis, swelling of the liver, jaundice, bloody dysentery and intestinal wounds. They are also used for constipation, indigestion, respiratory and throat disorders, asthma, pleuropneumonia and swelling of the mucous membranes in the respiratory tract and lungs. They are also used in skin disorders including ringworm, alopecia, eczema, urticaria, scabies, ticks and lice. Other minor indications include metritis, orchitis, tetanus, stoppage of urination, swelling of the kidney, mastitis, otitis, abscess in the ear, rinder pest and rheumatism.[2]

Major chemical constituents

Terpenes and limonoids

The major active components are the limonoids azadirachtin, 3-deacetyl-3-cinnamoylazadirachtin, 1-tigloyl-3-acetyl-11-methoxyazadirachtin, 22,23-dihydro-23β-methoxyazadirachtin, nimbanal, 3-tigloylazadirachtol, 3-acetyl-salannol,[3] nimbidiol,[4] margocin, margocinin, margocilin and others.[5] Terpenoids such as isoazadirolide,[6] nimbocinolide,[7] nimbonone, nibonolone, methylgrevillate,[8] margosinone, margosinolone,[9] nimosone, nimbosone, methyl nimbiol, methyl nimbionone, 13-acetyl-12-methoxy-8,11,13-podocarpatriene, sugiol, 12,13-dimethoxy-8,11,13-podocarpatriene-3,7-dione[10] and gedunin have been isolated.[11] The oil contains salannin, 1,3-diacetyl salannin, deacetyl salannin and salannol nimbidin, nimbidinin and nimbinin.[12] Meliacin cinnamates[13] have been isolated from root bark of the plant. Isonimolide, isolimbolide and isonimocinolide[14] have been reported from twigs.

Polysaccharides

The fruit pulp contains arabinogalatans and numerous other polysaccharides, referred to as G-IIa, G-IIIa, G-IIIb, $GIIIDO_2$'IIa and $GIIIDO_2$'IIb, etc.[15] Others, called CSP-II, III, CSSP-I, -II and -III, are present in the stem bark.[16]

Medicinal and pharmacological activities

Antifungal, antibacterial and antiviral activity: A leaf extract of neem showed significant inhibition of aflatoxin synthesis and fungal spore infection of *Aspergillus flavus* growing on the seeds of developing cotton bolls.[17] The oil extracted from the seeds exhibited significant antibacterial efficacy against *Bacillus subtilis, Salmonella typhosa* and *S. paratyphi*.[18] NIM-76, a spermicidal fraction prepared from neem oil, was investigated for its antimicrobial action against various bacteria, fungi and the polio virus. NIM-76 showed a stronger activity than whole neem oil and inhibited the growth of pathogens including *Escherichia coli* and *Klebsiella pneumoniae*, which were not affected by the whole oil. It also inhibited the growth of *Candida albicans* and replication of the polio virus. NIM-76 protected mice from systemic candidiasis, measured as an enhanced survival rate, and reduced colony formation in various tissues, demonstrating a potent, broad-spectrum, antimicrobial activity.[19] Neem leaf extract at a concentration of 3–4 mg/ml inhibited plaque formation of the chickungunya and measles viruses, together with a reduction in virus titre.[20]

Antiatherosclerotic activity: Administration of the mature leaf extract (IP) decreased serum cholesterol significantly without changing serum protein, blood urea and uric acid levels in rats.[21]

Antidiabetic activity: A significant reduction of insulin dosage (30–50%), without a significant effect on the blood glucose levels, was observed with the administration of 5 g of aqueous leaf extract or an equivalent amount of dried leaf. The same doses of insulin alone did not produce the effect when given without leaf preparation.[22] Oral administration of 10% w/v aqueous leaf extract to normoglycaemic animals at a dose 200 mg/kg resulted in marked hypoglycaemia. Intravenous administration of 0.15 mg/kg of a 50% w/v aqueous leaf extract in dogs resulted in a significant decrease in blood glucose levels in both normoglycaemic animals and adrenaline-induced hyperglycaemic animals.[23]

Antimalarial activity: The leaf extract containing the limonoid gedunin was examined for antimalarial activity using in vitro tests with two types of *Plasmodium falciparum*, one sensitive to chloroquine (W_2) and one chloroquine resistant (D_6). The extract was found to be more effective against the W_2 than the D_6 clone, suggesting there is no cross-resistance to chloroquine. Isolated gedunin was more potent than chloroquine against W_2.[24]

Antinociceptive activity: The analgesic potency of an aqueous extract was tested using experimental pain models in mice. In the glacial acetic acid (GAA)-induced writhing test, the extract (at 10, 30 and 100 mg/kg) dose-dependently reduced both the incidence and the number of writhes. It also enhanced tail withdrawal latencies in the tail flick test for nociception, at similar dose levels.[25]

Antipyretic activity: A 75% methanolic extract of leaf and bark showed antipyretic effects in rabbits when administered at a dose of 400 mg/kg. Similar effects were observed with the hexane, chloroform, 90% ethanol and water-soluble fractions at a dose of 150 mg/kg.[26]

Antiulcer activity: An aqueous extract of the leaf, at doses of 10, 40 or 160 mg leaf/kg body weight, in rats exposed to 2 hours of cold-restrained stress or given ethanol orally, caused a reduction in gastric ulcer severity and decreased ethanol-induced gastric mucosal damage. It prevented mast cell degranulation, which increased the amount of gastric mucus, in stressed animals.[27]

Anxiolytic activity: A single dose of freshly prepared leaf extract, given 45 minutes before behavioural testing in rats, showed that low doses (10, 20, 50, 100 and 200 mg/kg) of the extract produced a significant anxiolytic effect in both maze and open field tests. The effect induced by lower doses was comparable to that induced by diazepam (1 mg/kg), but was absent with higher doses.[28]

Cardiovascular activity: Administration of the leaf extract of *Azadirachta indica* was found to induce a potent and dose-dependent hypotension in rabbits (5–200 mg/kg, IP) and guinea pigs (5–40 mg/kg). The extract also exhibited antiarrhythmic activity (40 mg/kg IV) against ouabain-induced dysrhythmia in rabbits. The mechanism of action may be due to an effect on vascular smooth muscle, giving rise to vasodilation.[29]

CNS depressant activity: CNS depressant activity, evidenced by a reduction in locomotor activity and potentiation of pentobarbitone-induced hypnosis, was observed with the oral administration of an acetone extract of the leaf.[30]

Hepatoprotective activity: The leaf extract provided a hepatoprotective effect against paracetamol-induced hepatic cell damage in rats, findings supported by histopathological studies.[31]

Hypoglycaemic activity: Both the leaf extract and seed oil produced a hypoglycaemic effect in normal as well as diabetic rabbits, comparable to that of glibenclamide. The effect was more pronounced in the diabetic animals. Pretreatment with *A. indica* leaf extract or seed oil, given 2 weeks prior to alloxan, partially prevented the rise in blood glucose levels as compared to control diabetic animals.[32]

Antiinflammatory activity: Oral administration of 800 mg/kg of a 75% methanolic extract of bark and leaf produced inhibition of carrageenan-induced oedema in rats.[33] Sodium nimbate, administered IP at a dose of 40 mg/kg, also reduced carrageenan-induced oedema in rats, with an ED_{50} of 44.1 mg/kg. Formaldehyde-induced arthritis in rats was also inhibited by 20 mg/kg sodium nimbate.[34] Polysaccharides coded as G-IIa, G-IIIa, G-IIIb, $GIIIDO_2$'IIa and $GIIIDO_2$'IIb, isolated from stem bark, exhibited significant antiinflammatory activity at doses of 25, 0.40, 50, 10 and 10 mg/kg respectively.[35] Nimbidin, the crude bitter principle from the seed oil consisting of a mixture of limonoids, exhibited a dose-dependent inhibition of carageenan-induced oedema (ED_{50} = 79.4 mg/kg). Doses of 40 and 80 mg/kg also produced a significant inhibition of both kaolin-induced oedema and formaldehyde-induced arthritis. Inhibition of croton oil-induced granuloma formation was also observed (at 80 mg/kg).[36]

Antitumour activity: Antitumour effects were seen against Sarcoma-180 ascites tumour cells in mice following the IP administration of polysaccharides Gia and Gib, isolated from the stem bark of *Azadirachta indica*.[37]

Antifertility activity: Oral administration of a 50% ethanol extract of neem flower caused a marked decrease in the weight of testes and epididymis of male rats, by arresting spermatogenesis. Sperm motility and density were significantly reduced.[38] Depletion in the levels of androgen and spermatogenesis were also observed due to reduced testicular weight and protein, sialic acid and glycogen content. The seed extract caused degenerative changes in the ovarian follicles and led to a degeneration of endometrial epithelium, disorganisation of uterine glands, breakage and deterioration of luminal epithelium and a decrease in protein and glycogen contents.[39] No change in hormonal parameters was observed. An active fraction of the hexane extract of the seed (containing mono- and diunsaturated free fatty acids and their methyl esters) resulted in long-term, reversible, antifertility effect after a single intrauterine administration in female rats of proven fertility. The mechanism appeared to involve intervention of local cell-mediated immunity in the reproductive system.[40]

Insecticidal and growth regulatory activity: Aqueous and ethanol extracts of the seed, flower and leaves of *Azadirachta indica* were found to disrupt the growth and development of larvae of tobacco caterpillar and *Sodoptera litura* (E) at 0.25%, 0.5% and 1.0% concentrations. Various types of abnormality as well as a reduction in size and weight were observed. The seed kernel extract was found to have the highest activity, followed by that of the leaf, seed coat and flower.[41] Oral administration was more effective than topical application. Azadirachtin has been identified as the active compound against a range of insects. The seed kernel extract induced histological and histochemical alterations in the ovaries of *Caryedon gangara* (Caleoptera: Bruchidae), evaluated by comparing oogenesis in normal-maturing females reared on tamarind seed with those treated with neem kernel extract. Where oocytes were already developed, degenerative changes involving yolk deposition in oocytes of the treated females, and disturbance in the post-vitellogenic follicles, were observed.[42] The effects of azadirachtin, salannin, nimbin and 6-desacetylnimbin, isolated from seed kernels, have been studied on ecdysone 20-monooxygenase (E-20-M) activity using various preparations of *Drosophila melanogaster*, *Aedes aegypti* or *Manduca sexta*. They were incubated with radiolabelled ecdysone and increasing concentrations of the compounds. All were found to inhibit, in a dose-dependent fashion, the E-20-M activity in all three insect species. The concentration of compounds required to produce 50% inhibition ranged from 2×10^{-5} to 1×10^{-3} M.[43]

Antiulcer activity: Nimbidin exhibited a strong protective effect in tests against acetylsalicylic acid-, stress-, serotonin- or indomethacin-induced gastric lesions in rats, as well as histamine or cysteamine-induced duodenal lesions in guinea pigs and rats respectively. In ulcer-healing tests, the healing process was enhanced in acetic acid-induced chronic gastric lesions using rats and dogs, after oral doses of nimbidin.[44]

Immunomodulatory activity: An aqueous extract of the bark, leaf and seed showed an increase in phagocytic activity and induced expression of MHC-II antigens on macrophages, indicating enhancement of antigenic potency, stimulated lymphocyte proliferative response of splenocytes to mitogens and selectively activated TH1-type of T-cell response. A significant inhibition of intracellular multiplication of Chlamydia and cytopathic effect of Herpes was observed when mouse spleen cells were treated with neem extracts, indicating that these effects of neem are probably mediated by the immune system.[45]

Safety profile

No toxicity has been observed in moderate use, although toxic effects have been observed in the liver and kidneys of laboratory animals after the administration of concentrated aqueous suspensions of fresh and dried leaves. The LD_{50} of a 50% ethanolic extract of the stem bark was found to be >1000 mg/kg body weight when given IP to adult albino rats.[46]

Occasionally toxic effects have been reported, especially with the oil and seeds, but these may be due to infestation with mycotoxins.

Dosage

Infusion: 10–20 ml

Powder: 1–2 g

Oil: 0.2–1 ml

Ayurvedic properties

Rasa: *Tikta* (bitter), *kashaya* (astringent)

Guna: *Laghu* (light)

Vipaka: *Katu* (pungent)

Veerya: *Shita* (cold)

Dosha: Balances *kapha* and *pitta*

Further reading

Kapoor LD 1990 Handbook of Ayurvedic medicinal plants. CRC Press, Boca Raton

Pandey GS (ed) 1998 Indian materia medica. Chaukhambha Bharati Academy, Gokul Bhawan, Varanasi

Ross I 2000 Medicinal plants of the world, vol 2. Humana Press, New Jersey

Schmutterer H (ed) 1995 The neem tree. VCH Verlagsgesellschaft, Weinheim

Council of Scientific and Industrial Research 1985 The wealth of India. PID, CSIR, New Delhi

References

1 International Institute of Rural Reconstruction 1994 Ethnoveterinary medicine in Asia. An information kit on traditional animal health care practices, Part I, general information. IIRR, Silang, Philippines

2 Jha MK 1992 Folk veterinary medicine of Bihar – a research project. NDDB, Anand, Gujrat

3 Rojatkar SR, Bhat VS, Kulkarni MM, Joshi VS, Nagasampagi BA 1989 Tetranortriterpenoids from *Azadirachta indica*. Phytochemistry 28(1):203

4 Majumdar PL, Maiti DC, Kraus W, Bokel M 1987 Nimbidiol, a modified diterpenoid of the root bark of *Azadirachta indica*. Phytochemistry 26(11):3021

5 Ara I, Siddiqui BS, Faizi S, Siddiqui S 1990 Tricyclic diterpenoids from the root bark of *Azadirachta indica*. Phytochemistry 29(3):911

6 Siddiqui S, Siddiqui BS, Faizi S, Mahmood T 1986 Isoazadiorolide, a new tetratriterpenoid from *Azadirachta indica* A. Juss (Meliaceae). Heterocycles 24(11):3163

7 Siddiqui S, Siddiqui BS, Mahmood T, Faizi S 1989 Tetranortriterpenoids from *Azadirachta indica* A. Juss (Meliaceae). Heterocycles 29(1):87

8 Ara I, Siddiqui BS, Faizi S, Siddiqui S 1989 Diterpenoids from the stem bark of *Azadirachta indica*. Phytochemistry 28(4):1177

9 Ara I, Siddiqui BS, Faizi S, Siddiqui S 1989 Margosinone and margosinolone, two new polyacetate derivatives from *Azadirachta indica*. Fitoterapia 60(6):519

10 Ara I, Siddiqui BS, Faizi S, Siddiqui S 1989 Tricyclic diterpenoids from the stem bark of *Azadirachta indica*. Journal of Natural Products 51(6):1054

11 Khalid SA, Duddeck H, Gonzalez-Sherra M 1989 Isolation and characterization of an antimalarial agent from the neem tree *Azadirachta indica*. Journal of Natural Products 52(5):922

12 Tewari DN 1992 Monograph on neem. International Book Distributors, Dehradun, India

13 Ara I, Siddiqui BS, Faizi S, Siddiqui S 1989 Isolation of meliacin cinnamates from the root bark of *Azadirachta indica* A. Juss (Meliaceae). Heterocycles 29(4):729

14 Siddiqui S, Mahmood T, Siddiqui BS, Faizi S 1987 Isonimolide and isolimbolide, two new tetranortriterpenoids from the twigs of *Azadirachta indica* A. Juss (Meliaceae). Heterocycles 26(7):1827

15 Sen AK, Das AK, Banerji N 1993 A water soluble arabinogalactan from the fruit pulp of *Azadirachta indica*. Indian Journal of Chemistry 32B:862

16 Kurokawa Y, Takeda T, Ogihara Y 1990 Further studies on the structure of polysaccharides from the bark of *Melia azadirachta*. Shoyakugaku Zasshi 44(1):29

17 Zeringue HJ, Bhatnagar D 1990 Inhibition of aflatoxin production in *Aspergillus flavus* infected cotton bolls after treatment with neem (*Azadirachta indica*) leaf extracts. J. Am. Oil Chem. Soc. 67(4):215

18 Jain PP, Suri RK, Deshmukh SK, Mathur KC 1987 Fatty oils from oil seeds of forest origin as antibacterial agent. Indian Forestry 113(4):297

19 Sairam M, Ilavazhagan G, Sharma SK et al 2000 Anti-microbial activity of a new vaginal contraceptive NIM-76 from neem oil (*Azadirachta indica*). Journal of Ethnopharmacology 71(3):377

20 Gogate SS, Marathe AD 1989 Antiviral effects of neem leaf (*Azadirachta indica* Juss.). Journal of Research and Education in Indian Medicine 8(1):1

21 Chattopadhyay RR, Sarkar SK, Ganguly S, Banerjee RN 1992 Active effects of *Azadirachta indica* on some biochemical constituents of blood in rats. Science and Culture 58(1&2):39

22 Shukla R, Singh S, Bhandari CR 1973 Preliminary clinical trials on antidiabetic actions of *Azadirachta indica*. Medicine, Surgery 13:11

23 Luscombe DK, Taha SA 1974 Pharmacological studies on the leaves of *Azadirachta indica* extract on Chikungunya and measles virus. Journal of Pharmacy and Pharmacology 26S:111

24 MacKinnon S, Durst T, Arnason JT et al 1997 Antimalarial activity of tropical Meliaceae extracts and gedunin derivatives. Journal of Natural Products 60(4):336

25 Khanna N, Goswami M, Sen P, Ray A 1995 Antinociceptive action of *Azadirachta indica* (neem) in mice: possible mechanisms involved. Indian Journal of Experimental Biology 33:848

26 Khattak SG, Gilani SN, Ikram M 1985 Antipyretic studies on some indigenous Pakistani medicinal plants. Journal of Ethnopharmacology 14:45

27 Garg GP, Nigam SK, Ogle CW 1993 The gastric antiulcer effects of the leaves of the Neem tree. Planta Medica 59:215

28 Jaiswal AK, Bhattacharya SK, Acharya SB 1994 Anxiolytic activity of *Azadirachta indica* leaf extract in rats. Indian Journal of Experimental Biology 32(7):489

29 Thompson EB, Anderson CC 1978 Cardiovascular effects of *Azadirachta indica* extract. Journal of Pharmaceutical Science 67:1476

30 Singh PP, Junnarkar AY, Thomas GP, Tripathi RM, Varma RK 1990 A pharmacological study of *Azadirachta indica*. Fitoterapia 61(2):164

31 Chattopadhyay RR, Sarkar SK, Ganguly S, Banerjee RN, Basu TK, Mukherjee A 1992 Hepatoprotective activity of *Azadirachta indica* leaves on paracetamol induced hepatic damage in rats. Indian Journal of Experimental Biology 30(8):738

32 Khosla P, Bhanwra S, Singh J, Seth S, Srivastava RK 2000 A study of hypoglycaemic effects of *Azadirachta indica* (Neem) in normal and alloxan-diabetic rabbits. Indian Journal of Physiology and Pharmacology 44(1):69

33 Okpanyi SN, Ezeukwu GC 1981 Anti-inflammatory and antipyretic activities of *Azadirachta indica*. Planta Medica 41:34

34 Bhargava KP, Gupta MB, Gupta GP, Mitra CR 1970 Anti-inflammatory activity of saponins and other natural products. Indian Journal of Medical Research 58:724

35 Fujiwara T, Sugishita E, Takeda T et al 1984 Further studies on the structure of polysaccharides from the bark of *Melia azadirachta*. Chemical and Pharmaceutical Bulletin 32:1385

36 Pillai NR, Santhakumari G 1981 Antiarthritic and anti-inflammatory actions of nimbidin. Planta Medica 43:59

37 Fujiwara T, Takeda T, Ogihara Y, Shimizu M, Nomura T, Tomita Y 1982 Studies on the structure of polysaccharides from the bark of *Melia azadirachta*. Chemical and Pharmaceutical Bulletin 30:4025

38 Purohit A, Joshi VS, Dixit VP 1990 Contraceptive efficacy of *Azadirachta indica* (flower and bark) in male rats. A biochemical and sperm dynamics analysis. Journal of Bioscience 7(4):129

39 Prakash AO, Mishra A, Mathur R 1991 Studies on the reproductive toxicity due to the extract of *Azadirachta indica* (seeds) in adult cyclic female rats. Indian Drugs 28(4):163

40 Garg S, Talwar GP, Upadhyay SN 1998 Immunocontraceptive activity guided fractionation and characterization of active constituents of neem (*Azadirachta indica*) seed extracts. Journal of Ethnopharmacology 60(3):235

41 Prabhu ST, Singh RP 1993 Insect-growth regulatory activity of different parts of neem (*Azadirachta indica* Juss.) against tobacco caterpillar, *Sodoptera litura* (E). World Neem Conference, Bangalore, India, 24–28 February

42 Sufia B, Chatterjee NB 1991 Histological and histochemical alteration induced by extract of neem, *Azadirachta indica*, kernels in the ovaries of *Caryedon gangara* (Caleoptera: Bruchidae). International Journal of Toxicology, Occupational and Environmental Health 1(1):247

43 Mitchell MJ, Smith SL, Johnson S, Morgan ED 1997 Effects of the neem tree compounds azadirachtin, salanin, nimbin and 6-desacetylnimbin on ecdysone 20-monooxygenase activity. Archives of Insect Biochemistry and Physiology 35(1–2):199

44 Pillai NR, Santhakumari G 1984 Effects of nimbidin on acute and chronic gastroduodenal ulcer models in experimental animals. Planta Medica 50:143

45 Upadhyaya S, Dhawan S 1994 Neem (*Azadirachta indica*): immunomodulatory properties and therapeutic potential. Update Ayurveda, Bombay

46 Dhar ML, Dhar MM, Dhawan BN, Mehrotra BN, Ray C 1968 Screening of Indian plants for biological activity Part I. Indian Journal of Experimental Biology 6:232

Bacopa monniera L. (Scrophulariaceae) (syn. *Herpestis monniera* (L.) Penn., *Lysimachia monnieria* L., *Gratiola monnieria* L. and *Moniera cunefolia* Michx)

English: Thyme-leaved gratiola

Hindi: *Brahmi*

Sanskrit: *Barambhi, nirabarhmi*

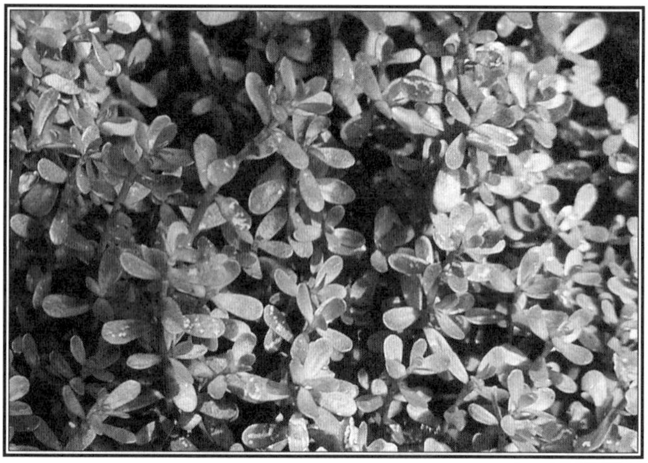

Brahmi forms the ingredient of a number of Ayurvedic prescriptions such as *Brahmighritam, Brahmirasayanam,* etc. and possesses numerous medicinal properties. Its use is documented in ancient Indian texts as far back as the 6th century and the herb has been widely used to promote the intellect and treat mental problems. It still occupies a predominant place in Hindu medicine and is used in Chinese medicine.

Habitat

The plant is commonly distributed in moist and damp areas on the edges of streams and water trenches. In India and other Asian countries it is found ascending to an altitude of 1320 m.

Botanical description

A small, prostrate, glabrous and fleshy herb (Plate 11). The leaves are sessile, soft, succulent, reniform, obovate-oblong or spatulate, up to 2.5 mm long, with obscure venation. The lower surface is punctate and entire. The stem is 10–30 cm long and 1–2 mm thick, with soft ascending branches. Flowers blue or white with purple veins, axillary and solitary on peduncles usually longer than the leaves, with linear bracteoles. Fruits ovoid, acute capsules included in the persistent calyx.

Parts used

Dried whole plant, mainly leaves and stems.

Traditional and modern use

The herb is used as an astringent, bitter and coolant. It is mainly used to promote the intellect and as a potent nervine, cardiotonic and diuretic, but is also said to have a positive effect in asthma, hoarseness and various types of insanity. It is included in many Ayurvedic formulations. It is recommended for children suffering from bronchitis and diarrhoea and the fresh juice of the plant is applied to inflamed joints to relieve pain.

Ethnoveterinary usage

Leaves and whole plants are used in tribal veterinary medicine, particularly in the treatment of epilepsy.[1]

Major chemical constituents

Saponins and triterpenes

Dammaranes such as the bacosides and bacosaponins, based on the bacogenins A_1–A_5, are the most important constituents. These include bacosides A, B and C, with bacoside A constituting about 2.5–3%. Bacoside A produces ebelin lactone on acid hydrolysis and yields jujubogenin on degradation. Bacopasaponin D (a pseudojujubogenin glycoside), the bacopasaponins E and F (based on jujubogenin), hersaponin and monnierin have also been reported, together with the triterpenes betulic acid, bacosine, β-sitosterol, stigmastanol and stigmasterol.[2–17]

Alkaloids

Brahmine and herpestine are present in the aerial parts.[18]

Flavonoids

Flavonoids such as glucuronyl-7-apigenin and glucuronyl-7-luteolin are present along with luteolin-7-glucoside and luteolin.[19]

Medicinal and pharmacological activities

Effect on cognitive function: Cognitive effects of *Bacopa monniera* extract were evaluated in healthy human subjects in a double-blind, placebo-controlled, independent group trial design. The randomly allocated subjects received either placebo or *brahmi* (300 mg). *B. monniera* significantly improved the speed of visual information processing, learning rate and memory consolidation and anxiety compared to placebo, with maximal effects evident after 12 weeks, suggesting the role of *brahmi* in improving higher-order cognitive processes.[20] It also produced a positive effect on passive-avoidance tasks, maximal electroshock seizures and locomotor activity in rats, by improving the cognitive effect. When administered along with phenytoin (PHT) for 2 weeks it significantly reversed PHT-induced impairment. Both acquisition and retention of memory showed improvement without affecting anticonvulsant activity.[21] The extract may provide a useful contribution to the restoration of cognitive function, possibly in conjunction with the judicious application of growth factors.[22]

Effect on learning: The effects on learning performance in rats were studied in different conditioning schedules by administering an aqueous suspension of an alcoholic extract (40 mg/kg, PO) for 3 or more days. The first schedule induced labile behaviour, using a shock-motivated brightness discrimination reaction. The treated group showed better acquisition, improved retention and delayed extinction. Similarly, in an active conditioned flight reaction, the drug-treated animals showed a shorter reaction time than the controls, which was confirmed in the continuous avoidance response.[23] Treatment with *brahmi* also produced an improvement in learning capability confirmed by a maze-learning experimental method.[24]

Anxiolytic activity: A standardised extract of *B. monniera* given to experimental models elicited a similar reaction to that of the benzodiazepine lorazepam and was dose dependent.[25]

Antioxidant properties: *Bacopa monniera* exerted antioxidant activity on rat brain frontal cortical, striatal and hippocampal regions by altering superoxide dismutase (SOD), catalase (CAT) and glutathione peroxidase (GPX) levels. The antioxidant activity was comparable to deprenyl. *Bacopa monniera* induced a dose-related activity in all brain regions, although deprenyl acted only on the frontal cortex and striatum. The effect was considered to be a result of the increase in oxidative free radical scavenging activity of the plant extract.[26] The alcoholic extract of the herb has protective action against ferrous sulphate and cumene hydroperoxide-induced experimental lipid peroxidation, equivalent to the antioxidants tris, EDTA and vitamin E. The effect extended to hepatic glutathione content and was found to be dose dependent.[27]

Spasmolytic activity: In animal studies, an ethanol extract of *brahmi* antagonised calcium channel activity. Spontaneous movement of smooth muscle induced by acetylcholine and histamine was inhibited by the plant extract, indicating a direct action. The effect of calcium chloride on blood vessels and jejunum was attenuated by the extract, implying a direct interference with influx of calcium ions. There was a lack of effect on either noradrenaline- or caffeine-induced contractions.[28]

Bronchodilatory activity: An ethanol extract dilated the bronchial smooth muscles of anaesthetised rats, counteracting bronchoconstriction induced by carbachol. This property reduced expiratory pressure, resembling salbutamol rather than isoprenaline in manner. The action may be mediation through both adrenoceptor-dependent and independent mechanisms.[29]

Analgesic activity: Bacosine was found to have analgesic activity but without barbiturate-type narcosis.[30]

Safety profile

The plant is safe in usual therapeutic doses and adverse reactions are rare.

Dosage

Infusion: 8–16 ml

Powder: 5–10 g

Ayurvedic properties

Rasa: *Tikta* (bitter)

Guna: *Laghu* (light), *snigdha* (unctuous)

Veerya: *Ushna* (hot)

Vipaka: *Katu* (pungent)

Dosha: Pacifies *kapha* and *vata*

Further reading

Chatterjee A, Prakashi SC 1997 The treatise of Indian medicinal plants, vol 5. PID, New Delhi

Handa SS, Kaul MK 1996 Supplement to cultivation and utilization of medicinal plants. Regional Research Laboratory, Jammu

Indian Drug Manufacturers' Association 1999 Indian herbal pharmacopoeia, vol 1. IDMA/Regional Research Laboratory, Jammu

Kapoor LD 2001 Handbook of Ayurvedic medicinal plants. CRS Press, Boca Raton

References

1 Jha MK 1992 Folk veterinary medicine of Bihar – a research project. NDDB, Anand, Gujrat

2 Mahato SB, Garai S, Chakravarty AK 2000 Bacopasaponins E and F: two jujubogenin bisdesmosides from *Bacopa monniera*. Phytochemistry 53(6):711

3 Rastogi S, Kulshreshtha DK 1999 Bacoside A2 – a triterpenoid saponin from *Bacopa monniera*. Indian Journal of Chemistry 38B(3):353

4 Garai S, Mahato SB, Ohtani K, Yamasaki K 1996 Bacopasaponin D-A pseudojujubogenin glycoside from *Bacopa monniera*. Phytochemistry 43(2):447

5 Garai S, Mahato SB, Ohtani K, Yamasaki K 1996 Dammarane-type triterpenoid saponins from *Bacopa monniera*. Phytochemistry 42(3):815

6 Rastogi S, Pal R, Kulshreshtha DK 1994 Bacoside A3, a triterpenoid saponin from *Bacopa monniera*. Phytochemistry 36(1):133

7 Jain PK, Dinesh K 1993 Bacoside A1, a minor saponin from *Bacopa monniera*. Phytochemistry 33(2):449

8 Rastogi S, Pal R, Kulshreshtha DK 1993 Bacogenin A5: a rearranged sapogenin from the saponins of *Bacopa monniera*. Indian Journal of Heterocyclic Chemistry 2(3):149

9 Kawai K, Shibata S 1978 Pseudojujubogenin, a new sapogenin from *Bacopa monniera*. Phytochemistry 17(2):287

10 Chandel RS, Kulshreshtha DK, Rastogi RP 1977 Bacogenin-A3: a new sapogenin from *Bacopa monniera*. Phytochemistry 16(1):141

11 Kulshreshtha DK, Rastogi RP 1975 Chemical examination of Bacopa monniera, VII. Absolute structures of the novel genins, bacogenins A1 and A2 from bacosides isolated from *Bacopa monniera*. Indian Journal of Chemistry 13(4):309

12 Kawai K, Akiyama T, Ogihara Y, Shibata S 1974 Chemical studies on Oriental plant drugs XXXVIII. New sapogenin in the saponins of *Zizyphus jujuba, Hovenia dulcis*, and *Bacopa monniera*. Phytochemistry 13(12):2829

13 Kawai K, Iitaka Y, Shibata S, Kulshreshtha DK, Rastogi RP 1973 Crystal and molecular structure of bacogenin-A1 dibromoacetate. Acta Crystallography, Section B 29(12):2947

14 Kulshreshtha DK, Rastogi RP 1973 Chemical examination of *Bacopa monniera*, V. Identification of ebelin lactone from bacoside A and the nature of its genuine sapogenin. Phytochemistry 12(8):2074

15 Kulshreshtha DK, Rastogi RP 1973 Chemical examination of *Bacopa monniera*, IV. Bacogenin-A1. Novel dammarane triterpene sapogenin from *Bacopa monniera*. Phytochemistry 12(4):887

16 Dutta T, Basu UP 1963 Triterpenoids. II. Isolation of a new triterpene saponin, monnierin, from *Bacopa monniera*. Indian Journal of Chemistry 1(9):408

17 Chakravarty AK, Sarker T, Masuda K, Shiojima K, Nakane T, Kawahara N 2001 Bacopaside I and II: two pseudojujubogenin glycosides from *Bacopa monniera*. Phytochemistry 58(4):553

18 Chatterjee N, Rastogi RP, Dhar ML 1963 Chemical examination of *Bacopa monnieri*, I. Isolation of chemical constituents. Indian Journal of Chemistry 1:212

19 Proliac A, Chabaud A, Raynaud J 1991 Two O-glucuronyl flavones in the stems and leaves of *Bacopa monnieri* L. (Scrofulariaceae). Pharmaceutica Acta Helvetica 66(5–6):153

20 Stough C, Lloyd J, Clarke J et al 2001 The chronic effects of an extract of *Bacopa monniera* (Brahmi) on cognitive function in healthy human subjects. Psychopharmacology 156(4):481

21 Vohora D, Pal SN, Pillai KK 2000 Protection from phenytoin-induced cognitive deficit by *Bacopa monniera*, a reputed Indian nootropic plant. Journal of Ethnopharmacology 71(3):383

22 Kidd PM 1999 A review of nutrients and botanicals in the integrative management of cognitive dysfunction. Alternative Medicine Review 4(3):144

23 Singh HK, Dhawan BN 1982 Effect of *Bacopa monniera* Linn. (Brahmi) extract on avoidance responses in rat. Journal of Ethnopharmacology 5(2):205

24 Dey CD, Bose S, Mitra S 1976 Effect of some centrally active phyto products on maze learning of albino rats. Indian Journal of Physiology and Allied Sciences 30(3):88

25 Bhattacharya SK, Ghosal S 1998 Anxiolytic activity of a standardized extract of *Bacopa monniera*. An experimental study. Phytomedicine 5(2):77

26 Bhattacharya SK, Bhattacharya A, Kumar A, Ghosal S 2000 Antioxidant activity of *Bacopa monniera* in rat frontal cortex, striatum and hippocampus. Phytotherapy Research 14(3):174

27 Tripathi YB, Chaurasia S, Tripathi E, Upadhyay A, Dubey GP 1996 *Bacopa monniera* Linn. as an antioxidant: mechanism of action. Indian Journal of Experimental Biology 34(6):523

28 Dar A, Channa S 1999 Calcium antagonistic activity of *Bacopa monniera* on vascular and intestinal smooth muscles of rabbit and guinea-pig. Journal of Ethnopharmacology 66(2):167

29 Dar A, Channa S 1997 Bronchodilatory and cardiovascular effects of an ethanol extract of *Bacopa monniera* in anesthetized rats. Phytomedicine 4(4):319

30 Vohora SB, Khanna T, Athar M, Bahar A 1997 Analgesic activity of bacosine, a new triterpene isolated from *Bacopa monniera*. Fitoterapia 68(4):361

Berberis aristata DC (Berberidaceae) (syn. *B. chitria* Lindl., *B. floribunda* Wall)

English: Indian barberry

Hindi: *Daruhaldi*

Sanskrit: *Daru haridra*

A crude extract, known as *rasaut* in Hindi, is prepared from the root bark and is used as a topical application in affections of the eyelids and chronic ophthalmia. It has a specific use in bacillary dysentery similar to that of other berberine-containing plants in various parts of the world. The literature often uses *B. chitria* as the name of the species and both are used here.

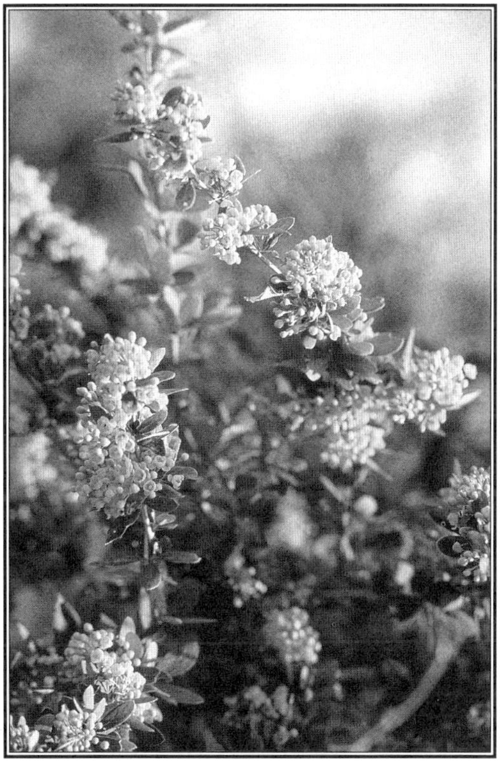

Habitat

Found mainly in the north-western Himalayas in open shrubby places, at altitudes of 2000–3500 m, and cultivated elsewhere.

Botanical description

An erect, glabrous spiny shrub, reaching 3–6 m in height (Plate 12). The leaves are obovate to elliptical, with a subacute or obtuse apex and an entire or toothed margin. The yellow flowers occur in corymbose racemes and the fruits are oblong or ovoid, bright red berries. The stem is externally greyish-brown, sometimes covered with lichen or moss, and internally is greenish-yellow, with bright yellow medullary rays.

Parts used

Roots, root bark, stem, wood, fruits.

Traditional and modern use

A tincture made from the stem and root bark is used as a bitter tonic, stomachic, cholagogue, antiperiodic and alterative and for periodic neuralgia. It is particularly important in the treatment of remittent and intermittent fevers and the consequent debility, and for fevers accompanied by bilious symptoms and diarrhoea. It is used to treat enlargement of the liver and spleen and a simple decoction sweetened with honey is often given in jaundice. In the treatment of bleeding piles it is administered as an ointment made with ghee. Externally, a decoction of the root bark is painted on the eyelids for eye infections and applied to other skin disorders. It may also be used to wash infected ulcers to improve healing and cicatrisation and a crude extract mixed with honey is a useful application to aphthous sores, abrasions and ulceration.

Ethnoveterinary usage

The roots, stem and berries are used in the treatment of diarrhoea, repeat oestrus in cows and buffaloes and for kidney stones.[1] The leaf and stem are used for eye disease of ruminants and swine.[2]

Major chemical constituents

Alkaloids

The root and stem bark contain berberine, berbamine, aromaline, karachine, palmatine, oxyacanthine, oxyberberine, taxilamine, jatrorrhizine[3–6] and others. Chitrianines A, B and C and dihydropalmatine-N-oxide have also been isolated from the root.[7]

Flavonoids and polyphenolics

The root and flowers contain quercetin and its 3-O-diglucoside, quercitrin, rutin, dihydro-kaempferol and others, and the flowers contain caffeic and chlorogenic acids.[8]

Fatty acids, hydrocarbons and phytosterols

Stearic palmitic, linoleic and oleic acids, n-triacontane and n-triacontanol, and β-sitosterol are present in the root.

Medicinal and pharmacological activities

Antichlamydial activity: The activity of an extract of *B. aristata* root (*'rasaut'*) was compared with penicillin, tetracycline, oxytetracycline and sodium sulphadiazine, using 7-day-old embryonated hen eggs (raised on an antibiotic-free diet) against 10 different *Chlamydia psittaci*, isolated originally from various clinical conditions of domestic animals. It exhibited considerable antichlamydial activity at a dose of 0.5 mg per embryo.[9]

Antiplatelet activity: An alcoholic extract of the root of *B. aristata* inhibited platelet-activating factor (PAF)-induced aggregation of rabbit platelets in a dose-dependent manner. A concentration of 38 μg/ml produced a 50% inhibition. The rate of aggregation was also reduced and the extract inhibited the binding of ^{3}H-PAF to rabbit platelets in a concentration-dependent manner, with an ID_{50} of 480 μg/ml. The results suggested that the alcoholic extract inhibited PAF binding to its receptor site, thereby reducing its cellular responses.[10]

Antimicrobial activity: Ethanolic and aqueous extracts of *B. chitria* roots were found to be useful in the treatment of eye infections or conjunctivitis.[11]

Hepatoprotective activity: The effect of an aqueous-methanol extract of *B. aristata* fruits was investigated against paracetamol and CCl_4-induced hepatic damage. Paracetamol (acetaminophen) caused a 100% mortality rate at a dose of 1 g/kg in mice, whereas pretreatment of animals with the crude extract (500 mg/kg) reduced the death rate to 10%. Pretreatment of rats with an extract of the fruit (500 mg/kg orally, twice daily) for 2 days also prevented both the paracetamol (640 mg/kg) and CCl_4 (1.5 ml/kg)-induced rise in serum transaminases (GOT, GPT). Posttreatment administration (with three successive doses of extract, 500 mg/kg, given 6-hourly) also reduced the hepatic damage induced by paracetamol. The plant extract caused a significant prolongation of pentobarbital-induced sleep (at 75 mg/kg), as well as increasing strychnine-induced lethality in mice, suggesting an inhibitory effect on microsomal drug-metabolising enzymes.[12] Acetominophen-induced liver damage was also prevented by an extract of the leaves of *Berberis aristata.*[13]

Actions of berberine

Hepatoprotective activity: Pretreatment of rodents with berberine (4 mg/kg, orally twice daily for 2 days) prevented both the acetaminophen and CCl_4-induced rise in serum levels of alkaline phosphatase and aminotransaminases, suggestive of hepatoprotection. Postdamage treatment with three successive oral doses of berberine (at 4 mg/kg 6-hourly) reduced the hepatic damage induced by acetaminophen, although CCl_4-induced hepatotoxicity was not modified, suggesting a different mode of action. Pretreatment of animals with a single oral dose of berberine (at 4 mg/kg) also prolonged the phenobarbitone-induced sleeping time (at 60 mg/kg IP phenobarbitone) as well as increasing the strychnine-induced toxicity (at 0.3 mg/kg strychnine). This indicates an inhibitory effect on microsomal drug-metabolising enzymes such as the cytochrome P450s.[14]

Antidiarrhoeal activity: Berberine prevented the death of young rabbits suffering from cholera when given at an early stage. The action of berberine on *Vibrio cholerae* was bacteriostatic during the early stages of growth and membrane damage during the initial static period, due to leakage of the intercellular constituents, was involved. The crude toxin made from berberine-treated *Vibrio cholerae* organisms failed to produce cholera symptoms in the infant rabbit model, suggesting that the toxin was either inactivated or neutralised.[15] Clinical studies with berberine have been conducted in 356 patients with cholera and compared with 264 patients treated with chloramphenicol. Berberine was found to be effective in both bacteriologically positive and negative patients. It reduced the mortality rate, volume and duration of diarrhoea, intake of intravenous fluid and convalescence period and was found to be superior to chloramphenicol in several respects.[16] Berberine also inhibited (by approximately 70%) the secretory responses of the heat-labile enterotoxins of *V. cholerae* and *Escherichia coli* in a rabbit ligated intestinal loop model. It was effective when given either before or after enterotoxin binding and both intraluminally and parenterally, and did not inhibit the stimulation of adenylate cyclase by cholera enterotoxin. There was no histological damage to intestinal mucosa. Berberine markedly inhibited the secretory response of *E. coli* heat-stable enterotoxin in the infant mouse model, although the mechanism of action of the drug is not yet known. These data provide a rationale for the clinical usefulness in treating acute diarrhoea of varying aetiology.[17] Berberine sulphate (100 mg/kg) protected rats from amoebic infection, in both short- and long-term study groups. However, the alkaloid at a dose of 50 mg/kg showed only partial protection (40–60%) of amoebic infection in rats. Diarrhoea, which was seen in four out of 10 rats, was reduced on the subsequent administration of berberine.[18]

A randomised, placebo-controlled, double-blind, clinical trial was carried out using 400 patients presenting with acute watery diarrhoea. Berberine or tetracycline, and both together, were given. Of the 185 patients with cholera, those given tetracycline or tetracycline with berberine had a considerably reduced volume and frequency of diarrhoeal stools, duration of diarrhoea in general and volume of required intravenous and oral rehydration fluid. Berberine alone did not produce an antisecretory effect, but analysis (by factorial design equations) showed a reduction in volume and cyclic AMP (adenosine monophosphate) concentration levels in stools (by 77%). However, after 24 hours, considerably fewer patients given tetracycline or tetracycline with berberine were found to excrete *V. cholerae* organisms in stools than those given berberine alone.[19]

Antiinflammatory activity: Berberine was found to effectively inhibit local inflammation induced by cholera toxin in a dose-dependent manner and was most effective when injected at the inflammation site. In contrast, hydrocortisone and cyproheptadine did not inhibit this type of inflammation and indomethacin inhibited the swelling only at toxic doses. Carrageenan- or formalin-induced swelling was inhibited by cyproheptadine and indomethacin but not by berberine, indicating an unusual mechanism of action. Berberine was also far less effective than hydrocortisone in inhibiting chronic cotton pellet-induced granuloma and possibly works against cholera toxin-induced inflammation by some form of selective antagonism.[20] It does, however, have significant antiinflammatory activity on acute, subacute and chronic types of inflammation produced by both immunological and non-immunological methods.[21]

Antileishmanial activity: Berberine has shown leishmanicidal properties on the promastigote form of *Leishmania donovani* when tested in vitro. The alkaloid, at 1 μg/ml, inhibited the growth of the promastigotes by 50%, whilst at 5 μg/ml complete inhibition was observed. Endogenous respiration of the organism was significantly inhibited (by 70%) at 10 μg/ml and glucose oxidation of the parasite was also inhibited (by about 46%). The mode of action was thought to be due to inhibition of nucleic acid and protein synthesis.[22] Berberine also markedly diminished the parasitic load and proved to be less toxic than pentamidine in both the 8-day and long-term models of *L. donovani* infection in hamsters. It rapidly improved the haematological picture of infected animals and inhibited both the in vitro multiplication of amastigotes in macrophage culture and their transformation to promastigotes in a cell-free culture. The mode of action was again thought to be an inhibitory action on macromolecular biosynthesis and a decrease in deoxyglucose uptake, probably due to interaction with DNA from *L. donovani* promastigotes.[23]

Antiplatelet activity: Berberine inhibited collagen-induced platelet aggregation in a dose-dependent manner in platelet-rich plasma prepared from normal human volunteers. It did not inhibit aggregation mediated by activation of thromboxane A_2, increase in calcium influx or stimulation of G-protein linked pathways, so it is likely that berberine selectively inhibits platelet aggregation by interfering with the collagen-mediated adhesion process.[24]

***Activity against* Entamoeba histolytica, Giardia lamblia *and* Trichomonas vaginalis:** Berberine sulphate inhibited the growth of *E. histolytica*, *G. lamblia* and *T. vaginalis* and induced morphological changes in the parasites. Exposure of *E. histolytica* to berberine caused a clumping of chromatin in the nucleus, the formation of autophagic vacuoles and aggregates of small vacuoles in the cytoplasm. In berberine-treated *G. lamblia*, an irregularly shaped vacuole appeared in the cytoplasm and gradually enlarged during culture; the trophozoites became swollen and deposits of glycogen were seen in the cytoplasm. Soon after exposure of *T. vaginalis* to berberine, autophagic vacuoles increased in number and one large vacuole appeared, which was characteristic of treated cells.[25]

Antibacterial activity: The effects of berberine chloride solution and Berberis tincture on large numbers of bacteria were studied in vitro. The tincture was more effective than solution, probably due to a higher concentration of berberine in the former or the presence of other compounds.[26] In veterinary medicine, five antibacterial intrauterine preparations were tested in 21 cows with second-degree endometritis. Five applications of each drug were given on alternate days over a 9-day period. The cure rate was 81% for a combination of oxytetracycline, oleandomycin, neomycin, prednisolone and chlorpheniramine maleate, 67% for tetracycline, 57% for Lugol's solution (0.5%), 52% for berberine hydrochloride and 33% for chlortetracycline.[27]

Safety profile

The LD_{50} for berberine sulphate in mice is 24.3 mg/kg IP[28] and for a 50% ethanolic extract of the roots has been reported as 200 mg/kg.[29]

Dosage

Decoction: 5–10 ml

Powdered root: 1–3 g

Ayurvedic properties

Rasa: *Tikta* (bitter), *kashiya* (astringent)

Guna: *Laghu* (light), *ruksha* (rough)

Veerya: *Ushna* (hot)

Vipaka: *Katu* (pungent)

Dosha: Balances *kapha* and *vata*

Further reading

Kapoor LD 1990 Handbook of Ayurvedic medicinal plants. CRC Press, Boca Raton

Ministry of Health and Family Welfare 1989 Ayurvedic pharmacopoeia of India. Government of India, New Delhi

Nadkarni AK 1976 Indian materia medica. Popular Prakshan PVT Ltd, Bombay

Pandey GS (ed) 1998 Indian materia medica. Chaukhambha Bharati Academy, Gokul Bhawan, Varanasi

Council of Scientific and Industrial Research 1985 The wealth of India. PID, CSIR, New Delhi

References

1 Jha MK 1992 Folk veterinary medicine of Bihar – a research project. NDDB, Anand, Gujrat

2 International Institute of Rural Reconstruction 1994 Ethnoveterinary medicine in Asia. An

information kit on traditional animal health care practices. IIRR, Silang, Philippines

3 Rahman A, Ansari AA 1983 Alkaloids of *Berberis aristata*. Isolation of aromoline and oxyberberine. Journal of the Chemical Society of Pakistan 5(4):283

4 Blasko G, Murugesan N, Freyer AJ, Sharma M, Ansari AA, Rahman A 1982 Karachine: an unusual protoberberine alkaloid. Journal of the American Chemistry Society 104:2039

5 Blasko G, Sharma M 1982 Taxilamine, a pseudobenzyl isoquinoline alkaloid. Heterocycles 19(2):257

6 Hussaini FA, Shoeb A 1985 Isoquinoline derived alkaloids from *Berberis chitria*. Phytochemistry 24(3):633

7 Chauhan AK, Dobhal MP 1989 Characterization of a new alkaloid from the roots of *Berberis chitria*. Pharmazie 44(7):510

8 Sivakumar R, Ramachandran Nair AG 1991 Polyphenolic constituents of the flowers of *Berberis aristata*. Journal of the Indian Chemical Society 68:531

9 Purohit VD, Gupta RKP, Khanna RNS 1988 *In vivo* studies on anti-chlamydial activity of some antibiotics and an indigenous drug (*Berberis aristata*) against *Chlamydia psittaci* isolates. Haryana Agriculture University, Journal of Research 18(4):253

10 Tripathi YB, Shukla SD 1996 *Berberis aristata* inhibits PAF-induced aggregation of rabbit platelets. Phytotherapy Research 10:628–630

11 Dobhal MP, Joshi PC 1992 *In-vitro* antimicrobial efficacy of *Berberis chitria*. Fitoterapia 63(1):69

12 Gilani AH, Janbaz KH 1995 Preventive and curative effects of *Berberis aristata* fruit extract on paracetamol and CCl_4 -induced hepatotoxicity. Phytotherapy Research 9:489

13 Gilani AH, Janbaz KH 1992 Prevention of acetaminophen-induced liver damage by *Berberis aristata* leaves. Biochemistry Society Transactions 20(4):347S

14 Janbaz KH, Gilani AH 2000 Studies on preventive and curative effects of berberine on chemical induced hepatotoxicity in rodents. Fitoterapia 71:25

15 Dutta NK, Panse MV 1962 Usefulness of berberine (an alkaloid from *Berberis aristata*) in the treatment of cholera (experimental). Indian Journal of Medical Research 50:732

16 Lahiri SC, Dutta NK 1967 Berberine and chloramphenicol in the treatment of cholera and severe diarrhea. Journal of the Indian Medical Association 48:1

17 Sack RB, Froehlich JL 1982 Berberine inhibits intestinal secretory response of *Vibrio cholerae* and *Escherichia coli* enterotoxins. Infection and Immunity 35(2):471

18 Kulkarni SK, Dandiya PC, Varandani NL 1972 Pharmacological investigations of berberine sulfate. Japanese Journal of Pharmacology 22:11

19 Khin-Maung U, Khin M, Nyunt-Nyunt W, Kyaw A, Tin U 1985 Clinical trial of berberine in acute watery diarrhoea. British Medical Journal 291:1601

20 Akhter MH, Sabir M, Bhide NK 1977 Antiinflammatory effect of berberine in rats injected locally with cholera toxin. Indian Journal of Medical Research 65(1):133

21 Halder RK, Neogi NC, Rathor RS 1970 Pharmacological investigations on berberine hydrochloride. Indian Journal of Pharmacy 2:26

22 Ghosh SK, Rakshit MM, Ghosh DK 1983 Effect of berberine chloride on *Leishmania donovani*. Indian Journal of Medical Research 78:407

23 Ghosh AK, Bhattacharya FK, Ghosh DK 1985 *Leishmania donovani:* amastigote inhibition and mode of action of berberine. Experimental Parasitology 60(3):404

24 Shah BH, Nawaz Z, Saeed SA, Gilani AH 1998 Agonist-dependent differential effects of berberine in human platelet aggregation. Phytotherapy Research 12S:S60–S62

25 Kaneda Y, Torii M, Tanka T, Aikawa M 1991 *In vitro* effects of berberine sulfate on the growth and structure of *Entamoeba histolytica, Giardia lamblia* and *Trichomonas vaginalis*. Annals of Tropical Medicine and Parasitology 85(4):417

26 Pepeljnjak S, Petricic J 1992 Anti-microbial effect of berberine and tinctura Berberidis. Pharmazie 47:307

27 Sinha AK, Singh BK, Arneja DV 1976

Comparative studies on the efficacy of drugs against endometritis in cattle. Indian Veterinary Journal 53(6):430

28 Blumenthal M 1998 The complete German Commission E monographs. Therapeutic guide to herbal medicines. American Botanical Council, Austin, Texas

29 Dhar ML, Dhar MM, Dhawan BN, Mehrotra BN Ray C 1968 Screening of Indian plants for medicinal activity. Indian Journal of Experimental Biology 6:237

Boerhaavia diffusa L. (Nyctaginaceae)(syn. *B. repens* Linn., *B. procumbens* Roxb.)

English: Spreading hogweed, pigweed

Hindi: *Gadahpurna*

Sanskrit: *Punarnava*

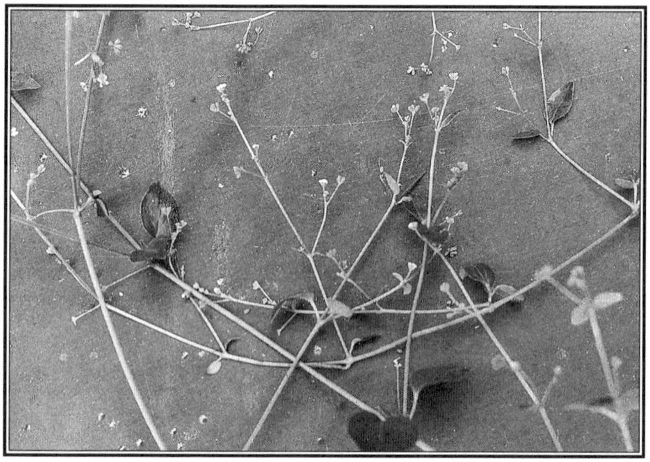

The plant has been used for diverse diseases for centuries. The term *punarnava* is also applied to other varieties of Boerhaavia.

Habitat

It is found growing wild all over India and other Asian countries, to an altitude of 2000 m, in sandy soil and on waste ground.

Botanical description

Profusely branched, pubescent or glabrous, prostrate herb with a creeping stem 1–2 m long and a stout woody root (Plate 13). The leaves are ovate, thick, with long petioles and entire margins. The lower surface is white and smooth and the upper surface green and rough. The flowers are small, pink, red or white in axillary or terminal panicles; fruits are oblong with glandular anthocarps.

Parts used

Roots, whole plant, leaves and flowers.

Traditional and modern use

It is widely used, particularly as a diuretic in dropsy and renal disease, and has been used to treat asthma, convulsions, dysentery, diarrhoea, dysmenorrhoea, epilepsy, fever, erysipelas, fistula, jaundice, prolapse, malaria, hysteria, gastritis and enteritis, and as an emetic and expectorant.

Ethnoveterinary usage

The whole plant is used in ruminants to treat difficulties in urinating.[1]

Major chemical constituents

Rotenoids

Roots contain the rotenoids boeravinone A, B, C2, D and F and punarnavoside has also recently been isolated.[2-6]

Lignans

Liriodendrin and syringaresinol mono-B-D-glucoside have been isolated from the methanol extract.

Xanthones

The benzene extract yielded boerhavine, a dihydroisofuranoxanthone.[7]

Medicinal and pharmacological activities

Hepatoprotective activity: An aqueous extract of the root (2 ml/kg) conferred a marked protection of the serum parameters GOT, GPT, ACP and ALP; however, no protection of GLDH and bilirubin was observed. The aqueous extract was more potent than the powdered drug. The chloroform and methanolic extract of roots also exhibited hepatoprotective activity and oral administration of an ethanolic extract of the whole plant of *B. diffusa* showed activity against carbon tetrachloride-induced hepatotoxicity in rats and mice. A strong choleretic action was observed which resulted in an increase in bile flow and no signs of toxicity were observed up to an oral dose of 2 g/kg body weight in mice. Three rotenoids, one steroid and one flavone isolated from the plant lowered the content of enzyme GOT.[8]

Ca^{2+} channel antagonism: Liriodendrin, a lignan isolated from the methanolic extract of the roots of *B. diffusa*, exhibited a significant Ca^{2+} channel antagonistic effect in frog heart single cells using the whole cell voltage clamp method.[5]

Antifibrinolytic activity: The root extract, administered to monkeys fitted with an intrauterine device (IUD), produced a noticeable reduction in the amount and duration of menstrual flow (124%) and menstrual iron loss, indicating a potent antifibrinolytic and antiinflammatory action and substantiating its use in IUD-induced menorrhagia. Punarnavoside has been identified as an antifibrinolytic agent.[4]

Inhibition of bone resorption: A methanolic extract of the whole plant, as well as two flavonoids isolated from it (eupalitin-3-0-B-D-galactopyranosyl-(1-2)-B-D-glucopyranoside and eupalitin-3-0-B-D-galactopyranoside), showed significant inhibitory action regarding bone resorption.[9]

Teratogenicity: Administration of an ethanolic extract of *B. diffusa* daily in a dose of 250 g/kg body weight PO to pregnant albino female rats during the entire period of gestation did not cause any teratogenic effects.[10]

Effect on levels of GABA: Differential effects on GABA levels in various regions of the brain of rats under stress were observed when treated with *Boerhaavia diffusa* and a reduction in stress and protection from haemorrhagic ulcers were observed. GABA-ergic involvement in the antistress activity of the drug was postulated.[11]

Diuretic action: Clinically, a diuretic effect comparable to furosemide was observed, with a reduction in urinary protein excretion and increase in serum protein level in patients with nephrotic syndrome. Immunoglobulins and immune complexes were increased after a month of medication and *punarnava* was considered to be a useful and safe drug. A seasonal variation was exhibited for the diuretic and antiinflammatory effects of the roots and leaves of the plant, with maximum activity observed in plants collected in the rainy season.[12]

Safety profile

Safe if used with appropriate clinical guidance but may raise blood pressure and affect the heart. The LD_{50} for a 50% ethanolic extract of the root and the whole plant was 1000 mg/kg body weight in adult albino rats.[13]

Dosage

Root juice: 9–12 g

Leaf juice: 12–25 g

Root powder: 8–15 g

Ayurvedic properties

Rasa: *Madhur* (sweet), *tikta* (bitter), *kashaya* (astringent)

Guna: *Laghu* (light), *ruksha* (dry)

Vipaka: *Madhur* (sweet)

Veerya: *Ushna* (hot)

Dosha: Pacifies the *tridosha*

Further reading

Bharatiya Vidya Bhavan's Swami Prakashanandra Ayurveda Research Centre 1992 Selected medicinal plants of India. Chemexcil, Mumbai

Ministry of Health and Family Welfare 1989 Ayurvedic pharmacopoeia of India. Government of India, New Delhi

Pandey GS (ed) 1998 Indian materia medica. Chaukhambha Bharati Academy, Gokul Bhawan, Varanasi

References

1 International Institute of Rural Reconstruction 1994 Ethnoveterinary medicine in Asia. An information kit on traditional animal health care practices. Part I. General information. IIRR, Silang, Philippines

2 Lami N, Kadota S, Tezuka Y, Kikuchi T 1990 Constituents of the roots of *Boerhaavia diffusa* L. II Structure and stereochemistry of a new rotenoid, boeravinone C2. Chemical and Pharmaceutical Bulletin 38(6):1558

3 Kadota S, Lami N, Tezuka Y, Kikuchi T 1989 Constituents of the roots of *Boerhaavia diffusa* L.I. Examination of sterols and structures of new rotenoids boeravinones A and B. Chemical and Pharmaceutical Bulletin 37(12):3214

4 Jain GK, Khanna NM 1989 Punarnavoside, a new antifibrinolytic agent from *Boerhaavia diffusa* Linn. Indian Journal of Chemistry 28B(2):163

5 Lami N, Kadota S, Kikuchi T, Momose Y 1991 Constituents of the roots of *Boerhaavia diffusa* L.III. Identification of Ca^{2+} channel antagonistic compound from the methanol extract. Chemical and Pharmaceutical Bulletin 39(6):1551

6 Lami N, Kadota S, Kikuchi T 1991 Constituents of the roots of *Boerhaavia diffusa* L. IV Isolation and structure determination of boeravinones D, E and F. Chemical and Pharmaceutical Bulletin 39(7):1863

7 Ahmed B, Chung-Ping Yu 1992 Boerhavine, a dihydroisofuranoxanthone from *Boerhaavia diffusa*. Phytochemistry 31(12):4382–4384

8 Chandan BK, Sharma AK, Anand KK 1991 *Boerhaavia diffusa*: a study of its hepatoprotective activity. Journal of Ethnopharmacology 31(3):299–307

9 Li J, Li H, Kadota S, Namba T, Miyahara T, Khan UG 1996 Effects on cultured neonatal mouse calvaria of the flavonoids isolated from *Boerhaavia repens*. Journal of Natural Products 59(11):1015

10 Singh A, Singh RG, Singh RH, Mishra N, Singh N 1991 An experimental evaluation of possible teratogenic potential in *Boerhaavia diffusa* in albino rats. Planta Medica 57(4):315

11 Sharma K, Pasha KV, Dandiya PC 1991 Effect of *Boerhaavia diffusa* Linn. on GABA levels of the brain during stress. Conference on Pharmacology and Symposium on Herbal Drugs, New Delhi, March

12 Mishra AS, Verma J, Kumari N 1995 Studies on medicinal properties of *Convolvulus pluricaulis* and *Boerhaavia diffusa*. Biojournal 6(1/2):31

13 Dhar ML, Dhar MM, Dhawan BN, Mehrotra BN, Ray C 1968 Screening of Indian medicinal plants for biological activity: Part I. Indian Journal of Experimental Biology 6:232

Boswellia serrata Roxb. (Burseraceae)

English: Indian olibanum tree

Hindi: *Salai*

Sanskrit: *Sallaki*

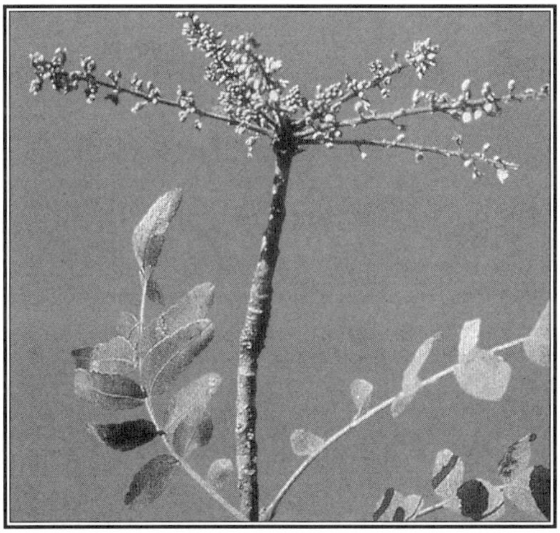

The plant has been used for cosmetic purposes since ancient times. It was associated with longevity and memory and burnt as an incense to drive away evil spirits. In the Bible, the gum exudate from the tree was offered to Adam as a consolation for losing the Garden of Eden. It is sometimes referred to as myrrh, although this in fact comes from *Commiphora abyssinica*. Frankincense comes from the related *B. sacra*.

Habitat

The plant grows in the drier parts of India, including the Deccan, central India, the eastern states and north of Gujrat.

Botanical description

It is a deciduous branching tree reaching 4–5 m in height and 1–1.5 m in girth (Plate 14). The leaves are opposite and sessile, variable in shape but usually ovate or lanceolate, obtuse, with a serrate margin and rounded base. The flowers are in racemes with long, ovate, cream-coloured petals. The oleo-gum resin is exuded by cuts made in the bark of the trunk.

Parts used

Oleo-gum resin, bark.

Traditional and modern use

The gum resin is used as a stimulant, antirheumatic, diaphoretic, in nervous and skin diseases, urinary disorders, obesity and scrofulous affections. The oil obtained from the resin is used as a demulcent, in colic, chronic and aphthous ulcers and for ringworm, dysmenorrhoea and bone disorders. Both the gum and oil have been used as a diuretic, astringent and emmenagogue and to treat gonorrhoea.

Ethnoveterinary usage

The gum resin is used in pox, rinder pest and diarrhoea.[1]

Major chemical constituents

Triterpenes

The gum resin contains a mixture of triterpene acids known as boswellic acids (α, β, γ-boswellic acids) and their derivatives.

It also yields a volatile oil (about 0.6%), containing anisaldehyde, α-pinene, α-phellandrene and sesquiterpene alcohols.[2–5]

Sugars

The gum contains arabinose, galactose, xylose, galacturonic acid and digitoxose. The main constituents isolated from the leaves are D-fructose, D-lactose, D-glucose, L-sorbose, raffinose, rhamnose and D-galactose.[6]

Medicinal and pharmacological activities

Antiinflammatory and antiarthritic activity: *B. serrata* is valued for its well-documented antiarthritic action, which is attributable to the boswellic acids. These acids inhibited leukotriene synthesis via 5-lipoxygenase, but did not affect either 12-lipoxygenase or cyclooxygenase. Boswellic acids did not impair the peroxidation of arachidonic acid by iron and ascorbate, indicating they are specific, non-redox inhibitors of leukotriene synthesis either interacting directly with 5-lipoxygenase or blocking its translocation.[7] The boswellic acids possessed varying degrees of activity in dose-related acute and chronic test models. In acute tests at a dose range of 50–200 mg/kg administered orally, an activity of between 26% and 43% was observed in rats and 20–34% in mice with carrageenan-induced oedema. In chronic tests using the developing adjuvant polyarthritis, doses of 50–200 mg/kg produced an antiarthritic activity of 32–50%.[8] A human clinical study involving 175 patients of both sexes and a mean age of 35 (about 70% of whom were bedridden), with duration of illness between 1 and 6 years, has been carried out. Parameters assessed were morning stiffness of joints, pain, loss of grip strength and difficulty in performance of routine jobs. Results were as follows: 67% showed a good or excellent effect, with 30% showing some improvement and 3% little or none.[9]

Analgesic activity: An extract of the gum resin showed sedative and analgesic properties in rats.[10]

Cholesterol-lowering effect: In vitro and in vivo experiments showed a dose-dependent fall in the cholesterol biosynthesis. Inhibition in vivo was at a dosage of 100 mg/kg.[11]

Immunomodulatory activity: A single dose of boswellic acids (50–200 mg/kg) inhibited the expression of the delayed hypersensitivity reaction and primary humoral response to sheep erythrocytes (SRBC) in mice. The secondary response was appreciably enhanced at lower doses. Prolonged oral administration of boswellic acids (25–100 mg/kg/day for 21 days) increased the body weight, total leucocyte counts and humoral antibody titres in rats.[12] Boswellic acids were also found to possess anticomplementary activity in both the classic and alternative complement pathways. A significant reduction in immunohaemolysis in vitro was observed at concentrations of 0.005–0.1 mM, with an IC_{50} value of about 10 μmol/l.[8]

Antitumour activity: 3-O-Acetyl-11-keto-β-boswellic acid, isolated from gum resin, inhibited the synthesis of DNA, RNA and protein in human leukaemia HL-60 cells in a dose-dependent manner. It showed pronounced inhibitory effects, with IC_{50} values of 0.6, 0.5 and 4.1 μM respectively.[13]

Antiasthmatic activity: In a double-blind, placebo-controlled study, 40 patients of both sexes in the age range 18–75 years, and with a mean duration of bronchial asthma of 9.58 years, were treated with a preparation of gum resin (300 mg thrice daily) for a period of 6 weeks. Seventy percent of patients showed some improvement as evidenced by the disappearance of physical symptoms such as dyspnoea and number of attacks. There was an improvement in biochemical parameters including a decrease in eosinophil count and ESR. The control group of 40 patients were treated with lactose (300 mg thrice daily) for 6 weeks and of these, 27% showed some improvement.[9]

Antifungal activity: The essential oil showed a significant antifungal activity against plant pathogens such as *Phytophthora parasitica*. It exhibited a weak antifungal action against human pathogens.[14]

Safety profile

During preclinical toxicological studies, primates and rats were fed with an ethanolic extract of gum resin for over 6 months, during which no adverse effects were observed.[15] The maximum tolerated doses in rats of the 50% ethanolic extracts of root, fruit and stem were 50 mg/kg, 500 mg/kg and 250 mg/kg body weight respectively given IP.[16] The boswellic acids have not been found to exhibit any toxic effects.[17]

Dosage

Gum resin: 2–3 g

Oil: 1–1.5 ml

Bark decoction: 56–112 ml

Ayurvedic properties

Rasa: *Kashaya* (astringent), *tikta* (bitter), *madhur* (sweet)

Guna: *Laghu* (light), *ruksha* (dry)

Veerya: *Ushna* (hot)

Vipaka: *Katu* (pungent)

Dosha: Balances *kapha* and *pitta*

Further reading

Ministry of Health and Family Welfare 1989 Ayurvedic pharmacopoeia of India. Government of India, New Delhi

Nadkarni AK 1976 Indian materia medica. Popular Prakashan PVT Ltd, Bombay

Pandey GS (ed) 1998 Indian materia medica. Chaukhambha Bharati Academy, Gokul Bhawan, Varanasi

Council of Scientific and Industrial Research 1985 The wealth of India. PID, CSIR, New Delhi

References

1 Jha MK 1992 Folk veterinary medicine of Bihar – a research project. NDDB, Anand, Gujrat
2 Mahajan B, Taneja SC, Sethi VK, Dhar KL 1995 Two triterpenoids from *Boswellia serrata* gum resin. Phytochemistry 39(2):453–455
3 Simpson JCE, Williams NE 1938 The triterpene group. Part I. β-Boswellic acid. Journal of the Chemical Society 686
4 Sharma RA, Varma KC 1980 Studies on gum obtained from *Boswellia serrata* Roxb. Indian Drugs 17:225
5 Bhuchar VM, Agrawal AK, Sharma SK 1982 Constituents of gum obtained from *Boswellia serrata* exudate. Indian Journal of Technology 20(1): 38
6 Gangwal ML, Vardhan DK 1995 Carbohydrate contents of *Boswellia serrata*. Asian Journal of Chemistry 7(3):677
7 Ammon HPT, Safayhi H, Mack T, Sabieraj J 1993 Mechanism of anti-inflammatory actions of curcumin and boswellic acids. Journal of Ethnopharmacology 38(2,3):113

8 Knaus U, Wagner H 1996 Effects of Boswellic acids of *Boswellia serrata* and other triterpenic acids on the complement system. Phytomedicine 3(1):77

9 Gupta I, Gupta V, Parihar A et al 1998 Effects of *Boswellia serrata* gum resin in patients with bronchial asthma: results of a double-blind, placebo-controlled, 6 week clinical study. European Journal of Medical Research 3(11):511

10 Menon MK, Kar A 1971 Analgesic and psychopharmacological effects of the gum resin of *Boswellia serrata*. Planta Medica 19(4):333

11 Zutshi U, Rao PG, Kaur S, Singh GB, Singh S, Atal CK 1986 Mechanism of cholesterol lowering effects of Salai guggul ex.*Boswellia serrata* Roxb. Indian Journal of Pharmacology 18(3):182

12 Sharma ML, Kaul A, Khajuria A, Singh S, Singh GB 1996 Immunomodulatory activity of Boswellic acids (pentacyclic triterpene acids) from *Boswellia serrata*. Phytotherapy Research 10(2):107

13 Shao Y, Ho CT, Chin CK, Badmaev V, Huang MT 1998 Inhibitory activity of boswellic acids from *Boswellia serrata* against human leukemia HL-60 cells in culture. Planta Medica 64(4):328

14 Gangwal ML, Vardhan DK 1995 Antifungal activity of essential oil of *Boswellia serrata*. Asian Journal of Chemistry 7(3):675

15 Singh GB, Singh S, Bani S, Kaul A 1992 Boswellic acids – a new class of anti-inflammatory drugs with a novel mode of action. International Seminar on Traditional Medicine, Calcutta, 7–9 November

16 Dhar ML, Dhar MM, Dhawan BN, Mehrotra BN, Ray C 1968 Screening of Indian plants for biological activity: Part I. Indian Journal of Experimental Biology 6:237

17 Singh GB, Atal CK 1986 Pharmacology of an extract of salai guggal ex-*Boswellia serrata*, a new non-steroidal anti-inflammatory agent. Agents and Actions 18:407

Caesalpinia bonducella Fleming (Leguminosae) (syn. *Caesalpinia crista* L., *C. bonduc* Roxb.)

English: Bonduc nut, fever nut

Hindi: *Katikaranja, kankarej*

Sanskrit: *Kuberakshi*

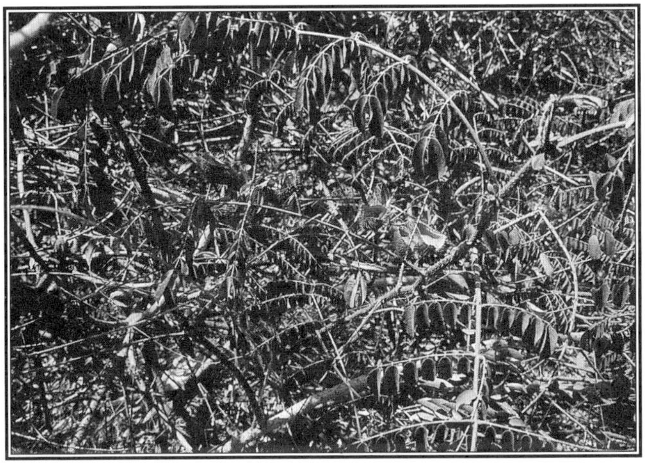

The seeds are grey coloured and resemble eyeballs, which explains the Sanskrit name *kuberakshi,* meaning eyes of Kubera, the Hindu god of wealth. It has also been called *vajrabijaka* which implies its diamond-like hard nature. The bark of the tree has been described as a purgative and recommended as a treatment for disturbed *kapha* and *vata*, gynaecological disorders, skin diseases, constipation, abdominal distension, piles and ulcers.

Habitat

It is found throughout the hotter parts of India, Burma and Sri Lanka, particularly on waste ground and along the coastal areas.

Botanical description

An extensive climber, with branches finely grey and downy, armed with both hooked and straight, hard yellow prickles (Plate 15). The leaves are bipinnate, 30–60 cm long with short prickly petioles; the stipules a pair of reduced pinnae at the base of the leaf each furnished with a long mucronate point. There are 6–8 pairs of pinnae, each 5.0–7.5 cm long, with a pair of hooked stipulary spines at the base. Leaflets 6–9 pairs, 2.0–3.8 cm long and 1.3–2.2 cm wide, membranous, elliptic to oblong, obtuse, strongly mucronate, glabrous above and more or less puberulous beneath. Flowers produced in dense terminal racemes (usually spicate) with long peduncles and supraaxillary racemes which are close at the top, looser downwards, 15–25 cm long. The pedicles are very short in the buds, elongating to 5 mm in flowers and 8 mm in fruits, brown and downy; bracts squarrose, linear, acute, reaching 1 cm long. The calyx is 6–8 mm long, fulvous and hairy; lobes obovate-oblong and obtuse. Petals oblanceolate, yellow; filaments declinate, flattened at the base, clothed with long white silky hairs. Pods shortly stalked, oblong, 5.0–7.5 by about 4.5 cm, densely armed with wiry prickles. Seeds 1–2, oblong, dark grey, up to 1.3 cm long.

Parts used

Seeds, roots, bark and leaves.

Traditional and modern use

Bonduc is antiperiodic, a febrifuge, tonic and anthelmintic and a powder of the roasted pods has been used as a substitute for quinine. The root bark is used to treat fever, intestinal worms, tumours, amenorrhoea, cough and for removing the placenta after childbirth. The leaves and their juice are used similarly and also traditionally for elephantiasis and smallpox, disorders of the liver and to destroy perspiration odour. In Sri Lanka, they are applied for toothache. The flower is bitter, with a warming effect on the body, ameliorates *kapha* and *vata* and the ash is used in ascites. The seeds are astringent and have been used to control contagious diseases, treat inflammation, colic, hydrocoele, skin diseases and leprosy. In Madras, an ointment is made from the powdered seeds with castor oil and applied externally. The seed sprouts have been used for tumours. The fruit is acrid, heating to the body, astringent to the bowels and is considered an aphrodisiac. It is also used to treat urinary disorders, leucorrhoea, piles and wounds. The oil from the fruit is applied to indolent ulcers and the oil from the seeds is used in convulsions and paralysis. In Guinea, the crushed seeds are considered vesicant and the boiled leaves used as a gargle for sore throat. The leaves and seeds, after roasting with castor oil, are applied externally to inflammatory swellings, especially to inflamed piles, hydrocoele, and orchitis.

Ethnoveterinary usage

The seeds, leaves and roots are used for the treatment of tachycardia, bradycardia, tuberculosis, tympanitis, pain in the abdomen, fever, cold and cough and liver fluke in ruminants.[1]

Major chemical constituents

Cassane diterpenes and furanoditerpenes

The root contains caesaldekarins C, F and G,[2] caesalpinin;[3] bonducellpins A,B,C and D;[4] the seed kernels contain α-caesalpin, β-caesalpin, γ-caesalpin,[5] ε-caesalpin[6] and caesalpin F.[7]

Steroidal saponin

Diosgenin[8] occurs in the root.

Fatty acids, hydrocarbons and phytosterols

Seed kernels contain palmitic, stearic, octadeca-4-enoic and octadeca-2,4-dienoic, lignoceric, oleic and linolenic acids, heptacosane and sitosterol.[9,10]

Isoflavones

Seed kernels contain bonducellin.[11]

Aminoacids

Aspartic acid, arginine and citrulline are present in the seed.[12]

Phenolics

Brazilin and bonducin have been isolated from the leaf.[13]

Medicinal and pharmacological activities

Antidiarrhoeal activity: The fruits were found to have significant antidiarrhoeal activity in mice.[14]

Antimalarial activity: An ethanolic extract of the defatted seed kernels showed promising antimalarial activity when screened using a *Plasmodium berghei*-infected mouse model by a blood schizontocidal test.[15]

Antiviral activity: An ethanolic extract of the root and stem exhibited activity against the Vaccinia virus.[16]

Antioestrogenic activity: Powdered seeds of *C. bonducella* were found to have anti-oestrogenic activity in mice and rabbits, and an antifertility action in mice and rats.[17]

Antifilarial activity: The ethanolic extract of the seed kernel showed antifilarial activity against *Litomosoides carinii* in the cotton rat. The hexane-soluble portion of the extract showed a 95.5% macrofilaricidal activity with a gradual fall in microfilaraemia up to day 42, at a dose of 1 g/kg daily given orally for 5 days. When tested against *Brugia malayi* in Mastomys, at the same dose, the hexane fraction produced gradual reduction in microfilaraemia up to day 91 but did not show any macrofilaricidal action. However, all female worms were sterilised.[18]

Hypoglycaemic and antihyperglycaemic activity: The hypoglycaemic activity of the seed powder has been studied fairly extensively. In normal and alloxan-diabetic rabbits, the drug was administered orally as a single dose of 0.5, 1 or 1.5 g/kg. The highest decrease (36.5%) in blood glucose levels was obtained with the 1.5 g/kg dose, 12 hours after administration, with a more moderate effect at 4 and 24 hours. In diabetic rabbits, the drug produced a significant antihyperglycaemic effect within 3 days when given 1.5 g/kg/day for 10 days.[19] In another study, in normal rats, the aqueous and 50% ethanolic extracts of the seeds exhibited a hypoglycaemic action as early as 4 hours after administration, at a dose of 100 mg/kg. The activity induced by the aqueous extract was of a more prolonged duration than the 50% ethanolic extract and both extracts produced a significant antihyperglycaemic effect in streptozotocin-diabetic rats from day 5 onwards.[20] The hypoglycaemic effect of an aqueous extract was also studied in fed, fasted, dextrose-loaded and streptozotocin- and alloxan-induced diabetic albino rats. It produced a significant hypoglycaemic effect in dextrose-loaded and streptozotocin- and alloxan-diabetic rats but the effects were less pronounced in the fed and fasted rats.[21] An aqueous extract administered intraperitoneally into diabetic rats also reduced fasting blood glucose concentration.[22]

Hypolipidaemic activity: The aqueous extract of the seeds showed antihypercholesterolaemic and antihypertriglyceridaemic effects in streptozotocin-induced diabetic rats.[25]

Uterine stimulant effect: The aqueous extract of the leaves of *C. bonducella* increased the contractile force in isolated strips of pregnant rat myometrium preparations in a concentration-dependent manner. The effect induced was comparable to that of acetylcholine and was inhibited by atropine. The extract produced a uterine contraction in calcium-free solutions, even in the presence of EDTA or EGTA. This suggests an interaction with cholinergic receptors which would influence the influx of calcium (phasic contraction) and mobilisation of calcium from cellular stores (tonic contraction), both of which are responsible for the increase of contractile activity and development of the contracture of uterine smooth muscle.[23]

Antiinflammatory activity: The antiinflammatory activity was studied in rats using the formalin arthritis and granuloma pouch methods. At a dose of 250 mg/kg the extract was found to be effective in the granuloma pouch model and compared favourably with phenylbutazone.[24] The seeds showed a 50% inhibitory activity against carrageenan-induced oedema in the rat hind paw, at an oral dose of 1000 mg/kg, when given 24 hours and 1 hour prior to carrageenan injection (IP). The activity (66.67% inhibition) was comparable to that of phenylbutazone at a dose of 100 mg/kg.[25]

Safety profile

The maximum tolerated dose of the 50% ethanolic extract was found to be more than 1000 mg/kg body weight when tested in adult male albino mice.[21]

Dosage

Powdered seed: 1–2 g

Powdered root: 1–2 g

Leaf infusion: 12–20 ml

Ayurvedic properties

Rasa: *Tikta* (bitter), *kashaya* (astringent)

Guna: *Laghu* (light), *ruksha* (dry), *tikshna* (sharp)

Veerya: *Ushna* (hot)

Vipaka: *Katu* (pungent)

Dosha: Pacifies *tridosha*

Further reading

Arya Vaidya Sala Kottakkal 1993 Indian medicinal plants, vol. 1. Orient Longman, Hyderabad

Chatterjee A, Chandra Pakrashi S 1992 Treatise on Indian medicinal plants, vol 2. PID, CSIR, New Delhi

Kapoor LD 1990 Handbook of Ayurvedic medicinal plants. CRC Press, Boca Raton

Kirtikar KR, Basu BD 1975 Indian medicinal plants, vol II. Lalit Mohan Basu, Allahabad

Pandey GS (ed) 1998 Indian materia medica. Chaukhambha Bharati Academy, Gokul Bhawan, Varanasi

Sivarajan VV, Balachandran I 1994 Ayurvedic drugs and their plant sources. Oxford and IBH Publishing, New Delhi

References

1 Jha MK 1992 Folk veterinary medicine of Bihar – a research project. NDDB, Anand, Gujrat

2 Peter S, Tinto WF, McLean S, Reynolds WF, Yu M 1998 Cassane diterpenes from *Caesalpinia bonducella*. Phytochemistry 47(6):1153

3 Peter SR, Tinto WF, Mclean S, Reynolds WF, Tay LL 1997 Caesalpinin, a rearranged cassane furoditerpene of *Caesalpinia bonducella*. Tetrahedron 38(33):5767

4 Sonia RP, Winston FT 1997 Bonducellpins A-D, new cassane furanoditerpenes of *Caesalpinia bonduc*. Journal of Natural Products 60(12):1219

5 Canonica L, Jommi G, Manitto P, Pelizzoni F 1963 Bitter principles of *Caesalpinia bonducella*. Tetrahedron 29:2079

6 Balmain A, Bjamer K, Connolly JD, Ferguson G 1967 The constitution and stereochemistry of E. caesalpin. Tetrahedron 49:5027

7 Pascoe KO, Burke BA, Chan WR 1986 Caesalpin F: a new furanoditerpene from *Caesalpinia bonducella*. Journal of Natural Products 49:913

8 Jain S, Saraf S, Kharya MD, Dixit VK 1991 First report of diosgenin from seed kernels of *Caesalpinia crista* Linn. Indian Drugs 28(4):202

9 Rastogi S, Shaw AK, Kulshreshtha DK 1996 Characterisation of fatty acids of the antifilarial triglyceride fraction from *Caesalpinia bonduc*. Fitoterapia 67(1):63

10 Tummin Katti MC 1930 Chemical examination of the seeds of *Caesalpinia bonducella* Flem. Journal of the Indian Chemical Society 7:207

11 Purushottaman KK, Kalyani K, Subramanian K, Shanmuganathan SP 1982 Structure of bonducellin, a new homoisoflavone from *Caesalpina bonducella*. Indian Journal of Chemistry 21B(4):383

12 Thanki RJ, Thakur KA 1980 Amino acid composition of the seeds of the plants *Caesalpinia crista* and *Holarrhena antidysenterica*. Journal of the Institute of Chemistry (India) 52(5):209

13 Watt JM, Breyer-Brandwijk MG 1962 The medicinal and poisonous plants of Southern and Eastern Africa, 2nd edn. Churchill Livingstone, Edinburgh

14 Iyengar MA, Pendse GS 1965 Anti-diarrhoeal activity of the nut of *Caesalpinia bonducella* (Flem.). Indian Journal of Pharmacology 27:307

15 Jain S, Saraf S, Kharya MD, Revapurkar DM, Dixit VK 1992 Antimalarial activity of *Caesalpinia crista* nuts. Indian Journal of Natural Products 8(1):13

16 Dhar ML, Dhar MM, Dhawan BN, Mehrotra BN, Ray C 1968 Screening of Indian plants for biological activity, Part I. Indian Journal of Experimental Biology 6:232

17 Bhide MB, Nikam ST, Chavan SR 1970 Effect of seeds of sagarghota (*Caesalpinia bonducella*) on some aspects of reproductive system. Proceedings of the 16th Annual Conference of Physiology and Pharmacology, Calcutta, India 28

18 Murphy PK, Farima N, Kulshreshtha DK, Chatterjee RK 1993 Proceedings of the Third Asian Congress of Parasitology. CDRI, Lucknow

19 Rao VV, Dwivedi SK, Swarup D 1994 Hypoglycaemic effect of *Caesalpinia bonducella* in rabbits. Fitoterapia 65(3):245

20 Sharma SR, Dwivedi SK, Swarup D 1997 Hypoglycaemic, antihyperglycaemic and hypolipidaemic activities of *Caesalpinia bonducella* seeds in rats. Journal of Ethnopharmacology 58(1):39

21 Biswas TK, Bandyopadhyay S, Mukherjee B, Sengupta BR 1997 Oral hypoglycaemic effect of *Caesalpinia bonducella*. International Journal of Pharmacognosy 35(4):261

22 Simon OR, Singh N, Smith K, Smith S 1987 Effect of an aqueous extract of Nichol (*Caesalpinia bonduc*) on blood glucose concentration: evidence of an antidiabetic action. Journal of the Science and Research Council of Jamaica 6(2):25

23 Datte JY, Traore A, Offoumou AM, Ziegler A 1998 Effects of leaf extract of *Caesalpinia bonduc* (Caesalpiniaceae) on the contractile activity of uterine smooth muscle of pregnant rats. Journal of Ethnopharmacology 60:149

24 Jetmalani M, Sabnis PB, Gaitonde BB 1966 Anti-inflammatory activity of *Caesalpinia bonducella* (Putikaranja). Indian Journal of Pharmacy 28(12):341

25 Vedavathy S, Narayana-Rao, K 1995 Anti-inflammatory activity o0f some indigenous medicinal plants of Chittoor District, Andhra Pradesh. Indian Drugs 32(9):427

Carica papaya L. (Caricaceae)

English: Papaya, pawpaw

Hindi: *Papita*

Sanskrit: *Chirbhita*

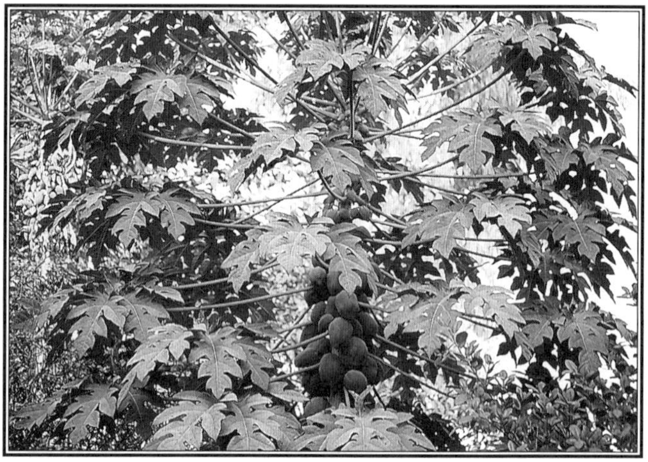

Papaya juice, shoots and latex were used in Mayan herbal medicine and it has been in global use as both food and medicine. It has been cultivated since pre-Columbian times and was introduced to India and Europe in the 17th century.

Habitat

Indigenous to Central America and Mexico, it is now naturalised in lowland tropical forests throughout the world and cultivated in gardens as a fruit and ornamental tree.

Botanical description

A fast-growing, short-lived, single-stemmed small tree, reaching up to 10 m in height with a straight, cylindrical, soft, hollow grey trunk marked by leaf and inflorescence scars (Plate 16). The leaves are glabrous, deeply palmatifid, alternate, with long petioles and crowded at the apex of the trunk, forming a crown. Flowers are fragrant, trimorphous, usually unisexual and dioecious. Male flowers occur in loose, densely pubescent cymes, at the tip of the pendulous, fistular rachis. Female flowers are large, solitary or in sparse racemes, with a short thick rachis. The fruit is a large berry, variable in size, globose or elongated with a large central cavity. The seeds are black and enclosed in a transparent aril.

Parts used

Milky juice, root, seeds, leaves and fruit pulp.

Traditional and modern use

The fruit juice is regarded as a medicine in all countries where the tree is found and the milky juice of the unripe fruit is thought to possess powerful anthelmintic properties, particularly against roundworms. In southern India it is also believed to be an emmenagogue and the fruit is eaten to induce menstruation. The latex has been applied to the neck of the womb to procure abortion[1] and a mixture of the root with the resin of *Ferula narthex* is also used for that purpose. The powdered seeds are taken in northern India as an anthelmintic[2] and their extract used as an antiinflammatory and analgesic. In Nigeria the leaf extract and latex of the raw fruit are also taken to treat worm infestations.[3] Other indications for which the plant is used include the ripe fruits as a diuretic and to treat flatulence[4] and the latex for indigestion, colic, haemorrhoids and liver or spleen enlargement. Extracts of the flower or leaves are used as a febrifuge and heart tonic and a decoction of the inner stem bark for the treatment of dental caries.[5]

Ethnoveterinary usage

The fruits are used as fodder. Fruit, leaves, latex and stem are used to treat indigestion, diarrhoea, swelling of the lungs, stoppage of urination, blindness, tachycardia, ringworm and alopecia.[6] The seeds are used as anthelmintics.

Major chemical constituents

Enzymes

The latex is a rich source of enzymes, including papain,[7] papaya glutamine cyclotransferase,[8] glutaminyl-peptide cyclotransferase,[9] chitinase,[10] chymopapain, caricain, glycyl endopeptidase,[11] papaya peptidases A and B,[12] α-D-mannosidase and N-acetyl-β-D-glucosaminidase.[13,14] The fruit contains β-galactosidases I, II and III[15] and 1-amino cyclopropane-1-carboxylate (ACC) oxidase,[16] phenol-D-glucosyltransferase.[17]

Carotenoids

The fruit contains β-carotene, cryptoxanthin, violaxanthin and zeaxanthin.[15,18]

Alkaloids

The leaves contain carpinine and carpaine, and the heartwood also contains pseudocarpaine.[19,20]

Monoterpenoids

4-Terpineol, linalool and linalool oxide are present in the fruit.[15]

Flavonoids

The shoots contain quercetin, myricetin and kaempferol.[21]

Minerals

The fruit contains calcium, potassium, magnesium, iron, copper, zinc and manganese.[22]

Vitamins

Thiamine, riboflavin, niacin, ascorbic acid and α-tocopherol are present in the shoots.[15,23]

Glucosinolates

Benzyl isothiocyanate has been isolated from the seed.[24]

Medicinal and pharmacological activities

Antifertility activity: The antifertility effects of *Carica papaya* were investigated by feeding adult cycling and pregnant rats with different components of the fruit. No attempt was made to force-feed the animals and the results indicated that the unripe fruit interrupted the oestrus cycle and induced abortion. This effect decreased as the fruit became stale or ripe and exogenous progesterone partially counteracted this effect; the surviving foetuses were without distinct malformations.[25] Adult male albino rats were administered 0.5 mg seed extract/kg body weight for 7 days and a significant reduction in total protein and sialic acid contents in both epididymal fluid and sperm pellet was observed. As compared with the control, lowered acid phosphatase activity was recorded in sperm pellet but higher levels in epididymal fluid after the treatment. The extract treatment also caused significant reduction in levels of inorganic phosphorus in the epididymal fluid.[26]

The chloroform extract, benzene, methanol and ethyl acetate subfractions of the seeds were tested on sperm motility immediately after addition of the extracts and every 5 minutes thereafter for 30 minutes. Results showed that there was a dose-dependent spermicidal effect, showing an instant fall in sperm motility to less than 20%, and many of the spermatozoa became vibratory. Total inhibition of motility was observed within 20–25 minutes at all concentrations. Scanning and transmission electron microscopy revealed deleterious changes in the plasma membrane of the head and mid-piece of the spermatozoa. Sperm viability tests and estimations of abnormal spermatozoa suggested that they were infertile. Effects were spermicidal rather than spermiostatic, as revealed by sperm revival test.[27] Contraceptive effects of the benzene fraction were reported in male albino rats. Body weight, weight of testis, epididymis, seminal vesicle and ventral prostate remained unaltered during the entire course of the investigation. Total suppression of cauda epididymal sperm motility coincided with a decrease in sperm count, viability and an increase in percentage of abnormal spermatozoa over 60–150 days. Minor changes in germ cell proliferation in the testis and vacuolisation and pyknotic nuclei in a few epithelial cells of the cauda epididymis were observed. Histology and biochemical composition of the testis and accessory sex organs, haematology and serum clinical biochemistry and serum testosterone levels remained unchanged throughout the course of the investigation. Tests also indicated mild oestrogenicity and monthly fertility tests revealed negative fertility. All altered parameters returned to normal levels 60 days following withdrawal of the treatment. These results suggested antifertility effects without undue adverse toxicity and that the effects may be directly rendered on the spermatozoa.[28]

Contraceptive efficacy, reversibility and toxicity of various fractions of the chloroform extract of the seeds were investigated in adult male rabbits at a dose regimen of 50 mg/amimal/day for 150 days of treatment. Body weight, semen analysis, haematology, serum clinical biochemistry and the fertility status of control and treated animals were evaluated in the study. The chloroform and ethyl acetate chromatographic fractions did not produce appreciable changes in these parameters; however, the benzene fraction resulted in uniform azoospermia after 15 days of treatment, which was maintained for the remainder of the 150-day observation period. The levels of fructose, glycerophosphocholine, acid phosphatase and lactate dehydrogenase in the seminal plasma were within the control range. Haematology and the serum clinical parameters showed no appreciable changes, indicating a lack of toxicity. The libido of the treated animals appeared to be normal although the fertility rate was zero. Normalcy of altered parameters was observed 60 days following withdrawal of treatment. It was concluded that this fraction of the seeds possesses reversible male contraceptive potential and the effects appear to be mediated through the testis.[29]

In another experiment, a crude aqueous extract of *Carica papaya* seeds was studied on semen profile, fertility, body and organ weight response and toxicology, in male albino rats. Cauda epididymal sperm motility and count were reduced significantly at low and high dose regimens, for both oral and intramuscular administration. Reduced sperm motility was associated with morphological defects. Testicular sperm counts were also reduced in all treatment groups except for the low-dose intramuscular group. Fertility tests showed a dose- and duration-dependent reduction, with zero fertility observed at high-dose regimens. Testicular weight was reduced in all treatment groups, whereas accessory sex organs showed a variable effect. Body weight and toxicological observations did not reveal any untoward response and fertility and associated changes returned to normal within 45 days of treatment cessation.[30] The antifertility effect of pawpaw seeds on the gonads of male albino rats was also demonstrated using an oral dose of 100 mg/kg body weight administered orally for 8 weeks. A degeneration of the germinal epithelium and germ cells, a reduction in the number of Leydig cells and the presence of vacuoles in the tubules were observed.[31]

Short-term administration of an aqueous extract of the seed manifested an androgen-deprived effect on the target organs and thereby caused the antifertility effect in adult male albino rats. The complete loss of fertility was attributed to a decline in sperm motility and alteration in morphology, as well as reduced contractile response of the vas deferens. The extract caused a slight alteration in the histoarchitecture and weight of the reproductive organs, mainly cauda and distal vas deferens. This appeared to be related to their greater androgen sensitivity in comparison to the other target organs or a diminished response to testosterone and its metabolites. Functional sterility was induced in male rats by the treatment, which shows potential as a male contraceptive.[12]

An aqueous extract of *Carica papaya* seeds (5 mg/kg/day IM and 20 mg/kg/day PO) was investigated in male mice treated for 60 days. Reversibility studies were carried out to see if the effects were transient. The extract did not manifest oestrogenic effects in male mice and LD_{50} studies indicated it to be non-toxic. Total body weight and weights of the reproductive organs, kidney and adrenal glands were not affected and serum SGOT, SGPT, protein and cholesterol levels remained within the normal range in the treated mice, suggesting that liver function and cholesterol and protein metabolism were not influenced by the extract.[32]

The chloroform extract of the seeds has also been screened for hormonal properties using ovariectomised female rats to test for oestrogenicity, oestrogen-primed immature rats to test for progestogenicity and castrated adult male rats to test for androgenicity. The results revealed that the extract lacked progestogenic and androgenic effects, but did possess mild oestrogenic activity. An increase in weight of the vagina and uterus and presence of cornified epithelial cells in vaginal smears were observed, together with hypertrophy of the uterine epithelium, endometrium and stroma.[33]

Uterotonic activity: Papaya latex extract (PLE) was tested on rat uterine preparations in vitro at various stages of the oestrus cycle and gestation periods. Uterine contractile activity was increased by PLE in the pro-oestrus and oestrus stages, rather than at the metoestrus and dioestrus stages. Maximum contractile activity was observed during the later stages of pregnancy, which corresponds to peak plasma levels of oestrogen. A direct, dose-dependent, spasmodic action with increased frequency and amplitude was observed with PLE in all non-gravid uterine preparations. Pretreatment of the tissue with phenoxybenzamine non-competitively inhibited the effect and blocking the 5-HT receptors with methylsergide partially inhibited the excitatory response to PLE. Pretreatment with indomethacin (a cyclooxygenase inhibitor) had no effect on the response. Mast cell degranulation (and subsequent release of heparin, biogenic amines or prostaglandins) was ruled out by pretreating the tissue with sodium cromoglycate, a mast cell stabiliser. Uterine contractions induced by pure papain were not sustained for a long period and at higher concentrations, the receptor proteins were denatured by its enzymatic action. From this study it appears that crude papaya latex contains a uterotonic principle, which may be a combination of enzymes, alkaloids and other substances acting mainly via the α-adrenergic receptor population of the uterus at different stages.[34]

Diuretic activity: Extracts of *Carica papaya* root, given orally to rats at a dose of 10 mg/kg, produced a significant increase in urine output ($p < 0.01$) comparable to that of hydrochlorothiazide and giving a similar profile of urinary electrolyte excretion. The analyses of urinary osmolality and electrolyte excretion per unit time suggested the observed effect may be a result of a high salt content of the extract.[35]

Hypotensive activity: Male albino Wistar rats were randomly divided into three batches (15 rats in each) of renal, DOCA-salt hypertensive and normotensive animals. Each batch was further divided into three groups: untreated, hydralazine-treated and extract-treated groups. The mean arterial blood pressure (MAP) and heart rate were measured in all groups. Both hydralazine (200 μg/100 g IV) and extract (20 mg/kg body weight IV) produced a significant depression of MAP in all groups ($p < 0.01$ v controls), but the extract produced about 28% more depression of MAP than hydralazine in the hypertensive groups. In another group of rats, the extract failed to depress the MAP in rats pretreated with propranolol, but atropine and noradrenaline pretreatment did not inhibit the action of the extract. In vitro studies using isolated rabbit arterial (aorta, renal and vertebral) strips showed that the extract (10 μg/ml) produced a relaxation of vascular muscle tone, which was, however, attenuated by phentolamine (0.5–1.5 μg/ml). It was concluded that the fruit juice contains antihypertensive agent(s), with mainy α-adrenoceptor activity.[36]

Hypolipidaemic activity: Pectin from *Carica papaya* showed a highly significant hypolipidaemic activity in albino rats, mainly due to a lower rate of absorption and higher rate of degradation and elimination of lipids. Increased plasma lecithin cholesterol acyl transferase (LCAT) activity could account for the decrease in cholesterol levels and increased activity of lipoprotein lipase in adipose tissue and the heart may be responsible for the decreased concentration of triglycerides in serum of rats fed with pectin.[37]

Antiulcerogenic activity: Effects on

exogenous ulcers and histamine-induced acid secretion were studied in rats. The latex of the unripe fruit was effective in protecting against exogenous ulcer and significantly lessened acid secretion induced by histamine in chronic gastric-fistulated rats. Crystalline papain was also highly effective and the conclusion was that papain is the active principle exerting ulcer-protective effects.[38]

Anthelmintic activity: Activity of papaya latex against *Heligmosomoides polygyrus* was demonstrated in experimentally infected mice. Five groups of BALB/C mice were infected with *H. polygyrus* (100 infective larvae per mouse). At day 22, four groups were given papaya latex suspended in water at dose levels of 2, 4, 6 and 8 g of latex/kg body weight. One group served as non-treated controls. All animals were necropsied on day 25, that is, 3 days after treatment, for post-mortem worm counts. The latex showed a dose-dependent effect, suggesting a potential role for papaya latex as an anthelmintic, against patent intestinal nematodes in mammalian hosts.[39]

In an investigation of the anthelmintic activity of papaya latex against infection of *Ascaris suum* in pigs, 16 naturally infected animals were allocated into four groups of four pigs on the basis of faecal egg counts and body weights. Three groups were given papaya latex orally at dose levels of 2, 4 and 8 g of papaya latex per kg body weight and the fourth group served as a non-treated control. Results of worm counts on day 7 post treatment revealed reductions of approximately 40%, 80% and 100% respectively. Some of the pigs receiving the highest dose of the latex showed mild diarrhoea on the day following treatment but otherwise, no clinical or pathological changes were observed.[40]

Papaya seeds were extracted and fractionated and aliquots tested for anthelmintic activity using viability assays of *Caenorhabditis elegans*. Benzyl isothiocyanate (BITC) was found to be the predominant or sole anthelmintic agent in papaya seed extracts and is active against nematodes.[24] Different parts of the plant were screened for in vitro anthelmintic activity against *Ascaridia galli* worms, which infect birds, and most were found to be more effective than piperazine.[41] The mechanism of action of BITC was also compared to that of mebendazole (MBZ) using *Ascaridia galli*. Both BITC (100 and 300 μM) and MBZ (3 and 10 μM) inhibited glucose uptake and depleted glycogen content in the presence of glucose. However, neither had any effect on glycogen content of the worms in the glucose-free incubation medium. MBZ enhanced lactic acid production but BITC had variable effects and neither BITC nor MBZ had any effect on acetylcholinesterase activity of *A. galli* in vitro. BITC per se contracted the toad rectus muscle and enhanced frequency and magnitude of spontaneous contractions. It reduced the gross visible motility of *A. galli* after 20 hours of incubation, and in conclusion, the mechanism of action of BITC seems to lie both in inhibiting energy metabolism and affecting motor activity of the parasite.[42]

Wound-healing activity: Pawpaw fruit is used by Jamaican nurses as a dressing for chronic skin ulcers and comments from them suggested that topical application of the unripe fruit promoted desloughing, granulation and healing and reduced odour in ulcers. It was cost effective and was considered to be superior to other topical application in the treatment of chronic ulcers. Although there was concern about the use of a non-sterile, non-standardised procedure, there were no reports of wound infection.[43]

Fruit of *Carica papaya* is also used in the paediatric unit of the Royal Victoria Hospital, Banjul (The Gambia) as a major component of burns dressings. Cheap and widely available, the pulp of the papaya fruit is mashed and applied daily to infected burns. It appears to be effective in desloughing necrotic tissue, reducing infection and providing a granulating wound suitable for the application of a split-thickness skin graft. Possible mechanisms of action include the activity of the proteolytic enzymes chymopapain and papain, as well as an antimicrobial activity.[44]

Antiamoebic activity: The seeds demonstrated in vitro antiamoebic activity.[45]

Antifungal activity: The latex inhibited the growth of *Candida albicans* when added to a culture during the exponential growth phase. This fungistatic effect appeared to be the result of cell wall degradation, due to a lack of polysaccharidic constituents in the outermost layers of the fungal cell wall, and release of cell debris into the culture medium.[46]

A mixture of *Carica papaya* latex (0.41 mg protein/ml) and fluconazole (2 μg/ml) showed a synergistic action on the inhibition of *Candida albicans* growth. This synergistic effect manifested in partial cell wall degradation, as indicated by transmission electron microscopy.[47]

Antimicrobial activity: The flesh, seed and pulp of *Carica papaya* was shown by the agar-cup method to be bacteriostatic against several enteropathogens such as *Bacillus subtilis, Enterobacter cloacae, Escherichia coli, Salmonella typhi, Staphylococcus aureus, Proteus vulgaris, Pseudomonas aeruginosa* and *Klebsiella pneumoniae*.[46] Ripe and unripe fruits (epicarp, endocarp and seeds) were extracted separately and all produced significant antibacterial activity against *Staphylococcus aureus, Bacillus cereus, Escherichia coli, Pseudomomas aeruginosa* and *Shigella flexneri*. The extracts were much more active against Gram-positive than Gram-negative bacteria.[48]

Antitumour activity: Flowers of *Carica papaya* showed strong in vitro antitumour-promoting activity when assayed by immunoblotting analysis of Raji cells carrying the Epstein–Barr virus (EBV) genome. The expresson of 'early antigens diffuse' (EA-D) and 'early antigens restricted' (EA-R) was determined by Western blotting of treated Raji cells with human sera of nasopharyngeal carcinoma patients. The extract was shown to suppress both EA-D and EA-R.[49] An ethanolic extract was screened in vitro for antitumour-promoting activity, using inhibition of EBV activation in Raji cells induced by phorbol 12-myristate 13 acetate and sodium-n-butyrate. It was found to be a strong inhibitor of EBV activation.[50]

Free radical scavenging activity: Antioxidant action of a fermented papaya preparation (PS-501) on free radicals and lipid peroxidation was evaluated using electron spin resonance (ESR) spectrometry. The preparation (50 mg/ml) scavenged 80% of hydroxyl radicals generated by Fenton reagents, with an IC_{50} value of 12.5 mg/ml. Oral administration for 4 weeks decreased elevated lipid peroxide levels in the ipsilateral cerebrum 30 minutes after injection of iron solution into the left cortex of rats. It also increased superoxide dismutase activity in the cortex and hippocampus, suggesting antioxidant activity and a possible prophylactic effect against some age-related and neurological diseases associated with free radicals. PS-501 was investigated on DNA damage and tissue injury in the brain, formed during iron-induced epilepsy in rats. 8-Hydroxy-2′-deoxyguanosine (8-OHdG) is a major product of oxidative DNA damage. 8-OHdG levels in the ipsilateral cerebrum increased 30 minutes after injection of ferric chloride solution into the left sensory motor cortex of rats, but administration of PS-501 in drinking water prevented the increase of 8-OHdG levels in the cerebrum. It also inhibited the generation of nitroxide radicals in an image of the rat brain.[51]

A Japanese health food, 'Bio-normaliser', prepared by the fermentation of *Carica papaya*, exhibited therapeutic properties against various pathologies including tumours and immunodeficiency. It efficiently inhibited the formation of oxygen radicals in cell free systems and partly decreased spontaneous and menadione-stimulated superoxide production by erythrocytes, but manifested both stimulatory and inhibitory effects on oxygen radical release by dormant and activated phagocytes (neutrophils and macrophages). Bio-normaliser was able to enhance intracellular production of the innocuous superoxide ion and, at the same time, diminished the formation of reactive hydroxyl radicals, perhaps by inactivation of ferrous ion, the catalyst for the superoxide-driven Fenton reaction.[52]

The seed and pulp were unequivocally demonstrated (by ESR spectrometry) to scavenge 1,1-diphenyl-2-picrylhydrazyl, hydroxyl and superoxide radicals. The seed gave the highest activity at concentrations (IC_{50}) of 2.1, 10.0 and 8.7 mg/ml, respectively and was comparable to that of soybean paste, miso, rice bran and baker's yeast. Vitamin C, malic acid, citric acid and glucose are thought to be possible antioxidative components in papaya.[53]

Safety profile

Papaya is used as a food in most tropical regions of the world and no health hazards have been noted in conjunction with designated therapeutic dosages. Papaya is contraindicated in pregnancy because of the uterine and antifertility effects. There is a possible interaction with warfarin and large quantities should be avoided in coagulation disorders. Allergic reactions have also been documented. The leaves are categorised Class 1 by the American Botanical Council, meaning that they are safe when used appropriately.[54] Oral administration of papain up to 800 mg/kg did not adversely affect prenatal development in rats and did not cause signs of maternal toxicity.[55] Ethanol/water (1:1) extracts of the aerial parts, when administered intraperitoneally to mice, gave an LD_{50} > 1.0 g/kg and a crude ethanol extract of the unripened fruit administered to mice intraperitoneally gave an LD_{50} of 325.2 mg/kg.[56]

Dosage

Dried leaves: 60–120 mg

Dried latex: 120–240 mg

Seed powder: 0.5–1 g

Ayurvedic properties

Rasa: *Katu* (pungent), *tikta* (bitter)

Guna: *Laghu* (light), *ruksha* (unctuous), *tikshna* (sharp)

Veerya: *Ushna* (hot)

Vipaaka: *Katu* (pungent)

Dosha: Pacifies *kapha* and *vata*. Ripe fruit pacifies *pitta*

Further reading

Blumenthal M et al (eds) 1999 The complete Commission E monographs. American Botanical Council, Austin, Texas

Bown D 1995 Encyclopaedia of herbs and their uses. Dorling Kindersley, London

Chevallier A 1996 The encyclopedia of medicinal plants. Dorling Kindersley, London

Kapoor LD 2001 Handbook of Ayurvedic medicinal plants. CRC Press, Boca Raton

Ross I 2000 Medicinal plants of the world, vol 2. Humana Press, Totowa, New Jersey

References

1 Tiwari KC, Majumder R, Bhattacharjee S 1982 Folklore information from Assam for family planning and birth control. International Journal of Crude Drug Research 20:133

2 Shah GL, Gopal GV 1985 Ethnomedical notes from the tribal inhabitants of the North Gujrat (India). Journal of Economic and Taxonomic Botany 6(1):193

3 Bhat RB, Eterjere EO, Oladipo VT 1990 Ethnobotanical studies from Central Nigeria. Economic Botany 44(3):382

4 Reddy MB, Reddy KR, Reddy MN 1989 A survey of plant crude drugs of Anantapur District, Andhra Pradesh, India. International Journal of Crude Drug Research 27(3):145

5 Nagaraju N, Rao KN 1990 A survey of plant crude drugs of Royalaseema, Andhrapradesh, India. Journal of Ethnopharmacology 29(2):137

6 Jha MK 1992 The folk veterinary system of Bihar – a research survey. NDDB, Gujrat, India

7 Kozak M, Kozian E, Grzonka Z, Jaskolski M 1997 Crystallization and preliminary crystallographic studies of a new crystal form of papain from *Carica papaya*. Acta Biochimica Polonica 44(3):601

8 Zerhouni S, Amrani A, Nijs M et al 1998 Purification and characterization of papaya glutamine cyclotransferase, a plant enzyme highly resistant to chemical, acid and thermal denaturation. Biochimica et Biophysica Acta 1387(1–2):275

9 Zerhouni S, Amrani A, Nijs M, Vandermeers A, Looze Y 1997 Purification and characterization of the plant glutaminyl-peptide cyclotransferase isolated from papaya latex. International Journal of Bio-Chromatography 3(3):189

10 Azarkan M, Amrani A, Nijs M et al 1997 *Carica papaya* latex is a rich source of a class II chitinase. Phytochemistry 46(8):1319

11 Maes D, Bouckaert J, Poortmans F, Wyns L, Looze Y 1996 Structure of chymopapain at 1.7 ANG resolution. Biochemistry 35(50):16292–16298

12 Ross I 1999 Medicinal plants of the world, vol 1. Humana Press, Totowa, New Jersey

13 Oberg KA, Ruysschaert J-M, Azarkan M et al 1998 Papaya glutamine cyclase, a plant enzyme highly resistant to proteolysis, adopts an all β-conformation. European Journal of Biochemistry 258(1):214

14 Giordani R, Siepaio M, Moulin-Traffort J, Regli P 1991 Antifungal action of *Carica papaya* latex: isolation of fungal cell wall hydrolysing enzymes. Mycoses 34(11–12):469

15 Ali ZM, Ng S-Y, Othman R; Goh L-Y; Lazan H 1998 Isolation, characterization and significance of papaya β-galactanases to cell wall modification and fruit softening during ripening. Physiology of Plants 104(1):105

16 Dunkley HM, Golden KD 1998 ACC oxidase from *Carica papaya:* isolation and characterization. Physiology of Plants 103(2):225

17 Keil U, Schreier P 1989 Purification and partial characterization of UDP-glucose:phenol-D-glucosyltransferase from papaya fruit. Phytochemistry 28(9):2281

18 John J, Munhambo AE 1982 Beta-carotene

content of two main varieties of pawpaw (*Carica papaya* – Family Caricaceae) grown in Tanzania. East African Medical Journal 59(6):410

19 Tang CS 1979 Macrocyclic piperidine and piperidine alkaloids in *Carica papaya*. Tropical Foods, Chemistry and Nutrition 1:55

20 Khuzhaev VU, Aripova SF 2001 Pseudocarpaine from *Carica papaya*. Chemistry of Natural Compounds 36(4):418

21 Miean KH, Mohamed S 2001 Flavonoid (myricetin, quercetin, kaempferol, luteolin and apigenin) content of edible tropical plants. Journal of Agriculture and Food Chemistry 49(6):3106

22 Hardisson A, Bubio C, Baez A, Martin MM, Alvarez R 2001 Mineral composition of the papaya (*Carica papaya*, variety 'Sunrise') from Tenerife Island. European Food Research and Technology 212(2):175

23 Ching LS, Mohamed S 2001 Alpha-tocopherol content in 62 edible tropical plants. Journal of Agriculture and Food Chemistry 49(6):3101

24 Kermanshai R, Mccarry BE, Rosenfeld J, Summers PS, Weretilnyk EA, Sorger GJ 2001 Benzyl isothiocyanate is the chief or sole anthelmintic in papaya seed extracts. Phytochemistry 57(3):427

25 Gopalakrishnan M, Rajasekharasetty MR 1978 Effect of papaya (*Carica papaya*) on pregnancy and estrus cycle in albino rats of Wistar strain. Indian Journal of Physiology and Pharmacology 22(1):66

26 Verma RJ, Chinoy NJ 2001 Effect of Papaya seed extract on microenvironment of cauda epididymis. Asian Journal of Andrology 3(2):143

27 Lohiya NK, Kothari LK, Manivannan B, Mishra PK, Pathak N 2000 Human sperm immobilization effect of *Carica papaya* seed extracts: an in vitro study. Asian Journal of Andrology 2(2):103

28 Pathak N, Mishra PK, Manivannan B, Lohiya NK 2000 Sterility due to inhibition of sperm motility by oral administration of benzene chromatographic fraction of the chloroform extract of the seeds of *Carica papaya* in rats. Phytomedicine 7(4):325

29 Lohiya NK, Mishra PK, Pathak N, Manivannan B, Jain SC 1999 Reversible azoospermia by oral administration of the benzene chromatographic fraction of the chloroform extract of the seeds of *Carica papaya* in rabbits. Advances in Contraception 15(2):141

30 Lohiya NK, Goyal RB, Jayaprakash D, Ansari AS, Sharma S 1994 Antifertility effects of aqueous extract of *Carica papaya* seeds in male rats. Planta Medica 60(5):400

31 Udoh P, Kehinde A 1999 Studies on antifertility effect of pawpaw seeds (*Carica papaya*) on the gonads of male albino rats. Phytotherapy Research 13(3):226

32 Chinoy NJ, D'Souza JM, Padman P 1994 Effects of crude aqueous extract of *Carica papaya* seeds in male albino mice. Reproductive Toxicology 8(1):75

33 Mishra PK, Pathak N, Manivannan B, Lohiya NK 2000 Screening for the hormonal properties of the chloroform extract of *Carica papaya* Linn. seeds for anti-fertility investigation. Natural Product Science 6(1):5

34 Cherian T 2000 Effect of papaya latex extract on gravid and non-gravid rat uterine preparations in vitro. Journal of Ethnopharmacology 70(3):205

35 Sripanidkulchai B, Wongpanich V, Laupattarakasem P, Suwansaksri J, Jirakulsomchok D 2001 Diuretic effects of selected Thai indigenous medicinal plants in rats. Journal of Ethnopharmacology 75(2–3):185

36 Eno AE, Owo OI, Itam EH, Konya RS 2000 Blood pressure depression by the fruit juice of *Carica papaya* (L.) in renal and DOCA-induced hypertension in the rat. Phytotherapy Research 14(4).235

37 Kumar GP, Sudheesh S, Ushakumari B et al 1997 A comparative study on the hypolipidemic activity of eleven different pectins. Journal of Food Science and Technology 34(2):103–107

38 Chen CF, Chen SM, Chow SY, Han PW 1981 Protective effects of *Carica papaya* Linn on exogenous gastric ulcer in rats. American Journal of Chinese Medicine 9(3):205

39 Satrija F, Nansen P, Murtini S, He S 1995 Anthelmintic activity of papaya latex against patent *Heligmosomoides polygyrus* infections in mice. Journal of Ethnopharmacology 48(3):161

40 Satrija F, Nansen P, Bjorn H, Murtini S, He S 1994 Effect of papaya latex against *Ascaris suum* in naturally infected pigs. Journal of Helminthology 68(4):343

41 Lal J, Chandra S, Raviprakash V, Sabir M 1976. *In vitro* anthelmintic action of some indigenous medicinal plants on *Ascardia galli* worms. Indian Journal of Physiology and Pharmacology 20(2):64

42 Kumar D, Mishra SK, Tripathi HC 1991 Mechanism of anthelmintic action of benzylisothiocyanate. Fitoterapia 62(5):403

43 Hewitt H, Whittle S, Lopez S, Bailey E, Weaver S 2000 Topical use of papaya in chronic skin ulcer therapy in Jamaica. West Indian Medical Journal 49(1):32

44 Starley IF, Mohammed P, Schneider G, Bickler SW 1999 The treatment of paediatric burns using topical papaya. Burns 25(7):636

45 Tona L, Kambu K, Ngimbi N, Cimanga K, Vlietinck AJ 1998 Antiamoebic and phytochemical screening of some Congolese medicinal plants. Journal of Ethnopharmacology 61(1):57

46 Giordani R, Cardenas ML, Moulin-Traffort J, Regli P 1996 Fungicidal activity of latex sap from *Carica papaya* and antifungal effect of D(+)-glucosamine on *Candida albicans* growth. Mycoses 39(3–4):103

47 Giordani R, Gachon C, Moulin TJ, Regli P 1997 A synergistic effect of *Carica papaya* latex sap and fluconazole on *Candida albicans* growth. Mycoses 40(11–12):429

48 Emeruwa AC 1982 Antibacterial substance from *Carica papaya* fruit extract. Journal of Natural Products 45(2):123

49 Ali AM, Mooi LY, Yih K et al 2000 Antitumor promoting activity of some Malaysian traditional vegetable (ulam) extracts by immunoblotting analysis of Raji cells. Natural Product Science 6(3):147

50 Mooi LY, Ali AM, Norhanom A et al 1999 Anti-tumor promoting activity of some Malaysian traditional vegetables (ulam). Natural Product Science 5(1):33

51 Imao K, Komatsu M, Wang H, Hiramatsu M 1999 Inhibitory effect of fermented papaya preparation on oxidative DNA damage and tissue injury in the brain formed during iron-induced epileptogenesis in rats. Journal of Brain Science 25(1–2):71

52 Osato JA, Korkina LG, Santiago LA, Afanas'ev IB 1995 Effects of 'Bio-normalizer' (a food supplementation) on free radical production by human blood neutrophils, erythrocytes, and rat peritoneal macrophages. Nutrition 11 (5 suppl):568

53 Osato JA, Santiago LA, Remo GM, Cuadra MS, Mori A 1993 Antimicrobial and antioxidant acivities of unripe papaya. Life Science 53(17):1383

54 McGuffin M, Hobbs C, Upton R, Goldberg A 1997 Botanical safety handbook. American Herbal Products Association. CRC Press, Boca Raton

55 Schmidt H 1995 Effect of papain on different phases of prenatal ontogenesis in rats. Reproductive Toxicology 9(1):49

56 Dhawan BN, Patnaik GK, Rastogi RP, Singh KK, Tandon JS 1977 Screening of Indian plants for biological activity. VI. Indian Journal of Experimental Biology 15:208

Cedrus deodara (D. Don) G. Don f. (Pinaceae) (syn. *Cedrus deodara* (Roxb.) Loud)

English: Himalayan cedar

Hindi: *Deodar*

Sanskrit: *Devadaru*

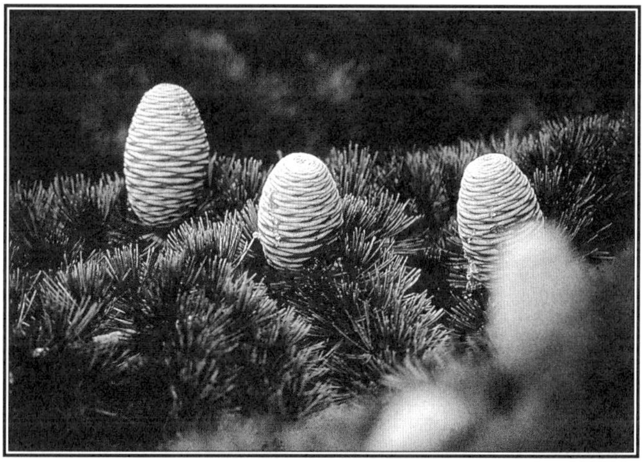

The Himalayan cedar, *deodar*, is a majestic and handsome tree, growing to a great height and wide girth and living to a great age. The name *devadaru* is sometimes applied to *Erythroxylon monogynum* or *Polyalthia longifolia* but these are not interchangeable with the true *deodar*.

Habitat

It is found throughout the western Himalayas, from Kashmir to Garhwal, at altitudes of 1200–3000 m. It is often cultivated as an ornamental.

Botanical description

A large evergreen conifer, reaching up to 85 m in height with ascending, spreading branches (Plate 17). The leaves, which are present in whorls, are triquetrous, needle-like, 2–4 cm long, dark green with a silver sheen. Male cones are cylindrical, female cones ovoid with overlapping thin woody placental scales; both are solitary, up to 12 cm long and 10 cm in thickness and occur at the ends of branchlets. Seeds are winged, up to 1.5 cm long and triangular in shape. The bark is blackish, rough, thick, furrowed, with vertical fissures. The heartwood is light yellowish-brown, darkening on exposure, scented and rich in oil.

Parts used

Heartwood, bark, leaves and oil.

Traditional and modern use

The oil is antiseptic and used in skin diseases, sores, wounds and ulcers and also for headache, fever, urogenital diseases, piles and as a carminative, antidiarrhoeal, diaphoretic, diuretic and insecticide. The heartwood is used for similar purposes and as an antiinflammatory, laxative, sedative, cardiotonic and for many other disorders. The leaves are bitter and acrid and used mainly in inflammation.

Ethnoveterinary usage

The wood and bark are used in bloody dysentery[1] and the oil in skin diseases and ulcers, against mange in buffaloes, calves, goats and camels and to treat sore hooves in cattle.

Major chemical constituents

Essential oil

The heartwood yields about 2.1% of essential oil, consisting mainly of the sesquiterpene hydrocarbons α-himachalene 6–7%, β-himachalene around 91% and other isomers including δ-himachalene,[2] with p-methyl acetophenone, p-methyl-Δ^3-tetrahydroacetophenone, atlantone and himachalol.[3]

Hydrocarbons

The petroleum ether extract of the bark oil yields saturated, straight chain and branched chain hydrocarbons (C_{14}–C_{20}).

Flavonoids

Stem bark contains deodarin (3′, 4′, 5, 7-tetrahydroxy-8-C-methyl dihydroflavonol), taxifolin and quercetin.

Medicinal and pharmacological activities

Treatment of skin disorders: A mixture of *Cedrus deodara* and *Ricinus communis* oils was found to be safe in the treatment of mange in animals.[4] In another study, the oil of *Cedrus deodara* (15% in castor oil base) cured 95.6% of sheep of *Sarcoptes scabiei* infection[5] after treatment with 10 applications. It was also found to be effective in demodectic mange and psoroptic mange in affected cattle and sheep.

Antimicrobial activity: The oil exhibits antifungal action and is used in the treatment of human and animal phycomycotic diseases.[6,7]

Molluscicidal activity: The oil of *Cedrus deodara* in Tween-80 proved 100% ovicidal and molluscicidal at 15–20 ppm (24-hour exposure) in the laboratory. Under field conditions the suspension at 30 ppm gave 100% mortality of snails and their eggs within 24 hours.[8]

Insecticidal activity: Low concentrations (0.45%) of the oil produced a mortality rate of around 50% in adult *Anopheles stephensi*. The toxicity of the steam-distilled oil was tested at 26°C against 4th instar larvae and the LD_{50} for larvae found to be 63.2 ppm.[9] It was effective against other insect pests such as cockroaches and houseflies.[10]

Anticancer activity: The ethanolic extract was found to have cytotoxicity against human epidermal carcinoma of the nasopharynx in tissue culture.[11]

Antispasmolytic activity: The major antispasmodic constituent in the wood of *Cedrus deodara* has been identified as himachalol. The spasmolytic action was similar to that of papaverine as observed by the effect of himachalol on various isolated smooth muscles and several agonists.[12]

Safety profile

A 15% mixture of *C. deodara* oil in castor oil was subjected to acute toxicity tests in mice and found to be non-toxic. The formulation was non-irritant to the skin of rabbit and sheep and did not alter blood urea nitrogen and blood glucose levels.[13] The LD_{50} was 500 mg/kg in adult albino mice.[11] Applied topically to rabbits, it was found to have no adverse effects on skin or any other vital organ.[4]

Dosage

Powdered wood: 3–6 g

Decoction: 28–56 ml

Oil: 0.5–3 ml

Ayurvedic properties

Rasa: *Tikta* (bitter)

Guna: *Laghu* (light), *snigdha* (unctuous)

Veerya: *Ushna* (hot)

Vipaka: *Katu* (pungent)

Dosha: Pacifies *vata* and *kapha*

Further reading

Pandey GS (ed) 1998 Indian materia medica. Chaukhambha Bharati Academy, Gokul Bhawan, Varanasi

References

1 International Institute of Rural Reconstruction 1994 Ethnoveterinary medicine in Asia. An information kit on traditional animal health care practices. Part I, General information. IIRR, Silang, Philippines

2 Nigam MC, Ahmad A, Misra LN 1990 Composition of the essential oil of *Cedrus deodara*. Indian Perfumer 34(4):278

3 Bisarya SC 1964 Allohimachalol, a new type of sesquiterpenoid. Tetrahedron 29:3761

4 Tandan SK, Singh S, Gupta S, Chandra S, Jawahar L 1989 Subacute dermal toxicity study of *Cedrus deodara* wood essential oil. Indian Veterinary Journal 66(11):1088

5 Kar K, Puri VN, Patnaik GK et al 1975 Studies on comparative efficacy of *Cedrus deodara* oil, benzyl benzoate and tetraethylthiuram monosulphide against sarcoptic mange in sheep. Journal of Pharmaceutical Science 64(2):258

6 Mall HV, Asthana A, Dubey NK, Dixit SN 1985 Toxicity of cedarwood oil against some dermatophytes. Indian Drugs 22(6):296

7 Dixit A, Dixit SN 1982 A promising antifungal agent. Indian Perfumer 26(2–4):216

8 Gupta SC, Yadav SC, Jawahar L, Chandra R, Lal J 1988 Molluscicidal activity of *Cedrus deodara* (wood essential oil) against *Lymnaea auricularia rufescens* Grey: laboratory and field evaluations. Journal of Veterinary Parasitology 2(2):109

9 Kumar A, Dutta, GP 1987 Indigenous plant oils as larvicidal agent against *Anopheles stephensi* mosquitoes. Current Science 56(18):959

10 Singh D, Rao SM, Tripathi AK 1984 Cedarwood oil as a potential insecticidal agent against mosquitoes. Naturwissenschaften 71(5):265

11 Dhar ML, Dhar MM, Dhawan BN, Mehrotra BN, Ray C 1968 Screening of Indian plants for biological activity, Part I. Indian Journal of Experimental Biology 6:232

12 Lal J, Sambasivarao K, Chandra S, Naithani RC, Chattopadhyay SK, Sabir M 1976 Spasmolytic constituents of *Cedrus deodara* (Roxb.) Loud: pharmacological evaluation of himachalol. Indian Veterinary Journal 53(7):543

13 Chandra S, Prasad MC, Tandon SK, Gupta S, Jawahar L 1989 Evaluation of a formulation of *Cedrus deodara* wood essential oil on blood urea nitrogen and blood glucose level and on skin irritation. Indian Veterinary Journal 66:30

Centella asiatica L. Urb. Apiaceae (Umbelliferae) (syn. *Hydrocotyle asiatica* L.)

English: Indian pennywort, gotu kola

Hindi: *Kula kudi*

Sanskrit: *Mandukparni*

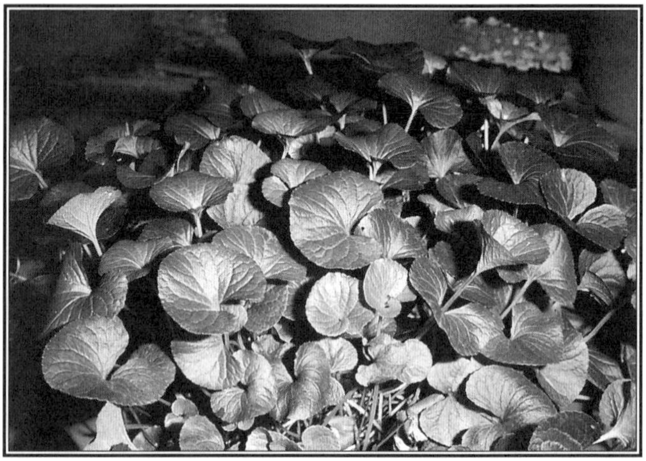

Centella asiatica has been employed as a medicinal plant in India and south-east Asia since prehistoric times.[1] The name hydrocotyle is derived from the Greek words for 'water' and 'cup', to describe the habitat, water, and the appearance of the leaves, cup-shaped.

Habitat

C. asiatica is the most ubiquitous species of Centella and is found in India, Sri Lanka, south-east Asia, China, Madagascar, South Africa, south-eastern USA, Mexico, Venezuela and Columbia. It grows in moist habitats at altitudes up to 2500 m.

Botanical description

A perennial, slender, herbaceous, creeper plant (Plate 18) flowering between August and September. The plant has a smell reminiscent of tobacco and a mildly bitter taste. The leaves are glabrous, kidney shaped, 2–5 cm in diameter, with long petioles, arising from the stem nodes in rosettes. The stems (stolons) are slender, prostrate and often reddish coloured. The flowers are pale violet. Each umbel bears 2–5 fruits, enclosed within a thick, hard pericarp.

Parts used

Aerial parts.

Traditional and modern use

Centella asiatica is commonly mentioned as a *rasayana* in Ayurveda and for various ailments including abdominal disorders. *Rasayanas* are advocated for use in rejuvenation therapy. Its use as a therapy for leprosy is also well documented and in folk medicine it is used particularly for treating wounds and for bronchitis, epilepsy, dysentery, fever, inflammation, leucoderma and as a nerve tonic.[2,3]

Ethnoveterinary usage

The whole plant is used in jaundice, contagious abortion, foot and mouth disease, colic and swelling of the respiratory tract.[4]

Major chemical constituents

Triterpenoids

Asiatic acid, 6-hydroxy asiatic acid, madecassic acid, betulinic acid, thankunic acid and isothankunic acid are present together with their glycosides (up to 8%), depending on the country of origin of the plant. The major saponins are asiaticoside, asiaticoside A, asiaticoside B, madecassoside, braminoside, brahmoside, brahminoside, thankuniside and isothankuniside.[5]

Essential oil

This constitutes about 0.1% of the aerial parts and contains sesquiterpenoids (up to about 80%), with β-caryophyllene, α-humulene and germacrene-D, elemene and bicycloelemene, trans-farnesene being the most abundant.[6]

Flavone derivatives

Quercetin and kaempferol glycosides and astragalin have been found.[5]

Phytosterols

Stigmasterol, sitosterol.[3]

Aminoacids

The leaf contains alanine, arginine, aspartic acid, glutamic acid, glycine, histidine, isoleucine, leucine, lysine, methionine, phenylalanine, proline, threonine and tryptophan.[5]

Medicinal and pharmacological activities

Antiulcerogenic activity: The antiulcerogenic activity of the fresh juice of *C. asiatica* was studied against ethanol-, aspirin-, cold restraint stress- and pyloric ligation-induced gastric ulcers in rats. When given orally at doses of 200 and 600 mg/kg twice daily for 5 days, the drug showed significant protection against all the above experimental ulcer models. This effect was thought to be due to the strengthening of mucosal defensive factors.[7] Oral administration of Centella extract (0.05, 0.25 and 0.50 g/kg) before ethanol administration significantly inhibited gastric lesion formation (by 58–82%) and decreased mucosal myeloperoxidase (MPO) activity in a dose-dependent manner. It prevented gastric mucosal lesions by strengthening the mucosal barrier and reducing the damaging effects of free radicals.[8]

Spasmolytic activity: Activity was demonstrated when tested in vitro on isolated guinea pig ileum.[9]

Wound-healing activity: A titrated extract of *Centella asiatica* (TECA), containing asiatic acid, madecassic acid and asiaticoside, and its separate components were evaluated for their effects in the wound chamber model. TECA-injected wound chambers were characterised by increased dry weight, DNA, total protein, collagen and uronic acid contents. Peptidic hydroxyproline was also increased, showing an increased remodelling of the collagen matrix in the wound. The three purified components of TECA were all able to reproduce the effects of the complete drug.[10,11] The activity of asiaticoside was studied in normal and delayed-type wound healing. In guinea pig punch wounds topical applications of a 0.2% solution of asiaticoside produced a 56% increase in hydroxyproline, 57% increase in tensile strength, increased collagen content and improved epithelialisation. In streptozotocin-diabetic rats, where healing is delayed, topical application of a 0.4% solution of asiaticoside over punch wounds increased hydroxyproline content, tensile strength, collagen content and epithelialisation, thereby facilitating healing. Asiaticoside was also active by the oral route at 1 mg/kg and is thought to be the main active constituent of *Centella asiatica*. Asiaticoside enhanced antioxidant levels at an initial stage of wound healing which may be an important contributory factor in the healing properties of this constituent.[12] The extract also protected skin against radiation injury.[13]

Immunomodulatory activity: An alcoholic extract showed stimulatory effect on the reticuloendothelial system (RES) in mice and an in vitro study of the aqueous extract demonstrated a positive effect on both the classic and alternative pathways of complement activation.[14,15]

Antitubercular activity: An injection of 0.5 ml of a 4% solution of hydroxyasiaticoside was given in guinea pigs, inoculated 15 days previously with tubercle bacillus. It reduced the number of tubercular lesions in the liver, lungs, nerve ganglions and spleen and decreased the volume of the spleen over that of untreated control animals, thereby displaying antitubercular activity.[16]

Psychoneurological activity: The alcoholic extract, when given orally to rats and mice treated with phenobarbitone, significantly prolonged sleeping time. In the maximum electroshock-induced convulsion test in rats, it significantly reduced the duration of individual convulsions. In a behavioural test it reduced the duration of the immobility phase, indicating sedative, antidepressive and analgesic actions.[17]

Antimicrobial activity: Asiaticoside at a concentration of 10 mg/ml showed antibacterial activity against *Pseudomonas pyocyaneus* and *Trichoderma mentagrophytes*.[18]

Antiviral activity: The alcoholic extract showed antiviral activity against Herpes simplex type II virus.[19]

Antilarval activity: A new triterpenoid glycoside 3-O-[α-L-arabinopyranosyl] 2α,3β,6β,23α-tetrahydroxyurs-12-ene-28-oic acid exhibited dose-dependent growth inhibitory activity against larvae of *Spilarctia obliqua*.[20]

Safety profile

The maximum tolerated dose of a 50% alcoholic extract in mice was found to be 250 mg/kg.[21] Allergic contact dermatitis and photosensitivity have been reported after topical application.[5] Occasional burning pain following injections, or the local application of powder, has been reported.[22]

Dosage

Dried leaves: 0.6 g

Extract: 60 mg/day

Ayurvedic properties

Guna: *Laghu* (light)

Rasa: *Tikta* (bitter), *kashaya* (astringent)

Veerya: *Shita* (cold)

Vipaka: *Katu* (pungent)

Dosha: Balances *kapha* and *pitta*

Further reading

Duke JA 1992 Handbook of phytochemical constituents of GRAS herbs and other economic plants. CRC Press, Boca Raton

Nadkarni AK 1976 Indian materia medica. Popular Prakashan PVT Ltd, Bombay

References

1 Karting T 1988 Clinical Application of *Centella asiatica* (L.) Urb. In: Craker LE (ed) Herbs, spices and medicinal plants. Recent advances in botany, horticulture and pharmacology, vol. 3. Oryx Press, Phoenix

2 Alam MK 1992 Medicinal ethnobotany of the Marma tribe of Bangladesh. Economic Botany 46:330

3 Ramaswamy AS, Periyasamy SM, Basu NK 1970 Pharmacological studies on *Centella asiatica*. Journal of Research and Education in Indian Medicine 4:160

4 Jha MK 1992 The folk veterinary system of Bihar – a research survey. NDDB, Anand, Gujrat

5 Newall CA, Anderson LA, Phillipson JD 1996 Herbal medicines. Pharmaceutical Press, London

6 Wong KC, Tan GL 1994 Essential oil of *Centella asiatica* (L.) Urb. Sch. Journal of Essential Oil Research 6(3):307

7 Sairam K, Rao CV, Goel RK 2001 Effect of *Centella asiatica* Linn. on physical and chemical factors of induced gastric ulceration and secretion in rats. Indian Journal of Experimental Biology 39(2):137

8 Cheng CL, Koo MWL 2000 Effects of *Centella asiatica* on ethanol-induced gastric mucosal lesions in rats. Life Sciences 67(21):2647

9 Singh B, Rastogi RP 1969 A reinvestigation of the triterpenes of *Centella asiatica.* Phytochemistry 8:917

10 Maquart FX, Chastang F, Simeon A, Birembaut P, Gillery P, Wegrowski Y 1999 Triterpenes from *Centella asiatica* stimulate extracellular matrix accumulation in rat experimental wounds. European Journal of Dermatology 9(4):289

11 Shukla A, Rasik AM, Jain GK, Shankar R, Kulshreshtha DK, Dhawan BN 1999 *In vitro* and *in vivo* wound healing activity of asiaticoside isolated from *Centella asiatica*. Journal of Ethnopharmacology 65(1):1

12 Shukla A, Rasik AM, Dhawan BN 1999 Asiaticoside-induced elevation of antioxidant levels in healing wounds. Phytotherapy Research 13(1):50

13 Chen Y-J, Dai Y-S, Chen B-F et al 1999 The effect of tetrandrine and extracts of *Centella asiatica* on acute radiation dermatitis in rats. Biological and Pharmaceutical Bulletin 22(7):703

14 DiCarlo FJ, Haynes LJ, Silver NJ, Phillips GH 1964 Reticuloendothelial system stimulants of botanical origin. Journal of the Reticuloendothelial Society 1:224

15 Labadie RP, Nat JM, Simons JM et al 1989 Ethnopharmacognostic approach to the search for immunomodulators of plant origin. Planta Medica 55:339

16 Boiteau P, Dureuil M, Rakoto-Ratsimamanga A 1949 Antitubercular properties of hydroxyasiaticoside (a water-soluble derivative of asiaticoside from *Centella asiatica* extracts). Comptes Rendus de l'Academie des Sciences (Paris, Serie D) 228:1165

17 Sakina MR, Dandiya PC 1990 A psycho-neuropharmacological profile of *Centella asiatica* extract. Fitoterapia 61:291

18 Tschesche W, Wulff G 1965 Uber die antimikrobielle Wirksamkeit von Saponinen. Zeitschrift fur Naturforschung 20b:543

19 Zheng MS 1989 An experimental study of the anti-HSV-II action of 500 herbal drugs. Journal of Traditional Chinese Medicine 9:113

20 Shukla YN, Srivastava R, Tripathi AK, Prajapati V 2000 Characterization of an ursane triterpenoid from *Centella asiatica* with growth inhibitory activity against *Spilarctia obliqua*. Pharmaceutical Biology 38(4):262

21 Dhar ML, Dhar MM, Dhawan BN, Mehrotra BN, Ray C 1968 Screening of Indian plants for biological activity. Indian Journal of Experimental Biology 6:232

22 Arpaia MR, Ferrone R, Amitrano M 1990 Effects of *Centella asiatica* extract on mucopolysaccharide metabolism in subjects with varicose veins. International Journal of Clinical Pharmacology Research 10(4):229

Cissus quadrangularis L. (Vitaceae) (syn. *Vitis quadrangularis* (L.) Wallich ex Wight)

English: Bone setter

Hindi: *Hajora*

Sanskrit: *Asthisanhari*

The name *asthisanhari* is derived from its use in healing bone fractures.

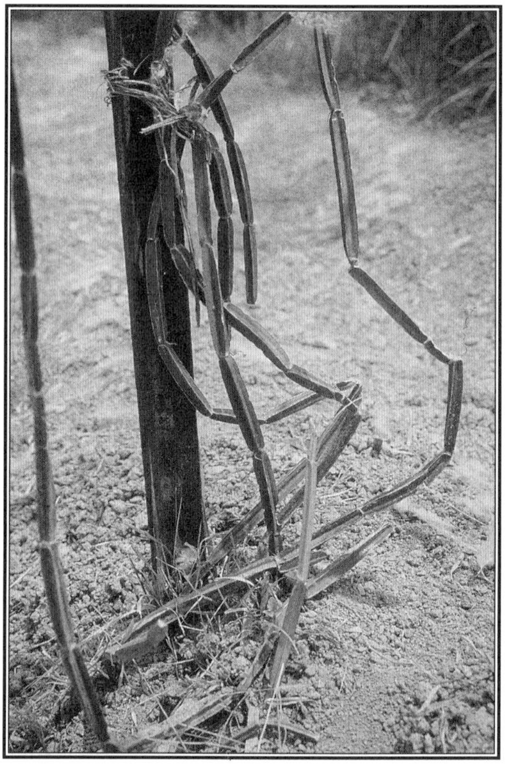

Habitat

The plant grows commonly in the hotter and drier regions of India, including the Deccan peninsula, extending west to the lower eastern slopes of the Western Ghats and south to Travencore. It is also widespread in the drier parts of Africa and Arabia.

Botanical description

A rambling shrub usually found climbing over bushes (Plate 19). The stem is thick, fleshy, glabrous, ridged and quadrangular, as the name suggests, and constricted at the nodes. The leaves are simple, alternate, thickened, broadly ovate to suborbicular, obtuse, with a serrate margin, about 8 cm long and 6 cm broad. There are numerous tendrils arising from the nodes; flowers small, in umbellate cymes occurring opposite the leaves, with a cup-shaped, lobed calyx; petals greenish-yellow and red tipped. The fruits are globose berries.

Parts used

Leaves, stems, roots.

Traditional and modern use

The leaves and stem are frequently eaten with curry in southern India. In Madras the young shoots of the plant are burnt to ashes in a closed vessel and administered in dyspepsia and indigestion. The juice of the stem is used in otorrhoea and epistaxis. A paste of the stem is used by traditional healers, applied as a poultice over bone fractures and swellings. The entire plant is considered to be an alterative, anthelmintic, aphrodisiac, antiasthmatic and is useful in gastrointestinal disorders such as colic and dyspepsia and irregular menstruation. It is also important in *Siddha* medicine where the plant is burnt to ash before being used for similar indications.

Ethnoveterinary usage

The herb is fed to cattle to induce flow of milk. The whole plant is used in fractures, sprains, rheumatism, irregular growth of teeth, broken horn, anthrax, haematuria, elephantiasis, dislocation of hip, various wounds and cracked tail.[1]

Major chemical constituents

Stilbene derivatives

Quadrangularins A, B and C, resveratrol, piceatannol, pallidol and parthenocissin are present in the stem.[2]

Lipids and phytosterols

4-Hydroxy-2-methyltricos-2-en-22-one, 9-methyl-octadec-9-ene, heptadecyl octadecanoate, icosanyl icosanoate, 31-methyltritriacontan-1-ol, 7-hydroxy-20-oxo-docosanyl cyclohexane and 31-methyltriacontanoic acid, 7-oxoonocer-8-ene-3-21-diol[3], onocer-7-ene-3-21-diol, onocer-7-ene-3-21-diol, α-amyrin, α-amyrone taraxeryl acetate, friedelan-3-one, taraxerol, β-sitosterol and isopentacosanoic acid[4] have been isolated from the stem.

Medicinal and pharmacological activities

Bone-healing activity: A phytosterol fraction isolated from *Cissus quadrangularis* showed bone-healing activity when tested in experimental bone fractures of the right humerus in young rats. Examination of the pituitary, thyroid and adrenal glands indicated no obvious abnormalities but an increase in wet weight was noted.[5] Daily injections of this fraction for 6 weeks in rats also produced a marked increase in body weight, mucopolysaccharide content of bone and uptake of ^{85}Sr and enhanced the rate of healing of the fractured bones by influencing the early regeneration process of connective tissue and mineralisation.[6] Studies involving tagging with radioactive ^{14}C in rats, using micro-autoradiography of various tissues, suggested that the probable pathway may be through the anterior pituitary and the adrenal glands. After metabolism in the liver, the sterol fraction reached the osteogenic cells at the fracture site and appeared to exert a stimulating effect on healing.[7]
Histopathological studies showed that the rate of healing was enhanced in experimental fractures of the right femur in dogs which had been treated with IM injections of an aqueous extract of *C. quadrangularis*. The rate of progress of ossification in the treated animals was faster than in untreated animals. After 3 weeks, the callus in the untreated animals contained cartilaginous tissue with a few, thin and sparse bony trabeculae, whereas treated animals had considerably advanced ossification and the callus consisted of a network of bony trabeculae. After 6 weeks ossification was complete and remodelling was advanced in the treated animals in comparison to the untreated animals where ossification was still in progress.[8] An aqueous extract of the plant, applied topically or given by IM injection, hastened healing of fractures as measured by a reduction in the convalescent period. It aided the

strengthening of the bones by up to 90% over 6 weeks and had an influence on both the organic and mineral phases of fracture healing. Ca^{45} uptake studies also demonstrated an earlier completion of the calciferous process, suggesting it may be useful not only in building up the bone but also in improving functional efficiency.[9] A total extract of the plant was found to neutralise the antianabolic effect of cortisone in healing of fractures, possibly due to its vitamin content.[10]

Safety profile

The fresh juice of the plant can irritate the skin and cause itching. A 50% ethanol extract of stem administered IP in mice showed an LD_{50} of 681 mg/kg body weight.[11]

Dosage

Decoction of dried stalks: 10–30 ml

Juice: 10–20 ml

Powder: 2.5 g

Ayurvedic properties

Guna: *Laghu* (light), *ruksha* (dry)

Rasa: *Madhur* (sweet)

Veerya: *Ushna* (hot)

Vipaka: *Amla* (sour)

Dosha: Pacifies *vata* and *pitta*

Further reading

Bharatiya Vidya Bhavan's Swami Prakashananda Ayurveda Research Centre 1992 Selected medicinal plants of India. Chemexcil, Mumbai

Chopra RN, Chopra IC, Handa KL, Kapoor LD 1958 Indigenous drugs of India, 2nd edn. Academic Publishers, Calcutta

Nadkarni AK 1976 Indian materia medica. Popular Prakashan PVT Ltd, Bombay

Sairam TV 1999 Home remedies, vol II. Penguin India, New Delhi

Sivarajan VV, Balachandran I 1994 Ayurvedic drugs and their plant sources. Oxford and IBH Publishing, New Delhi

References

1 Jha MK 1992 The folk veterinary system of Bihar – a research survey. NDDB, Anand, Gujrat

2 Adesanya SA, Nia R, Martin MT, Boukamcha N, Montagnac A, Paies M 1999 Stilbene derivatives from *Cissus quadrangularis*. Journal of Natural Products 62(12):1694

3 Gupta, MM, Verma RK 1990 Unsymmetric tetracyclic triterpenoids from *Cissus quadrangularis*. Phytochemistry 29(1):336

4 Gupta MM, Verma RK 1991 Lipid constituents of *Cissus quadrangularis*. Phytochemistry 30(3):875

5 Prasad GC, Chatterjee SC, Udupa KN 1970 Effect of phytogenic steroid of *Cissus quadrangularis* on endocrine glands after fracture. Journal of Research in Indian Medicine 4(2):132

6 Udupa KN, Prasad G, Sen SP 1965 The effect of phytogenic anabolic steroids of *Cissus quadrangularis* in the acceleration of fracture repair. Life Sciences 4(3):317

7 Prasad GC, Udupa KN 1972 Pathways and site of action of phytogenic steroids from *Cissus quadrangularis*. Journal of Research in Indian Medicine 7:29

8 Chopra SS, Patel MR, Awadhiya R 1976 Studies on *Cissus quadrangularis* in experimental fracture repair: a histopathological study. Indian Journal of Medical Research 64(9):136

9 Udupa KN, Prasad GC 1964 Biochemical and Ca^{45} studies on the effect of *Cissus quadrangularis* in fracture healing. Indian Journal of Medical Research 52(5):480

10 Prasad GC, Udupa KN 1963 Effect of *Cissus quadrangularis* on the healing of cortisone-treated fracture. Indian Journal of Medical Research 51:667

11 Dhawan BN, Dubey MP, Mehrotra BN, Rastogi RP, Tandon JS 1980 Screening of Indian medicinal plants for biological activity: Part IX. Indian Journal of Experimental Biology 18:594

Commiphora mukul Hook. ex Stocks (Burseraceae) (syn. *Balsamodendron mukul* Hook.)

English: Indian bdellium tree

Hindi: *Guggul*

Sanskrit: *Guggulu*

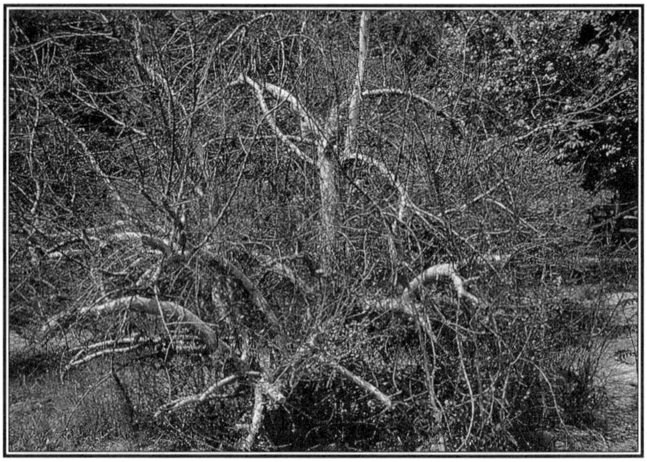

The gum exudate of *Commiphora mukul*, known as myrrh, has been considered an important medicament in the Middle East, India and China since biblical times for use in infected wounds, bronchial and digestive complaints. It is especially associated with women's health and purification rituals. The resin (myrrh) was one of the three gifts presented by the Magi to the infant Jesus and was used to embalm Christ's body after the crucifixion. Hindus use the resin as offering to gods and in prayers.

Habitat

It grows in the arid rocky tracts of Rajasthan, Gujrat, Maharashtra, Tamil Nadu, Karnataka, Assam and Bangladesh.

Botanical description

It is a small tree or shrub with spiny branches (Plate 20). The bark is ash-coloured and flaky, the underbark also peels off like paper. The gum resin is obtained by making incisions in the bark and is collected during the winter season.The resin is pale yellow, brown or dull green in colour. It has a bitter, aromatic taste and balsamic odour. The leaves are alternate, simple, smooth and shiny. The flowers are unisexual or bisexual, present as solitaries or in clusters. The drupe is round and fleshy.

Parts used

Gum resin, stem and leaves.

Traditional and modern use

Guggul is well known as an Ayurvedic drug and has been widely used in the treatment of various types of arthritis. Traditional usage of the gum resin has been described in the treatment of rheumatism, neurological disorders, obesity and related disorders, scrofula, syphilis, skin and urinary disorders. The gum is also used as an astringent, antiseptic, aperitif, carminative, diaphoretic, diuretic, emmenagogue, expectorant, stomachic, alterative, uterotonic and sedative. It is also used in the treatment of bronchitis, catarrh, gingivitis, inflammation, pyorrhoea, sores, tonsillitis, hysteria and mania. Fumes from burning *guggul* have also been recommended for hay fever, nasal catarrh, laryngitis, bronchitis and phthisis.

Ethnoveterinary usage

The gum resin is used in rheumatism, cold and cough.[1]

Major chemical constituents

Lignans

Guggullignan-I and guggullignan-II.[2]

Lipids

Long chain aliphatic tetrols: octadecan-1,2,3,4-tetrol, eicosan-1,2,3,4-tetrol and nonadecan-1,2,3,4-tetrol.[3]

Terpenes and phenylpropanoids

Cembrene-A and mukulol[4] were isolated from gum resin. An essential oil, prepared by the steam distillation of the gum resin, contains myrcene and eugenol.

Sterols

Z-guggulsterone, E-guggulsterone, guggulsterol I, II and III and β-sitosterol.[5]

Medicinal and pharmacological activities

Antiatherosclerotic activity: Significant prevention of experimental atherosclerosis in albino rats was observed by the ethyl acetate extract. The extract increased plasma fibrinolytic activity. Deteriorative changes were seen in serum cholesterol, triglycerides and in fibrinogen level.[6]

Antiinflammatory activity: The petroleum ether extract of the gum resin at a dose of 200 and 500 mg/kg PO significantly inhibited carrageenan-induced rat paw oedema.[7]

Antiobesity activity: In a clinical trial 22 patients with hypercholesterolaemia associated with obesity, ischaemic heart disease, hypertension and diabetes were administered oral *Commiphora mukul* at 6.12 g, in three divided doses for 15 days to one month. Decrease in the levels of serum cholesterol and serum lipid phosphorus was noted. The body weight was also significantly reduced.[8,9]

Hypolipidaemic activity: The effect of guggulsterone (mixture of Z- and E- guggulsterone isomers) on biogenic monoamine levels and dopamine β-hydroxylase activity of the rat brain and heart was studied. Guggulsterone administration to rats led to an inhibition of brain dopamine β-hydroxylase activity with marked stimulation of heart both in vitro and in vivo. Catecholamine levels were also similarly inhibited by guggulsterone whilst serotonin and histamine contents were enhanced in the brain but decreased in the heart. The results confirmed that alterations in biogenic amines and dopamine β-hydroxylase activity may be one of the possible mechanisms of the antilipaemic effect of guggulsterone.[10] The incorporation of the gum resin of *Commiphora mukul* (2%) in the adulterated (1% cholesterol) diet of Wistar rats lowered the serum cholesterol, liver cholesterol, serum triglycerides and serum phospholipids by 36%, 60%, 49%and 8%. The study compared the effects with those of *shilajit*, which lowered the above parameters in 39%, 55%, 47% and 25%

respectively.[11] The petroleum ether-soluble portion and alcoholic extracts of the gum resins lowered the serum cholesterol in hypercholesterolaemic chicks, rabbits and domestic pigs.[12] The alcoholic extract and a pure steroid of *guggul* also lowered serum cholesterol in Triton-treated rats. The steroid fraction of *guggul* also lowered LDL cholesterol by 65%, triglycerides by 39.4%, phospholipids and non-esterified fatty acids by 42.9% as compared to clofibrate (which lowered the same parameters by 47.6%, 51.0%, 41.7% and 31.0% respectively). This also lowered LDL cholesterol (76.1%) and VLDL cholesterol (40.6%) significantly. The ratio of HDL cholesterol to total cholesterol in the steroid-treated monkeys was significantly higher at all intervals, as compared with the initial values.[13]

A clinical trial with purified *guggul* was carried out on 35 patients in order to assess its efficacy, dose development, resistance development and side effects. The results revealed that the gum resin has digestive and analgesic action.[14] Purified gum resin at a dose of 4.5 g daily, in two divided doses, were administered for 16 weeks. Serum triglyceride and serum cholesterol levels were lowered at the end of the eighth and fourth week, respectively. Significant lowering of VDL and LDL was observed. However, a gradual increase in HDL cholesterol was seen.[15]

Fibrinolytic activity: In a study 21 patients with ischaemic heart disease were compared with 27 controls. Guggul gum (1.2 g) increased the fibrinolytic activity in the patients with heart disease, without any effect on platelet aggregation,[16] and a significant prolongation in clotting time, with changes in plasma fibrinogen level, was also observed.

Safety profile

Guggulipid does not appear to have any adverse effects when administered at a dose of 400 mg three times daily. It is contraindicated during pregnancy and internal inflammatory conditions and it may cause gastrointestinal discomfort. In clinical studies, the crude resin revealed mild side effects such as skin rashes, diarrhoea, menorrhagia and irregular menstruation.[8]

Dosage

Powdered gum resin: 0.4–1.5 g

Ayurvedic properties

Rasa: *Katu* (pungent), *tikta* (bitter)

Guna: *Laghu* (light), *ruksha* (dry), *tikshna* (sharp), *vishad* (conspicuous), *sukshma* (minute), *sugandhi* (aromatic), *snigdha-pichchhil* (unctuous-sticky)

Veerya: *Ushna* (hot)

Vipaka: *Katu* (pungent)

Dosha: Pacifies *tridosha*

Further reading

Bharatiya Vidya Bhavan's Swami Prakashananda Ayurveda Research Centre 1992 Selected medicinal plants of India. Chemexcil, Mumbai

Ministry of Health and Family Welfare 1989 Ayurvedic pharmacopoeia of India. Government of India, New Delhi

Sairam TV 1999 Home remedies, vol I. Penguin India, New Delhi

Council of Scientific and Industrial Research 1985 The wealth of India. CSIR, New Delhi

References

1 Jha MK 1992 Folk veterinary medicine of Bihar – a research project. NDDB, Anand, Gujrat

2 Chatterjee A, Pakrashi CS 1994 The treatise of Indian medicinal plants. PID, CSIR, New Delhi

3 Patil VD, Nayak UR, Sukh D 1973 Chemistry of Ayurvedic crude drugs – III, guggulu (resin from *Commiphora mukul*)-3, long chain aliphatic tetrols, a new class of naturally occurring lipids. Tetrahedron 29:1595

4 Patil VD, Nayak UR, Sukh D 1973 Chemistry of Ayurvedic crude drugs – II, guggulu (resin from *Commiphora mukul*)-2 diterpenoid constituents. Tetrahedron 29:341

5 Patil VD, Nayak UR, Sukh D 1972 Chemistry of Ayurvedic crude drugs – I, guggulu (resin from *Commiphora mukul*)-1 steroidal constituents. Tetrahedron 28:2341

6 Srivastava VK, Lata S, Saxena RS, Kumar A, Saxena AK 1991 Beneficial effects of ethyl acetate extract of *Commiphora mukul* (guggulu) in experimental atherosclerosis. Proceedings of a Conference on Pharmacology and Herbal Drugs 15 March, New Delhi

7 Sharma JN, Rajpal MN, Rao TS, Gupta SK 1988 Some pharmacological investigations on the alcoholic extract of Triphala alone and in combination with petroleum ether extract of oleogum resin of *Commiphora mukul*. Indian Drugs 25(6):220

8 Satyavati GV 1966 Effect of an indigenous drug on disorders of lipid metabolism with special reference to atherosclerosis and obesity (Medaroga). MD thesis (Doctor of Ayurvedic Medicine), Banaras Hindu University, Varanasi

9 Kuppurajan K, Rajagopalan SS, Koteswara Rao T, Vijayalakshmi AN, Dwarkanath C 1973 Effect of guggulu (*Commiphora mukul*-Engl) on serum lipids in obese subjects. Journal of Research in Indian Medicine 8:4

10 Srivastava M, Kapoor NK 1986 Guggulsterol induced changes in the levels of biogenic monoamines and dopamine β-hydroxylase activity of rat tissue. Journal of Bioscience 10:15

11 Saukhla A, Mathur PN, Saukhla AK, Dashora PK 1992 Comparative efficiency of Shilajeet and gum guggal (*Commiphora mukul*) in preventing diet induced hypercholesterolemia in Wistar rats. Indian Journal of Clinical Biochemistry 7(1):45

12 Sastry VVS 1967 Experimental and clinical studies on the effect of oleogum resin of *Commiphora mukul* on thrombotic phenomenon associated with hyperlipaemia (Snehavyapat). MD thesis (Doctor of Ayurvedic Medicine), Banaras Hindu University, Varanasi

13 Bhargava SK 1984 Hypolipidemic activity of a steroid fraction of guggal resin (*Commiphora mukul* Hook. Ex Stocks) in monkeys (*Presbytis entellus entellus* Dufresne). Plantes Medicinales et Phytotherapie 18:68

14 Vyas SN, Shukla CP 1987 A clinical study on the effect of Shuddha guggulu in rheumatoid arthritis. Rheumatism 23(1):15

15 Verma SK, Bordia A 1988 Effect of *Commiphora mukul* (gum guggul) in patients of hyperlipidemia with special reference to HDL-cholesterol. Indian Journal of Medical Research 87:356

16 Motani HA 1981 The effect of guggul (*Commiphora mukul*) on lipid profile and coagulation in ischaemic heart disease. PhD thesis, Nagpur University

Crataeva nurvala Buch. (Capparidaceae) (syn. *Crataeva religiosa* Hook. f. & Thoms. f., *Crataeva magna* (Lour.) D.C.)

English: Three-leaved caper

Hindi: *Barna, barun*

Sanskrit: *Varuna*

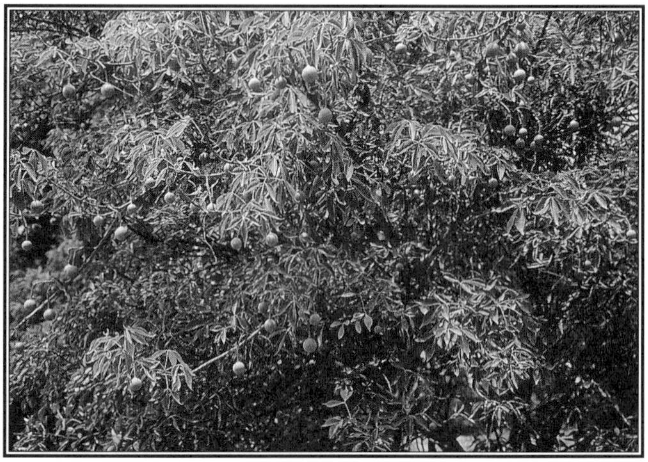

The name *Crataeva* derives from Crataevus, a Greek botanist, while the suffix 'religiosa' denotes its growth near places of worship. It was known to ancient Ayurvedic physicians who used it as a blood purifier and to maintain homeostasis.

Habitat

A small tree, often found wild along river banks and cultivated throughout India. It is distributed in sub-Himalayan tracts and is indigenous to Tamil Nadu, Kerala and Karnataka.

Botanical description

A deciduous and much-branched tree, with trifoliate, glabrous, ovate leaflets (Plate 21). The flowers are large, greenish-white in dense terminal corymbs and the fruits fleshy, ovoid with a tough rind and brown seeds embedded in the fleshy pulp. The mature bark is wrinkled and rough with visible lenticels; the outer surface is greyish to greyish-brown in colour.

Parts used

Stem bark, root bark, leaves.

Traditional and modern use

It is used mainly in the treatment of urinary calculi, crystalluria and urinary infections, but is valued as a bitter, antiperiodic, aperitif, astringent, demulcent, laxative, rubefacient, tonic, liver stimulant and vesicant. It has also been used for malaria and tumours.

Ethnoveterinary usage

The stem bark is used in the treatment of renal lithiasis, swelling of the liver and diarrhoea.

Major chemical constituents

Alkaloids

Cadabicine and cadabicine diacetate are present in the stem bark.

Tannins

(–) Epiafzelechin, (–) epiafzelechin-5-O-β-D glucoside and catechin in bark.[1]

Triterpenes

Diosgenin has been isolated from the stem bark,[1] β-sitosterol, lupeol and their acetates, varunol, spinasterol acetate, taraxasterol, 3-epilupeol and lupenone from stem, root and seeds.

Flavonoids

Rutin, quercetin, isoquercetin and glucocapparin are also present.[2,3]

Medicinal and pharmacological activities

Antiinflammatory activity: Lupeol and its linoleate ester, when administered orally at a dose of 50 mg/kg for 8 days in a model of adjuvant-induced rat inflammation, reduced the alterations in the enzyme levels found in arthritic rats compared to normal rats.[4]

Antilithiatic activity: The effect of lupeol on calcium oxalate stones was measured. Ammonium oxalate was administered to the adult male rats of Wistar strain to induce a hyperoxaluric condition, resulting in increased excretion of oxalate and elevation of the urinary marker enzymes, indicating renal tissue damage. Lupeol, at a dose of 25 mg/kg, reduced the levels of these enzymes. This suggests a beneficial effect in reducing deposition of stone-forming constituents in the kidney.[5,6] In another experiment the effect of a *Crataeva nurvala* bark decoction was studied in inbred male albino rats predisposed to calcium oxalate stone formation. In the control, calculogenic, group, there was a significant increase in activities of the major oxalate-synthesising enzymes in the liver, namely glycollate oxidase (GAO) and lactate dehydrogenase (LDH). However, a significant decrease in liver GAO activity was observed in rats treated with the bark decoction. A marginal decrease in Na+, K+ -ATPase and an increase in aspartate aminotransferase activities (without altering other enzymes) were produced by the decoction in rats fed with the calculi-producing diet. The decrease in liver GAO activity seen during decoction treatment may prove beneficial as a prophylactic measure in preventing stone recurrence.[7] The bark decoction also lowered levels of small intestinal Na+, K+ -ATPases. The action on the small intestinal tract seems to be mediated through these, which in turn may affect the transport of metabolites.[8] Clinically, the antilithic effect was studied in patients with calcium oxalate and calcium phosphate nephrolithiasis. Treatment with *Crataeva nurvala* provided symptomatic relief of pain and dysuria and the disappearance of urinary crystals in 65–70% patients in the calcium oxalate group and 50–70% in the calcium phosphate group. Radiological reduction in size was also observed.[9]

Safety profile

The leaves are reported to cause reddening and even blistering of the skin when applied topically. The decoctions of the root bark and stem bark appear to be well tolerated. The LD_{50} of a 50% ethanolic extract of stem bark was found to be >1000 mg/kg administered IP to adult rats.[10]

Dosage

Leaf paste: topical use

Decoction: 50 ml bd

Ayurvedic properties

Rasa: *Tikta* (bitter), *kashaya* (astringent)

Guna: *Laghu* (light), *ruksha* (dry)

Veerya: *Ushna* (hot)

Vipaka: *Katu* (pungent)

Dosha: Pacifies *kapha* and *vata*, promotes *pitta*

Further reading

Bharatiya Vidya Bhavan's Swami Prakashananda Ayurveda Research Centre 1992 Selected medicinal plants of India. Chemexcil, Mumbai

Indian Drug Manufacturers' Association 1998 Indian herbal pharmacopoeia, vol 1. IDMA/Regional Research Laboratory, Jammu

References

1 Ahmed VU, Fizza K, Amber AUR, Arif S 1987 Cadabicine and cadabicine diacetate from *Crataeva nurvala* and *Cadaba farinosa*. Journal of Natural Products 50(6):1186

2 Sharma V, Pandhya MA 1989 Screening of *Crataeva nurvala* for glucosinolate-glucocapparin. Indian Drugs 26(10):572

3 Prabhakar YS, Suresh KD 1990 The varuna tree, *Crataeva nurvala*, a promising plant in the treatment of urinary stones – a review. Fitoterapia 61(2):99

4 Geetha T, Varalakshmi P, Latha RM 1998 Effects of triterpenes from *Crataeva nurvala* stembark on lipid peroxidation in adjuvant induced arthritis in rats. Pharmacological Research 37(3):191

5 Malini MM, Bhaskar R, Varalakshmi P 1995 Effect of lupeol, a pentacyclic triterpene, on urinary enzymes in hyperoxaluric rats. Japanese Journal of Medical Science and Biology 48(5–6):211

6 Varalakshmi P, Shamila Y, Latha E 1990 Effect of *Crataeva nurvala* in experimental urolithiasis. Journal of Ethnopharmacology 28(3):313

7 Bhaskar R, Saravanan N, Varalakshmi P 1995 Effect of *Crataeva nurvala* bark decoction on enzymatic changes in liver of normal and stone forming rats. Indian Journal of Clinical Biochemistry 10(2):98

8 Varalakshmi P, Latha E, Shamila Y, Jayanthi S 1991 Effect of *Crataeva nurvala* on the biochemistry of the small intestinal tract of normal and stone forming rats. Journal of Ethnopharmacology 31:67

9 Singh RG, Usha D, Kapoor S 1991 Evaluation of antilithic properties of Varuna (*Crataeva nurvala*): an indigenous drug. Journal of Research and Education in Indian Medicine 1092:35

10 Bhakuni DS, Dhar ML, Dhar MM, Dhawan BN, Gupta B, Srimal RC 1971 Screening of Indian plants for biological activity. Indian Journal of Experimental Biology 9:92

Curcuma longa L. (Zingiberaceae) (syn. *Curcuma domestica* Valeton)

English: Turmeric

Hindi: *Haldi*

Sanskrit: *Haridra*

In the 16th century it was known as *Crocus indicus*, Turmeracke and Curcuma and Dioscorides originally referred to it as Cyperus. The name comes from *kurkum*, the Arabic name for these plants. There are several varieties, of which Bengal turmeric is considered best for dyeing silk and wool. The orange-yellow robes of Buddhists are often dyed with it. It is considered to be auspicious for Hindus and is a part of all religious occasions.

Habitat

It is native to south Asia, especially India, but is cultivated in many of the warmer regions of the world. It is found in all states of India but particularly in Tamil Nadu, West Bengal and Maharashtra.

Botanical description

It is a perennial, stemless herb, reaching up to 1.5 m in height, with large, pale green, elongated and tufted leaves (Plate 22). The rhizome is short, branched and bright yellow within. The pale yellow flowers are present in dense, cylindrical inflorescences, 10–15 cm long, which develop in the centre of the leaves.

Parts used

Rhizomes, leaves.

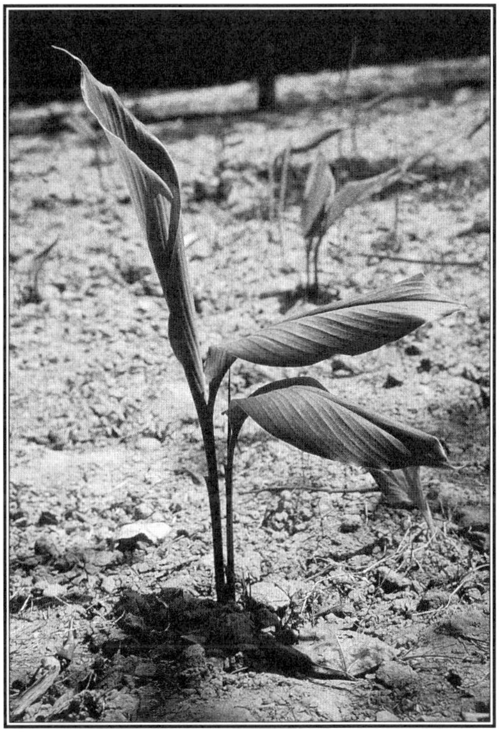

Traditional and modern use

It is used as a general tonic and blood purifier and as an antiinflammatory agent and analgesic in arthritis and rheumatism and for the common cold. It finds a particular use in diseases of the liver such as jaundice and as a cholagogue and has also been used as an anodyne, antimalarial, antiepileptic, aperitif, carminative, diuretic and vermifuge. Externally it can be applied to insect bites and wounds as an antiseptic.[1]

Ethnoveterinary usage

The rhizome of the plant is used as an application for abscesses, ulcers, ticks, castration wounds, bleeding, eye disorders and fungal diseases. It is also used to treat diarrhoea, rheumatism, intestinal worms in poultry, constipation, udder infection and swollen teats, sprains, coughs and colds in ruminants and poultry, jaundice and for swinepox. The rhizome is used in digestive disorders including *E. coli* bacillosis, glossitis, threadworm, indigestion, as well as irregular growth of teeth, holes in the hard palate, loss of appetite and colic. It has been used in respiratory disorders, swelling in the throat, tonsillitis, leeches in the nostrils, asthma, pneumonia and renal disorders such as polyurea. Other minor indications are lumbar and compound fractures, haemorrhagic septicaemia, rinder pest, sprain, haematuria, anthrax and baldness.

Major chemical constituents

Phenylpropanoids

Curcumin, the main active principle, is present as 2–5% dry weight in the rhizome. Curcumenone, curlone, bis-desmethoxycurcumin, bis-(para-hydroxy-cinnamoyl)methane, L-α-curcumene, cyclocurcumin, curcumenol, curdione, curzerenone, dehydroturmerone, dihydrocurcumin, eugenol, turmerin, turmerone, turmeronol and others are present.[1,2]

Monoterpenes

More than 20 components have been identified from the leaf oil of *Curcuma longa*, of which the major monoterpenes are α-phellandrene, 1,8-cineole, p-cymene and β-pinene.[2] Others are α-terpinene, γ-terpinene and terpinolene.

Glycans

Ukonans A,B,C and D.[3]

Sesquiterpenes

Zingiberene, bisabolol, germacrone, sabinene and others.[2,3]

Others

Arabinose, ascorbic acid, α and γ-atlantone, ortho and p-coumaric acid, phytosterols, etc.[1,2,3]

Medicinal and pharmacological activities

Antiallergic activity: Antiallergic activity in Curcuma extract has been reported.[4]

Antiinflammatory activity: Antiinflammatory activity has been exhibited by several fractions.[5] In carrageenan-induced rat paw oedema, the volatile oil at a dose of 1.6 ml/kg exhibited activity comparable to that of phenylbutazone at 100 mg/kg.[6] Isolated curcumin also showed significant activity in carrageenan-induced rat paw oedema, equivalent to phenylbutazone; however, it was only half as potent in chronic models.[7] Clinically, patients suffering from rheumatoid arthritis were subjected to a short-term double-blind trial where curcumin was compared with phenylbutazone. A significant improvement in symptoms was observed with curcumin, although phenylbutazone was more potent, probably because it also has analgesic action.[8] In a postoperative inflammation model for evaluating antiinflammatory activity, curcumin was found to have greater activity than phenylbutazone or placebo in a double-blind clinical trial.[8]

Antimicrobial activity: The essential oil showed activity against Gram-negative bacteria and pathogenic fungi at a dilution of

1:32.[9] The alcoholic extract and curcumin inhibited the growth of Gram-positive bacteria in several in vitro studies.

Antimutagenic activity: Antimutagenic activity has been observed for *C. longa* extract and the isolated curcumins in a number of assays,[1] for example against 7,12-dimethylbenz(a)anthracene-induced mutagenesis in *Salmonella typhimurium* TA 98. The most active was the isomer curcumin III. A para hydroxy group in the benzene ring seems to be essential and additional hydroxyl groups add to the activity.[1,10] Curcumin also showed a dose-dependent inhibition of the in vitro mutagenicity of cayenne extract and capsaicin.[7,8]

Antioxidant activity: Various extracts of the rhizome are active as antioxidants and the curcuminoids are the main active compounds.[1] Curcumin was the most potent when tested against air oxidation of linoleic acid and showed better activity than dl-α-tocopherol at the same concentration.[11] Another antioxidant principle is a heat-stable protein isolated from the water extract; it has an approximate molecular weight of 24000 Da.[12] Three curcuminoids from turmeric, namely curcumin, demethoxy curcumin and bisdemethoxycurcumin, were found to protect PC12 rat phaeochromocytoma and normal human umbilical vein endothelial cells from β-amyloid (1–42) insult, as measured by the 3-[4,5-dimethylthiazol-2-yl]-2,5-diphenyltetrazolium bromide reduction assay.[13] Oxidative stress induced by β-amyloid is a well-established pathway of neuronal cell death in Alzheimer's disease.

Antispasmodic activity: Curcumin exhibited antispasmodic action.[5]

Antiulcer activity: Ethanolic extracts of *C. longa* were given to rats with ulceration induced by hypothermic restraint stress, pyloric ligation, indomethacin and reserpine. The extract showed significant antiulcer action, thought to be by increasing gastric mucus and restoring non-protein sulfhydryl content in the stomach.[14]

Antiviral activity: Curcumin showed inhibitory activity against purified human immunodeficiency virus type 1 (HIV-1) integrase.[8]

Hepatoprotective activity: Curcumin and turmeric were tested against CCl_4, aflatoxin-B1, paracetamol, iron and cyclophosphamide-induced liver damage in the mouse, rat and ducklings.[8] Administration over 10 days was found to be protective. *C. longa* also prevented CCl_4-induced liver damage when given in combination with *Phyllanthus niruri* and *Eclipta alba*. Elevated levels of lipids in the liver and serum bilirubin were decreased to normal but an increase in levels of serum triglycerides, pre-β-lipoproteins and cholesterol was noted, together with levels of glycogen.[15]

Hypoglycaemic activity: A 50% ethanolic extract of the rhizome produced a lowering of blood sugar (by 37.2% and 54.5% at 3 and 6 hours after administration) in alloxan-diabetic rats.[16] When given together with *Momordica charantia* and *Phyllanthus emblica* (all in powder form), it exhibited an even more pronounced antidiabetic action.[17]

Immunostimulant activity: Ukonans A, B, C and D, glycans isolated from a hot water extract of *C. longa*, exhibited reticuloendothelial system-potentiating activity in a carbon clearance test.[18,19] Another immunostimulant polysaccharide, similar to bacterial lipopolysaccharide, has also been isolated.[20]

Antiasthmatic activity: Oral administration of the volatile oil was found to be clinically effective in cases of bronchial asthma.[21] A protective effect by curcumin (200 mg/kg for 7 days) on rat lung, against toxicity induced by cyclophosphamide, has been observed.[22]

Hypocholesterolaemic effects: A clinical trial carried out on 16 patients in China showed that administration of an extract equivalent to 50 g/day of rhizome for 12 weeks lowered plasma cholesterol levels by 49 mg/dl and triglyceride by 62 mg/dl. This therapeutic efficacy was almost equivalent to clofibrate. Another study on 90 subjects showed the reduction of cholesterol and triglycerides in nearly all cases. Both studies also showed an amelioration of the symptoms of angina pectoris.[8]

Safety profile

Safe for oral use as per Commission E monograph. The use is contraindicated in biliary obstruction, duodenal and gastric ulcers. Use with caution during pregnancy. It can cause contact allergy; in one case a positive patch test was observed which was most intense at 48 hours.[23] The maximum tolerated dose of a 50% ethanolic extract of rhizome was 250 mg/kg and the LD_{50} was 500 mg/kg when given IP to adult mice.[24] The oral LD_{50} in mice, however, was more than 2.0 g/kg.

Dosage

Infusion: 5–10 ml

Powder: 1–4 g

Ayurvedic properties

Rasa: *Tikta* (bitter), *katu* (pungent)

Guna: *Laghu* (light), *ruksha* (dry)

Veerya: *Ushna* (hot)

Vipaka: *Katu* (pungent)

Dosha: Balances *tridosha*

Further reading

Kapoor LD 1990 Handbook of Ayurvedic medicinal plants. CRC Press, Boca Raton

Ministry of Health and Family Welfare 1966 The Indian pharmacopoeia. Government of India, New Delhi

Ministry of Health and Family Welfare 1989 Ayurvedic pharmacopoeia of India. Government of India, New Delhi

Nadkarni AK 1976 Indian materia medica. Popular Prakashan PVT Ltd, Bombay

References

1 Ross I 1999 Medicinal herbs of the world, vol 1. Humana Press, Totowa, New Jersey

2 Dung NX, Tuyet NTB, Leclercq PA 1995 Constituents of the leaf oil of *Curcuma domestica* L. from Vietnam. Journal of Essential Oil Research 7(6):701

3 Duke JA 1992 Handbook of phytochemical constituents of GRAS herbs and other economic plants. CRC Press, Boca Raton

4 Yano S, Terai M, Shimizu KI et al 1996 Proceedings of the 2nd International Congress on Phytomedicine, Munich, September 11–14

5 Ammon HPT, Wahl MA 1991 Pharmacology of *Curcuma longa*. Planta Medica 57(1):1

6 Iyengar MA, Rama Rao MP, Gurumadhva Rao S, Kamath MS 1994 Anti-inflammatory activity of volatile oil of *Curcuma longa* leaves. Indian Drugs 31(11):528

7 Srimal RC, Dhawan BN 1973 Pharmacology of diferuloyl methane (curcumin), a non-steroidal anti-inflammatory agent. Journal of Pharmacy and Pharmacology 25:447

8 Srimal RC 1997 Turmeric: a brief review of medicinal properties. Fitoterapia 68:483

9 Iyengar MA, Rama Rao M, Bairy I, Kamath MS 1995 Antimicrobial activity of the essential oil of *Curcuma longa* leaves. Indian Drugs 32(6):249

10 Mulky N, Amonkar AJ, Bhide SV 1987 Antimutagenicity of curcumins and related compound: the structural requirement for the antimutagenicity of curcumins. Indian Drugs 25(3):91

11 Toda S, Miyase T, Arichi H, Tanizawa H, Takino Y 1985 Natural antioxidants. III. Antioxidative components isolated from rhizome of *Curcuma longa*. Chemical and Pharmaceutical Bulletin 33:1725

12 Selvam R, Subramanian L, Gayathri R, Angayarkanni N 1995 The anti-oxidant activity of turmeric (*Curcuma longa*). Journal of Ethnopharmacology 7(2):59

13 Kim DS, Park SY, Kim JK 2001 Curcuminoids from *Curcuma longa* L. (Zingiberaceae) that protect PC12 rat pheochromocytoma and normal human umbilical vein endothelial cells from beta-amyloid (1→42) insult. Neuroscience Letters 303(1):57

14 Rafatullah S, Tariq M, Al-Yahya MA, Mossa JS Ageel AM 1990 Evaluation of turmeric (*Curcuma longa*), for gastric and duodenal antiulcer activity in rats. Journal of Ethnopharmacology 29(1):25

15 Chandra T, Sadique J 1987 A new recipe for liver injury. Ancient Science of Life 7(2):99

16 Tank R, Sharma N, Sharma I, Dixit VP 1990 Antidiabetic activity of *Curcuma longa* in alloxan induced diabetic rats. Indian Drugs 27(11):587

17 Sankaranarayanan J, Jolly CI 1993 Phytochemical, antibacterial and pharmacological investigations on *Momordica charantia* Linn., *Emblica officinalis* and *Curcuma longa* Linn. Indian Journal of Pharmaceutical Sciences 55(1):6

18 Tomoda M, Gonda R, Shimizu N, Kimura M, Kanari M 1990 A reticuloendothelial system activating glycan from the rhizomes of *Curcuma longa*. Phytochemistry 29(4):1083

19 Gonda R, Tomoda M, Shimizu N, Kanari M 1990 Characterization of polysaccharides having activity on the reticuloendothelial system from the rhizome of *Curcuma longa*. Chemical and Pharmaceutical Bulletin 38(2):482

20 Inagawa H, Nishizawa T, Tsukioka D et al 1992 Homeostasis as regulated by activated macrophage. Chemical and Pharmaceutical Bulletin 40:994

21 Jain JP, Naqvi SMA, Sharma KD 1990 A clinical trial of volatile oil of *Curcuma longa* Linn.(Haridra) in cases of bronchial asthma (Tamaka Swasa). Journal of Research in Ayurveda and Siddha 11(1–4):20

22 Venkatesan N, Chandrakasan G 1995 Modulation of cyclophosphamide-induced early lung injury by curcumin, an anti-inflammatory antioxidant. Molecular and Cellular Biochemistry 142:79

23 Goh CL, Ng SK 1987 Allergic contact dermatitis to *Curcuma longa* (turmeric). Contact Dermatitis 17(3):186

24 Dhar ML, Dhar MM, Dhawan BN, Mehrotra BN, Ray C 1968 Screening of Indian plants for biological activity: Part I. Indian Journal of Experimental Biology 6:232

Cyperus rotundus L. (Cyperaceae)

English: Nutgrass, sedge weed, nutsedge, chido

Hindi: *Motha*

Sanskrit: *Mustak*

It is widely used throughout the tropics for a variety of uses; the dried tubers are used in perfumery and for the preparation of fragrant sticks called 'agarbatties'.

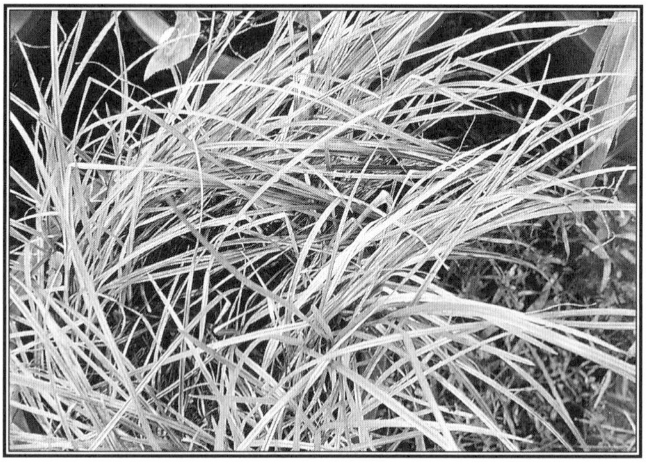

Habitat

Indigenous to India but now found all over the world, it is considered to be among the world's most invasive weeds and is especially prevalent in damp places.

Botanical description

A perennial sedge grass (Plate 23), with slender, scaly creeping rhizomes, bulbous at the base, arising singly from the tubers which are about 1–3 cm long, externally blackish in colour and reddish white inside, with a characteristic odour. The stem is up to 25 cm tall and the leaves linear, dark green and grooved on the upper surface. Inflorescences are small, with 2–4 bracts, consisting of tiny flowers with a red-brown husk. The nut is three-angled, oblong-ovate, yellow in colour and black when ripe.

Parts used

Tubers or rhizomes.

Traditional and modern use

The tuber and rhizome are used to treat abdominal problems, particularly peptic ulcer, diarrhoea and dyspepsia, and as a carminative, demulcent, analgesic and diuretic, as well as for amenorrhoea and dysmenorrhoea. It is used also for skin conditions including scorpion bite, inflammation, wounds, sores and oedema; cold and congestion, impotence and hypertension. It has anthelmintic, antibacterial and fungicidal activities and has been used for many other complaints.

Ethnoveterinary usage

The tubers are used to treat wounds, tuberculosis, pneumonia, scabies and pox and to help heal cracked tail.[1]

Major chemical constituents

Essential oil

Steam distillation of the tubers and bulbous rhizome yields about 0.5–0.9% of an essential oil consisting mainly of sesquiterpene hydrocarbons (25%), epoxides (12%) and ketones (20%) and monoterpene and aliphatic alcohols (25%).[2] These include isocyperol, cyperone rotundines A–C,[3] cyperene, cyperol, cyperlolonecyperotundone, rotundene, β-selinene, patchoulenone, isopatchoula-3,5-diene, caryophyllene-6,7 oxide, caryophyllene-α-oxide, caryophylla-6-one, caryophyllene and 10,12-peroxycalamenene, 4,7-dimethyl-1-tetralone and many other common monoterpenes such as cineole, limonene and camphene.

Triterpenes

β-Sitosterol, oleanolic acid and others.

Miscellaneous

Flavonoids, sugars and minerals have also been isolated from the tuber.[4]

Medicinal and pharmacological activities

Antiemetic activity: An ethanolic extract of the rhizome exhibited antiemetic activity in dogs, as shown by antagonism of apomorphine-induced vomiting.[5]

Antiinflammatory and antipyretic activities: Significant antiinflammatory activity against carageenan-induced oedema in albino rats was observed in the petroleum ether extract (75% inhibition), chloroform (60.6%) and methanol extracts (57.7%) of the roots of *C. rotundus* at doses of 10 mg/kg, compared to hydrocortisone (57.7%). The alcoholic extract of the tubers showed antipyretic action, which compared well with sodium salicylate in suppressing yeast-induced pyrexia. These activities were traced to the β-sitosterol content and the antiinflammatory activity of this compound is known to be independent of the pituitary adrenal system. β-Sitosterol has a wide margin of safety with minimal ulcerogenic activity and may have therapeutic value.[6]

Antimalarial activity: 10,12-Peroxycalamenene, an endoperoxide sesquiterpene, isolated from the tubers of *C. rotundus* exhibited antimalarial activity[7] at EC_{50} 2.33×10^{-6} M.

Antiobesity activity: A pilot study was carried out on 30 obese people who were administered the powdered tuber of *C. rotundus* for 90 days. A reduction in weight along with a decrease in serum cholesterol and triglycerides were observed.[8]

Cytoprotective activity: A decoction of the rhizome of *C. rotundus* was evaluated against ethanol-induced gastric damage. The extract, which was orally administered at a dose of 1.25, 2.5 and 4.0 g crude drug/kg, exhibited antiulcer activity in a dose-dependent manner. The protective action was related to its inhibition of gastric motility and endogenous prostaglandins may play an important role.[9]

Effects on pigmentation: The lyophilised methanolic extract of the plant stimulated the growth of cultured melanocytes, substantiating its use in the preparation of several formulations for the treatment of skin and hair pigmentation.[10]

Oestrogenic activity: The essential oil exhibited mild oestrogenic activity.[11]

Tranquillising, hypotensive and muscle relaxant activity: Tranquillising, hypotensive and muscle relaxant activity was observed in the ethanolic extract of the rhizome of *C. rotundus*.[5]

Antibacterial activity: The essential oil inhibited the growth of *Staphylococcus aureus* but was ineffective against *E.coli, E. typhosum, Vibrio cholerae* and various strains of *Shigella*. Of the fractions, cyperone was completely inert, while the hydrocarbon fractions cyperene I and II were more potent than the oil and cyperol.[12] Other types of extract were found to be active on various types of bacteria.[13]

Safety profile

The LD_{50} of β-sitosterol is >3 g/kg IP in mice and the minimum ulcerogenic dose 600 mg/kg IP in rats.[6] The LD_{50} of the ethanolic extract of rhizome was found to be 1500 mg/kg.[5]

Dosage

Powder: 1–3 g

Decoction: 56–112 ml

Ayurvedic properties

Rasa: *Tikta* (bitter), *kashaya* (astringent)

Guna: *Laghu* (light), *ruksha* (dry)

Veerya: *Shita* (cold)

Vipaka: *Katu* (pungent)

Dosha: Pacifies *kapha* and *pitta*

Further reading

Pandey GS (ed) 1998 Bhavprakash Nighantu. Chaukhambha Bharati Academy, Gokul Bhawan, Varanasi

Council for Scientific and Industrial Research 1985 The wealth of India. PID, CSIR, New Delhi

References

1 Jha MK 1992 Folk veterinary medicine of Bihar – a research project. NDDB, Anand, Gujrat

2 Kapadia VH, Naik VG, Wadia MS, Sukhdev S 1967 Sesquiterpenes from essential oils from *Cyperus rotundus*. Tetrahedron 47:4661

3 Jeong SJ, Miyamoto T, Inagaki M, Kim YC, Higuchi R 2000 Rotundines A-C, three novel sesquiterpene alkaloids from *Cyperus rotundus*. Journal of Natural Products 63(5):673

4 Kalsi PS, Sharma A, Singh A, Singh IP, Chhabra BR 1995 Biogenetically important sesquiterpenes from *Cyperus rotundus*. Fitoterapia 66(1):94

5 Singh N, Kulshreshtha VK, Gupta MB and Bhargava KP 1970 A pharmacological study of *Cyperus rotundus*. Indian Journal of Medical Research 58(1):103

6 Gupta MB, Nath R, Srivastava N, Shanker K, Kishor K, Bhargava KP 1980 Anti-inflammatory and antipyretic activities of β-sitosterol. Planta Medica 39:157

7 Thebtaranonth C, Thebtaranonth Y, Wanauppathamkul S, Yuthavong Y 1995 Antimalarial sesquiterpenes from tubers of *Cyperus rotundus*: structure of 10,12-peroxycalamenene, a sesquiterpene endoperoxide. Phytochemistry 40(1):125

8 Karnick CR 1992 Clinical evaluation of *Cyperus rotundus* Linn (Motha) on obesity: a randomised double blind placebo controlled trial on Indian patients. Indian Medicine 4(2):7

9 Zhu M, Luk HH, Fung HS, Luk CT 1997 Cytoprotective effects of *Cyperus rotundus* against ethanol induced gastric ulceration in rats. Phytotherapy Research 11:392

10 Alain M, Frederic B, Marc D 1992 Cosmetic or pharmaceutical composition containing a *Cyperus* extract for pigmentation of the skin or hair. International Patent Application 92,20,322

11 Indira M, Sirsi M, Radomir S, Dev S 1956 Occurrence of estrogenic substances in plants I. Estrogenic activity of *Cyperus rotundus*. Indian Journal of Science Research 15:202

12 Radomir S, Sukh D, Sirsi M 1956 Chemistry and antibacterial activity of nut grass. Current Science 4:118

13 Ross I 1999 *Cyperus rotundus.* In: Medicinal plants of the world, Vol 1. Humana Press, Totowa, New Jersey

Eclipta alba (L.) Hassak. (Asteraceae) (syn. *E. prostrata* L.)

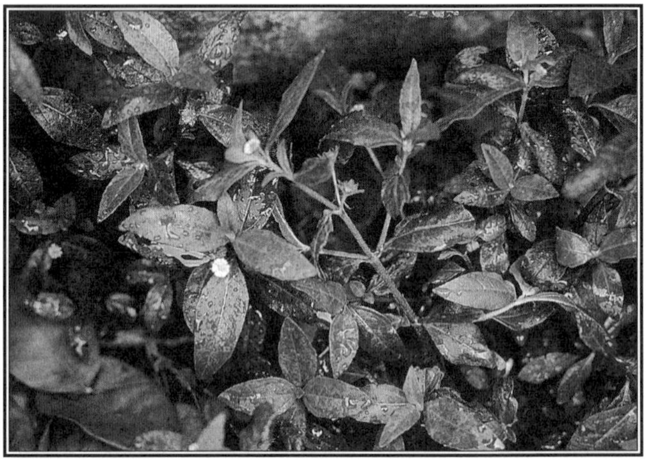

English: Trailing eclipta, false daisy

Hindi: *Bhangra, babri*

Sanskrit: *Bhringaraja, tekarajah*

One of the Ten Auspicious Flowers (*Dasapushpam*), it has been used in cosmetic preparations for hair and skin since ancient times and is a well-regarded remedy in Ayurvedic medicine. It is the source of a black dye used for the hair and is thought to impart a glowing complexion. The leaves are used as food in Java.

Habitat

It is a common weed growing throughout India on waste ground, up to an altitude of 2000 m.

Botanical description

An erect or prostrate, much-branched annual herb (Plate 24). Leaves are opposite with appressed hairs on both surfaces, sessile to subsessile, up to 10 cm long. Composite flowers are white with compressed rays.

Parts used

Whole plant, roots, seeds and seed oil.

Traditional and modern use

The herb is used particularly for alopecia, ringworm and as a hair dye and for liver and spleen enlargement, hepatitis and jaundice and as a general tonic. It has been used for catarrh, cough, enterorrhagia, haemorrhage, indigestion, vertigo, to aid parturition and for toothache, giddiness and as an antiseptic and wound-healing agent. The root is used as an emetic and purgative and a paste of leaves is considered to be an excellent remedy for scorpion sting.

Ethnoveterinary usage

The leaves, herb and root are used for wounds, blisters, broken horns, cracked tail, scratching, scabies, abscess in the ear, haemorrhagic septicaemia, mastitis, rabies, jackal bites, glossitis, oral lesions, jaundice, leeches in the nostril, pneumonia, swelling of the throat and nasal mucus membranes, epistaxis and tetanus.[1]

Major chemical constituents

Triterpene glycosides and saponins

Six new oleanane glycosides, the eclalbasaponins I–VI, as well as β-amyrin and other sterols have been isolated from the aerial parts.[2]

Flavonoids and isoflavonoids

Apigenin, luteolin and their glucosides have been isolated from the leaves and stem; and the isoflavonoids wedelolactone, desmethylwedelolactone and its 7-0-glucoside from the whole plant.[4]

Others

Ecliptal, a terthienyl aldehyde, has been isolated from the whole plant and L-terthienyl methanol and wedelic acid from leaves and stem, and the sesquiterpene lactone columbin.[4]

Medicinal and pharmacological activities

Antiinflammatory activity: An extract of *Eclipta alba*, tested in both acute and chronic antiinflammatory models, inhibited chronic inflammation up to 58.67%.[3]

Antinociceptive activity: In mice, a hydroalcoholic extract inhibited acetic acid-induced writhing by 35–55%, at a dose of 200 mg/kg PO. At the same dose, the effect ranged from 41% to 77% using the formalin test in mice, and the extract preferentially inhibited the second phase of the response.[4]

Hepatoprotective activity: An ethanol:water 1:1 extract was studied in carbon tetrachloride-induced hepatotoxicity in rats and it was found that the extract provided protection by regulating the levels of hepatic microsomal drug-metabolising enzymes.[5] *Eclipta alba* exhibited activity in the same model when administered in combination with *Phyllanthus niruri* and curcumin (from *Curcuma longa*) at a ratio of 25:15:10 (*Phyllanthus niruri*:*Eclipta alba*:curcumin). Elevated levels of lipids in the liver and serum bilirubin were decreased and normalised. The preparation increased the levels of serum triglyceride, pre-β-lipoproteins and cholesterol and decreased levels of glycogen were elevated.[6] An ethanolic extract of the fresh plant of *Eclipta alba* showed dose-dependent significant hepatoprotective activity in CCl_4-induced liver damage in rats and mice with no signs of toxicity observed up to a level of 2.0 g/kg given either orally or IP in mice.[7] In another study using albino rats, significant hepatoprotective action was observed at 100 mg/kg body weight.[8]

The hepatoprotective effects of the freeze-dried aqueous extract of the plant were also studied in acute hepatitis induced in mice by a single dose of CCl_4 or acetaminophen (paracetamol) and in rats by β-D-galactosamine. The extract showed significant inhibition of the acute elevation of serum transaminases induced by CCl_4 in mice and by β-D-galactosamine in rats, but no significant improvement was observed in acetaminophen-induced liver damage.[9]

Hypotensive activity: A mixture of polypeptides from *Eclipta alba* exhibited hypotensive activity in dogs and columbin, isolated from the ethanolic extract of the whole plant, showed remarkable antihypertensive action on anaesthetised rats.[10]

Safety profile

The maximum tolerated dose of the 50% ethanolic extract of the whole plant was found to be 1000 mg/kg body weight when given IP to adult albino mice.[11]

Dosage

Infusion: 4–12 ml

Powder: 3–6 g

Ayurvedic properties

Rasa: *Katu* (pungent), *tikta* (bitter)

Guna: *Laghu* (light), *ruksha* (dry)

Veerya: *Ushna* (hot)

Vipaka: *Katu* (pungent)

Dosha: Balances *kapha* and *vata*

Further reading

Kapoor LD 1990 Handbook of Ayurvedic medicinal plants. CRC Press, Boca Raton

Nadkarni AK 1976 Indian materia medica. Popular Prakashan PVT Ltd, Bombay

Pandey GS (ed) 1998 Bhavprakash Nighantu. Chaukhambha Bharati Academy, Gokul Bhawan, Varanasi

Sairam TV 1999 Home remedies, vol II. Penguin India, New Delhi

Council of Scientific and Industrial Research 1985 The wealth of India. PID, CSIR, New Delhi

References

1 Jha MK 1992 Folk veterinary medicine of Bihar – a research project. NDDB, Anand, Gujrat

2 Yahara S, Ding N, Nohara T 1994 Oleanane glycosides from *Eclipta alba*. Chemical and Pharmaceutical Bulletin 42(6):1336

3 Reddy KRK, Tehara SS, Goud PV, Alikhan MM 1990 Comparison of the anti-inflammatory activity of *Eclipta alba* (Bhangra) and *Solanum nigrum* (Mako Khushk) in rats. Journal of Research and Education in Indian Medicine 9(4):43

4 Leal LK, Ferreira AA, Bezerra GA, Matos FJ, Viana GS 2000 Antinociceptive, anti-inflammatory and bronchodilator activities of Brazilian medicinal plants containing coumarins: a comparative study. Journal of Ethnopharmacology 70(2):151

5 Saxena AK, Singh B, Anand KK 1993 Hepatoprotective effects of *Eclipta alba* on subcellular levels in rats. Journal of Ethnopharmacology 40(3):155

6 Chandra T, Sadique J 1987 A new recipe for liver injury. Ancient Science of Life 7(2):99

7 Singh B, Saxena AK, Chandan BK, Agarwal SG, Bhatia MS, Anand KK 1993 Hepatoprotective effect of ethanolic extract of *Eclipta alba* on experimental liver damage in rats and mice. Phytotherapy Research 7(2):154

8 Murthy TS, Rao BG, Satyanarayana T, Rao RVK 1993 Hepatoprotective activity of *Eclipta alba*. Journal of Research and Education in Indian Medicine 12(2):41

9 Lin S-C, Yao C-J, Lin C-C, Lin Y-H 1996 Hepatoprotective activity of Taiwan folk medicine: *Eclipta prostrata* Linn. against various hepatotoxins induced acute hepatotoxicity. Phytotherapy Research 10:483

10 Rashid MD, Karim V, Ahmed M, Choudhury AR 1992 Antihypertensive activity of *Eclipta alba*. International Seminar on Traditional Medicine, Calcutta, 7–9 November

11 Dhar ML, Dhar MM, Dhawan BN, Mehrotra BN Ray C 1968 Screening of Indian plants for biological activity: Part I. Indian Journal of Experimental Biology 6:232

Embelia ribes Burm. (Myrsinaceae)

English: Embelia

Hindi: *Viranga*

Sanskrit: *Vidanga*

The drug is esteemed as an anthelmintic, as the synonym *vidanga* suggests, and it is an important ingredient of a number of formulations for this purpose, many of them from ancient Ayurvedic or Unani texts. More recently, it has been gaining importance for its potential as a contraceptive. In other parts of the world it is eaten as a vegetable.

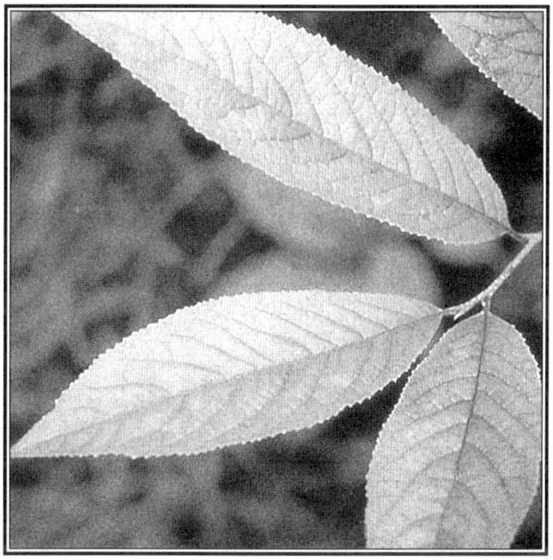

Habitat

The plant is native to India and south-east Asia and found in hilly regions from the central and lower Himalayas as far as Sri Lanka and Singapore.

Botanical description

It is a large climbing shrub (Plate 25), with simple, alternate, narrowly elliptical to lanceolate, coreaceous leaves, obtusely acute, up to 14 cm long and 4 cm wide. They are glossy green on the upper surface and more silvery on the lower, with scattered, minute, sunken glands. The flowers are small, white or greenish, in terminal or axillary panicles; calyx five-lobed, corolla puberulous, with five stamens. Fruits are globose berries, up to 4 mm in diameter, dull red or brownish-black when dried, with a wrinkled or warty surface. The thin pericarp encloses a single red seed, which is enveloped in a delicate membrane. The berries have a faint spicy odour and a pungent and astringent taste.

Parts used

Fruit, leaves.

Traditional and modern use

The powdered berries are used to expel worms. They are used as an astringent, alterative and nervine tonic and for constipation, colic, dyspepsia, flatulence and piles. The pulp is purgative and a paste is applied to skin diseases such as ringworm. The fresh juice is cooling, diuretic and laxative. The leaves are used for sore throats and mouth ulcers. The root has been used to improve digestion and alleviate flatulence and colic and the dried powdered root bark was a remedy for toothache.

Ethnoveterinary usage

The fruits are used in ruminants for the treatment of bloat.[1]

Major chemical constituents

Quinones

The fruit contains embelin (embelic acid), which is considered to be the major active principle, and vilangin.[2]

Fatty acids

Seed oil contains palmitic, oleic and linoleic acids.[3]

Alkaloid

The fruit contains christembine.[2,3]

Medicinal and pharmacological activities

Anthelmintic activity: The alcoholic and aqueous extracts of the berries were tested on 40 children infested with ascarides. The alcoholic extract cured 80% of cases, whilst the aqueous extract cured 55%, expelling the worms and rendering the stool free from ova. No toxicity was observed during and after the treatment.[4]

Contraceptive activity: Embelin has demonstrated significant antifertility activity.[5] It has been evaluated as a contraceptive agent in dogs after administration of 80 mg/kg, given orally. After 100 days, the epididymides were devoid of spermatozoa and histological, tissue biochemistry and blood chemistry results were consistent with a complete inhibition of spermatogenesis. Blood serum parameters revealed normal liver and kidney function. Without embelin, after 250 days a complete recovery of spermatogenesis occurred, suggesting it could be used as a promising, reversible, male contraceptive.[6] Powdered berries of *E. ribes*, when administered orally for 3 months at a dose of 100 mg/day to male bonnet monkeys, adversely affected the quantity and quality of semen and produced a reduction in circulating testosterone levels. Testicular biopsy revealed normal spermatogenesis, but a reduction in testosterone levels may be responsible for a reduced secretory activity of the accessory glands, resulting in a decrease in the volume of the semen.[7] The effect of embelin as an oral contraceptive was demonstrated in female mated rats, by studying the biochemical changes in the uterus and uterine fluid. Embelin (10 mg/kg), when administered orally from days 1 to 5 of pregnancy, decreased the glycogen content of the uterus and lactic acid in uterine fluid and increased alanine aminotransferase activity, suggesting an antiimplantation effect by decreasing the energy available to the blastocyst for survival.[8] When administered daily 20 mg/kg SC to male albino rats for 15 or 30 days, embelin caused an inhibition of epididymal motile sperm count, fertility parameters such as pregnancy attainment and litter size. These changes were reversible. Addition of embelin to epididymal sperm suspensions caused a dose- and duration-dependent inhibition of spermatozoal motility and the activities of the enzymes of carbohydrate metabolism. Light and SEM microscopy revealed that both in vivo and in vitro treatment caused profound morphological changes in spermatozoa, such as decapitation of the spermatozoal head, discontinuity of the outer membranous sheath in the mid-piece and the tail region and alteration in the shape of cytoplasmic droplets in the tail.[9] Embelin also significantly reduced the sperm count and motility and the weight of the testes in rats[10] and has been shown to alter rat testicular histology and glycogen levels, gametogenic counts and accessory sex gland fructose levels at doses of 0.3, 0.4 and 0.5 mg/kg when administered SC for 35 days.[11] In female rats, embelin demonstrated 57.9% and 55.5% antifertility activity at doses of 100 and 50 mg/kg respectively.[12]

Antitumour activity: The cytotoxicity of *Embelia ribes* was demonstrated when a fibrosarcoma cell line was exposed in vitro to increasing concentrations of embelin and simultaneously inoculated with [3H]-thymidine. A dose-dependent decrease in labelled thymidine uptake, lipid peroxide and glutathione levels was observed.[13] Embelin decreased tumour size and prevented an increase in the activity of serum enzymes in rats with experimental fibrosarcoma, indicating that it interfered with carbohydrate and aminoacid metabolism in tumour-bearing animals.[14]

Insecticidal activity: The efficacy of embelin against *Tribolium castaneum* was demonstrated in wheat samples. Embelin at 0.18% brought about adult mortality even after 8 months of storage. The reproduction of the insect was also reduced significantly.[15] Embelin as protectant of wheat against other insect pests, *Sitophilus oryzae*, *Rhyzopertha dominica* and *Ephestia cautella*, has also been shown at low doses after 14 days exposure. The mortality was increased, the number of progeny of *S. oryzae* and *R. dominica* reduced and adult emergence of *E. cautella* significantly lowered as compared with the controls. Protection against larvae of *Corcyra cephalonica* and *E. cautella* and *Trogoderma granarium* was maintained even after 8 months storage.[16]

Antiplaque activity: Extracts of the fruits of *Embelia ribes* showed antibacterial effects and prevented adherence of viable cells of *Staphylococcus mutans* to smooth surfaces with a 50% inhibitory concentration (IC_{50}) of 10–30 μg/ml. It also had antienzymatic action against glucosyltransferase. The active principle was identified as embelin, which inhibited the bacterial growth at a minimum inhibitory concentration of 62.5 μg/ml and glucan synthesis with an IC_{50} of 125 μg/ml.[17]

Antimicrobial activity: Embelin showed antibacterial activity at 800 μg/ml against *Staphylococcus aureus*, *S. albus* and *S. citreus*.[18]

Analgesic activity: Potassium embelate was found to be a centrally acting analgesic in mice and rats. Mixed μ- and κ- binding sites in the brain may be involved in the analgesic action of this compound.[19] The results compared well with morphine, although it was not antagonised by naloxone, indicating a central site of action different from the opiates.[20]

Trypsin inhibition: Embelin was found to be a non-competitive, reversible inhibitor of trypsin.[21]

Safety profile

The 50% alcoholic extract of the seed showed an LD_{50} value of 750 mg/kg body weight when administered IP in mice.[22]

Dosage

Powder: 6–12 g (adult), 2–3 g (children)

Decoction: 14–28 ml

Ayurvedic properties

Guna: *Laghu* (light), *ruksha* (dry), *tikshna* (sharp)

Rasa: *Katu* (pungent)

Veerya: *Ushna* (lukewarm)

Vipaka: *Katu* (pungent)

Dosha: Balances *kapha* and *vata*

Further reading

Chevallier A 1996 The encyclopedia of medicinal plants. Dorling Kindersley, London

Kapoor LD 1990 Handbook of Ayurvedic medicinal plants. CRC Press, Boca Raton

Ministry of Health and Family Welfare 1989 Ayurvedic pharmacopoeia of India. Government of India, New Delhi

Nadkarni AK 1976 Indian materia medica. Popular Prakashan PVT Ltd, Bombay

Sarin YK 1996 Illustrated manual of herbal drugs used in Ayurveda. CSIR & ICMR, Lucknow

Sivarajan VV, Balachandran I 1994 Ayurvedic drugs and their plant sources. Oxford and IBH Publishing, New Delhi

References

1 International Institute of Rural Reconstruction 1994 Ethnoveterinary medicine in Asia. An information kit on traditional animal health care practices. IIRR, Silang, Philippines

2 Rao TV, Padmanabha VV 1965 Some natural and synthetic methylenebisbenzoquinones. Bulletin of the National Institute of Science of India 28:14

3 Ahmad,R, Ahmad I, Mannan A, Ahmad F, Osman SM 1986 Studies on minor seed oils XI. Fette Seifen Arzneimittel 88(4):147

4 Guru LV, Mishra DN 1966 Effect of the alcoholic and aqueous extractives of *Embelia ribes* (Burm.) in patients infested by ascarides. Journal of Research in Indian Medicine 1:47

5 Bhargava SK 1988 Antifertility agents from plants. Fitoterapia 59(3):163

6 Dixit VP, Bhargava SK 1983 Reversible contraception-like activity of embelin in male dogs (*Canis indicus* Linn). Andrologia 15(5):486

7 Purandare TV, Kholkute SD, Gurjar A et al 1979 Semen analysis and hormonal levels in bonnet macaques administered *Embelia ribes* berries, an indigenous plant having contraceptive activity. Indian Journal of Experimental Biology 17(9):935

8 Seshadri C, Suganthan D, Santhakumari G, Iyer GYN 1978 Biochemical changes in the uterus and uterine fluid of mated rats treated with embelin – a nonsteroidal oral contraceptive. Indian Journal of Experimental Biology 16(11):1187

9 Gupta S, Sanyal SN, Kanwar U 1989 Antispermatogenic effect of embelin, a plant benzoquinone, on male albino rats *in vivo* and *in vitro*. Contraception 39(3):307

10 Seth SD, Johri N, Sundaram KR 1982 Antispermatogenic effect of embelin from *Embelia ribes*. Indian Journal of Pharmacology 14(2):207

11 Agrawal S, Chauhan S, Mathur R 1986 Antifertility effects of embelin in male rats. Andrologia 8(2):125

12 Krishnaswamy M, Purushothaman KK 1980 Antifertility properties of *Embelia ribes* (embelin). Indian Journal of Experimental Biology 18(11):1359

13 Chitra M, Sukumar E, Shyamala Devi CS 1995 [3H]-Thymidine uptake and lipid peroxidation by tumor cells on embelin treatment: an *in vitro* study. Oncology 52(1):66

14 Chitra M, Sukumar E, Suja V, Shyamala Devi CS 1994 Effect of embelin on enzyme profile in experimental fibrosarcoma. Indian Journal of Medical and Scientific Research 22(12):877

15 Chander H, Ahmed SM 1989 Comparative evaluation of fungicidal quinones and natural embelin against some insect pests of storage. Journal of Stored Products Research 25(2):87

16 Chander H, Ahmed SM 1985 Efficacy of natural embelin against the red flour beetle, *Tribolium castaneum* Herbst. Insect Science and its Application 6(2):217

17 Namba T, Tsunezuka M, Dissanayake DMRB et al 1985 Studies on dental caries prevention by traditional medicines (Part VII). Screening of

Ayurvedic medicines for anti-plaque action. Shoyakugaku Zasshi 39(2):146

18 Gopal RH, Purushothaman KK 1986 Effect of new plant isolates and extracts on bacteria. Bulletin of Medical Ethnobotany Research 7(1–2):78

19 Zutshi U, Johri RK, Atal CK 1989 Possible interaction of potassium embelate, a putative analgesic agent, with opiate receptors. Indian Journal of Experimental Biology 27(7):656

20 Atal CK, Siddiqui MA, Zutshi U et al 1984 A non-narcotic, orally effective, centrally acting analgesic from an Ayurvedic drug. Journal of Ethnopharmacology 11(3):309

21 Vijaya S, Vasudevan TN 1994 Trypsin inhibitor in *Embelia ribes*. Indian Journal of Pharmaceutical Science 56(4):156

22 Dhawan BN, Dubey MP, Mehrotra BN, Rastogi RR, Tandon JS 1980 Screening of Indian medicinal plants for biological activity: Part-IX. Indian Journal of Experimental Biology 18:594

Eucalyptus globulus Labill. (Myrtaceae)

English: Blue gum tree, Australian fever tree

Hindi: *Nilgiri*

Sanskrit: *Tailparna*

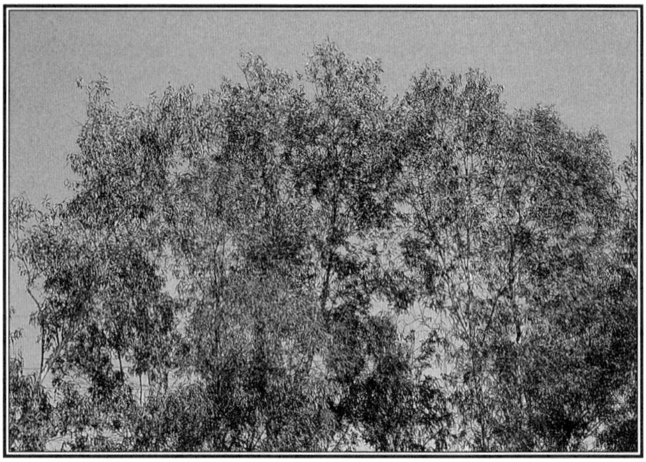

The eucalyptus was first brought to India by the Sultan of Tippu in around 1790. It was grown initially in the Nandi hills of Karnataka and then extended to the Nilgiri hills of southern India. The species *Eucalyptus iereticornis*, popularly known as eucalyptus hybrid or Mysore gum, was then the most widely cultivated plantation species.[1] Now, *E. globulus* and *E. citriodora* are grown in the Nilgiris for their essential oil, distilled from the leaves, for use in the fragrance industry. *E. globulus* trees are coppiced once in every ten years and the timber used for the production of viscose fibre. The eucalyptus was only introduced to the west from Australia in the 19th century. Commercial production of the oil began in about 1860 in Victoria, Australia.

Habitat

Native to Australia and Tasmania, eucalyptus species are cultivated in many tropical, subtropical and temperate areas of the world. Planting can cause ecological problems because the trees absorb large amounts of water, which can inhibit the growth of native plants. Eucalyptus are among the world's fastest growing and tallest trees, the largest recorded at 99 m (326 ft).

Botanical description

A deciduous tree, usually reaching up to 40 m, with a twisted trunk and silver-grey bark (Plate 26). The juvenile leaves differ from the mature leaves, being ovate, cordate or broadly lanceolate, up to 16 cm long by 9 cm wide, and glaucus. The mature leaves are narrower, lanceolate, acuminate or asymmetrical rounded, up to 13 cm long by 4 cm, and glossy green. The flowers are solitary on short pedicles. There are no sepals but numerous long, split stamens, turned inwards. The fruit is globose, up to 3 cm long, somewhat tapering toward the base, with four main ribs. Eucalyptus oil is obtained by steam distillation, followed by rectification, of the fresh leaves and branch tops.[2,3]

Parts used

Oil, leaves, bark.

Traditional and modern use

Eucalyptus, a traditional Aboriginal remedy, is a powerful antiseptic still used all over the world for relieving coughs and colds, sore throats and other infections, including bronchitis. The diluted essential oil may be applied to the skin as a chest rub and has a decongestant and warming effect, which helps to relieve respiratory congestion. The diluted oil is also used to relieve aching pain and stiffness of rheumatic joints. The leaves and oil have been used as a febrifuge, expectorant and stimulant and for wounds, burns, ulcers and cancers. In Chinese medicine it is used for similar purposes and an aqueous extract of the leaves is used to treat aching joints, bacterial dysentery, ringworm and pulmonary tuberculosis. The steam produced by pouring boiling water on eucalyptus leaves has been used as a simple and useful disinfectant, for purifying the air of the sick room in cases of diphtheria, for example. The extract of the fresh leaves, suitably diluted, can also be employed as a disinfectant lotion in skin diseases, ulcers and offensive discharges of all kinds and as a gargle in mouth infections and bleeding gums.

Ethnoveterinary usage

The flowers, leaves and roots are used in the treatment of peeling of skin in ruminants, and the leaves in ruminants and poultry for the treatment of fever, sprains and wounds. The whole plant is insect repellent.[3,4]

Major chemical constituents

Essential oil

1,8-Cineole, α-pinene, β-pinene, limonene, p-cymene, globulol, aromadendrene,[5] α-terpineol, γ-terpinene, terpinen-4-ol, terpinolene,[6] allo-aromadendrene,[7] β-caryophyllene, citronellal, ocimene, fenchone, geraniol and many others in the volatile oil of the leaf and fruit.[8]

Flavonoids

Rutin, quercitrin and many other quercetin glycosides are present in the leaf,[9,10] and rhamnetin, quercetin, taxifolin, engeletin, naringenin and eriodictoyol in the stem bark.[8,11]

Tannins and polyphenols

Macrocarpals H, I, and J, euglobals I–VII, tellimagrandin I, eucalbanin C, gallic acid glucosides, and (+)-catechin have been isolated from the leaf,[12,13] and ellagic acid, with a number of rhamnosides, from the stem bark.[8,14] Rutin is present in the root[15] and gallic, vanillic and ellagic acids in the wood.[16]

Triterpenoids

Oleanolic, acetyloleanolic, betulinic, acetylbetulinic, ursolic, acetylursolic, 23-hydroxyursolic and trans-p-methoxycinnamoyloxy-ursolic acids are present in the wood, as well as their derivatives such as methyl cis-p-methoxycinnamoyloxyoleanolate and methyl cis-p-methoxycinnamoyloxyursolate, β-amyrin, uvaol and β-sitosterol.[17,18]

Others

(2-O-α-D-galactopyranosyl-4-O-methyl-α-D-glucurono)-D-xylan[19] is present in the stem bark and pinoresinol in the wood.[11]

Medicinal and pharmacological activities

Antioxidant activity: The antioxidant activity of eucalyptus oil was investigated using iron or EDTA-mediated oxidation of linoleic acid and compared with that of butylated hydroxytoluene and α-tocopherol. Eucalyptus oil showed antioxidant activity against linoleic acid autoxidation and did not show any prooxidant activity.[20] The antioxidant activities of the ellagic acid rhamnosides were demonstrated by measuring the inhibition of lipid peroxidation using rat liver microsomes, with IC_{50} values of 10.0–14.0 μg/ml.[13] Phenolic compounds including pinoresinol, methyl gallate, rhamnazin, rhamnetin, eriodictyol, quercetin, taxifolin, engelitin and catechin extracted from the wood and stem bark also showed antioxidant activity.[11,21]

Antibacterial activity: The activity of the ethyl acetate extract obtained from acid hydrolysates of the wood was demonstrated against a selection of bacteria and yeasts. Minimum inhibitory concentrations (MIC) in the range of 102–105 μg/ml were obtained.[22] The macrocarpals, which are phloroglucinol-sesquiterpene coupled constituents isolated from the leaves, demonstrated antibacterial activity against oral pathogens with MIC values ranging from 0.20 to 6.25 μg/ml. Inhibition of glucosyltransferase activity by these compounds was also noted.[13] Callus cultures initiated from *E. globulus* produced intracellular activity against the Gram-negative bacteria *Proteus vulgaris* and *Pseudomonas aeruginosa*, but the extract did not show activity against the yeasts *Candida albicans* or *C. tropicalis*.[23] Extracts of eucalyptus leaves were found to be as effective against *Trichophyton mentagrophytes, Propionibacterium acnes* and methicillin-resistant *Staphylococcus aureus* (MRSA)[24] and, together with chitosan, showed synergistic antimicrobial activity against *Staph. aureus, Bacillus subtilis, Escherichia coli, Aspergillus niger* and *Penicillium citrinum*. Application of the microbicides to chicken eggs, beef, wet tissues and disposable diapers was also described.[25] The macrocarpals were active against oral bacteria and had an inhibitory effect on glucosyltransferase (GTase). 60% ethanol extracts, containing mostly macrocarpals, were evaluated for their cariostatic effects in vitro and were found to significantly inhibit the growth of cariogenic bacteria, although their activity against intestinal bacteria was relatively low. The anticariogenic effect is enhanced by the strong inhibition of glucan synthesis (especially adhesive insoluble glucan) by GTase.[26]

The essential oil from eight species of eucalyptus leaves was investigated and the most active compounds found to be 1,8-cineole, caryophyllene, citronellal and cryptone. The antimicrobial activity was evaluated against five species of Gram-positive bacteria, four species of Gram-negative bacteria and seven species of fungi. Clarithromycin (antibacterial) and nystatin (antifungal) were used as standard reference compounds. The oil was effective against all the microorganisms used except *Penicillium digitatum* and 1,8-cineole appeared to be more potent against both bacteria and fungi than the other components of the oil.[27] The methanolic extract showed strong in vitro antimicrobial activity against

Staphylococcus aureus, Escherichia coli, Pseudomonas aeruginosa and *Candida albicans*.[28]

Hypoglycaemic activity: Eucalyptus is used as a traditional treatment for diabetes. Incorporation of leaves of eucalyptus into the diet (62.5 g/kg) and drinking water (2.5 g/l) reduced the hyperglycaemia of streptozotocin-treated mice. This was associated with reduced polydipsia, development of hyperphagia and hypoinsulinaemia and a reduced rate of body weight loss.[29] An aqueous extract of eucalyptus (AEE) (0.5 g/l) enhanced 2-deoxy-glucose transport by 50%, glucose oxidation by 60% and incorporation of glucose into glycogen by 90% in mouse abdominal muscle and evoked a stepwise enhancement of insulin secretion from the clonal pancreatic β-cell line (BRIN-BD11). The stimulatory effect was unaltered by the presence of 400 μmol diazoxide and prior exposure to AEE did not alter subsequent insulin secretory response to L-alanine, thereby negating a detrimental effect on cell viability. The effect of AEE was not potentiated by glucose or demonstrable in cells exposed to a depolarising concentration of KCl. The active principle was heat stable, acetone insoluble, stable to acid but abolished by exposure to alkali. Sequential extraction with solvents revealed activity in both the methanol and water fractions and indicated the presence of more than one biological active extract constituent.[30]

Antiinflammatory activity: The seed reduced oedematous swelling of the ear, inhibited the proliferation of granuloma and reduced blood capillary permeability in mice and inhibited cotton pellet granuloma and carrageenan-induced oedema in rats.[31]

Collagenase inhibition: 50% ethanol extract inhibited collagenase activity which was attributed to the polyphenol compounds present.[32,33]

Antihypertensive and diuretic activity: The hydroalcoholic extract containing phloroglucinols produced 94.9% inhibition of angiotensin-converting enzyme (ACE)[34] and a decoction of the dried leaf, administered nasogastrically to rats at a dose of 1.0 g/kg, showed diuretic activity.[35]

Insect repellant and insecticidal activity: The oil has insect repellant, acaricidal and pediculicidal effects.[8]

Larvicidal activity: The crude aqueous extract derived from fresh leaves demonstrated lethal activity against *Aedes aegypti* and *Culex quinquefasciatus* larvae, with a maximum effect after 48 hours exposure.[36]

Antitumour activity: The euglobals and related compounds demonstrated strong inhibitory effects on Epstein–Barr virus activation by a short-term in vitro assay.[37,38]

Safety profile

Eucalyptus globulus is listed as a Class 2d herb by the American Herbal Products Association. It is contraindicated in inflammatory diseases of the bile ducts and gastrointestinal tract and in severe liver diseases.[39] Overdose leads in rare cases to nausea, vomiting and diarrhoea. Eucalyptus oil induces liver enzymes, so may affect other drugs administered concurrently,[40] and can be dangerous if taken internally. Likewise, infants and children should not have preparations containing the oil applied directly to the face, as it can lead to glottal or bronchial spasms and asthma-like attacks.

Mice treated subcutaneously with eucalyptus oil at a dose of 135 mg/kg body weight during the period of organogenesis (days 6–15 of gestation) showed no evidence of embryotoxicity or foetotoxicity.[41] The oral LD_{50} of eucalyptus oil in the rat is 4.44 g/kg body weight[42] and 3.32 g/kg in mice.[43]

Dosage

Internal, average daily dose: leaf 4–6 g, oil 0.3–0.6 g

External: 5–20% in oil and semi-solid preparations, 5–10% in aqueous alcoholic preparations[44]

Ayurvedic properties

Rasa: *Katu* (pungent), *tikta* (bitter)

Guna: *Laghu* (light), *snighda* (unctuous)

Veerya: *Ushna* (hot)

Vipaka: *Katu* (pungent)

Dosha: Pacifies *kapha* and *vata*

Further reading

Blumenthal M, Busse WR, Goldberg A et al (eds) 1999 The complete Commission E monographs. American Botanical Council, Austin, Texas

Bown D 1995 Encyclopaedia of herbs and their uses. Dorling Kindersley, London

Chevallier A 1996 The encyclopedia of medicinal plants. Dorling Kindersley, London

European Scientific Cooperative on Phytochemistry 1999 Monographs on the medicinal uses of plant drugs. Fascicule 6. ESCOP, Exeter, UK

Ross I 1999 Medicinal plants of the world, vol 1. Humana Press, Totowa, New Jersey

References

1 Kandasamy OS, Yassin MM, Babu RC 2000 Biology, ecology, silviculture, and potential uses of Eucalyptus – an overview. Journal of Medicinal and Aromatic Plants 22(1B):330

2 Sastry KP, Kumar S 2000 Cultivation of economically important Eucalyptus species in the Western Ghats of Tamil Nadu. Journal of Medicinal and Aromatic Plants 22(1B):528

3 Jha MK 1992 The folk veterinary system of Bihar – a reseach survey. NDDB, Gujrat, India

4 International Institute of Rural Reconstruction 1994 Ethnoveterinary medicine in Asia. An information kit on traditional animal health care practices. IIRR, Silang, Philippines

5 Renedo J, Otero JA, Mira JR 1990 Huile essentielle d'*Eucalyptus globulus* L. d'Cantabrie (Espagne). Variation au cours de la distillation. Plantes Medicinales et Phytotherapie 24:31

6 Dethier M, Nduwimana A, Cordier Y, Menut C, Lamaty G 1994 Aromatic plants of tropical central Africa. XVI. Studies on essential oils of five eucalyptus species grown in Burundi. Journal of Essential Oil Research 6(5):469

7 Erazo S, Bustos C, Erazo AM et al 1990 Comparative study of the twelve species of Eucalyptus acclimatized in Quilpue Region, Chile. Plantes Medicinales et Phytotherapie 24(4):248

8 Ross I 2001 Medicinal plants of the world, vol. 2. Humana Press, Totowa, New Jersey

9 Manguro LOA, Mukonyi KW, Githiomi JK 1995 A new flavonol glycoside from *Eucalyptus globulus* subsp. *Maidenii.* Natural Products Letters 7(3):163

10 Conde E, Cadahia E, Garcia-Vallejo MC 1997 Low molecular weight polyphenols in leaves of *Eucalyptus camaldulensis, E. globulus* and *E. rudis*. Phytochemical Analysis 8:186

11 Yun BS, Lee IK, Kim JP, Chung SH, Shim GS, Yoo ID 2000 Lipid peroxidation inhibitory activity of some constituents isolated from the stem bark of *Eucalyptus globulus*. Archives of Pharmaceutical Research 23(2):147

12 Hou AJ, Liu YZ, Yang H, Lin ZW, Sun HD 2000 Hydrolyzable tannins and related polyphenols from *Eucalyptus globulus*. Journal of Asian Natural Products and Research 2(3):205

13 Osawa K, Yasuda H, Morita H, Takeya K, Itokawa H 1996 Macrocarpals H, I and J from the leaves of *Eucalyptus globulus*. Journal of Natural Products 59(9):823

14 Kim JP, Lee IK, Yun BS et al 2001 Ellagic acid rhamnosides from the stem bark of *Eucalyptus globulus*. Phytochemistry 57(4):587

15 Lagrange H, Jay-Allgemand C, Lapeyrie F 2001 Rutin, the phenolglycoside from eucalyptus root exudates, stimulates *Pisolithus hyphal* growth at picomolar concentrations. New Phytology 149(2):349

16 Conde E, Cadahia E, Garcia-Vallejo MC, Fernandez de Simon MB 1995 Polyphenolic composition of wood extracts from *Eucalyptus camaldulensis, E. globulus* and *E. rudis*. Holzforschung 49(5):411

17 Martinez-Inigo MJ, Gutierrez A, del Rio JC, Martinez MJ, Martinez AT 2000 Time course of fungal removal of lipophilic extractives from *Eucalyptus globulus* wood. Journal of Biotechnology 84(2):119

18 Santos GG, Alves JCN, Rodilla JML, Duarte AP, Lithgow AM, Urones JG 1997 Terpenoids and other constituents of *Eucalyptus globulus*. Phytochemistry 44(7):1309

19 Shatalov AA, Evtuguin DV, Pascoal Neto C 1999 (2-O-α-D-galactopyranosyl-4-O-methyl-α-D-glucurono)-D-xylan from *Eucalyptus globulus* Labill. Carbohydrates Research 320(1–2):93

20 Dessi MA, Deiana M, Rosa A et al 2001 Antioxidant activity of extracts from plants growing in Sardinia. Phytotherapy Research 15(6):511

21 Cruz JM, Dominguez JM, Dominguez H, Parajo JC 1999 Solvent extraction of hemicellulosic wood hydrolysates: a procedure useful for obtaining both detoxified fermentation media and polyphenols with antioxidant activity. Food Chemistry 67(2):147

22 Cruz JM, Dominguez JM, Dominguez H, Parajo JC 2001 Antioxidant and antimicrobial effects of extracts from hydrolysates of lignocellulosic materials. Journal of Agricultural and Food Chemistry 49(5):2459

23 Khafagi IK 1999 Screening *in vitro* cultures of some Sinai medicinal plants for their antibiotic activity. Egyptian Journal of Microbiology 34(4):613

24 Sakaino M, Takahashi T, Kokubo I 1999 Eucalyptus extracts as antibacterial agents. Japanese Patent JP 11080012

25 Takahashi T 2000 Microbiocides containing Eucalyptus leaf extract and chitosan. Japanese Patent JP 2000154109

26 Osawa K, Saeki T, Yasuda H, Morita H, Takeya K, Itokawa H 1998 Antibacterial activity of *Eucalyptus globulus* on cariogenic bacteria and its inhibitory effect on glucosyltransferase. Natural Medicines (Tokyo) 52(1):32

27 Saeed MA, Sabir AW 1995 Anti-microbial studies of the constituents of Pakistani eucalyptus oils. Journal of the Faculty of Pharmacy, Gazi University 12(2):129

28 Navarro V, Villarreal L, Rojas G, Lozoya X 1996 Anti-microbial evaluation of some plants used in Mexican traditional medicine for the treatment of infectious diseases. Journal of Ethnopharmacology 53:143

29 Swanston-Flatt SK, Day C, Bailey CJ, Flatt PR 1990 Traditional plant treatments for diabetes. Studies in normal and streptozotocin diabetic mice. Diabetologia 33(8):462

30 Gray AM, Flatt PR 1998 Antihyperglycemic actions of *Eucalyptus globulus* (Eucalyptus) are associated with pancreatic and extra-pancreatic effects in mice. Journal of Nutrition 128(12):2319

31 Jiao S, Chen B, Gao W, Song H 1996 Studies on the anti-inflammatory and analgesic action of Tasmanian blue-gum (*Eucalyptus globulus*) seed. Zhongcaoyao 27(4):223

32 Kyotani D, Obayashi K, Okano Y, Masaki H 1999 Inhibitory effect of *Eucalyptus globulus* on collagenase type I (MMP-1). Nippon Koshohin Kagakkaishi 23(2):83

33 Obayashi K, Kyotani T, Masuda K, Okano Y, Masaki H 1998 Inhibitory effects of plant extracts

on matrix proteinases. Nippon Koshohin Gijusush a Kaishi 32(3):272

34 Saeki T, Osawa K, Yasuda H 1999 Angiotensin-converting enzyme inhibitors and foods and beverages containing them. Japanese Patent JP 11060498

35 Caceres A, Giron LM, Martinez AM 1987 Diuretic activity of plants used for the treatment of urinary ailments in Guatemala. Journal of Ethnopharmacology 19(3):233

36 Monzon RB, Alvior JP, Luczon LL, Morales AS, Mutuc FE 1994 Larvicidal potential of five Philippine plants against *Aedes aegypti* (L.) and *Culex quinquefasciatus* (Say). Southeast Asian Journal of Tropical Medicine and Public Health 25(4):755

37 Takasaki M, Konoshima T, Fujitani K et al 1990 Inhibitors of skin-tumor promotion. VIII. Inhibitory effects of euglobals and their related compounds on Epstein-Barr virus activation 1. Chemical and Pharmaceutical Bulletin 38(10):2737

38 Takasaki M, Konoshima T, Kozuka M, Haruna M, Ito K, Shingu T 1995 Structures of euglobals from Eucalyptus plants. Toronkai Koen Yoshishu 37:517

39 McGuffin M, Hobbs C, Upton R, Goldberg A 1997 Botanical safety handbook. American Herbal Products Association. CRC Press, Boca Raton, USA

40 Blumenthal M, Busse WR, Goldberg A et al 1998 The complete German Commission E monographs. American Botanical Council, Austin, Texas

41 Pages N, Fournier G, Le Luyer F, Marques MC 1990 Les huiles essentielles et leur proprietes teratogenes potentielles: example de l'huile essentielle d'*Eucalyptus globulus*, etude preliminaire chez la souris. Plantes Medicinales et Phytotherapie 24:21

42 Von Skramlik E 1959 Uber die giftigkeit und vertraglichkeit von atherischen olen. Pharmazie 14:435

43 Ohsumi T, Kuroki K, Kimura T, Murakami Y 1984 Study on acute toxicities of essential oils used in endodontic treatment. Kyushu Shika Gakki Zasshi 38:1064

44 European Scientific Cooperative on Phytochemistry 1999 Monographs on the medicinal uses of plant drugs. Fascicule 6. ESCOP, Exeter

Euphorbia hirta L. (Euphorbiaceae)

English: Snakeweed

Hindi: *Dudhi*

Sanskrit: *Dugadhika*

According to the Doctrine of Signatures, the plant has a reputation for increasing milk flow in women, because of its milky latex, and is used for other female complaints as well as diseases of the respiratory tract. Other species of Euphorbia are sometimes substituted but this should be done with great care as many of these contain poisonous diterpene esters.[1]

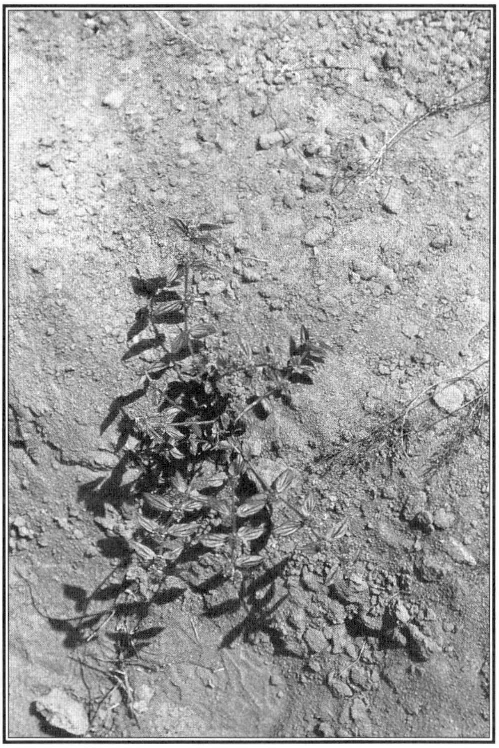

Habitat

The plant is native to India but is a pantropical weed, found especially on roadsides and wasteland.

Botanical description

A small, erect or ascending annual herb reaching up to 50 cm, with hairy stems (Plate 27). The leaves are opposite, elliptical, oblong or oblong-lanceolate, with a faintly toothed margin and darker on the upper surface. The flowers are small, numerous and crowded together in dense cymes about 1 cm in diameter. The fruits are yellow, three-celled, hairy, keeled capsules, 1–2 mm in diameter, containing three brown, four-sided, angular, wrinkled seeds.

Parts used

Whole plant.

Traditional and modern use

The plant has been used for female disorders but is now more important in treating respiratory ailments, especially cough, coryza, bronchitis and asthma. In India it is used to treat worm infestations in children and for dysentery, gonorrhoea, jaundice, pimples, digestive problems and tumours.

Ethnoveterinary usage

The fresh milky latex is applied to wounds and warts and the root of the plant is used in sprains and inflammation, miscarriage, epilepsy, maggots in wounds and irregular growth of teeth.[2]

Major chemical constituents

Flavonoids

Euphorbianin, leucocyanidol, camphol, quercitrin and quercitol.[3,4]

Polyphenols

Gallic acid, myricitrin, 3,4-di-O-galloylquinic acid, 2,4,6-tri-O-galloyl-D-glucose, 1,2,3,4,6-penta-O-galloyl-β-D-glucose.[5,6]

Tannins

Euphorbins A, B, C, D, E.[7]

Triterpenes and phytosterols

β-Amyrin, 24-methylenecycloartenol, and β-sitosterol.[8]

Alkanes

Heptacosane, n-nonacosane and others.[9]

Medicinal and pharmacological activities

Antiamoebic activity: The polyphenolic extract of the whole plant inhibited the growth of *Entamoeba histolytica* with a minimum active concentration of less than 10 μg/ml.[10]

Antispasmodic activity: The same extract, at a concentration of 80 μg/ml in an organ bath, also exhibited more than 70% inhibition of acetylcholine and/or KCl solution-induced contractions on isolated guinea pig ileum.[9]

Antidiarrhoeal activity: The antidiarrhoeal activity of a lyophilised decoction of the whole plant was investigated in mice. It demonstrated activity in experimental models of diarrhoea induced by castor oil, arachidonic acid and prostaglandin E_2.[11] Quercitrin, a flavonoid glycoside isolated from *Euphorbia hirta*, showed antidiarrhoeal activity, at doses of 50 mg/kg, against castor oil- and PGE_2-induced diarrhoea in mice, but not when magnesium sulphate was used as a cathartic agent. It also delayed small intestinal transit in the rat if this was accelerated with castor oil, but did not modify the fluid transport across the colonic mucosa when administered intraluminally. However, quercetin, the aglycone of quercitrin, increased colonic fluid absorption in the presence of secretagogue compounds, suggesting that the antidiarrhoeal activity of quercitrin is due to its aglycone, which is released by the glycoside in the intestine.[12]

Antiinflammatory activity: The n-hexane extract of the aerial parts of *E. hirta* and its main constituent triterpenes, β-amyrin, 24-methylenecycloartenol, and β-sitosterol were evaluated for antiinflammatory effects in mice. Both the extract and the triterpenes exerted significant and dose-dependent anti-inflammatory activity in the model of phorbol acetate-induced ear inflammation in mice.[8,13] The lyophilised aqueous extract showed analgesic, antipyretic and antiinflammatory activity in mice and rats. A central depressant activity, expressed by a strong sedative effect associated with anxiolytic effect, was also observed.[14]

Anticancer activity: Extracts of *Euphorbia hirta* have been found to show selective cytotoxicity against several cancer cell lines. The plant is useful in effective treatment of cancers, particularly malignant melanomas and squamous cell carcinomas.[14]

Antibacterial activity: The antibacterial effects of a methanol extract of *E. hirta* was demonstrated in vitro using species of

Shigella. The extract was non-cytotoxic and antibacterial.[15]

Immunomodulatory activity: Aqueous and aqueous-alcoholic extracts, containing flavonoids, polyphenols, sterols and terpenes, demonstrated immunostimulant activity. The aqueous extract affected lectin-induced lymphoblast transformation in vitro.[16]

Antifungal activity: An ethanolic extract displayed antifungal activity when tested against the plant pathogens *Colletotrichum capsici, Fusarium pallidoroseum, Botryodiplodia theobromae, Alternaria alternata, Penicillium citrinum, Phomopsis caricae-papayae* and *Aspergillus niger* using the paper disc diffusion technique.[17]

Aflatoxin inhibition activity: An aqueous extract significantly inhibited aflatoxin production on rice, wheat, maize and groundnut.[18]

Galactogenic activity: The powdered plant, given to female guinea pigs before puberty, increased the development of the mammary glands and induced secretion.[19]

Antifertility activity: *Euphorbia hirta* at a dose level of 50 mg/kg body weight reduced the sperm motility and density of cauda epididymal and testis sperm suspension significantly, leading eventually to 100% infertility.[20]

Antiasthmatic activity: The drug is reported to have a relaxation effect on the bronchial tubes and a depressant action on respiration.[21]

Safety profile

Maximum tolerated dose of 50% alcoholic extract of whole plant when given IP to mice was found to be 1000 mg/kg body weight.[22]

Dosage

Dried plant: 120–300 mg or as infusion

Liquid extract (1:1 in 45% alcohol): 0.1–0.3 ml

Ayurvedic properties

Guna: *Snigdha* (unctuous)

Rasa: *Madhur* (sweet)

Veerya: *Shita* (cold)

Vipaka: *Madhur* (sweet)

Dosha: Pacifies *pitta*

Further reading

Chevallier A 1996 The encyclopedia of medicinal plants. Dorling Kindersley, London

Duke JA 1992 Handbook of phytochemical constituents of GRAS herbs and other economic plants. CRC Press, Boca Raton

Leung DY, Foster S 1996 Encyclopedia of common natural ingredients used in food, drugs and cosmetics. John Wiley, New York

Council of Scientific and Industrial Research 1985 The wealth of India. PID, CSIR, New Delhi

References

1 Evans FJ, Taylor SE 1983 Proinflammatory, tumour-promoting and anti-tumour diterpenes of the plant families Euphobiaceae and Thymeliaceae. Fortschritte der Chemie Organischer Naturstoffe 44:27–72

2 Jha MK 1992 The folk veterinary system of Bihar – a research survey. NDDB, Anand, Gujrat

3 Blanc P, De Saqui-Sannes G 1972 Flavonoids of *Euphorbia hirta* (Euphorbiaceae). Plantes Medicinales et Phytotherapie 6(2):106

4 Aqil M, Khan IZ 1999 Euphorbianin, a new flavonol glycoside from *Euphorbia hirta* Linn. Global Journal of Pure and Applied Science 5(3):371

5 Chen L 1991 Polyphenols from leaves of *Euphorbia hirta* L. Zhongguo Zhongyao Zazhi 16(1):38

6 Yoshida T, Chen L, Shingu T, Okuda T 1988 Tannins and related polyphenols of Euphorbiaceous plants. IV. Euphorbins A and B, novel dimeric dehydroellagitannins from *Euphorbia hirta* L. Chemical and Pharmaceutical Bulletin 36(8):2940

7 Yoshida T, Namba O, Yokoyama K, Okuda T, Chen L 1989 Hydrolyzable tannin oligomers from Euphorbiaceae. Tennen Yuki Kagobutsu Toronkai Koen Yoshishu 31:601

8 Martinez V, Mariano A, Teresa OR, Lazcano ME, Bye R 1999 Anti-inflammatory active compounds from the n-hexane extract of *Euphorbia hirta.* Reviews Sociedad Quimica de Mexico 43:103

9 Gnecco S, Perez C, Bittner M, Becerra J, Silva YM 1996 Distribution pattern of n-alkanes in Chilean species from the Euphorbiaceae family. Bolletino Sociedad Chilena de Quimica 41(3):229

10 Tona L, Kambu K, Ngimbi N et al 2000 Antiamoebic and spasmolytic activities of extracts from some antidiarrhoeal traditional preparations used in Kinshasa, Congo. Phytomedicine 7(1):31

11 Galvez J, Zarzuelo A, Crespo ME, Lorente MD, Ocete MA, Jimenez J 1993 Antidiarrheal activity of *Euphorbia hirta* extract and isolation of an active flavonoid constituent. Planta Medica 59(4):333

12 Galvez J, Crespo ME, Jimenez J, Suarez A, Zarzuelo A 1993 Antidiarrheic activity of quercitrin in mice and rats. Journal of Pharmacy and Pharmacology 45(2):157

13 Lanhers MC, Fleurentin J, Dorfman P, Mortier F, Pelt JM 1991 Analgesic, antipyretic and anti-inflammatory properties of *Euphorbia hirta*. Planta Medica 57(3):225

14 Aylward JH, (Peplin Pty. Ltd., Australia). Patent. Appl. WO 9908994, 1999

15 Vijaya K, Ananthan S, Nalini R 1995 Antibacterial effect of theaflavin, polyphenon 60 (*Camellia sinensis*) and *Euphorbia hirta* on *Shigella* spp. – a cell culture study. Journal of Ethnopharmacology 49(2):115

16 Tamas Szenasi E (Hung.) 1992 *Euphorbia hirta* extracts as immunostimulants. German Patent DE 4102054

17 Mohamed S, Saka S, El-Sharkawy SH, Ali AM, Muid S 1996 Antimycotic screening of 58 Malaysian plants against plant pathogens. Pesticide Science 47(3):259

18 Singh P, Sinha KK 1986 Inhibition of aflatoxin production on some agricultural commodities through aqueous plant extracts. Journal of the Indian Botanical Society 65(1):30

19 Blanc P, Bertrand P, de Saqui-Sannes G, Lescure R 1963 Galactogenic properties of plants of the African flora: *Sersalisia djalonensis* and *Euphorbia hirta*. Annales de Biologie Clinique (Paris) 21(10–12):829

20 Mathur A, Dixit VP, Dobal MP 1995 Antifertility plant product: *Euphorbia hirta* in males. Proceedings of the International Symposium on Male Contraception: Present and Future, New Delhi

21 Chopra RN, Chopra IC, Handa KL, Kapur LD 1994 Indigenous drugs of India. Academic Publishers, Calcutta

22 Dhar ML, Dhar MM, Dhawan BN, Mehrotra BN, Ray C 1968 Screening of Indian plants for biological activity: Part-I. Indian Journal of Experimental Biology 6:232

Ficus religiosa L. (Moraceae)

English: Sacred fig, bo-tree, peepul, peepal

Hindi: *Pipal*

Sanskrit: *Pippala, ashwattha*

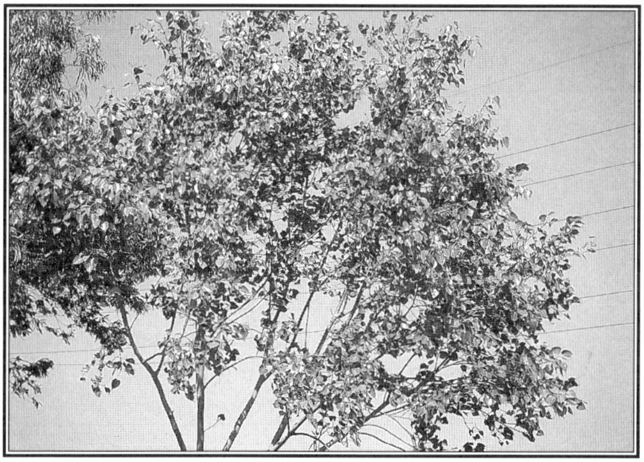

The peepul is worshipped all over India and is sacred to Hindus and Buddhists. Siddhartha sat in meditation under the peepal tree and attained enlightenment to become the Buddha. For this reason it is sometimes known as the Bodha (or 'awakening') tree. Brahmins offer prayers under it whilst facing East. It is long living: a peepul in Sri Lanka is reputed to be over 2000 years old. The bark forms an important ingredient in many Ayurvedic formulations.

Habitat

Peepul grows in northern and central India, in forests and alongside water. It is also widely cultivated throughout the subcontinent and south-east Asia, especially in the vicinity of the temples.

Botanical description

A large, glabrous tree, with a characteristic, milky latex and the trunk often covered with epiphytes (Plate 28). The bark is light grey and peels off in patches. The leaves are large, up to 16 cm in length, alternate, with long petioles (up to 12 cm) and a broadly ovate, subcoriacious lamina. The tip is long, lanceolate and cuspidate, the margin sinuate and the base truncate. The female fruit (figs) are small, axillary, paired, sessile, obovoid or globose, purplish when ripe. The male fruits are osteolar, sessile, ovate-lanceolate.

Parts used

Fruits, bark, seeds, leaves and latex.

Traditional and modern use

The bark and leaves are taken for diarrhoea and dysentery and the leaves for constipation. The leaves are sometimes applied with clarified butter as a poultice to boils and to swollen salivary glands in mumps. The powdered fruit is taken for asthma and the latex is used to treat warts. The bark is astringent, cooling, haemostatic and laxative. It is used in diabetes, diarrhoea, leucorrhoea, menorrhagia, nervous disorders, for vaginal and other urinogenital disorders and to improve the complexion. It has also been used in earache, bone fractures, glandular diseases (especially suppurating glands in the neck), scabies and other skin diseases and for ulcers and soreness in the mouth. An infusion or decoction of bark with a little honey has been used in gonorrhoea. Water in which the freshly burnt ashes of the bark have been steeped is said to cure obstinate cases of hiccups and to alleviate vomiting, and milk boiled with dried bark is a reputed aphrodisiac. Medicated oil made from the root bark is applied externally to skin diseases such as eczema, leprosy and is also used in rheumatism. The seeds and fruits are cooling, laxative and refrigerant. Leaves and young shoots are purgative.

Ethnoveterinary usage

In folk veterinary medicine it is used for swelling of the lung, opacity of the cornea and epilepsy. It is also used to treat blisters, abscesses and wounds in the mouth, at the root of the tail and near the hoof. It is recommended for throat diseases, kidney stones, blindness, otitis, rheumatism, bone dislocations, sprains and fractures, mastitis, jaundice, bloody dysentery, diarrhoea, glossitis, haematuria, miscarriage, indigestion, hernia, holes in the hard palate, broken horn and bee sting. In cows and buffaloes it is administered to treat repeat oestrus.[1] The fruits are a nutritious food for cattle.

Major chemical constituents

Sterols

Lanosterol, β-sitosterol and its glucoside, stigmasterol, lupen-3-one are present in the bark[2,3] and campestrol, stigmasterol, 28-isofucosterol, α-amyrin, β-amyrin and lupeol in the leaf.[4]

Coumarins

Bergapten and bergaptol have been isolated from the bark.[4]

Tannins

The leaves contain significant amounts of tannic acid.[5]

Aminoacids

Asparagine and tyrosine have been isolated from the fruit; alanine, threonine, tyrosine and valine from the seed[6] and arginine, serine, aspartic acid, glycine, threonine, alanine, proline, tryptophan, tyrosine, methionine, valine, isoleucine, leucine and others from the leaf.[7]

Vitamin

Vitamin K1 has been found in the stem bark.[4]

Hydrocarbons and aliphatic alcohols

n-Nonacosane, n-hentriacontanen-hexacosanol, n-octacosanol in the leaf.[8]

Minerals

Calcium, iron, copper, manganese and zinc are present in the leaf.[9]

Medicinal and pharmacological activities

Hypoglycaemic activity: β-sitosteryl-D-glucoside, isolated from the dried powdered bark and given by IV injection, produced a dose-dependent decrease in blood sugar. This compound, when given orally at 25 mg/kg body weight, caused a gradual reduction in blood sugar with a maximum at 4 hours. Tolbutamide, at the same dose, caused a maximal hypoglycaemic response in

3 hours.[3] An extract of *Ficus religiosa* has also shown hypoglycaemic activity, which was less than tolbutamide.[10]

Hypolipidaemic activity: Fibre from *Ficus religiosa*, fed at 10% dietary levels to rats, produced a greater resistance to hyperlipidaemia than did cellulose. It influenced total lipid, cholesterol, triglyceride and phospholipid levels in the liver to varying extents.[11]

Antiulcer activity: An aqueous extract of the bark, at 500 mg/kg, was studied for its effect on various models of gastroduodenal ulcers in rats, when given orally for 3 days. It was found to protect the animals against 2 hour cold-restraint stress and pylorus ligation-induced gastric ulcers and cystamine-induced duodenal ulcers. However, it was not effective against acute aspirin-induced gastric ulcers. The antiulcerogenic effect was thought to be due to an inhibitory effect on acid-pepsin secretion and augmentation of mucosal defensive factors, leading to enhanced mucin secretion and decreased cell shedding.[12]

Parasympatholytic and antiasthmatic activity: A 95% ethanolic extract of the bark relaxed the intestines of the rat, guinea pig, rabbit and dog and the uterus of the rat. It antagonised the spasmolytic effects of acetylcholine (Ach), histamine, barium chloride and serotonin, blocked the cardiovascular effects of Ach and protected guinea pigs against Ach and histamine-induced asthma.[13] When tested on the blood pressure of anaesthetised dog, it had vagolytic activity and antagonised Ach, but not histamine. The extract also relaxed the bronchial musculature and antagonised Ach-induced spasm in tracheal chain of the dog.[14]

The dried, powdered interior bark of *Ficus religiosa* has been suggested as a treatment for the symptoms of bronchial asthma in humans.[15]

Antitumour activity: The fruit extract demonstrated antitumour activity in the potato disc bioassay.[16]

Antibacterial activity: The fruit extract possesses significant antibacterial activity.[15] Bergapten and bergaptol, isolated from the bark, also showed antimicrobial activity.[2]

Antiprotozoal activity: The 50% alcoholic extract of stem bark showed in vitro antiamoebic activity against *Entamoeba histolytica* strain STA.[17]

Antiviral activity: The 50% alcoholic extract of the stem bark, at a dose of 0.05 mg/ml, also demonstrated antiviral activity against Ranikhet disease virus. It produced a 75% reduction in viral progeny in chorio-allantoic membrane cultures or chick embryo fibroblasts monolayers incubated at 37°C. The viral progeny was measured by noting the HA titre of the culture fluid after 48-hour incubation.[16]

Anthelmintic activity: The same extract was effective against *Ascaridia galli* when tested in vitro. The pH of the medium was adjusted to 7.2 and the period of incubation was 48 hours.[16]

Oestrogenic activity: The leaves of *Ficus religiosa* have shown oestrogenic activity.[18]

Dietary supplementation: The effects of incorporating the whole plant parts on feed intake, weight gain, feed efficiency ratio (FER), dry matter digestibility (DMD) and true protein digestibility (TPD) were studied in weanling rats. Their inclusion did not affect weight gain significantly, although all other parameters were influenced to a varying extent.[11] Leaves containing around 0.7% tannic acid were fed ad libitum to goats and found to be a useful fodder. All the goats showed positive balances of nitrogen, calcium and phosphorus.[5]

Safety profile

An alcoholic extract of the bark gave an oral LD_{50} in albino rats of 2.24 g/kg and an intravenous LD_{50} of 0.80 g/kg.[14] The LD_{50} of β-sitosterol D-glucoside was found to be 62 mg/kg in mice when given intraperitoneally.[3] The maximum tolerated dose (MTD) of a 50% alcoholic extract of stem bark was found to be 500 mg/kg when administered intraperitoneally to albino mice.[17]

Dosage

Powdered bark: 1–3 g

Decoction: 60–120 ml

Latex: applied topically

Ayurvedic properties

Rasa: *Kashaya* (astringent)

Guna: *Guru* (heavy), *ruksha* (dry)

Veerya: *Shita* (cold)

Vipaka: *Katu* (pungent)

Dosha: Pacifies *kapha* and *pitta*

Further reading

Bharatiya Vidya Bhavan's Swami Prakashanandra Ayurveda Research Centre 1992 Selected medicinal plants of India. Chemexcil, Mumbai

Chevallier A 1996 The encyclopedia of medicinal plants. Dorling Kindersley, London

Kapoor LD 2001 Handbook of Ayurvedic medicinal plants. CRC Press, Boca Raton

Sairam TV 1998 Home remedies, vol I. Penguin India, New Delhi

Sivarajan VV, Balachandran I 1994 Ayurvedic drugs and their plant sources. Oxford and IBH Publishing, New Delhi

References

1 Jha MK 1992 The folk veterinary system of Bihar – a research survey. NDDB, Gujrat, India

2 Swami KD, Malik GS, Bisht NPS 1989 Chemical investigation of stem bark of *Ficus religiosa* and *Prosopis spicigera*. Journal of the Indian Chemical Society 66(4):288

3 Ambike SH, Rao MRR 1967 Studies on a phytosterolin from the bark of *Ficus religiosa* Part I. Indian Journal of Pharmacy 29(3):91

4 Swami KD, Bisht NPS 1996 Constituents of *Ficus religiosa* and *Ficus infectoria* and their biological activity. Journal of the Indian Chemical Society 73(11):631

5 Panda SK, Panda NC, Sahu BK 1983 Effect of tree leaf tannin on dry matter intake by goats. Indian Veterinary Journal 60(8):660

6 Ali M, Qadry JS 1987 Amino acid composition of fruits and seeds of medicinal plants. Journal of the Indian Chemical Society 64(4):230

7 Verma RS, Bhatia SK 1986 Chromatographic study of aminoacids of the leaf protein concentrates of *Ficus religiosa* Linn. and *Mimusops elengi* Linn. Indian Journal of Hospital Pharmacy 23(5):231

8 Behari M, Rani K, Usha MT, Shimizu N 1984 Isolation of active principles from the leaves of *Ficus religiosa*. Current Agriculture 8(1–2):73

9 Desai HB, Desai MC, Patel BM, Patel BH, Shukla PC 1980 Proximate and trace elements content of the forest tree leaves of Dangs district collected during summer season. Gujrat Agricultural University Research Journal 6(1):34

10 Brahmachari HD, Augusti KT 1962 Orally effective hypoglycemic agents. Journal of Pharmacy and Pharmacology 14:254

11 Agarwal V, Chauhan BM 1988 A study on

composition and hypolipidemic effect of dietary fiber from some plant foods. Plant Foods and Human Nutrition 38(2):189

12 Bipul D, Maiti RN, Joshi VK, Agrawal VK, Goel RK 1997 Effect of some Sitavirya drugs on gastric secretion and ulceration. Indian Journal of Experimental Biology 35:1084

13 Malhotra CL, Das PK, Dhalla NS 1960 Parasympatholytic activity of *Ficus religiosa*. Indian Journal of Medical Research 48:734

14 Malhotra CL, Das PK, Dhalla NS 1960 Effect of *Ficus religiosa* on smooth muscles. Indian Journal of Physiology and Pharmacology 4:130

15 Patel JR, Patel DR 2000 Compositions for treatment of asthma containing *Ficus religiosa* bark admixed with rice pudding. US Patent No. 6149914

16 Mousa O, Vuorela P, Kiviranta J, Wahab SA, Hiltunen R, Vuorela H 1994 Bioactivity of certain Egyptian *Ficus* species. Journal of Ethnopharmacology 41(1–2):71

17 Dhar ML, Dhar MM, Dhawan BN, Mehrotra BN, Ray C 1968 Screening of Indian plants for biological activity. Part 1. Indian Journal of Experimental Biology 6:232

18 Ray BN, Pal AK 1967 Estrogenic activity of tree leaves as animal feed. Indian Journal of Physiology and Allied Sciences 20(1):6

Fumaria indica Pugsley (Fumariaceae) (syn. *F. parviflora* Lamk., *F. vallantii* Loisel.)

English: Fumitory

Hindi: *Pitpapra, khetpapra*

Sanskrit: *Parpata*

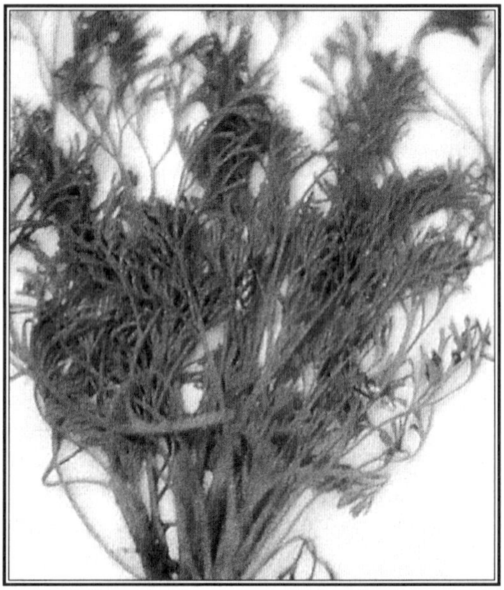

Fumaria indica is found throughout India and is one of the more commonly used herbs in Indian medicine. The plant is sold under the name *pitpapra* in Ayurvedic bazaars and used in the preparation of various traditional formulae such as *parpatadya kawatha* and *parpatadya arista*. It is also used in the Unani system of medicine and incorporated into *trifala shahtara*.

Habitat

The plant is distributed throughout India, particularly on the banks of the Ganges and in the Himalayas up to an altitude of 2700 m. It is also distributed in the higher elevations of the Mysore plateau and Nilgiris. It is also found in Europe, Africa and many other Asian countries.

Botanical description

It is an annual, diffuse herb, up to 30 cm high, with grooved branchlets (Plate 29). The leaves are pale green, 2–3 pinnatisect, 5–7 cm long. Flowers are asymmetrical, pale pink or white with purple tips, in terminal or leaf-opposed racemes, with a filiform style and a two-lobed stigma. The calyx consists of two lanceolate sepals which are much smaller than the corolla tube. The fruit is a small, indehiscent nutlet, rugose when dry, rounded at the top with two pits and containing one seed.

Parts used

Whole plant.

Traditional and modern use

Fumaria indica is used in aches and pains, diarrhoea, fever, influenza and liver complaints. The herb mixed with honey may be taken internally to prevent vomiting. A cold infusion of the plant is used to treat wasting diseases of children and to help cooling during fever and in the treatment of constipation and dyspepsia. It is used as a blood purifier for skin diseases and applied externally in leucoderma and as a fomentation for swollen joints. The dried plant is also used as an anthelmintic, diuretic and diaphoretic and, in combination with black pepper, for jaundice.

Ethnoveterinary usage

It is a very common plant in veterinary medicine and is used to overcome constipation and urinary problems in cattle.[1] It is used as a fodder in many parts of India, particularly in Assam. The leaf is used in udder infection of ruminants.

Major chemical constituents

Alkaloids

Protopine, cryptopine, dl-bicuculline, aldumine, fumaridine, fumarizine, spiroisoquinoline and d-hydrastine are chief alkaloids of the plant. Other, minor, alkaloids include parfumidine, parfumine, coptisine, tetrahydrocoptisine, fumariline, fumarilicine, narceimine, 8-methoxydihydrosanguinarine, oxysanguinarine, fumariflorine, lastourvilline, N-methyl corydaldine, oxycoptisine, raddeanine, N-methyl-hydrasteine, dehydrocheilanthifoline, narlumidine, papraine and paprazine.[2–10]

Others

Tannins and fumaric acid and other non-alkaloidal constituents such as nonacosanol and sitosterol, 19-methyloctacosanol and 3-methyloctacosanol have also been isolated from the plant.[11,12]

Medicinal and pharmacological activities

Hepatoprotective activity: A methanolic extract of the plant yielded monomethyl fumarate, which showed significant protection against hepatotoxicity induced by carbon tetrachloride, paracetamol and rifampicin in vivo. In an in vitro screening using thioacetamide-induced hepatotoxicity, the drug exhibited similar activity.[13]

Anticonvulsant activity: Fumariline, a spirobenzylisoquinoline alkaloid from the herb, showed a significant, dose-dependent anticonvulsant activity when tested using maximal electroshock-induced seizures.[14]

Analgesic and antiinflammatory activity: Fumariline showed antinociceptive activity in experimental animals, producing a dose-dependent activity measured as an increase in the latent period of the tail flick response (analgesic index). Alkaloids including narceimine, narlumidine and adlumidine exhibited antiinflammatory activity.[9] Protopine nitrate, an alkaloidal salt present in the plant, is a natural central nervous system stimulant.[15]

Antipsychotic activity: l-Tetrahydrocoptisine present in *Fumaria indica* exhibited neuroleptic activity. The antipsychotic activity of the constituent is like that of chlorpromazine in laboratory animals.[14]

Antifungal activity: Protopine, l-tetrahydrocoptisine, narlumidine and narlumicine from *Fumaria indica* were assessed against a number of spore-germinating plant pathogenic fungi. Narlumidine and protopine showed the most potent antifungal activity.[14]

Hypotensive activity: An extract of the plant was found to have a relaxant effect and produced a moderate fall in blood pressure in experimental animals. The major alkaloid protopine had a similar potency to that of papaverine.[16] In another study protopine exhibited marked relaxation on ileum and intestine of the experimental animals.[14]

Hypoglycaemic activity: *Fumaria indica*, administered orally to alloxan-induced diabetic animals, resulted in a significant reduction of the blood sugar levels.[17]

Safety profile

Fumaria indica has been used safely for many years in Ayurveda and Unani systems of medicine but no data are available.

Dosage

Decoction: 28–56 ml

Powder: 4–6 g

Ayurvedic properties

Rasa: *Tikta* (bitter)

Guna: *Laghu* (light)

Veerya: *Shita* (cold)

Vipaka: *Katu* (pungent)

Dosha: Pacifies *kapha* and *pitta*

Further reading

Gogte VM 1997 Ayurvedic pharmacology and therapeutic uses of medicinal plants. Bharatiya Vidya Bhavan, Mumbai

Husain A, Virmani OP, Popli SP et al 1992 Dictionary of Indian medicinal plants. CIMAP, Lucknow

Kapoor Ld 1990 Handbook of Ayurvedic medicinal plants. CRC Press, Boca Raton

Kaul MK 1997 Medicinal plants of Kashmir and Ladakh. Indus Publishing, New Delhi

Sivarajan VV, Balachandran I 1994 Ayurvedic drugs and their plant sources. Oxford and IBH Publishing, New Delhi

Thakur RS, Puri HS, Husain A 1989 Major medicinal plants of India. CIMAP, Lucknow

References

1 Jha MK 1992 Folk veterinary medicine of Bihar – a research project. NDDB, Anand, Gujrat

2 Sener B 1988 Turkish species of *Fumaria* L. and their alkaloids. IX. Alkaloids of *F. parviflora* Lam., *F. petteri* Reichb. Subsp. *thuretii* (Boiss.) Pugsley and *F. kralikii* Jardan. International Journal of Crude Drug Research 26(1):61

3 Temizer A, Kir S, Sener B, Orbey MT 1987 Determination of alkaloids by differential pulse polarography. II. *Fumaria* L. alkaloids. Journal de Pharmacie de Belgique 42(6):382

4 Atta-ur-Rahman, Ali SS, Qureshi MM, Hassan S, Bhatti K 1989 Fumarizine – a new benzylisoquinoline alkaloid from *Fumaria indica*. Fitoterapia 60(6):552

5 Atta-ur-Rahman, Bhatti MK, Ahmad H, Habib-ur-Rehman, Rycroft DS 1989 A new isoquinoline alkaloid papraine from *Fumaria indica*. Heterocycles 29(6):1091

6 Atta-ur-Rahman, Bhatti MK, Choudhary MI, Sener B 1992 Chemical constituents of *Fumaria indica*. Fitoterapia 63(2):129

7 Tripathi VK, Pandey VB 1992 Stem alkaloids of *Fumaria indica*. Phytochemistry 31(6):2188

8 Atta-ur-Rahman, Bhatti MK, Akhtar F, Choudhary MI 1992 Alkaloids of *Fumaria indica*. Phytochemistry 31(8):2869

9 Tripathi VK, Pandey VB 1992 Stem alkaloids of *Fumaria indica* and their biological activity. Planta Medica 58 (suppl. 1):A651

10 Kuryakov KH, Panov P 1976 On the alkaloids of *Fumaria parviflora* Lam. Chemical Abstracts 85:43724

11 Susplugas J, Privat G, Sarada JP 1967 The presence and distribution of choline in various organs of *Fumaria officinalis*, *F. parviflora* and *F. vaillanti*. Chemical Abstracts 67:97681s

12 Wahid MA 1961Chemical studies on *Fumaria parviflora*. I. Non-alkaloid constituents of the plant. Pakistan Journal of Scientific and Industrial Research 4:121

13 Rao KS, Mishra SH 1998 Antihepatotoxic activity of monomethyl fumarate isolated from *Fumaria indica*. Journal of Ethnopharmacology 60(3):207

14 Kumar A, Pandey VB, Seth KK, Dasgupta B, Bhattacharya SK 1986 Pharmacological actions of

fumariline isolated from *Fumaria indica*. Planta Medica 4:324

15 Tripathi YC, Dwivedi RK 1990 Central nervous system and anti-inflammatory activities of alkaloids of *Fumaria indica*. National Academy of Science Letters 13(6):231

16 Bhattacharya SK, Lal R, Sanyal AK, Das PK 1969 Pharmacological studies on *Fumaria parviflora* Lam. Indian Journal of Pharmacy 1:8

17 Akhtar MS, Khan QM, Kaliq T 1984 Effects of *Euphorbia prostrata* and *Fumaria parviflora* in normoglycaemic and alloxan-treated hyperglycaemic rabbits. Planta Medica 50:138

Gardenia gummifera L. (Rubiaceae)

English: Dikamali, cumbi-resin

Hindi: *Dikamali*

Sanskrit: *Nadi-hingu*

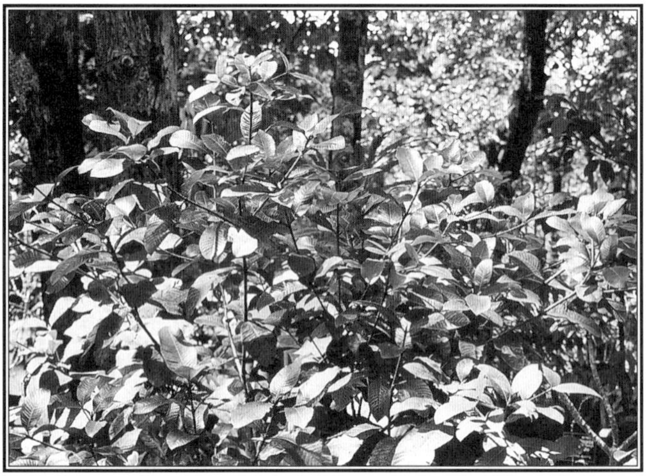

The gum of *dikamali* is one of the more important drugs in Ayurveda. The genus Gardenia is commonly grown for its attractive foliage and fragrant, showy flowers.

Habitat

It is found throughout the Deccan peninsula extending northwards to parts of Bihar. The shrub is common in deciduous forests of Tamil Nadu and Kerala and in some areas of Assam.

Botanical description

A large handsome shrub or small tree, reaching up to 2 m in height, often with a crooked stem and rough twisted branches (Plate 30). The leaves are sessile, cuneate or obovate and the flowers large, cream or yellowish, the fruits ovoid and fleshy. The leaf buds and the young shoots yield a resinous exudation, known in commerce as 'dikamali' or 'cumbi' gum, which is secreted freely in the form of tears. The shoots and buds are broken off with tears of resin attached and marketed either in this form or after agglutination into irregular masses. The resin is transparent, greenish-yellow, with a sharp taste and a peculiar odour.

Parts used

Gum resin.

Traditional and modern use

The oleoresin has a pungent odour resembling that of asafoetida and is occasionally used as a substitute for it, sometimes being known by the same name, i.e. *hing*. A decoction is prescribed in fevers, flatulent dyspepsia and as a stimulant and vermifuge. The gum may also be applied to open wounds and ulcers as an occlusive dressing, antiseptic, to keep flies away and to clean infected ulcers. Cumbi gum is used to treat nervous disorders in children, diarrhoea at the time of dentition ('teething') and rubbed on the gums to alleviate irritation.

Ethnoveterinary usage

The resin is extensively employed to keep away flies from sores, destroy maggots in wounds and as sheep wash. It is used for treating indigestion, bloat in ruminants and intestinal worms.[1,2]

Major chemical constituents

Triterpenes and phytosterols

Oleanonic aldehyde, erythrodiol, 19-α-hydroxyerythrodiol and β-sitosterol are present in the stem.

Flavonoids

Demethyltangeretin, nevadensin, gardenin, isoscutellarein, apigenin, numerous hydroxylated and methoxylated flavone derivatives including 5,7,3′,4′-tetrahydroxy-8-methoxyflavone and 5,7,3′,4′,5′-pentahydroxy-8-methoxyflavone, wogonin, 3′,4′-dihydroxywogonin, 3′,4′,5′-trihydroxywogonin and demethoxysudachitin.[3–8]

Medicinal and pharmacological activities

Antiseptic activity: The plant is reported to have demonstrable antiseptic activity.[9]

Insecticidal activity: Insecticidal effects have been reported.[10]

Hypothermic activity: A 50% ethanolic extract of the aerial parts of the plant showed CNS depressant activity and induced hypothermia and anticonvulsant activity against strychnine-induced seizures when tested in mice.[11]

Digestive and anthelmintic activity: It is reportedly an appetiser, digestive, carminative and anthelmintic and useful in anorexia, indigestion, constipation, flatulence and worms, particularly for treating tapeworm.[12]

Safety profile

A 50% alcoholic extract of the plant (excluding root), when administered IP to mice, showed LD_{50} of 1000 mg/kg body weight.[10]

Dosage

Gum resin: 250–500 mg

Ayurvedic properties

Guna: *Laghu* (light), *ruksha* (dry), *tikshna* (sharp)

Rasa: *Katu* (bitter), *tikta* (pungent)

Veerya: *Ushna* (lukewarm)

Dosha: Pacifies *kapha*

Further reading

Nadkarni AK 1976 Indian materia medica. Popular Prakashan PVT Ltd, Bombay

Thakur RS, Puri HS, Husain A 1989 Major medicinal plants of India. CIMAP, Lucknow

Council for Scientific and Industrial Research 1985 The wealth of India. PID, CSIR, New Delhi

References

1 Jha MK 1992 The folk veterinary system of Bihar – a research survey. NDDB, Anand, Gujrat

2 International Institute of Rural Reconstruction 1994 Ethnoveterinary medicines in Asia. An information kit on traditional animal health care practices. IIRR, Silang, Philippines

3 Gupta SR, Seshadri TR, Sharma CS, Sharma ND 1975 Chemical investigation of Dikamali gum. Isolation of a new flavone, 4′-hydroxywogonin. Indian Journal of Chemistry 13:785

4 Chhabra SC, Gupta SR, Sharma ND 1977 A new flavone from *Gardenia* gum. Phytochemistry 16(3):399

5 Krishnamurti M, Seshadri TR, Sharma ND 1971 Minor components of Dikamali gum. Indian Journal of Chemistry 9(2):189–190

6 Krishnamurti M, Seshadri TR, Sharma ND 1972 Chemical investigation of Dikamali gum:

isolation of two new flavones, dimethoxy and trimethoxy wogonins. Indian Journal of Chemistry 10:23

7 Chhabra SC, Gupta SR, Seshadri TR, Sharma ND 1976 Chemical investigation of Dikamali gum: isolation of two new flavones – 3′,4′-dihydroxy and 3′,4′,5′-trihydroxywogonin. Indian Journal of Chemistry 14B:651

8 Chhabra SC, Gupta SR, Sharma CS, Sharma ND 1977 A new wogonin derivative from *Gardenia* gum. Phytochemistry 16:1109

9 Chopra RN, Chopra LCC, Handa KL, Kapur LD 1994 Chopra's indigenous drugs of India. Academic Publishers, Calcutta

10 Mehta RK, Shilaskar DV 1967 Preliminary study on the insecticidal property of *Annona squamosa* L. and *Gardenia gummifera* L. Indian Medical Gazette 6(12):56

11 Dhar ML, Dhar MM, Dhawan BN, Mehrotra BN, Srimal RC, Tandon JS 1973 Screening of Indian medicinal plants for biological activity. Indian Journal of Experimental Biology 11:43

12 Gogte VVM 2000 Ayurvedic pharmacology and therapeutic uses of medicinal plants. Bharatiya Vidya Bhavan, Mumbai

Glycyrrhiza glabra L. (Papilionaceae)

English: Liquorice

Hindi: *Mulethi*

Sanskrit: *Yashtimadhu, madhuka*

The name 'glycyrrhiza' was coined by Dioscorides in the first century, by combining the Greek words *glukos* meaning sweet and *rhiza* meaning root. Theophrastus also referred to it as Radix Dulcis from the Latin equivalent. Liquorice has been used for centuries to treat various ailments throughout Europe and Asia; Pliny (23 AD) and Hippocrates (400 BC) both described the use of the plant. In Ayurveda it is considered to be a *rasayana* and is an important ingredient of many formulae, especially for bronchial conditions. Western herbalists use it for ulcers, as an antiinflammatory and expectorant and the Chinese ascribe rejuvenative and aphrodisiac powers to liquorice.

Habitat

It is a native of the Mediterranean region and the Near East and can now be found throughout the subtropical and temperate regions of the world. Liquorice is cultivated throughout Russia, Turkey, Greece, the Middle East, China and most of Asia and Europe and is readily commercially available as transversely cut pieces of root.

Botanical description

G. glabra is a hardy perennial shrub, attaining a height up to 2.5 m (Plate 31). The leaves are compound, imparipinnate, alternate, having 4–7 pairs of oblong, elliptical or lanceolate

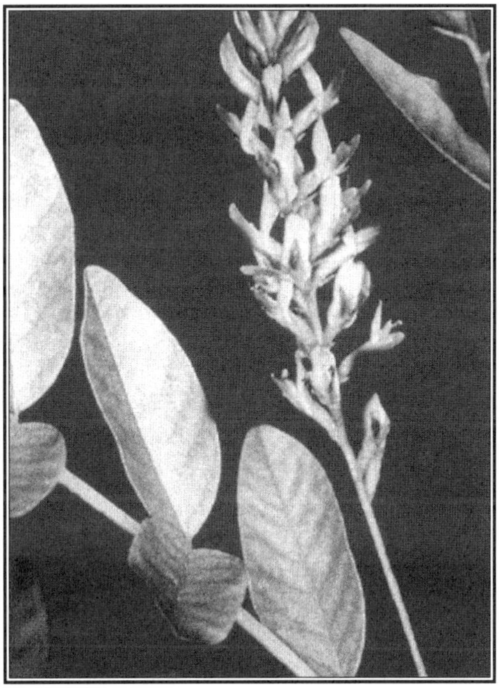

leaflets. The flowers are narrow, typically papilionaceous, borne in axillary spikes, lavender to violet in colour. The calyx is short, campanulate, with lanceolate tips and bearing glandular hairs. The fruit is a compressed legume or pod, up to 1.5 cm long, erect, glabrous, somewhat reticulately pitted, and usually contains 3-5 brown, reniform seeds. The taproot is approximately 1.5 cm long and subdivides into 3–5 subsidiary roots, about 1.25 cm long, from which the horizontal woody stolons arise. These may reach 8 m and when dried and cut, together with the root, constitute commercial liquorice. It may be found peeled or unpeeled. The pieces of root break with a fibrous fracture, revealing the yellowish interior with a characteristic odour and sweet taste.

Parts used

Dried roots and stolons, peeled or unpeeled.

Traditional and modern use

It is used as a tonic, laxative, demulcent, expectorant and emollient in many traditional systems of medicine. It finds particular use in cough, catarrh, bronchitis, fever, gastritis, gastric and duodenal ulcers and skin diseases and as a general tonic. It has been applied externally to cuts and wounds and used in the treatment of hyperdipsia, genitourinary diseases and many other minor indications, including as a corticosteroid replacement agent.

Ethnoveterinary usage

In India, *Glycyrrhiza glabra* has been used extensively for the treatment of various ailments of domestic animals from ancient times, for similar purposes to those in humans. For example, it is used for coughs and colds, as an expectorant and wound-healing agent in ruminants.[1,2]

Major chemical constituents

Triterpene saponins

Glycyrrhizin (glycyrrhizic acid) is the major saponin, responsible for the sweet taste of liquorice, and its aglycone, glycyrrhetinic acid; together with other derivatives and glycosides such as glycyrrhizol, glabrins A and B, glycyrrhetol, glabrolide, isoglabrolide and others.[4,5]

Flavonoids and isoflavonoids

Liquiritin, which during drying and storage undergoes partial conversion to isoliquiritin; their aglycones, liquiritigenin and isoliquiritigenin, isolicoflavonol, licoagrodione, glucoliquiritin apioside, prenyllicoflavone A, shinflavone, shinpterocarpin, 1-methoxyphyaseollin and rhamnoliquirilin.[5] A variety of isoflavones are also reported form the plant, including formononetin, glabrene, neoliquiritin, hispaglabridin A and B, glabridin, glabrol, 3-hydroxyglarol, glycyrrhisflavone, 4-O-methylglabridin, 3′-hydroxy-4′-O-methylglabridin and many 2-methyl isoflavones.[4,5,8]

Coumarins and coumestan derivatives

Herniarin, umbelliferone, C-liqucoumarin, 6-acetyl-5,hydroxy-4-methyl coumarin, glycycoumarin and licopyanocoumarin have been identified.[4,5,8]

Phytosterols

Stigmasterol, onocerin, β-sitosterol and β-amyrin.[4,5,8]

Volatile oil

Liquorice contains a trace amount (0.5%) of volatile oil, containing anethole, estragole, eugenol and hexanoic acid as the main constituents.[8]

Medicinal and pharmacological activities

Antiulcer activity: Liquorice has a well-documented antiulcer action, being as effective as cimetidine and pirenzapine in curing peptic ulcer.[6,7] An Ayurvedic preparation containing liquorice increased β-glucuronidase activity in the Brunner's glands, offering protection against duodenal ulcer.[8]

Hepatoprotective activity: Liquorice is used traditionally for the prevention of liver diseases.[9] Administration to experimental animals increased the duration of the lag phase of ascorbate free radical oxidation in the liver and myocardium, the antioxidant activity of the root powder being comparable to that of β-carotene, and markedly decreased lipid peroxides in liver.[10] An alcoholic extract increased the cumulative biliary and urinary excretion of acetaminophen without affecting the thioether or sulphate conjugates and also increased glucuronidation in rats, suggesting it may influence detoxification of xenobiotics.[11]

Antioxidant activity: An investigation using the isoflavonoids of liquorice focused on their ability to protect the liver mitochondria against oxidative stresses. This effect was linked with the inhibition of mitochondrial lipid peroxidation-related respiratory electron transport.[12] Glabridin and its derivatives contributed to the antioxidant activity induced by heavy metal ions and macrophages against low density lipoprotein (LDL) oxidation. LDL oxidation is a major factor in the production aetiology of early arteriosclerosis. The isoflavans also showed a potent scavenging effect on the DPPH radical and were able to chelate heavy metals. This action was associated with the 2′ hydroxy functional group as well as the hydrophobic moiety of the isoflavans.[13] Glabridin also inhibited the susceptibility of LDL to oxidation in an atherosclerotic apolipoprotein E deficient and in vitro human LDL oxidation model and prevented the consumption of β-carotene and lycopene.[14] Further experiments with glabridin and accompanying isoflavans suggested that glabridin is a potent inhibitor of cholesterol linoleate hydroperoxide formation.[15]

Antimicrobial activity: Extracts containing flavonoids showed significant antimycotic activity when evaluated using strains of *Candida albicans* isolated from clinical samples of acute vaginitis.[16] Flavonoid constituents isolated from liquorice hairy root cultures also exhibited antimicrobial activity when tested by the disc diffusion method.[17] Hispaglabridin A and B, glabridin, glabrol, 3-hydroxyglabrol and 4′-O-methylglabridin have demonstrated significant antimicrobial activity.[18]

Antiviral activity: Glycyrrhizin showed antiviral activity against Japanese encephalitis virus (JEV), with the inhibition of plaque formation at a concentration of 500 μg.[19] It also inhibits virus growth and inactivates virus particles.[20]

Anticancer activity: Liquorice potentiated the antitumour and antimetastatic activity of cyclophosphamide when tested in metastasising Lewis lung carcinoma.[21] Extracts have been assayed for cytotoxicity in vitro using the Yoshida ascites sarcoma, the petroleum ether extract exhibited a more potent activity than other solvent extracts.[22] Liquorice has also been shown to protect against skin tumorigenesis caused by DMBA (7,12-dimethyl-benz [a] anthracene) initiation and 12-O-tetradecanoylphorbol-13-acetate (TPA) promotion. The latency period of tumour onset was increased and the number of tumours decreased, possibly by inhibiting the carcinogen metabolism after DNA adduct formation.[23]

Antimutagenic activity: *Glycyrrhiza glabra* root and its isolated constituents were tested against ethyl methanesulphonate, N-methyl-N′-nitro-N-nitrosoguanidine and ribose-lysine Maillard models of mutagenesis using a Salmonella microsome reversion assay. The extract showed antimutagenic activity against ethyl methanesulphonate and 18-β glycyrrhetinic acid exhibited a significant desmutagenic activity against ribose-lysine mutagenic browning mixture.[24]

Antiinflammatory activity: Glycyrrhizin inhibited thrombin-induced platelet aggregation, which indicates antiinflammatory activity. It also prolonged plasma recalcification and fibrogen clotting times.[25] Glyderinine, a derivative of glycyrrhizic acid, reduced inflammation via the adrenal cortex, suppressed vascular permeability and allergic and antipyretic activity, without causing haemopoiesis or ulceration.[26]

Safety profile

Liquorice is considered safe within the designated therapeutic dosage. Excessive consumption may lead to hypertension and the potentiation of diuretic and corticosteroid activity. Its use in cardiovascular and renal patients is contraindicated as it may lead to disturbance of electrolytic balance and increased sensitivity to cardiac glycosides due to excess excretion of potassium. Use during breastfeeding is also not recommended.[27,28,29]

Dosage

Root powder: 1–5 g tid

Root extract: 1–1.5 g tid

Infusion: 2–4 g in 150 ml of hot water (after meals)

Ayurvedic properties

Rasa: *Madhur* (sweet)

Guna: *Guru* (heavy), *snigdha* (unctuous)

Veerya: *Shita* (cold)

Vipaka: *Madhur* (sweet)

Dosha: Pacifies *vata* and *pitta*

Further reading

Arya Vaidya Sala Kottakkal 1993 Indian medicinal plants, vol. 1. Orient Longman, Hyderabad

Bharatiya Vidya Bhavan's Swami Prakashanandra Ayurveda Research Centre 1992 Selected medicinal plants of India. Chemexcil, Mumbai

Bradley PR 1992 British herbal compendium, vol 1. British Herbal Medicine Association, Bournemouth

Duke JA 1992 Handbook of phytochemical constituents of GRAS herbs and other economic plants. CRC Press, Boca Raton

European Directorate for the Quality of Medicines 2001 European pharmacopoeia. EDQA, Strasbourg

Kapoor LD 1990 Handbook of Ayurvedic medicinal plants. CRC Press, Boca Raton

Kirtikar KR, Basu BD 1981 Indian medicinal plants, vol III. International Book Publishers, Dehradun

Leung DY, Foster S 1996 Encyclopedia of common natural ingredients used in food, drugs and cosmetics. John Wiley, New York

Wichtl M, Bisset NG 1994 Herbal drugs and phytopharmaceuticals. Medpharm Scientific Publishers, Stuttgart

References

1 Mathias E, Rangnekar DV, McCorkle CM 1988 Ethnoveterinary medicine, alternative for livestock development. Proceedings of an International Conference, BAIF Development Research Foundation, Pune, India

2 International Institute of Rural Reconstruction 1994 Ethnoveterinary medicine in Asia. An information kit on traditional animal health care practices. IIRR, Silang, Philippines

3 Blumenthal M 1997 German Commission E monographs: therapeutic monographs on medicinal plants for human use. American Botanical Council, Austin, Texas

4 Ross I 2001 Medicinal plants of the world, vol 2. Humana Press, Totowa, New Jersey

5 Kitagawa I, Chen WZ, Hori K et al 1994 Chemical studies of Chinese licorice-roots. I. Elucidation of five new flavonoid constituents from the roots of *Glycyrrhiza glabra* L. collected in Xinjiang. Chemical and Pharmaceutical Bulletin 42(5):1056

6 Morgan AG, McAdam WAF, Pacsoo C 1982 Comparison between cimetidine and Caved-S in the treatment of gastric ulceration, and subsequent maintenance therapy. Gut 23:545

7 Bianchi PG, Petrillo M, Lazzaroni M 1985 Comparison of pirenzepine and carbenoxolone in the treatment of chronic gastric ulcer: a double-blind endoscopic trial. Hepatogastroenterology 32:293

8 Nadar TS, Pillai MM 1989 Effect of Ayurvedic medicines on beta-glucuronidase activity of Brunner's glands during recovery from cysteamine induced duodenal ulcers in rats. Indian Journal of Experimental Biology 27(11):959

9 Luper S 1999 A review of plants used in the treatment of liver disease: part two. Alternative Medicine Review 4(3):178

10 Konovalova GG, Tikhaze AK, Lankin VZ 2000 Antioxidant activity of parapharmaceuticals containing natural inhibitors of the free radical process. Bulletin of Experimental Biology and Medicine 130(7):658

11 Moon A, Kim SH 1997 Effect of *Glycyrrhiza glabra* roots and glycyrrhizin on the glucuronidation in rats. Planta Medica 63(2):115

12 Haraguchi H, Yosida N, Ishikawa H, Tamura Y, Mizutani K, Kinoshita T 2000 Protection of mitochondrial functions against oxidative stresses by isoflavans from *Glycyrrhiza glabra*. Journal of Pharmacy and Pharmacology 52(2):219

13 Belinky PA, Aviram M, Fuhrman B, Rosenblat M, Vaya J 1998 The antioxidative effects of the isoflavan glabridin on endogenous constituents of LDL during its oxidation. Atherosclerosis 137(1):49

14 Belinky PA, Aviram M, Mahmood S, Vaya J 1998 Structural aspects of the inhibitory effect of glabridin on LDL oxidation. Free Radical Biology and Medicine 24(9):1419

15 Vaya J, Belinky PA, Aviram M 1997 Antioxidant constituents from licorice roots: isolation, structure elucidation and antioxidative capacity toward LDL oxidation. Free Radical Biology and Medicine 23(2):302

16 Trovato A, Monforte MT, Forestieri AM, Pizzimenti F 2000 *In vitro* anti-mycotic activity of some medicinal plants containing flavonoids. Bolletino Chimico Farmaceutico 139(5):225

17 Li W, Asada Y, Yoshikawa T 1998 Antimicrobial flavonoids from *Glycyrrhiza glabra* hairy root cultures. Planta Medica 64(8):746

18 Mitscher LA, Park YH, Clark D, Beal JL 1980 Antimicrobial agents from higher plants. Antimicrobial isoflavonoids and related substances from *Glycyrrhiza glabra* L. var. *typica*. Journal of Natural Products 43(2):259

19 Badam L 1997 *In vitro* antiviral activity of indigenous glycyrrhizin, licorice and glycyrrhizic acid (Sigma) on Japanese encephalitis virus. Journal of Communicable Diseases 29(2):91

20 Pompei R, Flore O, Marccialis MA, Pani A, Loddo B 1979 Glycyrrhizic acid inhibits virus growth and inactivates virus particles. Nature 281(5733):689

21 Razina TG, Zueva EP, Amosova EN, Krylova SG 2000 Medicinal plant preparations used as adjuvant therapeutics in experimental oncology.

Eksperimental'naia i Klinickaia Farmakologia 63(5):59

22 Trovato A, Monforte MT, Rossitto A, Forestieri AM 1996 *In vitro* cytotoxic effect of some medicinal plants containing flavonoids. Bolletino Chimico Farmaceutico 135(4):263

23 Agarwal R, Wang ZY, Mukhtar H 1991 Inhibition of mouse skin tumor-initiating activity of DMBA by chronic oral feeding of glycyrrhizin in drinking water. Nutrition and Cancer 15(3–4):187

24 Zani F, Cuzzoni MT, Daglia M, Benvenuti S, Vampa G, Mazza P 1993 Inhibition of mutagenicity in *Salmonella typhimurium* by *Glycyrrhiza glabra* extract, glycyrrhizinic acid, 18 alpha- and 18 beta-glycyrrhetinic acids. Planta Medica 59(6):502

25 Francischetti IM, Monteiro RQ, Guimaraes JA, Francischetti B 1997 Identification of glycyrrhizin as a thrombin inhibitor. Biochemistry and Biophysics Research Communications 235(1):259

26 Azimov MM, Zakirov UB, Radzhapova SD 1988 Pharmacological study of the anti-inflammatory agent glyderinine. Farmakologika Toksikologica 51(4):90

27 De Smet PAGM 1993 Adverse effects of herbal drugs. Springer Verlag, Berlin

28 McGuffin M, Hobbs C, Upton R, Goldberg A 1997 Botanical safety handbook. CRC Press, Boca Raton

29 World Health Organization 1999 Monographs on selected medicinal plants, vol 1. WHO, Geneva

Gossypium herbaceum L. (Malvaceae)

English: Cotton

Hindi: *Kapas*

Sanskrit: *Tundakesi*

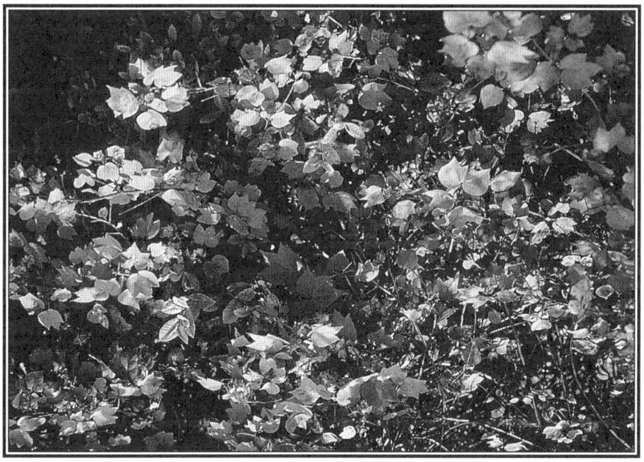

Cotton has been cultivated since ancient times mainly for its fibre, but also for its medicinal properties. It was originally valued for its ability to induce menstruation and its contraceptive effect which was first discovered in China when men became infertile after eating food cooked in the oil. It was introduced from India to Egypt and China around 500 BC and then to the USA in 1774.

Habitat

Cotton is native to the Indian subcontinent and the Arabian peninsula and thrives in warm humid temperatures and tropical climates. It is widely cultivated for the fibre, particularly in the southern USA, and the root and seeds are harvested in the autumn.

Botanical description

It is a small shrub, up to 2.5 m in height, with thick and rigid stems (Plate 32). The twigs and young leaves are sparsely hairy, rarely glabrous; the leaves flat, cleft up to halfway in 3–7 lobes, which are ovate or round and only slightly constricted at the base. The bracteoles are broadly triangular, flaring widely from the flower or capsule, and usually broader than long, with 6–8 serrated teeth on the margin. The flowers are yellow with a purple centre or, more rarely, white; the capsules rounded, beaked, rarely with prominent shoulders, with a smooth surface and very few oil glands and 3–4 loculae, which open slightly when ripe. The seeds usually have two coats of hairs; the lint hairs being white, grey or red-brown in colour, and the fuzz hairs (which may rarely be absent) are distributed uniformly over the seed.

Parts used

Bark, seeds, leaves, flowers and root bark.

Traditional and modern use

The emmenagogue properties of the root bark were first observed by Bouchelle in Mississippi, who noted that it was used to procure abortion. It is still used for this purpose in India, the USA and Mexico but it is most often used nowadays for amenorrhoea, dysmenorrhoea and dysentery. It has also been used for rejuvenation, treating tumours, throat infections, as a laxative and expectorant. In traditional medicine the seeds are considered to be an effective remedy against rheumatism and are used as an aphrodisiac and galactogogue. It gives strength to the body, dispels diseases caused by the morbidity of the *tridosha* and is said to alleviate thirst, burning sensation, oedema, uterine disorders, anaemia and genitourinary diseases. The leaves are diuretic and thought to be beneficial in mental disorders and skin diseases. The flowers are antiseptic and used to purify the blood and heal leprous ulcers.

Ethnoveterinary usage

The leaf of the plant is used to remove retained placenta in swine and the seeds in the treatment of decreased milk flow in ruminants. It is also used as a food in ruminants and poultry. The plant has been used for holes in the hard palate, tympanitis, cough, orchitis and fissures.[1]

Major chemical constituents

Sesquiterpenes

The seeds contain gossypol, a dimeric sesquiterpene, with gossyfulvin, gossypurpurin and gossycaerulin.

Flavonoids

The flowers contain gossypitrin, gossypin, gossypetin, herbacitrin, isoquercitrin, quercimeritrin, herbacetin and quercetin, and the root bark gossypetin and dihydroxybenzoic acid.[2]

Aminoacids

The seeds contain glycinebetaine,[3] aspartic acid, glutamic acid, arginine, lysine, histidine, serine, glycine, tyrosine, alanine, methionine, phenylalanine, leucine.[4]

Medicinal and pharmacological activities

Antifertility activity: Large-scale clinical trials in men have found gossypol to be orally active and relatively safe and effective; it acts by inhibiting sperm production and motility in a variety of male animal species. Gossypol appears to exert its contraceptive activity by inhibiting lactate dehydrogenase which plays a crucial role in energy metabolism in sperm and spermatogenic cells.[5] The effects of *Gossypium herbaceum* on fecundity were studied on sexually mature catfish (*Clarias batarachus*). Treatment resulted in reduced fecundity in female fish.[6] Treatment of pseudopregnant rats with gossypol acetic acid (GAA) at a dosage of 40 or 80 mg/kg for 5 days caused a decrease of cytoplasmic protein and oestrogen receptor level per uterus in the treated animals. Analysis showed that in immature rats, GAA at 40 mg/kg for 8 days reduced the number of oestrogen receptors per uterus. At high concentrations it was capable of inhibiting the binding of 3H-oestradiol with the receptor.[7] Gossypol has been shown to be an active antifertility agent in male hamsters and rats.[8] When given intramuscularly to female rats, gossypol inhibited implantation and the maintenance of normal pregnancy, probably by affecting luteinising hormone levels.[9]

Antibacterial activity: A pectin-rich extract of *Gossypium herbaceum* was shown to induce prolactin release and milk synthesis when administered orally to rats. Administration of an oral extract to women 2 days after parturition enhanced the concentration of complement C3 and C4 in colostrum, but did not modify the total haemolytic complement activity. These results suggest that the extract favours transfer of C3 and C4 from blood to colostrum, by an unknown mechanism, and hence could be used to reinforce the antibacterial activity of human colostrum.[10] 2,7-Dihydroxycadalene and its optically active oxidation products, isolated from cotton leaves, demonstrated an inhibitory activity towards *Xanthomonas campestris*, indicating that these sesquiterpenoids may form aqueous solutions capable of inhibiting bacterial pathogens.[11]

Antiviral activity: Gossypol and its derivatives have been shown to be active against the HIV virus.[12]

Antimutagenic activity: An extract of Gossypium had a moderate antimutagenic activity against benzo[a]pyrene when studied using the Salmonella microsomal system.[13]

Antitumour activity: Gossypol (at 25–100 µg/mouse/day IP) prolonged the survival time of Ehrlich ascites tumour-bearing mice.[14] Pretreatment of nude mice transplanted with SW-13 cells with oral gossypol (30 mg/kg/day) for 7 days delayed onset of visible tumours in subsequent weeks.[15]

Safety profile

A 50% ethanolic extract of the plant (excluding root) showed an LD_{50} of >1000 mg/kg body weight when administered IP in mice.[16]

Dosage

Root powder: 1–4 g

Decoction: 28–56 ml

Leaf infusion: 5–10 ml

Ayurvedic properties

Guna: *Laghu* (light), *snigdha* (unctuous)

Rasa: *Madhur* (sweet), *kasaya* (astringent)

Veerya: *Ushna* (hot)

Vipaka: *Madhur* (sweet)

Dosha: Pacifies *vata*

Further reading

Bown D 1995 Encyclopaedia of herbs and their uses. Dorling Kindersley, London

Chevallier A 1996 The encyclopedia of medicinal plants. Dorling Kindersley, London

Duke JA 1992 Handbook of phytochemical constituents of GRAS herbs and other economic plants. CRC Press, Boca Raton

Kapoor LD 1990 Handbook of Ayurvedic medicinal plants. CRC Press, Boca Raton

Ministry of Health and Family Welfare 1989 Ayurvedic pharmacopoeia of India. Government of India, New Delhi

Nadkarni AK 1976 Indian materia medica. Popular Prakashan PVT Ltd, Bombay

References

1 Jha MK 1992 The folk veterinary system of Bihar – a research survey. NDDB, Anand, Gujrat

2 Chander K, Seshadri TR 1996 Leucoanthocyanidins in cotton seed. Journal of Science and Indian Research 16A:319

3 Gorham J 1996 Glycinebetaine is a major nitrogen-containing solute in the Malvaceae. Phytochemistry 43(2):367

4 Nguyen KPP, Nguyen NX 1996 Determination of amino acids of the aqueous extract of *Gossypium herbaceum* seeds by HPLC with pre-column o-phthaldialdehyde derivatization. Hoa Hoc Cong Nghiep Hoa Chat 3:29

5 Der Marderosian A (ed) 2000 The review of natural products, facts and comparisons. Kluwer, Missouri

6 Menon RP, Reddy PUM 1993 Fecundity studies under Gossypium treatment in the fresh water cat fish *Clarias batarachus* (L.). Journal of Environmental Research 3(1):15

7 Wang NG, Guan MZ, Li HP, Lei HP 1987 Effect of gossypol acetic acid (GAA) and its 2-alpha-methyl ester (PG05) on estrogen receptor of rat uteri. Acta Pharma Sinica 22(2):103

8 Waller DP, Fong HHS, Cordell GA, Soejarto DD 1981 Antifertility effects of gossypol and its impurities on male hamsters. Contraception 23:653

9 Lin YC, Fukaya T, Rikishisa Y, Walton A 1985 Gossypol in female fertility control: ovum implantation and early pregnancy inhibited in rats. Life Sciences 37:39

10 Sepehri H, Roghani M, Houdebine, M-L 1998 Oral administration of pectin-rich plant extract enhances C3 and C4 complement concentration in woman colostrum. Reproduction, Nutrition and Development 38(3):255

11 Essenberg M, Grover PBJ, Cover EC 1990 Accumulation of antibacterial sesquiterpenoids in bacterially inoculated *Gossypium* leaves and cotyledons. Phytochemistry 29(10):3107

12 Prusoff W 1993 Effect of gossypol on HIV. Pharmacology and Therapeutics 60:315

13 Lee H, Lin JY 1988 Antimutagenic activity of extracts from anticancer drugs in Chinese medicine. Mutation Research 204(2):229

14 Tso WW 1984 Gossypol inhibits Erhlich ascites tumor cell proliferation. Cancer Letters 24:257

15 Wu, YW, Chik CL, Knazek RA 1989 An *in vitro* and *in vivo* study of antitumor effects of gossypol on human SW-13 adrenocortical carcinoma. Cancer Research 49:3754

16 Dhawan ML, Dhawan BN, Prasad CR, Rastogi RP, Singh KK, Tandon JS 1974 Screening of Indian medicinal plants for biological activity: Part-V. Indian Journal of Experimental Biology 12:512

Gymnema sylvestre R. Br. (Asclepiadaceae)

English: Periploca of the wood

Hindi: *Gurmar*

Sanskrit: *Meshasringi*

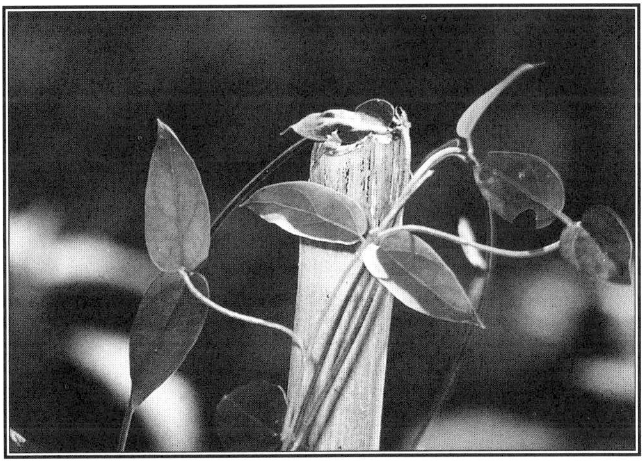

Gymnema has been used in India for the treatment of diabetes mellitus for over 2000 years. It also has the unusual property that when leaves of this plant are chewed, the taste of sugar and all sweet substances is abolished, hence the name *gurmar* meaning 'sugar destroying'.

Habitat

It is found commonly in the Deccan peninsula and extending to parts of northern and western India and also in Sri Lanka and tropical Africa.

Botanical description

A large, more or less pubescent, woody climber (Plate 33). Leaves opposite, usually elliptic or ovate, with both surfaces pubescent. Flowers small, yellow, in umbellate cymes; follicles terete, lanceolate, up to 8 cm in length.

Parts used

Leaves, root.

Traditional and modern use

The leaves of this plant have been used in India to treat *madhu meha* or 'honey urine', as well as a variety of other disorders such as indigestion, cough, constipation and malaria. Use as a cardiotonic, diuretic, laxative, stimulant, stomachic and uterine tonic has also been noted in traditional Ayurvedic literature. The leaves are applied topically to wounds and, mixed with castor oil, are applied to swollen glands and for the enlargement of the liver and spleen. The powdered root also has a reputation as a remedy for snakebite. The fruits are bitter and carminative and have been used to treat leprosy, diabetes, bronchitis, worms, ulcers and poisoning. The whole plant is taken orally in dysentery. The plant is used as a constituent of many traditional Ayurvedic preparations including *ayaskrti*, *varunadi kasayam* and *varunadi ghrtam*.

Ethnoveterinary usage

Leaves are fed to cattle as a galactagogue by the Irula people.

Major chemical constituents

Saponins and triterpenes

'Gymnemic acid' is the main active principle of *Gymnema sylvestre*;[1] it is a complex mixture of at least nine closely related glycosides, gymnemic acids A–D and V–Z.[2] The leaves contain many other dammarane saponins including the gymnemasins A–D, gymnemasides I–VII, gymnemosides a–f, gymnestrogenin and gymnemagenin.[3–8]

Polypeptide

The sweetness-suppressing polypeptide gurmarin consists of 35 aminoacid residues and contains three intramolecular disulphide bonds.[9]

Nitrogenous compounds

The leaves contain adenine, choline, betaine and other aminoacids including aminobutyric acid,[10] and a trace alkaloid gymnamine.[11]

Medicinal and pharmacological activities

Antihyperglycaemic activity: The antihyperglycaemic action of a crude saponin fraction and five isolated glycosides (gymnemic acids I–IV and gymnemasaponin V) derived from the methanol extract of leaves was studied in streptozotocin (STZ)-diabetic mice. The saponin fraction (60 mg/kg) reduced blood glucose levels 2–4 hours after the IP administration. Gymnemic acid IV, at doses of 3.4–13.4 mg/kg, reduced the blood glucose levels by 13.5–60.0% after 6 hours and was comparable to glibenclamide. It did not change blood glucose levels in normal mice. Gymnemic acid IV at 13.4 mg/kg increased plasma insulin levels in STZ-diabetic mice, indicating that release of insulin may contribute to the antidiabetic effects.[12] In another study, two gymnemic acid-enriched alcoholic fractions (GS4) were investigated for effects on insulin secretion from rat islets of Langerhans and several pancreatic β-cell lines. GS4 stimulated insulin release from HIT-T15, MIN6 and RINm5F β-cells and from islets in the absence of any other stimulus and this was inhibited by 1 mM EGTA. Examination of islet and β-cell integrity after exposure to GS4, by the trypan blue exclusion test, indicated that concentrations of GS4 which stimulated insulin secretion also caused an increase in uptake of dye. These results confirm the stimulatory effects of *G. sylvestre* on insulin release but indicate that it may act by increasing cell permeability, rather than stimulating exocytosis by regulated pathways.[13] It is also believed to delay glucose absorption in the small intestine[6] and increase the number of islets of Langerhans and β-cells in rats.[14] Gymnemic acid has been shown to inhibit sodium ion-dependent active glucose transport in the rat small intestine.[15]

Inhibitory effect on palatal taste response: Gymnema leaves prevent the perception of the sweet taste in all regions of the mouth. Administration of 5 mM of gymnemic acid to the human tongue raised the sweetness threshold of sucrose from 0.01 M to 1 M. It is thought to involve direct interaction with the apical side of the taste cells, possibly by binding to the sweet taste receptor protein.[16] Gurmarin (10 μg/ml) significantly depressed (by 40–50%) the phasic taste response to sugars and saccharin sodium in the rat, recorded from the greater superficial petrosal nerve, which innervates the taste buds. Phasic responses to D-aminoacids that taste sweet to humans were also depressed.[17] A recent genetic study using inbred strains provided evidence that the dpa gene, which probably controls sweet receptors, is inhibited by gurmarin.[18]

Hypolipidaemic activity: An aqueous extract of the leaf was effective in reducing serum lipids in 27 insulin-dependent diabetic patients taking insulin only, when treated with 400 mg/day. Serum levels of lipids returned to near normal.[19] Another study in rats showed that treatment with Gymnema leaf extract reduced elevated serum triglycerides, total cholesterol, very low density lipoprotein cholesterol and low density lipoprotein cholesterol in a dose-dependent manner.[20]

Smooth muscle relaxant activity: Water extracts containing gymnemic acids were evaluated for their effects on a high K^+-induced muscle contraction of the rat intestinal circular muscle. They inhibited the contraction in a dose-dependent manner and spontaneous contraction of the muscle was also diminished or abolished. It is thought this may be due to nitric oxide and endothelium-derived hyperpolarising factor participation.[21]

Antioxidant activity: Gymnema shows an antioxidant activity comparable to α-tocopherol.[22]

Prevention of dental caries: The decomposition of sugar and production of glucan by *Streptococcus mutans*, which causes plaque formation and dental caries, was prevented by gymnemic acid.[23]

Antiviral activity: Gymnemic acids A, B, C and D were tested for antiviral activity against influenza virus. Gymnemic acid A (75 mg/kg/day, IP) showed the greatest activity, moderate inhibition was obtained with gymnemic acid B and none with gymnemic acids C and D.[24]

Hepatoprotective activity: An alcoholic extract of the leaf at a dose of 300 mg/kg against CCl_4-induced liver damage was found to be effective.[25]

Safety profile

Gymnemic acids appear to be non-toxic to humans but diabetic patients taking hypoglycaemic agents may need to reduce doses of medication if treatment with Gymnema is added. The LD_{50} of a 50% alcoholic extract of whole plant (excluding root) when given intraperitoneally to mice was found to be 375 mg/kg body weight.[26]

Dosage

Decoction: 14–28 ml daily

Leaf powder: 2–4 g daily

Extract: 400 mg daily

Ayurvedic properties

Guna: *Laghu* (light), *ruksha* (dry)

Rasa: *Kashaya* (astringent), *katu* (bitter)

Veerya: *Ushna* (hot)

Vipaka: *Katu* (bitter)

Dosha: Pacifies *kapha* and *pitta*

Further reading

Chopra RN, Chopra IC, Handa KL, Kapoor LD 1994 Indigenous drugs of India. Academic Publishers, Calcutta

Kapoor LD 1990 Handbook of Ayurvedic medicinal plants. CRC Press, Boca Raton

Nadkarni AK 1976 Indian materia medica. Popular Prakashan PVT Ltd, Bombay

Council for Scientific and Industrial Research 1985 The wealth of India. PID, CSIR, New Delhi

References

1 Stoecklin W, Weiss E, Reichstein T 1967 Glycosides and aglycons CCLXXXVIII. Gymnemic acid, the antisaccharine principle of *Gymnema sylvestre*. Isolation and identification. Helvetica Chimica Acta 50(2):474

2 Sinsheimer JE, Rao G, Subba M, Huga M 1970 Constituents of *Gymnema sylvestre* leaves V: isolation and preliminary characterization of gymnemic acids. Journal of Pharmaceutical Science 59(5):622

3 Qin MJ, Ye WC, Zhang J, Tanaka T 1998 Determination of gymnemic acid content in leaves of *Gymnema sylvestre*. Zhiwu Ziyuan Yu Huanjing 7(1):59

4 Yoshikawa K, Arihara S, Matsuura K, Miyase T 1991 Dammarane saponins from *Gymnema sylvestre*. Phytochemistry 31(1):237

5 Yoshikawa M, Murakami T, Kadoya M et al 1997 Medicinal food stuffs IX. The inhibitors of glucose absorption from the leaves of *Gymnema sylvestre* R. Br. (Asclepiadaceae): structures of gymnemosides a and b. Chemical and Pharmaceutical Bulletin (Tokyo) 45(10):1671

6 Yoshikawa M, Murakami T, Matsuda H 1997 Medicinal foodstuffs X. Structures of new triterpene glycosides, gymnemosides-c,-d, and -f, from the leaves of *Gymnema sylvestre* R. Br.: influence of Gymnema glycosides on glucose uptake in rat small intestinal fragments. Chemical and Pharmaceutical Bulletin 45(12):2034

7 Stoecklin W 1968 Glycosides and aglycones CCCIX. Gymnestrogenin, a new penta-hydroxytriterpene from *Gymnema sylvestre* leaves. Helvetica Chimica Acta 51(6):1235

8 Stoecklin W 1969 Glycosides and aglycones. CCCXIII. Structure and O-isopropylidene derivatives of gymnemagenin. Helvetica Chimica Acta 52(2):365

9 Ota M, Shimizu Y, Tonosaki K, Ariyoshi Y 1998 Role of hydrophobic amino acids in gurmarin, a sweetness-suppressing polypeptide. Biopolymers 45(3):231

10 Sinsheimer JE, McIlhenny HM 1967 Constituents from *Gymnema sylvestre* leaves II. Nitrogenous compounds. Journal of Pharmaceutical Science 56(6):732

11 Rao GS, Sinsheimer JE, McIlhenny HM 1972 Structure of gymnamine, a trace alkaloid from *Gymnema sylvestre* leaves. Chemical Industry (London)13:537

12 Sugihara Y, Nojima H, Matsuda H, Murakami T, Yoshikawa M, Kimura I 2000 Antihyperglycemic effects of gymnemic acid IV, a compound derived from *Gymnema sylvestre* leaves in streptozotocin-diabetic mice. Journal of Asian Natural Product Research 2(4):321

13 Persaud SJ, Al-Majed H, Raman A, Jones PM 1999 *Gymnema sylvestre* stimulates insulin release *in vitro* by increased membrane permeability. Journal of Endocrinology 163(2):207

14 Shanmugasundaram ER, Gopinath KL, Shanmugasundaram KR 1990 Possible regeneration of the islets of Langerhans in streptozotocin-diabetic rats given *Gymnema sylvestre* leaf extracts. Journal of Ethnopharmacology 30(3):265

15 Yoshioka S 1986 Inhibitory effects of gymnemic acid and an extract from the leaves of *Ziziphus jujuba* on glucose absorption in the rat small intestine. Journal of the Yonago Medical Association 37:142

16 Miyasaka A, Imoto T 1995 Electrophysiological characterization of the inhibitory effect of a novel peptide gumarin on the sweet taste response in rats. Brain Research 676(1):63

17 Harada S, Kasahara Y 2000 Inhibitory effect of gurmarin on palatal taste responses to amino acids in the rat. American Journal of Physiology 6(2):278

18 Ninomiya Y 1999 Genetic approaches for taste receptor and transduction mechanisms. Shinkei Kenkyu no Shinpo 43(5):674

19 Shanmugasundaram ERB, Rajeswary B, Bagkaran L, Rajesh K, Ahmath BK 1990 Use of *Gymnema sylvestre* leaf extract in the control of blood glucose in insulin-dependent diabetes mellitus. Journal of Ethnopharmacology 30:281

20 Bishayee A, Chatterjee M 1994 Hypolipidaemic

and antiatherosclerotic effects of oral *Gymnema sylvestre* R.Br. leaf extract in albino rats fed on a high fat diet. Phytotherapy Research 8:118

21 Luo H 1999 Possible participation of NO and EDHF in the relaxation of rat intestinal circular muscle induced by *Gymnema* water extracts containing gymnemic acids. Yonago Igaku Zasshi 50(1):22

22 Inoue T, Ohfuji M, Komatsu M 1997 Antioxidative effect of infusions of green tea and 'Health Tea'. Kyoto-fu Hoken Kankyo Kenkyusho Nenpo 42:7

23 Hiji Y 1990 Gymnemic acid for prevention of dental caries. U.S. Patent 4,912,089

24 Sinsheimer JE, Rao GS, McIlhenny HM, Smith RV, Maassab HF, Cochran KW 1968 Isolation and antiviral activity of the gymnemic acids. Experientia 24(3):302

25 Rana AC, Avadhoot Y 1992 Experimental evaluation of hepatoprotective activity of *Gymnema sylvestre* and *Curcuma zedoaria*. Fitoterapia 63(1):60

26 Bhakuni DS, Dhar ML, Dhar MM, Dhawan BN, Gupta B, Srimal RC 1971 Screening of Indian plants for biological activity. Part III. Indian Journal of Experimental Biology 9:91

Holarrhena antidysenterica R. Br. (Apocynaceae)

English: Tellicherry, conessi

Hindi: *Kurchi*

Sanskrit: *Kutaja*

The seeds are called 'Indra's seeds' in Sanskrit and are said to have sprung from drops of the 'Amrita of life' which fell on the ground from the bodies of the monkeys of Lord Rama, who were then restored to life by Indra. *Holarrhena antidysenterica* has frequently been adulterated with *Wrightia tinctoria*; however, the seeds of the former herb are bitter in taste, compared to the seeds of the latter which are tasteless. The bark is collected from trees over 10 years old.

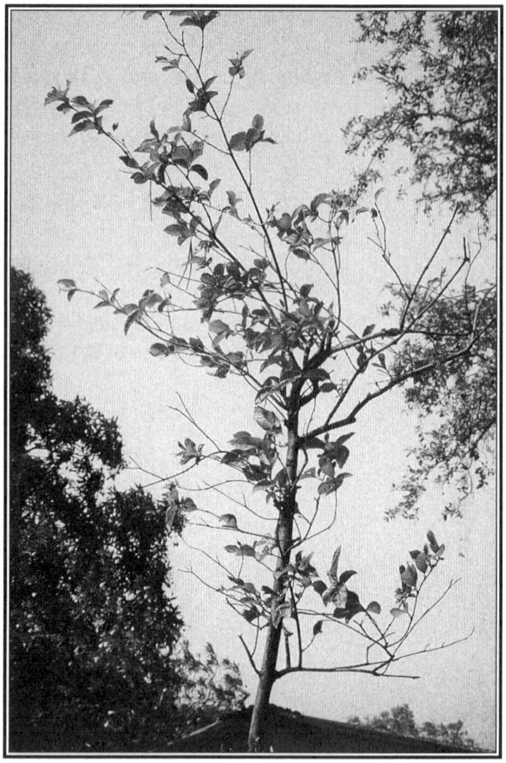

Habitat

It is found all over India and other Asian countries up to an altitude of 1300 m, especially in the sub-Himalayan tract, in deciduous forests and open wastelands.

Botanical description

A small shrub or deciduous tree, up to 13 m in height, with a milky latex (Plate 34). The bark peels off in flakes and is grey to pale brown in colour. The leaves are shiny on the upper surface, dull and hairy on the lower, opposite, subsessile and elliptic. The flowers are white, in terminal corymbose cymes, the fruits are cylindrical, dark grey with white specks, and occur in pairs; the seeds are light brown, 0.5–1.5 cm long, with long tufts of hair.

Parts used

Stem, root bark and seeds.

Traditional and modern use

Kutaja is primarily used for the treatment of dysentery but has several other therapeutic usages. It is particularly useful in bleeding disorders such as menorrhagia, haemorrhoids, diabetes and oedema[1] and has been used for tumours, abscesses, aches and pains, bronchitis, colic, diarrhoea, splenitis and as a vermifuge, laxative and astringent.

Ethnoveterinary usage

The seeds and bark are used in diarrhoea in ruminants.[2] The bark and seeds have been used for wounds, maggots in wounds, pox and anthrax. It is also used to treat jaundice, colic, bloody dysentery, cold and cough, diseases of skeletal system such as lumbar, rib, compound fractures and dislocation of hips, stoppage of urination and prolapse of the uterus.[3]

Major chemical constituents

Alkaloids

These are sometimes present as the tannates and include conessine (about 0.4%), conessimine, kurchine, conamine, conimine, conessidine, conarrhimine, holarrhimine, holarrhine and kurchicine. The steroidal alkaloids regholarrhenine A, B, C, D, E and F have been isolated from the stem bark of *Holarrhena antidysenterica*[4,5] and antidysentericine from the seeds.[6] The alkaloid content of the bark was found to be at a maximum when the plant was between 8–12 years old, and during the months of July to September.

Medicinal and pharmacological activities

Antibacterial activity: The methanolic extract of stem bark was tested for antibacterial efficacy against *Staphylococcus aureus, Staph. epidermidis, Streptococcus faecalis, Bacillus subtilis, Escherichia coli* and *Pseudomonas aeruginosa* using both the microdilution broth method as well as the disc diffusion method. The extract was active against all tested bacteria. Further studies revealed that the antibacterial activity was mainly associated with alkaloids, which showed remarkable activity against *Staph. aureus* (MIC = 95 µg/ml).[7] The seeds also exhibited antibacterial activity, particularly the chloroform and methanol extracts.[8]

Antidysentery and antidiarrhoeal activity: The efficacy of *Holarrhena antidysenterica* in chronic and amoebic dysentery has been established. Conessine was reported to be the most effective of the alkaloids.[9] In a small clinical trial of 25 patients suffering from diarrhoea and dysentery, relief for about 80% was observed after 3 days of treatment with an Ayurvedic formulation. This consisted of *Holarrhena antidysenterica* seeds, *Berberis aristata* wood, *Embelia ribes* fruits, *Cyperus rotundus* bulbous roots, *Aegle marmelos* fruit pulp and *Butea monosperma* seeds.[10]

Immunomodulatory activity: An ethanolic extract stimulated phagocytic functions while inhibiting the humoral component of the immune system in mice.[11]

Hypoglycaemic activity: This has been reported in the aqueous and alcoholic extracts of the seeds of *Holarrhena antidysenterica*. In a study conducted in rats in three models, a significant decrease in blood glucose level was observed both in normal and diabetic rats.[12]

Safety profile

The maximum tolerated dose of the 50% ethanolic extract of the stem bark and fruits was found to be 1000 mg/kg and 250 mg/kg body weight (IP in adult albino rats), respectively.[13]

Dosage

Seed powder: 2–4 g

Decoction and infusion: 28–74 ml

Tincture: 2–4 ml

Powder: 2–4 g

Ayurvedic properties

Rasa: *Tikta* (bitter), *kashaya* (astringent)

Guna: *Laghu* (light), *ruksha* (dry)

Veerya: *Shita* (cold)

Vipaka: *Katu* (pungent)

Dosha: Pacifies *kapha* and *pitta*

Further reading

Bharatiya Vidya Bhavan's Swami Prakashananda Ayurveda Research Centre 1992 Selected medicinal plants of India. Chemexcil, Mumbai

Kapoor LD 1990 Handbook of Ayurvedic medicinal plants. CRC Press, Boca Raton

Ministry of Health and Family Welfare 1989 Ayurvedic pharmacopoeia of India. Government of India, New Delhi

Pandey GS (ed) 1998 Bhavprakash Nighantu. Chaukhambha Bharati Academy, Gokul Bhawan, Varanasi

Sairam TV 1999 Home remedies, vol II. Penguin India, New Delhi

References

1 Singh KP, Chaturvedi GN 1988 Traditional research potentialities of Kutaja (*Holarrhena antidysenterica* Wall.) Journal of Research in Ayurveda and Siddha 4(1–4):6

2 International Institute of Rural Reconstruction 1994 Ethnoveterinary medicine in Asia. An information kit on traditional animal health care practices. Part I, General information. IIRR, Silang, Philippines

3 Jha MK 1992 Folk veterinary medicine of Bihar – a research project. NDDB, Anand, Gujrat

4 Bhutani KK, Ali M, Sharma SR, Vaid RM, Gupta DK 1988 Three new steroidal alkaloids from the bark of *Holarrhena antidysenterica*. Phytochemistry 27(3):925

5 Bhutani KK, Vaid RM, Ali M, Kapoor S, Soodan SR, Kumar D 1990 Steroidal alkaloids from *Holarrhena antidysenterica*. Phytochemistry 29(3):969

6 Kumar A, Ali M 2000 A new steroidal alkaloid from the seeds of *Holarrhena antidysenterica*. Fitoterapia 71(2):101

7 Chakraboorty A, Brantner AH 1999 Antibacterial steroid alkaloids from the stem bark of *Holarrhena pubescens*. Journal of Ethnopharmacology 68(1–3):339

8 Jolly CI, Mechery NR 1996 Comparative pharmacognostical, physicochemical and antibacterial studies on seeds of *Holarrhena antidysenterica* Wall. and *Wrightia tinctoria* R.Br. Indian Journal of Pharmaceutical Science 58(2):51

9 Basu NK, Jayaswal SB 1968 Amoebicidal activity of alkaloids of *Holarrhena antidysenterica in vitro*. Indian Journal of Pharmacy 30:289

10 Javalgekar RR 1982 Efficacy of a compound solid-extract in Ayurvedic treatment. Indian Journal of Pharmaceutical Science 44:25

11 Atal CK, Sharma ML, Kaul A, Khajuria A 1986 Immunomodulating agents of plant origin I. Preliminary screening. Journal of Ethnopharmacology 18(2):133

12 Gopal V, Chauhan MG 1993 *Holarrhena antidysenterica* – a novel herbal antidiabetic seed drug. Indian Journal of Pharmaceutical Science 56(4):156

13 Dhar ML, Dhar MM, Dhawan BN, Mehrotra BN, Ray C 1968 Screening of Indian plants for biological activity: Part I. Indian Journal of Experimental Biology 6:232

Leptadenia reticulata Wight & Arn. (Asclepiadaceae)

English: Leptadenia

Hindi: *Dori*

Sanskrit: *Jivanti*

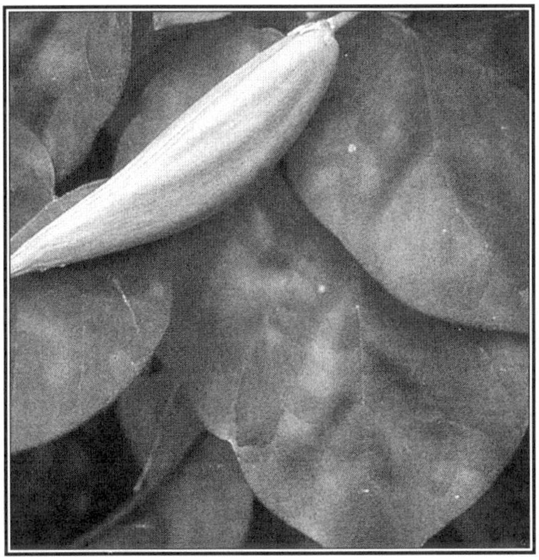

Known as *jivanti* (or *svarnajivanti*) in Sanskrit literature, the name (*jiv* = life) indicates that the plant is considered to have the ability to bestow health and vigour. It is considered to be a *rasayana* and included among the 10 drugs constituting the *Jivaniya gana* or 'vitalising group'.

Habitat

Found in the sub-Himalayan tracts of Punjab and Uttar Pradesh and throughout the Deccan peninsula up to an altitude of 900 m and found particularly in hedges. It is also distributed throughout Mauritius, Madagascar, Sri Lanka, the Himalayas and Burma.

Botanical description

A twining shrub, with numerous branches, the stems of which have a cork-like, deeply cracked bark, glabrous in the younger ones (Plate 35). Leaves coriaceous, ovate, acute, glabrous above, finely pubescent below. Flowers greenish-yellow, in lateral or subaxillary cymes, often with small hairs. Fruit follicles may be woody. The external surface of the root is rough, white or buff coloured with longitudinal ridges and furrows, and in transverse section, the wide cork, lignified stone cell layers and medullary rays can be seen.[1] In commerce, the root samples vary from 3 to 10 cm in length and 1.5 to 5 cm in diameter.

Parts used

Leaf, root, whole plant.

Traditional and modern use

The plant is a stimulant and restorative. The leaves and roots are used in skin affections such as ringworm, wounds, nose and ear disorders, asthma, cough and in the treatment of habitual abortion in women.

Ethnoveterinary usage

The bark, leaves and the whole plant are used to improve decreased milk flow in ruminants. The whole plant is also used to stimulate heat and prevent abortion. The leaves are used to treat eye diseases in swine.[2,3]

Major chemical constituents

Phytosterols and triterpenoids

The leaves and twigs contain stigmasterol, β-sitosterol,[4] leptadenol,[2] hentriacontanol, α-amyrin, β-amyrin and tocopherols.[5,8]

Flavonoids

Diosmetin and luteolin are present in the leaves and twigs and quercetin, isoquercitrin, rutin and hyperoside in the pericarp of the follicles.[6]

Medicinal and pharmacological activities

Antibacterial activity: Aqueous and ethanolic extracts of *L. reticulata* roots showed antibacterial activity against various pathogens including *Streptococcus pyogenes* var. *α*- and *β-haemolyticus*, *Salmonella typhi*, *S. paratyphi*, *S. schottmulleri* and *Escherichia coli*.[7]

Antifungal activity: Activity was observed in the aqueous and 50% ethanolic extracts of the leaf and root of *L. reticulata* against *Trichophyton rubrum*. The alcoholic extract was the more active.[9]

Hypotensive activity: An aqueous extract of *L. reticulata* showed potent and prolonged hypotensive action in anaesthetised dogs, the initial hypotension followed by a complete recovery and a secondary progressive hypotension. It did not possess parasympathomimetic or adrenolytic actions but blocked pressor response to nicotine.[8]

Spasmogenic activity: The alcoholic extract of *L. reticulata* showed spasmogenic action on isolated guinea pig ileum and uterus.[9]

Lactogenic activity: Stigmasterol and the ether fraction of *L. reticulata* were tested on lactating rats. Both showed lactogenic properties as assessed by parameters including pup weights, body weight of mother rats, protein and glycogen contents of mammary glands, photomicrographic studies and secretory rating of lactating mammary glands.[10] In another study *L. reticulata* powder was administered to goats, sheep, cows and buffaloes to assess its lactogenic properties. The powdered drug was administered at a dose of 536 mg per day in goats and sheep, 1840 mg per day in cows and buffaloes, and produced a significant galactopoietic response. No significant changes were observed in the composition of milk or blood in goats.[11]

Increased egg production in hens: *L.reticulata* powder and stigmasterol were found to increase egg yield.[12]

Safety profile

The LD_{50} of the 50% alcoholic extract of whole plant of *L. reticulata* (excluding root), when given to mice via the IP route, was found to be >1000 mg/kg body weight.[13]

Dosage

Root powder: 1–3 g

Decoction: 30–60 ml

Ayurvedic properties

Rasa: *Madhur* (sweet)

Guna: *Laghu* (light), *snigdha* (unctuous)

Veerya: *Shita* (cold)

Vipaka: *Madhur* (sweet)

Dosha: Balances *tridosha*

Further reading

Bharatiya Vidya Bhavan's Swami Prakashananda Ayurveda Research Centre 1992 Selected medicinal plants of India. Chemexcil, Mumbai

Pandey GS (ed) 1998 Bhavprakash Nighantu. Chaukhambha Bharati Academy, Gokul Bhawan, Varanasi

Sivarajan VV, Balachandran I 1994 Ayurvedic drugs and their plant sources. Oxford and IBH Publishing, New Delhi

References

1 Gupta RC, Kapoor LD 1971 Pharmacognostical studies on Jivanti. Part-II. *Leptadenia reticulata* Wight and Arn (Syn. *Gymnema aurantiacum* Wall. Ex Hook. F., *Asclepias tuberosa* Roxb.). Bulletin of the Botanical Survey of India 13:53

2 International Institute of Rural Reconstruction 1994 Ethnoveterinary medicine in Asia. An information kit on traditional animal health care practices. IIRR, Silang, Philippines

3 Jha MK 1992 Folk veterinary medicine of Bihar – a research project. NDDB, Anand, Gujrat

4 Krishna PVG, Rao EV, Rao DV 1975 Crystalline principles from the leaves and twigs of *Leptadenia reticulata*. Planta Medica 27(4):395

5 Anjaria JV, Mankad BN, Gulati OD 1974 Isolation of stigmasterol and tocopherols from *Leptadenia reticulata* by a short cut method. Indian Journal of Pharmacy 36:148

6 Subramanian SS, Nair AGR 1968 Chemical components of the follicles of *Leptadenia reticulata*. Current Science 37:373

7 Patel RP, Dantwala AS 1958 Antimicrobial activity of *Leptadenia reticulata*. Indian Journal of Pharmacy 20:241

8 Agarwal SL, Deshmankar BS, Verma SCL, Saxena SP 1960 Studies on *Leptadenia reticulata*, Part I. Pharmacological actions of aqueous extract. Indian Journal of Medical Research 48(4):457

9 Shrivastava PN, Shrivastava DN, Ahmad A 1974 Pharmacological studies on indigenous drugs – *Leptadenia reticulata, Bryenia patens* and Leptaden. Indian Veterinary Journal 51:554

10 Anjaria JV, Varia MR, Janakiraman K, Gulati OD 1975 Studies on *Leptadenia reticulata*. Lactogenic effects on rats. Indian Journal of Experimental Biology 13(5):448

11 Anjaria JV, Gupta I 1974 Studies on lactogenic property of *Leptadenia reticulata* (Jivanti) and Leptaden tablets in goats, sheep, cows and buffaloes. Indian Veterinary Journal 51:967

12 Anjaria JV, Naphade MS, Tripathi M, Gulati OD 1975 Studies on *Leptadenia reticulata*; Effects on egg yield in hens. Gujrat Agricultural University Research Journal 1:59

13 Dhar ML, Dhawan BN, Prasad CR, Rastogi RP, Singh KK, Tandon JS 1974 Screening of Indian plants for biological activity: Part V. Indian Journal of Experimental Biology 12:518

Mangifera indica L. (Anacardiaceae)

English: Mango tree

Hindi: *Aam*

Sanskrit: *Aamra*

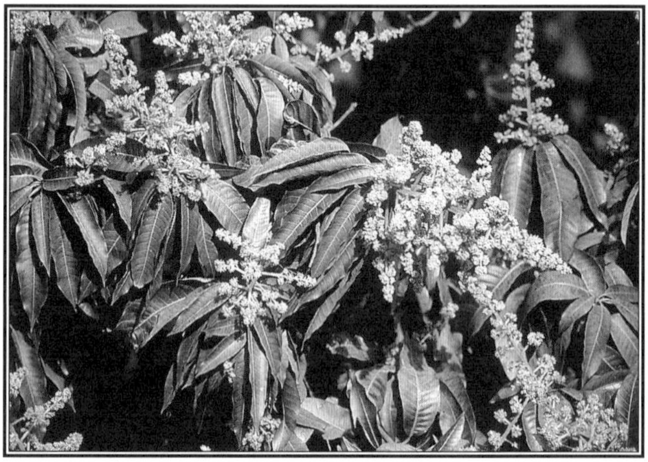

The mango is one of the most popular of all tropical fruits. Most parts of the tree are used medicinally and the bark also contains tannins, which are used for the purpose of dyeing.

Habitat

It is native to tropical Asia and has been cultivated in the Indian subcontinent for over 4000 years and is now found naturalised in most tropical countries.

Botanical description

A large evergreen tree which grows to a height of 10–45 m, dome shaped with dense foliage (Plate 36). The leaves are linear-oblong and release an aromatic odour when crushed. The bark is thick, grey to brown in colour and with age exfoliates in the form of flakes. The inflorescence occurs in panicles consisting of about 3000 tiny whitish-red or yellowish-green flowers. The fruit is a well-known large drupe, but shows a great variation in shape and size. It contains a thick yellow pulp, single seed and thick yellowish-red skin when ripe. The seed is solitary, ovoid or oblong, encased in a hard, compressed fibrous endocarp.

Parts used

Fruit, seeds, pulp, stem bark, roots, leaves.

Traditional and modern use

Ripe mango fruit is considered to be invigorating and freshening. The juice is a restorative tonic and used in heat stroke. Various parts of the plant are used as a dentifrice, antiseptic, astringent, diaphoretic, stomachic, vermifuge, tonic, laxative and diuretic and to treat diarrhoea, dysentery, anaemia, asthma, bronchitis, cough, hypertension, insomnia, rheumatism, toothache, leucorrhoea, haemorrhage and piles. The seeds are used in asthma and as an astringent.

Ethnoveterinary usage

The bark is used in haemorrhage and the seed kernel, leaf, fruit and pulp are used as feed in ruminants. All parts are used to treat abscesses, broken horn, rabid dog or jackal bite, tumour, snakebite, stings, datura poisoning, heat stroke, miscarriage, anthrax, blisters and wounds in the mouth, tympanitis, colic, diarrhoea, glossitis, indigestion, bacillosis, bloody dysentery, liver disorders, excessive urination, tetanus and asthma.

Major chemical constituents

Saponins, hydrocarbons and triterpenes

Indicoside A and B, manghopanal, mangoleanone, taraxerol, friedelin, cycloartan-3β-30-diol and derivatives, mangsterol, manglupenone, mangcoumarin, n-tetacosane, n-heneicosane, n-triacontane and mangiferolic acid methyl ester and others have been isolated from the stem bark of *Mangifera indica*.[1]

Xanthones and phenolics

Mangostin, 29-hydroxymangiferonic acid and mangiferin have been isolated from the stem bark,[2] together with common flavonoids. The flowers yielded alkyl gallates such as gallic acid, ethyl gallate, methyl gallate, n-propyl gallate, n-pentyl gallate, n-octyl gallate, 4-phenyl-n-butyl gallate, 6-phenyl-n-hexyl gallate and dihydrogallic acid.[3]

Chromones

The root contains the chromones, 3-hydroxy-2-(4′-methylbenzoyl)-chromone and 3-methoxy-2-(4′-methylbenzoyl)-chromone.[4]

Fatty acids

An unusual fatty acid, cis-9, cis-15-octadecadienoic acid was isolated from the pulp lipids of mango.[5]

Essential oil

The leaf and flower yield an essential oil containing humulene, elemene, ocimene, linalool, nerol and many others[4].

Vitamins and carotenoids

The fruit pulp contains vitamins A and C, β-carotene and xanthophylls.[4]

Medicinal and pharmacological activities

Antiinflammatory activity: An alcoholic extract of the seed kernel of *Mangifera indica* exhibited significant antiinflammatory activity in acute, subacute and chronic cases of inflammation.[6]

Antimicrobial activity: Moderate antibacterial activity has been observed in the seed kernel extracts. The leaf extract exhibited antibacterial activity against *Bacillus subtilis*, *Staphylococcus albus* and *Vibrio cholerae*.[6]

Antioxidant activity: The extract showed a powerful scavenging activity of hydroxyl radicals and acted as a chelator of iron. It also showed a significant inhibitory effect on the peroxidation of rat brain phospholipid and prevented DNA damage caused by bleomycin or copper-phenanthroline systems.[7]

Antiviral activity: Mangiferin was effective in controlling herpes simplex virus type 2, in vitro. Virus replication was significantly reduced and the study indicated that mangiferin did not act directly on the virus but inhibited the late events in HSV-2 replication.[8]

Effect on α-amylase: Ethanolic extracts of *Mangifera indica* were tested on α-amylase activity in vitro and showed an effect.[9]

Hepatoprotective activity: Mangiferin exhibited protection of liver against CCl_4-induced liver damage.[2]

Immunomodulatory action: Mangiferin induced both in vivo and in vitro activation of peritoneal macrophages by a mechanism not yet clear. The induction of interferon release from the macrophages by mangiferin, its potent metal-chelating activity, inhibitory effect on monoamine oxidase and lymphoproliferative effect on macrophage activation established the therapeutic potential of mangiferin as an immunomodulator and possible anticancer agent.[10]

Hypoglycaemic activity: A 50% ethanolic extract of the leaves produced a significant hypoglycaemic effect at a dose of 250 mg/kg, both in normal and streptozotocin-induced diabetic animals. The stimulation of β-cells to release insulin was thought to be part of the mechanism of action.[11]

Anticancer activity: Significant cytolytic activities were demonstrated by the stem bark extract against the breast cancer cell lines MCF 7, MDA-MB-435 and MDA-N, as well as against a colon cancer cell line (SW-620) and a renal cancer cell line (786-0).[12]

Antiinflammatory activity: The aqueous extract of stem bark (50–1000 mg/kg PO) exhibited a potent and dose-dependent antinociceptive effect using the acetic acid test in mice. The extract (20–1000 mg/kg PO) also dose dependently inhibited the second phase of formalin-induced pain, although not the first phase, being more potent than indomethacin at doses of 20 mg/kg. It inhibited oedema formation of both carrageenan- and formalin-induced oedema in rats, guinea pigs and mice, in a similar manner to that produced by indomethacin and sodium naproxen. The polyphenols found in the extract were thought to account for the activity reported.[13]

Safety profile

Exposure to mangoes, their skin, sap or trees may give rise to mango dermatitis. Four patients with urticaria and eczematous rash developed with exposure to mangoes or the trees were observed.[14] The LD_{50} of the 50% ethanolic extract of the leaves was found to be greater than 4.64 g/kg.[11]

Dosage

Pulp: As required
Bark: 3–6 g

Ayurvedic properties

Rasa: *Kashaya* (astringent)
Guna: *Laghu* (light), *ruksha* (dry)
Veerya: *Shita* (cold)
Vipaka: *Katu* (pungent)
Dosha: Pacifies *kapha* and *pitta*

References

1 Khan MNI, Nizami SS, Khan MA, Ahmed Z 1993 New saponins from *Mangifera indica*. Journal of Natural Products 56(5):767

2 Shankarnarayanan D, Gopalakrishnan C, Kameswaran L, Arumugum S 1979 The effect of mangostin, mangostin-3,6-di-O-glucoside and mangiferin in carbon tetrachloride liver injury. Mediscope 22:65

3 Khan MA, Khan MNI 1989 Alkyl gallates of flowers of *Mangifera indica*. Fitoterapia 60(3):284

4 Ross I 1999 Medicinal plants of the world, vol 1. Humana Press, Totowa, New Jersey

5 Shibahara A, Yamamoto K, Shinkai K, Nakayama T, Kajimoto G 1993 cis-9,cis-15-octadecadienoic acid: a novel fatty acid found in higher plants. Biochimica et Biophysica Acta 1170(3):245

6 Das PC, Das A, Mandal S et al 1989 Antiinflammatory and antimicrobial activities of the seed kernel of *Mangifera indica*. Fitoterapia 60(3):235

7 Martinez G, Delgado R, Perez G, Garrido G, Nunez Selles AJ, Leon OS 2000 Evaluation of the *in vitro* antioxidant activity of *Mangifera indica* L. extract (Vimang). Phytotherapy Research 14 (6):424

8 Zhu XM, Song JX, Huang ZZ, Wu YM, Yu MJ 1993 Antiviral activity of mangiferin against *Herpes simplex* virus type 2 *in vitro*. Chung Kuo Yao Li, Hsueh Pao 14(5):452

9 Prashanth D, Padmaja R, Samiulla DS 2001 Effect of certain plant extracts on alpha-amylase activity. Fitoterapia 72(2):179

10 Guha S, Chattopadhyay U, Ghosal S 1993 Activation of peritoneal macrophages by mangiferin, a naturally occurring xanthone. Phytotherapy Research 7:107

11 Sharma SR, Dwivedi SK, Swarup D 1997 Hypoglycaemic potential of *Mangifera indica* leaves in rats. International Journal of Pharmacognosy 35(2):130

12 Muanza DN, Euler KL, Williams L, Newman DJ 1995 Screening for antitumor and anti-HIV activities of nine medicinal plants from Zaire. International Journal of Pharmacognosy 33(2):98

13 Garrido G, Gonzalez D, Delporte C et al 2001 Analgesic and anti-inflammatory effects of *Mangifera indica* L. extract (Vimang). Phytotherapy Research 15(1):18

14 Calvert ML, Robertson I, Samaratunga H 1996 Mango dermatitis: allergic contact dermatitis to *Mangifera indica*. Australian Journal of Dermatology 37(1):59

Momordica charantia L. (Cucurbitaceae)

English: Bitter melon, bitter gourd

Hindi: *Karela*

Sanskrit: *Karavellaka, angarvelli*

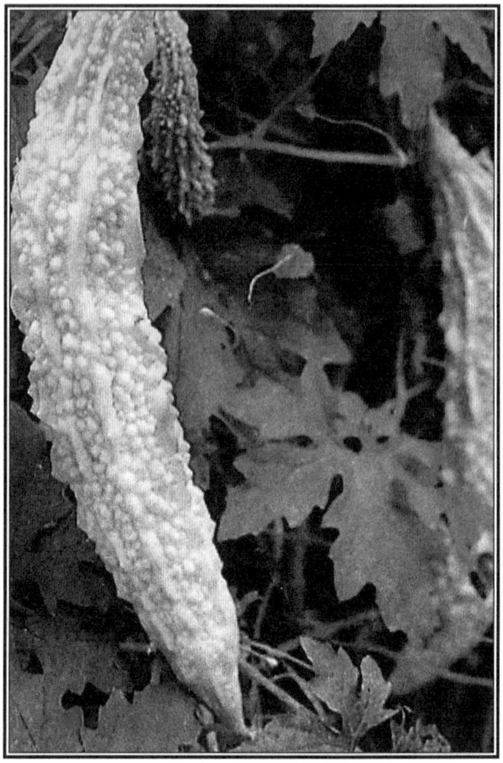

Karela has been used in the folk medicine in China, India, Africa, the West Indies and elsewhere, from ancient times. The fruits are pickled and used as a relish and the seed as a condiment. The bitterness can be reduced by steeping them in salt water, removing the outer skin and cooking. For use out of season, the fruits are preserved after slicing and drying.

Habitat

The plant is common throughout India and grown widely as a vegetable crop all over the tropics, especially in India, China, Africa and parts of America.

Botanical description

Karela is an annual creeper with branched stems, twining and slender (Plate 37). The leaf blades are 5–12 cm in diameter, reniform or suborbicular, prominently nerved, 5–7 lobed with irregular margins. Tendrils simple, slender and pubescent. Flowers monoecious, yellow in colour; male flowers solitary and female flowers bracteate at the base with a fusiform and muricate ovary. Fruits muricate or tuberculate, oblong, 2.5–7 cm long with tapering ends, green or yellowish in colour with numerous soft triangular spikes on the surface. Seeds 1.3 cm long, compressed, with a sculptured surface.

Parts used

Whole plant, leaves, but mainly fruits.

Traditional and modern use

The plant is highly recommended for the treatment of diabetes, both as part of the general diet and in the form of an extract or as a herbal tea made from the leaf. It is also used in asthma, skin infections, gastrointestinal problems and hypertension.

Ethnoveterinary usage

The herb is used widely in veterinary medicine for tetanus, eye disorders, abdominal pain, liver fluke and constipation. It is given to animals to promote digestion and urination. In cattle, it is used to expel the placenta and stop lactation after the death of a calf.[1] The prophylactic effects of *karela* were compared to those of salinomycin and bakin (*Melia azedarach*) against coccidiosis. Broiler chicks inoculated with mixed species of coccidia showed a better gain in body weight with the *karela* treatment.[2]

Major chemical constituents

Terpenoids

A series of cucurbitane-type triterpene glycosides called goyaglycosides a–h have been isolated along with the momordicosides A–L. Oleanane-type triterpene saponins, termed goyasaponins I, II and III, were also identified in the herb. The pyrimidine arabinopyranosides charine, vicine and others, along with the triterpenes momordicin, momordicinin and cucurbitanes I, II and III, have also been reported.[3–16]

Proteins

α, β and γ Momorcharins, with N-glycosidase activity, and momordins a and b, were identified along with ribosome-inactivating proteins (RIPs) and lectins.[17–23]

Sterols and fatty acids

Palmitic and oleic acids are the major components, with minor constituents such as stearic, lauric, linoleic, arachidic, myristic and capric acids. Conjugated octadecatrienoic acids form 63–68% of the oil content, together with β-sitosterol, campesterol, daucosterol, stigmasterol and momordenol (3-β-hydroxystigmasta-5,14-dien-16-one). The 4-monomethylsterols obtusifoliol, cycloeucalenol, 4-α-methylzymosterol, lophenol and the desmethylsterols spinasterol (chondrillasterol), and others were also identified.[3,24,25]

Volatile constituents

Valeric acid, aldehydes (mainly pentanal, 2-hexenal, 2-heptenal and nonadienal), amyl formate, amylvalerate, 2-butylfuran and 2-hexanone, p-cymene, menthol, nerolidol, pentadecanol, hexadecanol, myrtenol, 3-hexenol, benzyl alcohol, 1-penten-3-ol, cis-2-penten-1-ol, trans-2-hexenal, cis-sabinol and others have been identified.[3,26]

Medicinal and pharmacological activities

Anticancer activity: The aqueous extract killed human leukaemic lymphocytes in a dose-dependent manner, whilst not affecting the viability of normal human lymphocytes. A partially purified factor showed an inhibitory action on both viral and host cell RNA and on protein synthesis. This factor was found to be a single component with a molecular weight of 40 000 daltons.[27] The crude extract acted rapidly on human lymphocytes and leukaemic lymphocytic cells[28] and was reported to inhibit guanylate cyclase activity, preventing the growth of concanavalin A-stimulated rat splenic lymphocytes.[29] An injection of the extract resulted in cytotoxicity against YAC-1 targets in a short-term assay and implicated a non-adherent cell population, which was capable of killing NK-sensitive cell lines.[30] In experimental studies the ribosome-inactivating protein momordin was found to be specifically cytotoxic to the Thy 1.1-expressing mouse lymphoma cell line AKR-A in vitro.[31] A glycoprotein from the seeds inhibited protein synthesis by mitogen-stimulated normal and leukaemic lymphocytes, with a subsequent decrease in DNA formation and cell viability, which was more potent than haemagglutinin, possibly due to a greater penetration of lymphocytes by the lectin.[3] Application of Momordica proteins to MDA-MB-231 breast cancer cells resulted in inhibition of cell proliferation as well as the inhibition of the expression of the HER2 gene in vitro, suggesting a potential therapeutic use against carcinoma of the breast.[32]

Momordin 1 and momordin 2 from the seeds inhibited protein synthesis in rabbit reticulocyte lysate and showed potent cytotoxic activity against target Molt-4 cells, making them useful in allogenic bone marrow transplantation.[33] Momordin 2, conjugated to H65 monoclonal antibody, recognised human T lymphocyte CD5 surface antigen using a heterobifunctional crosslinking reagent, 2-iminothiolane. The resulting immunotoxins had no effect on human haematopoietic cells, but suppressed tumour growth.[33] α-Momorcharin inhibited the incorporation of [3H]leucine and [3H]uridine into P388 (mouse monocyte-macrophage), J774 (Balb/c macrophage), JAR (human placental choriocarcinoma) and sarcoma S180 cell lines. The most potent inhibitory effect was exerted on the P388 cell line, with the enhancement of the tumoricidal effect on mouse mastocytomal (P815) cells.[34] Tumour cell lines from renal, non-small cell lung and breast responded better to the proteins isolated from the plant.[35] A comparative study evaluating the inhibitory potential of *Momordica charantia* peel, pulp, seed and whole fruit extract on mouse skin papillomagenesis indicated that the peel is the most effective. Topical application also produced a significant elevation of sulfhydryl (-SH), cytosolic glutathione S-transferase (GST) and microsomal cytochrome b5.[36]

An anti-CD5 monoclonal antibody (mAb), linked to momordin (a type-1 ribosome-inactivating protein), was studied for in vitro cytotoxicity, measured as the inhibition of protein and/or DNA synthesis using isolated human peripheral blood mononuclear cells (PBMC) and neoplastic T lymphocytes. The potency of the immunotoxin on PBMC was very high and it was very efficient in the inhibition of the proliferative response in a mixed lymphocyte reaction, suggesting a possible use of anti-CD5-momordin conjugate in the treatment of some leukaemias and lymphomas.[37]

Hypoglycaemic activity: Extracts of *Momordica charantia* rapidly decreased and normalised blood sugar levels in alloxan- or streptozotocin-induced diabetes mellitus. The water-soluble peptide fraction (named MC6) was found to be effective on oral administration.[38] The effect of the insulin-like peptide on the lipid profile is not clear since it had no action on steroidogenesis, but other studies showed fractions with antilipolytic activity.[39] Fruit extracts reversed some of the complications of diabetes in the liver and kidney in experimental diabetes, with effective glucose control,[40] and reversed the effect of chronic diabetes on the modulation of both P450-dependent monooxygenase activities and GSH-dependent oxidative stress.[41] In a clinical study of Momordica in diabetic patients, hypoglycaemic effects were accompanied by significant adaptogenic properties indicated by a delay in the appearance of cataracts and other secondary complications of diabetes.[42]

Antifertility activity: The momorcharins are effective in inducing early and mid-term abortions, but have teratogenic effects.[43] Intraperitoneal administration to mice of β-momorcharin on days 4 and 6 of pregnancy led to an inhibition of pregnancy with the disturbance of periimplantation development.[44] The termination of early pregnancy in the mouse may have resulted from an inhibitory effect of the abortifacient protein on the differentiating endometrium.[45] α and β-momorcharin inhibit embryonic implantation, probably by inhibiting cell free protein synthesis.[46]

Antilipolytic activity: Different fractions of the fruits and seeds exhibited antilipolytic activity, resembling insulin by inhibiting hormone-induced lipolysis.[47] Two of the active compounds were identified as peptides with similar aminoacid compositions.[48]

Antigenotoxic activity: *Momordica charantia* decreased the genotoxic activity of methylnitrosamine, methanesulfonate and tetracycline, as shown by the decrease in chromosome breakage.[49]

Anthelmintic activity: Momordica was more effective than piperazine in the treatment of *Ascaridia galli.*[50]

Antimicrobial activity: *M. charantia* has shown antibacterial effects in several standard test systems.[3] Extracts of the dried powder alone, and in combination with the fruits of *Emblica officinalis* and rhizomes of *Curcuma longa* (qv), showed antibacterial activity.[51]

Antiviral activity: Proteins MAP30 and GAP30, isolated from *M. charantia*, are active against the infection and replication of Herpes simplex virus, comparable in effect to aciclovir.[52] MAP30 inactivated viral DNA and specific cleavage of 28 S rRNA, which may regulate HIV replication in conjunction with steroidal and non-steroidal inhibitors of prostaglandin synthesis. The use of the plant protein, in combination with dexamethasone and indomethacin, was therefore suggested for anti-HIV therapy.[53] The inhibition of HIV-1 integrase suggests that impediment of viral DNA integration may play a key role in the anti-HIV activity and the effect on cell-free HIV-1 infection and replication was proportionate to the dose.[54,55]

Hepatoprotective activity: Feeding *karela* to diabetic rats brought levels of aminopyrene N-demethylase close to that of control animals, while ethoxycoumarin-O-deethylase was further reduced to 60% of the control value, with the normalisation of cytosolic glutathione.[56] It involved in vitro metabolic activation of aflatoxin B1 and benzo[a]pyrene and demonstrates that the fruits contain monofunctional phase II enzyme inducers and compounds capable of repressing some monooxygenases, especially those involved in the metabolic activation of chemical carcinogens. This shows potential as a chemopreventive agent.[57]

Safety profile

As it is used so widely as a food, the fruit is thought to be reasonably safe, although the cytotoxic and other effects indicate that caution is required; hence it should not be taken by pregnant women. Overdosage may induce emesis and some of the toxic proteins will be degraded during cooking. Momordin 1 was shown to have an LD_{50} value of 8.8 mg/kg in mice.[58] The insulin-like polypeptide did not have any crossreaction with bovine insulin.[59] When used as an antiobesity agent, no side effects were observed.[60]

Dosage

Expressed juice of the whole plant or fruit: 10–30 ml

Ayurvedic properties

Rasa: *Tikta* (bitter), *katu* (pungent)

Guna: *Ruksha* (dry), *laghu* (light)

Veerya: *Ushna* (hot)

Vipaka: *Katu* (pungent)

Dosha: Pacifies *pitta* and *kapha*

Further reading

Chatterjee A, Prakashi SC 1997 Treatise of Indian medicinal plants, vol. 5. PID, New Delhi

Gogte VM 1997 Ayurvedic pharmacology and therapeutic uses of medicinal plants. Bharatiya Vidya Bhavan, Mumbai

Ross I 1999 Medicinal plants of the world, vol. 1. Humana Press, Totowa, New Jersey

References

1 Jha MK 1992 Folk veterinary medicine of Bihar – a research project. NDDB, Anand, Gujrat

2 Hayat B, Jabeen F, Hayat CS, Akhtar M 1996 Comparative prophylactic effects of salinomycin and some indigenous preparations against Coccidiosis in broiler chicks. Pakistan Veterinary Journal 16(4):164

3 Ross I 1999 Medicinal plants of the world, vol. 1. Humana Press, Totowa, New Jersey

4 Murakami T, Emoto A, Matsuda H, Yoshikawa M 2001 Medicinal foodstuffs. XXI. Structures of new cucurbitane-type triterpene glycosides, goyaglycosides-a, -b, -c, -d, -e, -f, -g, and -h, and new oleanane-type triterpene saponins, goyasaponins I, II, and III, from the fresh fruit of Japanese *Momordica charantia* L. Chemical and Pharmaceutical Bulletin 49(1):54

5 Begum S, Ahmed M, Siddiqui BS, Khan A, Saify ZS, Arif M 1997 Triterpenes, a sterol and a monocyclic alcohol from *Momordica charantia*. Phytochemistry 44(7):1313

6 Yuwai KE, Rao KS, Kaluwin C, Jones GP, Rivett DE 1991 Chemical composition of *Momordica charantia* L. fruits. Journal of Agricultural and Food Chemistry 39(10):1762

7 Fatope MO, Takeda Y, Yamashita H, Okabe H, Yamauchi T 1990 New cucurbitane triterpenoids from *Momordica charantia*. Journal of Natural Products 53(6):1491

8 El-Gengaihi S, Karawya MS, Selim MA, Motawe HM, Ibrahim N, Faddah LM 1995 A novel pyrimidine glycoside from *Momordica charantia* L. Pharmazie 50(5):361

9 Guevara AP, Lim-Sylianco CY, Dayrit FM, Finch P 1989 Acylglucosyl sterols from *Momordica charantia*. Phytochemistry 28(6):1721

10 Okabe H, Miyahara Y, Yamauchi T 1982 Studies on the constituents of *Momordica charantia* L. IV. Characterization of the new cucurbitacin glycosides of the immature fruits. (2). Structures of the bitter glycosides, momordicosides K and L. Chemical and Pharmaceutical Bulletin 30(12):4334

11 Okabe H, Miyahara Y, Yamauchi T 1982 Studies on the constituents of *Momordica charantia* L. III. Characterization of new cucurbitacin glycosides of the immature fruits. (1). Structures of momordicosides G, F1, F2 and I. Chemical and Pharmaceutical Bulletin 30(11):3977

12 Miyahara Y, Okabe H, Yamauchi T 1981 Studies on the constituents of *Momordica charantia* L. II. Isolation and characterization of minor seed glycosides, momordicosides C, D and E. Chemical and Pharmaceutical Bulletin 29(6):1561

13 Okabe H, Miyahara Y, Yamauchi T, Miyahara K, Kawasaki T 1980 Studies on the constituents of *Momordica charantia* L. I. Isolation and

characterization of momordicosides A and B, glycosides of a pentahydroxy-cucurbitane triterpene. Chemical and Pharmaceutical Bulletin 28(9):2753

14 Okabe H, Miyahara Y, Yamauchi T 1982 Structures of momordicosides F1, F2, G, I, K, and L, novel cucurbitacins in the fruits of *Momordica charantia* L. Tetrahedron Letters 23(1):77

15 Yasuda M, Iwamoto M, Okabe H, Yamauchi T 1984 Structures of momordicines I, II and III, the bitter principles in the leaves and vines of *Momordica charantia* L. Chemical and Pharmaceutical Bulletin 32(5):2044

16 Dutta PK, Chakravarty AK, Chowdhury US, Pakrashi SC 1981 Studies on Indian medicinal plants. Part-64. Vicine, a favism-inducing toxin from *Momordica charantia* Linn. seeds. Indian Journal of Chemisty 20B(8):669

17 Pu Z, Lu B, Liu W, Jin S 1996 Characterization of the enzymic mechanism of gamma-momorcharin, a novel ribosome-inactivating protein with lower molecular weight of 11,500 purified from the seeds of bitter gourd (*Momordica charantia*). Biochemistry and Biophysics Research Communications 229(1):287

18 Mock JWY, Ng TB, Wong RNS, Yao QZ, Yeung HW, Fong WP 1996 Demonstration of ribonuclease activity in the plant ribosome-inactivating proteins alpha- and beta-momorcharins. Life Sciences 59(22):1853

19 Wang H, Ng TB 1998 Ribosome inactivating protein and lectin from bitter melon (*Momordica charantia*) seeds: sequence comparison with related proteins. Biochemistry and Biophysics Research Communications 253(1):143

20 Fong WP, Poon YT, Wong TM et al 1996 A highly efficient procedure for purifying the ribosome-inactivating proteins alpha- and beta-momorcharins from *Momordica charantia* seeds, N-terminal sequence comparison and establishment of their N-glycosidase activity. Life Sciences 59(11):901

21 Minami Y, Nakahara Y, Funatsu G 1992 Isolation and characterization of two momordins, ribosome-inactivating proteins from the seeds of bitter gourd (*Momordica charantia*). Bioscience Biotechnology and Biochemistry 56(9):1470

22 Yeung HW, Ng TB, Li WW, Cheung WK 1987 Partial chemical characterization of alpha- and beta-momorcharins. Planta Medica 53(2):164

23 Feng Z, Li WW, Yeung HW et al 1990 Crystals of alpha-momorcharin. A new ribosome-inactivating protein. Journal of Molecular Biology 214(3):625

24 Armougom R, Grondin I, Smadja J 1998 Composition of fatty acids in lipid extracts of seeds of tropical Cucurbitaceae. Lipides 5(4):323

25 Chang MK, Conkerton EJ, Chapital DC, Wan PJ, Vandhwa OP, Spiers JM 1996 Chinese melon (*Momordica charantia* L.) seed; composition and potential use. Journal of the American Oil Chemistry Society 73(2):263

26 Binder RG, Flath RA, Mon TR 1989 Volatile components of bitter melon. Journal of Agricultural and Food Chemistry 37(2):418

27 Takemoto DJ, Jilka C, Rockenbach S, Hughes JV 1983 Purification and characterization of a cytostatic factor with anti-viral activity from the bitter melon. Preparative Biochemistry 13(5):391

28 Takemoto DJ, Dunford C, McMurray MM 1982 The cytotoxic and cytostatic effects of the bitter melon (*Momordica charantia*) on human lymphocytes. Toxicon 20(3):593

29 Takemoto DJ, Kresie R, Vaughn D 1980 Partial purification and characterization of a guanylate cyclase inhibitor with cytotoxic properties from the bitter melon (*Momordica charantia*). Biochemistry and Biophysics Research Communications 94(1):332

30 Cunnick JE, Sakamoto K, Chapes SK, Fortner GW, Takemoto DJ 1990 Induction of tumor cytotoxic immune cells using a protein from the bitter melon (*Momordica charantia*). Cellular Immunology 126(2):278

31 Stirpe F, Wawrzynczak EJ, Brown ANF et al 1988 Selective cytotoxic activity of immunotoxins composed of a monoclonal anti-Thy 1.1 antibody and the ribosome-inactivating proteins bryodin and momordin. British Journal of Cancer 58(5):558

32 Lee-Huang S, Huang PL, Sun Y et al 2000 Inhibition of MDA-MB-231 human breast tumor xenografts and HER2 expression by anti-tumor

agents GAP31 and MAP30. Anticancer Research 20(2A):653

33 Wang R, Chen X, Li Y, Shen P 1992 Immunotoxins composed of monoclonal antihuman T lymphocyte antibody and single chain ribosome-inactivating proteins: antitumor effects in vitro and in vivo. Zhongguo Mianyixue Zazhi 8(6):356

34 Ng TB, Liu WK, Sze SF, Yeung HW 1994 Action of α-momorcharin, a ribosome inactivating protein, on cultured tumor cell lines. General Pharmacology 25(1):75

35 Rybak SM, Lin JJ, Newton DL et al 1994 In vitro antitumor activity of the plant ribosome inactivating proteins MAP 30 and GAP 31. International Journal of Oncology 5(5):1171

36 Singh A, Singh SP, Bamezai R 1998 *Momordica charantia* (Bitter Gourd) peel, pulp, seed and whole fruit extract inhibits mouse skin papillomagenesis. Toxicology Letters 94(1):37

37 Porro G, Bolognesi A, Caretto P et al 1993 In vitro and in vivo properties of an anti-CD5-momordin immunotoxin on normal and neoplastic T lymphocytes. Cancer Immunology and Immunotherapy 36(5):346

38 Ng TB, Li WW, Yeung HW 1987 Effects of ginsenosides, lectins and *Momordica charantia* insulin-like peptide on corticosterone production by isolated rat adrenal cells. Journal of Ethnopharmacology 21(1):21

39 Ng TB, Wong CM, Li WW, Yeung HW 1986 Insulin-like molecules in *Momordica charantia* seeds. Journal of Ethnopharmacology 15(1):107

40 Baquer NZ, Gupta D, Raju J 1998 Regulation of metabolic pathways in liver and kidney during experimental diabetes: effects of antidiabetic compounds. Indian Journal of Clinical Biochemistry 13(2):63

41 Raza H, Ahmed I, John A, Sharma AK 2000 Modulation of xenobiotic metabolism and oxidative stress in chronic streptozotocin-induced diabetic rats fed with *Momordica charantia* fruit extract. Journal of Biochemical and Molecular Toxicology 14(3):131

42 Srivastava Y, Venkatakrishna-Bhatt H, Verma Y, Venkaiah K, Raval BH 1993 Antidiabetic and adaptogenic properties of *Momordica charantia* extract: an experimental and clinical evaluation. Phytotherapy Research 7(4):285

43 Chan WY, Tam PPL, Choi HL, Ng TB, Yeung HW 1986 Effects of momorcharins on the mouse embryo at the early organogenesis stage. Contraception 34(5):537

44 Chan WY, Tam PPL, Yeung HW 1984 The termination of early pregnancy in the mouse by β-momorcharin. Contraception 29(1):91

45 Chan WY, Tam PPL, So KC, Yeung HW 1985 The inhibitory effects of β-momorcharin on endometrial cells in the mouse. Contraception 31(1):83

46 Ng TB, Tam PPL, Hon WK, Choi HL, Yeung HW 1988 Effects of momorcharins on ovarian response to gonadotropin-induced superovulation in mice. International Journal of Fertility 33(2):123

47 Wong CM, Ng TB, Yeung HW 1985 Screening of *Trichosanthes kirilowii*, *Momordica charantia* and *Cucurbita maxima* (family Cucurbitaceae) for compounds with antilipolytic activity. Journal of Ethnopharmacology 13(3):313

48 Ng TB, Wong CM, Li WW, Yeung HW 1987 Peptides with antilipolytic and lipogenic activities from seeds of the bitter gourd *Momordica charantia* (family Cucurbitaceae). General Pharmacology 18(3):275

49 Balboa JG, Lim-Sylianco CY 1992 Antigenotoxic effects of drug preparations Akapulko and Ampalaya. Philippine Journal of Science 121(4):399

50 Lal J, Chandra S, Raviprakash V, Sabir M 1976 *In vitro* anthelmintic action of some indigenous medicinal plants on *Ascaridia galli* worms. Indian Journal of Physiology and Pharmacology 20(2):64

51 Sankaranarayanan J, Jolly CI 1993 Phytochemical, antibacterial, and pharmacological investigations on *Momordica charantia* Linn., *Emblica officinalis* Gaertn. and *Curcuma longa* Linn. Indian Journal of Pharmaceutical Science 55(1):6.

52 Bourinbaiar AS, Lee-Huang S 1996 The activity of plant-derived antiretroviral proteins MAP30 and GAP31 against herpes simplex virus infection

in vitro. Biochemistry and Biophysics Research Communications 219(3):923

53 Bourinbaiar AS, Lee-Huang S 1995 Potentiation of anti-HIV activity of the anti-inflammatory drugs dexamethasone and indomethacin by MAP30, the antiviral agent from bitter melon. Biochemistry and Biophysics Research Communications 208(2):779

54 Lee-Huang S, Huang PL, Huang PL, Bourinbaiar AS, Chen HC, Kung HF 1995 Inhibition of the integrase of human immunodeficiency virus (HIV) type 1 by anti-HIV plant proteins MAP30 and GAP31. Proceedings of the National Academy of Science of the USA 92(19):8818

55 Lee-Huang S, Huang PL, Nara PL et al 1990 MAP 30: a new inhibitor of HIV-1 infection and replication. FEBS Letters 272(1–2):12

56 Raza H, Amed I, Lakhani MS, Sharma AK, Pallot D, Montague W 1996 Effect of bitter melon (*Momordica charantia*) fruit juice on the hepatic cytochrome P-450-dependent monooxygenases and glutathione S-transferases in streptozotocin-induced diabetic rats. Biochemistry and Pharmacology 52(10):1639

57 Kusamran WR, Ratanavila A, Tepsuwan A 1998 Effects of neem flowers, Thai and Chinese bitter gourd fruits and sweet basil leaves on hepatic monooxygenases and glutathione S-transferase activities, and *in vitro* metabolic activation of chemical carcinogens in rats. Food Chemistry and Toxicology 36(6):475

58 Khanna P, Jain SC, Panagariya A, Dixit VP 1981 Hypoglycemic activity of polypeptide from a plant source. Journal of Natural Products 44(6):648

59 Dhar ML, Dhar MM, Dhawan BN, Mehrotra BN, Ray C 1968 Screening of Indian plants for biological activity-I. Indian Journal of Experimental Biology 6:232

60 Yamahara J 1998 D-Xylose and pharmaceutical natural products as anti-obesity agents. Japanese Patent application: JP 97-108130 19970409

Mucuna pruriens Bak. (Papilionaceae) (syn. *Macuna pruriens* (L.) DC.)

English: Cowhage, cowitch

Hindi: *Kavach*

Sanskrit: *Atmagupta, vanari*

The use of this species as an anthelmintic was first recorded by Patrick Browne in his *Civil and Natural History of Jamaica,* 1756, and it has also been mentioned in other books on traditional medicine. Ancient Sanskrit texts indicate that it was used as an aphrodisiac and its use in a formulation for tremors is recorded. L-dopa, the major constituent of the seeds, revolutionised the treatment of Parkinson's disease in the 1960s. The seeds have been used as promoters of virility.

Habitat

Originally from India, it is widely grown in the tropics as a fodder crop and naturalised in many other countries including Sri Lanka, south-east Asia and Malaysia.

Botanical description

A tender, evergreen, twining climber, reaching 3 m, with downy leaves up to 45 cm long, divided into three ovate, pointed leaflets (Plate 38). Clusters of purple or white, pea-like flowers, about 5 cm long, appear in summer, followed by flattened pods, up to 9 cm long and 2 cm wide, with a pointed, often hooked, apex. The pods contain 3–6 seeds, about 1 cm long, and are covered in orange or dark brown, irritant bristles.

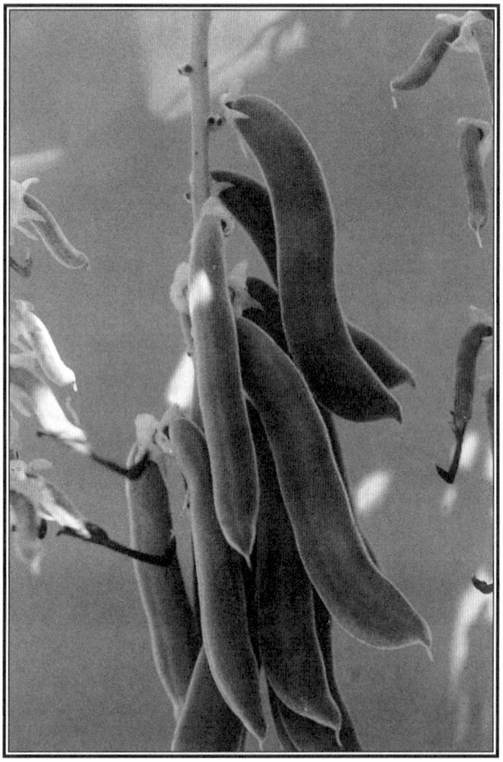

Parts used

Seeds, root, legumes.

Traditional and modern use

The traditional use centres mainly on its use as an antiparkinsonian agent, anthelmintic and aphrodisiac. A hot water extract of the dried fruit is administered to children in cases of intestinal worms and the powdered trichomes of the pod have been taken orally for this purpose, along with milk or buttermilk.[1] However, this can be dangerous and should be avoided. A water extract of leaves is used as an aphrodisiac, nerve tonic, for scorpion stings and in dysentery.[2] The seeds are taken orally by men to cure night dreams and impotency, to promote fertility and as an aphrodisiac to increase seminal fluid and vigour. In this case, two seeds are powdered and taken with a cup of cow's milk.[3] A powdered seed, taken with milk, is also used for diarrhoea.[4] Hot water extracts of the dried seeds are taken orally as a nervine[5] and to procure abortion.[6] The dried powdered root has been taken with honey as a blood purifier, diuretic and to dissolve kidney stones[7] and for persistent coughs, the seeds are sometimes placed over a hot plate or burning charcoal and the fumes inhaled through the mouth.[8] Several of these effects have been substantiated by recent scientific investigations.

Ethnoveterinary usage

It is used in urinary complaints, for elephantiasis, snake bite, anthrax, tympanitis and lumbar fracture.[9]

Major chemical constituents

Alkaloids

Prurienene, prurieninine, prurienidine, mucunine, mucunadine, mucuadine, mucuadinine, mucuadininine and nicotine are reported in the whole plant.[10,11]

Triterpenes and sterols

β-Sitosterol, stigmasterol, β-amyrin acetate, ursolic acid and betulinic acid are present in the root.[12]

Proteins and aminoacids

L-dopa, methionine, phenylalanine, tyrosine, lysine, aspartic acid, glutamic acids, glycine, leucine, isoleucine, and serine,[13] together with globulins and albumins, have been isolated from the seed.[14,15]

Fatty acids, carbohydrates and related compounds

Oleic acid, linoleic acid, palmitic acid, lecithin, lauric acid, linolenic acid and others, D-galactose and D-mannose are present in the seed.[16,17]

Medicinal and pharmacological activities

Antiparkinsonian activity: L-dopa has long been used for the treatment of Parkinson's disease in both modern medicine and ancient Indian therapeutics. In a recent study, rats fed with *Mucuna pruriens* endocarp (MP, 2.5 or 5.0 g/kg) showed superior activity to synthetic L-dopa (125 or 250 mg/kg). L-dopa, or MP at the same levels, plus carbidopa (50 mg/kg; controls received only carbidopa) was administered via gavage 1 h prior to testing, using a rotometer method as a measure of antiparkinsonian activity. Over 4 hours, dose for dose, MP was twice as potent as synthetic L-dopa in inducing contralateral rotation in the parkinsonian animal model. Thus, MP may contain unidentified antiparkinsonian compounds in addition to L-dopa or it may have adjuvants that enhance the efficacy of L-dopa.[18]

Comparison of the CNS profiles of L-dopa at 100 mg/kg and *M. pruriens* seed powder (3 g, containing 100 mg of L-dopa) showed equivalent hypothermic and anti-parkinsonian activity in rats and mice. MP had a faster onset of action and was significantly more active than LD. Both LD and MP significantly increased motor activity and both potentiated low-dose apomorphine-induced hypomotility. However, at high dose apomorphine-induced hypermotility LD had no effect but MP antagonised it. This differential effect suggests a different mode of action at dopamine post- and presynaptic receptor sites. In cardiovascular studies in animals, both L-dopa and MP caused a marginal potentiation of the pressor responses to adrenaline and antagonism of the carotid occlusion-induced pressor response to adrenaline. In haloperidol- and metoprolol-treated animals the adrenaline response was significantly potentiated by L-dopa but not by MP. The study showed that at equivalent doses, MP resembles L-dopa with respect to modulation of dopaminergic pathways, while the presence of other constituents in MP appears to contribute to improved anti-parkinsonian activity and greater tolerability.[19]

Efficacy and tolerability of HP-200, a preparation derived from *M. pruriens*, in treating patients with Parkinson's disease was demonstrated. Sixty patients with Parkinson's disease (46 male and 14 female) with a mean (± SD) age of 59±9 years were treated in an open study for 12 weeks. Of these, 26 patients were taking synthetic levodopa/carbidopa formulations before treatment with HP-200 and the remaining 34 were levodopa naive. HP-200 was mixed with water and given orally. The Unified Parkinson's Disease Rating Scale (UPDRS) was used periodically during the 12-week evaluation. Statistically significant reductions in UPDRS and other scores were seen from baseline to the end of the 12-week treatment. Adverse effects were mild and mainly gastrointestinal in nature and no adverse effects were seen in clinical laboratory reports.[20]

Hypoprolactinaemic effects: After oral pretreatment of patients with 15 g of the seed powder, chlorpromazine-induced hyperprolactinaemia was inhibited (by 40%) and was as effective as 0.5 g of L-dopa. No side effects were observed in the study.[21]

Hypoglycaemic activity: Oral feeding of MP (at a dose of 200 mg per kg body weight per day for 40 days) to streptozotocin-induced diabetic mice reduced plasma glucose concentrations by 9%. It also prevented polyuria and partially but significantly ($p < 0.05$) prevented renal hypertrophy as compared to diabetic controls.[22] Powdered seeds significantly decreased blood glucose levels in normal as well as alloxan-diabetic rabbits. It is not yet known whether the seeds act indirectly by stimulating the release of insulin or by a direct insulin-like action.[23]

Antihaemorrhagic activity: The properties of the seed extract were demonstrated against *Echis carinatus* venom (EV). This venom affects the coagulative cascade, causing severe bleeding and haemorrhage. The extract attentuated the increased prothrombin activation induced by EV in vitro and could explain the protective effect in vivo.[24] An aqueous extract of the leaves also showed a dose-dependent reduction in the time taken to clot for blood treated with a standardised dose of the same venom.[25]

Spermatogenic activity: The total alkaloidal extract from the seeds produced an increase in the numbers of spermatozoa and the weights of the testes, seminal vesicles and prostate of treated rats. A stimulation of testosterone-induced androgenic activity was also observed in treated animals.[26]

CNS activity: Indolealkylamines isolated from *Mucuna pruriens* showed hallucinogenic activity, as measured by marked behavioural changes, antagonism of pentobarbitone-induced hypnosis, inhibition of reserpine-induced ptosis, hypothermia and sedation. It also reduced chlorpromazine-induced catatonia, and enhanced amphetamine toxicity in rats.[27]

Aphrodisiac activity: The drug has been used to improve cases of depressed libido and potency of both organic and psychogenic origin and management of premature ejaculation in humans. This is supported by experiments in rats in which the effect of the seeds on the general mating behaviour, potency (penile reflex test) and libido (mounting frequency) were studied. The drug produced a striking and sustained increase of sexual activity and androgenic activity was demonstrated. All the parameters of mating behaviour, including ejaculatory latency, were augmented and penile reflexes as well as mounting frequency were increased.[28,29]

Anabolic activity: Plant administered orally to castrated adult and young male mice at a dose of 7.70 mg/animal was active. There was increased maltase activity of dorsoventral prostate and increase in fructose content of seminal vesicles.[30]

Analgesic, antiinflammatory and antipyretic activity: An ethanol (95%) extract of the dried trichomes, administered intragastrically to rats, was active against acetic acid-induced writhing. It also showed analgesic activity as demonstrated by the hot plate method and was active against carrageenan-induced rat paw oedema, as was a similar extract of the leaves. Both extracts inhibited yeast-induced pyrexia.[31]

Safety profile

Pods, hairs and powder are externally irritant to the skin, eyes and mucous membranes. The stinging hairs produce extremely aggressive itching and burning, accompanied by long-lasting inflammation, caused by serotonin and mucunain, a proteolytic enzyme. The intake of the hairs should therefore be avoided, although administration of the herb in the form of extract is probably fairly harmless. The ethanol/water (1:1) extract of the fruit, when administered intraperitoneally to mice, was tolerated at a maximum dose of 1 g/kg[32] and that of the root was 250 mg/kg.[33]

Dosage

Powdered seeds: 1.5–2.5 g

Ayurvedic properties

Rasa: *Madhur* (sweet), *tikta* (bitter)

Guna: *Guru* (heavy), *snigdha* (unctuous)

Veerya: *Ushna* (hot)

Vipaka: *Madhur* (sweet)

Dosha: *Rasayana*

Further reading

Bharatiya Vidya Bhavan's Swami Prakashananda Ayurveda Research Centre 1992 Selected medicinal plants of India. Chemexcil, Mumbai

Bown D 1995 Encyclopaedia of herbs and their uses. Dorling Kindersley, London

Kapoor LD 1990 Handbook of Ayurvedic medicinal plants. CRC Press, Boca Raton

Ministry of Health and Family Welfare 1989 Ayurvedic pharmacopoeia of India, vol III. Government of India, New Delhi

Ross I 2000 Medicinal plants of the world, vol 2. Humana Press, Totowa, New jersey

References

1 Joshi MC, Patel MB, Mehta PJ 1980 Some folk medicines of Dangs, Gujrat state. Bulletin of Medical and Ethnobotanical Research 1:8

2 Nagaraju N, Rao KN 1990 A survey of plant crude drugs of Rayalaseema, Andhra Pradesh, India. Journal of Ethnopharmacology 29(2):137

3 Bhandary MJ, Chandrashekar KR, Kaveirappa KM 1995 Medical ethnobotany of the Siddis of Uttar Kannada District, Karnataka, India. Journal of Ethnopharmacology 47(3):149

4 Girach RD, Aminuddin PA, Siddioui R, Khan SA 1994 Traditional plant remedies among the Kondh District of Dhenkanal (Orissa). International Journal of Pharmacognosy 32(3):274

5 Kapoor SL, Kapoor LD 1980 Medicinal plant wealth of the Karimnagr District of Andhra Pradesh. Bulletin of Medical and Ethnobotanical Research 1:120

6 Nath D, Sethi N, Singh RK, Jain AK 1992 Commonly used Indian abortifacient plants with special reference to their teratologic effects in rats. Journal of Ethnopharmacology 36(2):147

7 Pushpangadan P, Atal CK 1984 Ethno-medico-botanical investigations on Kerala 1. Some primitive tribals of Western Ghats and their herbal medicine. Journal of Ethnopharmacology 11(1):59

8 Dixit RS, Pandey HC 1984 Plants used as folk-medicine in Jhansi and Lalitpur sections of Bundelkhand, Uttar Pradesh. International Journal of Crude Drug Research 22(1):47

9 Jha MK 1992 The folk veterinary system of Bihar – a research survey. NDDB, Anand, Gujrat

10 Ross I 1999 *Mucuna pruriens*. In: Medicinal plants of the world. Humana Press, Totawa, New Jersey

11 Santra DK, Majumdar DN 1953 *Mucuna pruriens*. II, Isolation of water-insoluble alkaloids. Indian Journal of Pharmacy 15:60

12 Aruna V, Naidu KC, Satyanarayana T, Ganapaty S 1998 Phytochemical studies on the roots of *Mucuna pruriens* Baker. Indian drugs 35(6):356

13 Pant R, Singh KS 1969 Amino-acids of some wild legumes. Current Science 38(9):213–214

14 Prakash D, Niranjan A, Tewari SK 2001 Some nutritional properties of the seeds of three *Mucuna* species. International Journal of Food Science and Nutrition 52(1):79

15 Siddhuraju P, Vijayakumari K, Janardhanan K 1996 Chemical composition and protein quality of the little-known legume, velvet bean (*Mucuna pruriens*). Journal of Agricultural and Food Chemistry 44(9):2143

16 Singh RB 1999 Water soluble polysaccharide of Garhwal region flora: *Mucuna pruriens* Bak. seeds. Oriental Journal of Chemistry 15(1):187

17 Panikkar KR, Majella VL, Pillai PM 1987 Lecithin from *Mucuna pruriens*. Planta Medica 53(5):503

18 Hussain G, Manyam BV 1997 *Mucuna pruriens* proves more effective than L-DOPA in Parkinson's disease animal model. Phytotherapy Research 11(6):419

19 Rajendran VJ, Thangam DJ 1996 Reappraisal of dopaminergic aspects of *Mucuna pruriens* and comparative profile with L-DOPA on cardiovascular and central nervous system in animals. Indian Drugs 33(9):465

20 An alternative medicine treatment for Parkinson's disease: results of a multicenter clinical trial. HP-200 in Parkinson's Disease Study Group. Journal of Alternative and Complementary Medicine 1(3):249

21 Vaidya RA, Sheth AR, Aloorkar SD et al 1978 The inhibitory effect of the cowhage plant – *Mucuna pruriens* – and L-dopa on chlorpromazine-induced hyperprolactinemia in man. Neurology (India) 26(4):177

22 Grover JK, Vats V, Rathi SS, Dawar R 2001 Traditional Indian anti-diabetic plants attenuate progression of renal damage in streptozotocin induced diabetic mice. Journal of Ethnopharmacology 76(3):233

23 Akhtar MS, Qureshi AQ, Iqbal J 1990 Antidiabetic evaluation of *Mucuna pruriens*. Journal of the Pakistan Medical Association 40(7):147

24 Guerranti R, Aguiyi JC, Errico E, Pagani R, Marinello E 2001 Effects of *Mucuna pruriens* extract on activation of prothrombin by *Echis carinatus* venom. Journal of Ethnopharmacology 75(2–3):175

25 Houghton PJ, Skari KP 1994 The effect on blood clotting of some west African plants used against snakebite. Journal of Ethnopharmacology 44(2):99

26 Saksena S, Dixit VK 1987 Role of total alkaloids of *Mucuna pruriens* Baker in spermatogenesis in albino rats. Indian Journal of Natural Products 3(1):3

27 Bhattacharya SK, Sanyal AK, Ghosal S 1971 Hallucinogenic activity of indole alkylamines isolated from *Mucuna pruriens*. Indian Journal of Physiology and Allied Sciences 25(2):53

28 Rao MRR, Parakh SR 1978 Effect of some indigenous drugs on the sexual behavior of male rats. Indian Journal of Pharmaceutical Sciences 40:236E

29 Amin KMY, Khan NA, Rahman SZ 1993 The sexual function improving effect of 'Tukhm-e-Konch' (*Mucuna pruriens*) and its mechanism of action – an experimental study. Proceedings of the First National Seminar on Ilmul Advia, Beenapara, India. 23–25 April

30 Jayatilak PG, Pardanani DS, Murthy BD, Sheth AR 1976 Effect of an indigenous drug (Speman) on accessory reproductive functions of mice. Indian Journal of Experimental Biology 14:170

31 Jauk L, Galati EM, Kirjavainen S, Forestieri AM, Trovato A 1993 Analgesic and antipyretic effect of *Mucuna pruriens*. International Journal of Pharmacognosy 31(3):213–216

32 Dhar ML, Dhar MM, Mehrotra BN, Ray C 1968 Screening of Indian medicinal plants for biological activity. Part I. Indian Journal of Experimental Biology 6:232–247

33 Kapoor LD 1985 Handbook of Ayurvedic medicinal plants. CRC Press, Boca Raton

Nigella sativa L. (Ranunculaceae)

English: Black cumin, small fennel

Hindi: *Kalonji, kalajira*

Sanskrit: *Kalajaji*

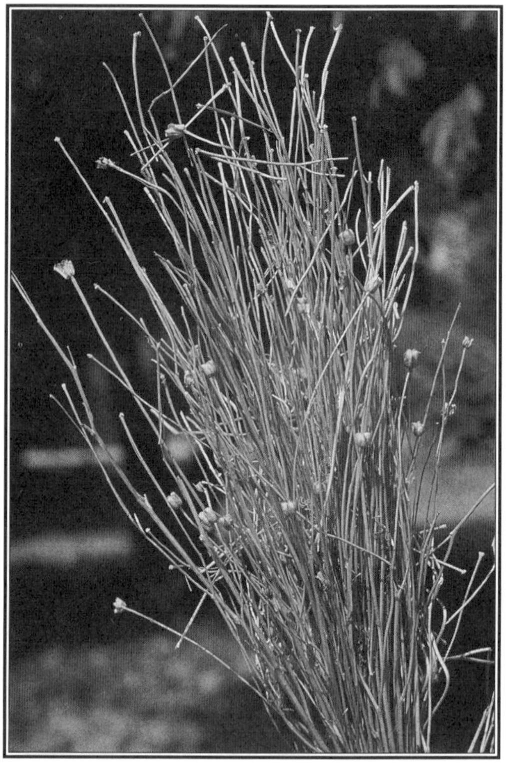

Kalonji seeds and their oil have a long history of folklore usage in Arabian and Indian civilisation and are used in food as well as medicine. The seeds are used as flavouring, to improve digestion and produce warmth, especially in cold climates. They are sometimes scattered in the folds of woollen fabrics to preserve them from insect damage.

Habitat

The plant is indigenous to the Mediterranean region but now found widely in Jammu, Kashmir, Himachal Pradesh, Bihar, Assam and Punjab. The herb is also cultivated in Bengal and north-east India.

Botanical description

A small prostrate annual herb about 45 cm high (Plate 39), 2–3 slender leaves pinnatisect, 2–4 cm long cut into linear segment, segments oblong-lanceolate. Flowers pale, blue on solitary long peduncles, seeds trigonous and black in colour.

Parts used

Seeds.

Traditional and modern use

Kalonji seeds are used as a carminative, aromatic, stimulant, diuretic, anthelmintic, galactagogue and diaphoretic. They are used as a condiment in curries. A tincture prepared from the seeds is useful in indigestion, loss of appetite, diarrhoea, dropsy, amenorrhoea and dysmenorrhoea and in the treatment of worms and skin eruptions. Externally the oil is used as an antiseptic. To arrest vomiting, seeds are roasted and given internally.

Ethnoveterinary usage

In ruminants seeds are used as a galactagogue in cases of reduced milk flow and as an antioxytocic agent during pregnancy and birthing to retain placenta.[1]

Major chemical constituents

Alkaloids

The major alkaloids are nigellidine, nigellicine and nigellimine.[2,3]

Flavonoid glycosides

A number of quercetin and kaempferol glycosides have been isolated.[4]

Saponins

The seeds have been reported to contain a hederagenin saponin, melanthin and melanthigenin.[5]

Sterols

Cholesterol, campesterol, stigmasterol, β-sitosterol and α-spinasterol.[6]

Volatile oil

Thymoquinone, thymol, carvone dithymoquinone, monoterpenes including d-limonene, p-cymene and (+) citronellol have been isolated.[7,8]

Fixed oil

Linoleic acid, palmitic acid, stearic acid and oleic acid are present.[7]

Medicinal and pharmacological activities

Antimicrobial activity: *Nigella sativa* exhibited strong antimicrobial activity against *Salmonella typhi*, *Pseudomonas aeruginosa* and others.[9] The essential oil has been shown to have activity against Gram-positive and Gram-negative bacteria. However, sensitivity against Gram-positive bacteria such as *Staphylococcus aureus* and *Vibrio cholerae* was found to be stronger. Bacteria like *Staph. aureus*, *Strep. pyogenes* and *Strep. viridans* are more susceptible to *Nigella sativa*. In an in vitro study, volatile oil showed activity comparable to ampicillin. The activity of the volatile oil also extended to drug-resistant strains of Shigella spp, *Vibrio cholerae* and *Escherichia coli* and was found to have a synergistic action with streptomycin and gentamicin.[10]

Hepatoprotective activity: Thymoquinone, one of the active constituents of *Nigella sativa*, is reported to have hepatoprotective activity.[11] An in vitro study showed the protective effect against tert-butyl hydroperoxide (TBHP)-induced oxidative damage to hepatocytes. The activity was demonstrated by a decreased leakage of alanine transaminase (ALT), aspartic transaminase (AST) and decreased trypan blue uptake, in comparison to the control TBHP-treated hepatocytes.[12]

Antidiabetic activity: Significant hypoglycaemic activity has been reported and is thought to be due to the essential oil present.[13,14] Clinical studies have confirmed these results and suggest that the antidiabetic action of the plant extract may be mediated partly through decreased hepatic gluconeogenesis.[15]

Antiinflammatory activity: Asthma and arthritis are chronic inflammatory disorders involving a variety of inflammatory mediators and different pathways. The fixed oil and thymoquinone from the seeds were found to inhibit eicosanoid generation in leucocytes and membrane lipid peroxidation and a significant reduction in rat paw oedema and a reduction in granuloma pouch weight were also observed.[16,17] Nigellone in low concentration is effective in inhibiting the histamine release from the mast cells, which supports an antiasthmatic role for the plant.[18]

Antifertility activity: The antifertility activity of *Nigella sativa* in male rats has been established, shown by an inhibition of spermatogenesis and a significant reduction in sialic acid content of the testis, epididymis, seminal vesicles and prostate.[19,20] A weak oestrogenic activity of the seeds was indicated with antiimplantational effects in experimental models.[21,22]

Antioxytocic activity: Preliminary reports suggest antioxytocic properties, in that a reversible inhibition of spontaneous smooth muscle contraction and inhibition of uterine smooth muscle contraction induced by oxytocin stimulation have been observed in rat and guinea pig.[23]

Cytotoxic activity: Cytotoxic and immunopotentiating effects of *Nigella sativa* have been established.[24,25] The long chain fatty acids are thought to contribute to the antitumour activity.[26] The extract shows a modulatory effect in cisplatin-induced toxicity in mice and a protective effect against cisplatin-induced falls in haemoglobin levels and leucocyte counts.[27] A cytotoxic effect of *Nigella sativa* was observed by the retardation of ascites growth in a Dalton's lymphoma ascites model.[28]

Anthelmintic activity: *Nigella sativa* was found to have an anthelmintic activity against tapeworm comparable to that of piperazine.[29] The pure essential oil showed activity against Monezia in sheep comparable to niclosamide.[30]

Analgesic activity: The essential oil produced significant analgesic activity using chemical and thermal noxious stimuli methods such as acetic acid-induced writhing, hot plate and tail flick tests. The activity was antagonised by naloxone, suggesting that the effects were mediated through opioid receptors.[31]

Other activites: Other reports include hypocholesterolaemic, antihypertensive and galactagogue effects.[32,33]

Safety profile

Seeds of *Nigella sativa* have a long history of use for food and medicinal purposes. No adverse or side effects have been reported when used within the recommended dosage, although dermatitis has been reported.[34]

Dosage

Powder: 1–3 g

Ayurvedic properties

Rasa: *Katu* (pungent), *tikta* (bitter)

Guna: *Laghu* (light), *ruksha* (dry), *tikshna* (sharp)

Veerya: *Ushna* (hot)

Vipaka: *Katu* (pungent)

Dosha: Pacifies *vatta* and *kapha*

Further reading

Duke JA 1992 Handbook of phytochemical constituents of GRAS herbs and other economic plants. CRC Press, Boca Raton

Kapoor LD 1990 Handbook of Ayurvedic medicinal plants. CRC Press, Boca Raton

Nadkarni AK 1976 Indian materia medica. Popular Prakashan PVT Ltd, Bombay

References

1 International Institute of Rural Reconstruction 1994 Ethnoveterinary medicine in Asia. An information kit on traditional animal health care practices. IIRR, Silang, Philippines

2 Rahman AU, Sohail M, Sadiq HSI, Choudhary M, Chao-Zhou N, Clardy J 1995 Nigellidine – a new indazole alkaloid from the seeds of *Nigella sativa*. Tetrahedron Letters 36(12):1993

3 Rahman AU, Sohail M, Zaman K 1992 Nigellimine: a new isoquinoline alkaloid from the seeds of *Nigella sativa*. Journal of Natural Products 55(5):676

4 Merfort I, Wray V, Barakat HH, Hussein SAM, Nawwar MAM, Willuhn G 1997 Flavonol triglycosides from seeds of *Nigella sativa*. Phytochemistry 46(2):359

5 Akbar AA, Hassan S, Kenne L, Rahman AU, Wehler T 1988 Structural studies on a saponin isolated from *Nigella sativa*. Phytochemistry 27(12):3977

6 Ustun G, Kent L, Cekin N, Civelekoglu H 1990 Investigation of the technological properties of *Nigella sativa* (Black Cumin) seed oil. J. Am. Oil Chem. Soc. 67(12):958

7 Rathee PS, Mishra SH, Kaushal R 1992 Antimicrobial activity of essential oil, fixed oil and unsaponifiable matter of *Nigella sativa* Linn. Indian Journal of Pharmaceutical Science 54:8

8 Hassan Y, Aboul-Enein, Abou-Basha LI 1995 Simple HPLC method for the determination of thymoquinone in black cumin seed oil (*Nigella sativa* Linn). Journal of Liquid Chromatography 18(5):895

9 Hasan CM, Ahsan M, Islam SKN 1989 In-vitro antibacterial screening of the oils of *Nigella sativa* seeds. Bangladesh Journal of Botany 18(2):171

10 Ferdous AJ, Islam SN, Ahsan M, Hasan CM 1992 *In-vitro* antibacterial activity of the volatile oil of *Nigella sativa* seeds against multiple drug-resistant isolates of *Shigella spp.* and isolates of *Vibrio cholerae* and *Escherichia coli*. Phytotherapy Research 6:137

11 Daba MH, Abdel-Rahman MS 1998 Hepatoprotective activity of thymoquinone in isolated rat hepatocytes. Toxicology Letters 95(1):23

12 Tennekoon KH, Jeevathayaparan S, Kurukulasooriya AP, Karunanayake EH 1991 Possible hepatotoxicity of *Nigella sativa* seeds and *Dregea volubilis* leaves. Journal of Ethnopharmacology 31(3):283

13 Hader AA, Agel M, Hasan Z 1993 Hypoglycemic effects of the volatile oil of *Nigella sativa*. International Journal of Pharmacognosy 31(2):96

14 Bamosa AO, Ali BA, Sowayan SA 1997 Effect of oral ingestion of *Nigella sativa* seeds on some blood parameters. Saudi Pharmaceutical Journal 5(2–3):126

15 Al-Awadi F, Fatania H, Shamte U 1991 The effect of a plant mixture extract on liver gluconeogenesis in streptozotocin induced diabetic rats. Diabetic Research 18(4):163

16 Mutabagani A, El-Mahdy SA 1997 Study of anti-inflammatory activity of *Nigella sativa* L. and thymoquinone in rats. Saudi Pharmaceutical Journal 5(2–3):110

17 Houghton PJ, Zarka R, Heras B, Hoult JRS 1995 Fixed oil of *Nigella sativa* and derived thymoquinone inhibit eicosanoid generation in leukocytes and membrane lipid peroxidation. Planta Medica 61:33

18 Chakravarty N 1993 Inhibition of histamine release from mast cells by nigellone. Annals of Allergy 70(3):237

19 Jacob D, Dhir RN, Vyas DK 1986 Effect of *Nigella sativa* Linn. seeds on the sialic acid concentration and fertility control. Indian Zoology 10:85

20 Agarwal C, Narula A, Vyas DK, Jacob D 1990 Effect of seeds of Kalaunji (*Nigella sativa* L.) on the fertility and sialic acid content of the reproductive organs of the male rat. GEOBIOS 17:269

21 Bhatt S, Jacob D 1989 Effect of pregnancy interceptory dose of chloroform acetone (9:1v/v) fraction of petroleum ether extract of *Nigella sativa* (Ranunculaceae) seeds on the uterine glycogen of the rat. Indian Zoology 13:57

22 Keshri G, Singh MM, Lakshmi V, Kamboj VP 1995 Post coital contraceptive efficacy of the seeds of (*Nigella sativa*) in rats. Indian Journal of Physiology and Pharmacology 39(1):59

23 Aqel M, Shaheen R 1996 Effects of the volatile oil of *Nigella sativa* seeds on the uterine smooth muscle of rat and guinea pig. Journal of Ethnopharmacology 52:23

24 Worthen DR, Ghosheh OA, Crooks PA 1998 The *in-vitro* anti-tumor activity of some crude and

purified components of black seed, *Nigella sativa* L. Anticancer Research 18(3A):1527

25 Swamy SMK, Tan BKH 2000 Cytotoxic and immunopotentiating effects of the ethanolic extract of *Nigella sativa* L. seeds. Journal of Ethnopharmacology 70:1

26 Salomi JJ, Nair SC, Jayawardanan KK, Varghese CD, Panikkar KR 1992 Antitumor principles from *Nigella sativa* seeds. Cancer Letters 63:41

27 Nair SC, Salomi MJ, Pannikar B, Pannikar KR 1991 Modulatory effects of *Crocus sativus* and *Nigella sativa* extracts on cisplatin induced toxicity in mice. Journal of Ethnopharmacology 31:75

28 Salomi MJ, Pannikar KR 1989 Anticancer activity of *Nigella sativa*. Ancient Science of Life 8(3/4):262

29 Agarwal R, Kharya MD, Shrivastava R 1979 Antimicrobial and anthelmintic activity of essential oil of *Nigella sativa* Linn. Indian Journal of Experimental Biology 17:1264

30 Akhtar MS, Javed I 1991 Efficacy of *Nigella sativa* Linn. seeds against *Moniezia* infection in sheep. Indian Veterinary Journal 68:726

31 Khanna T, Zaidi FA, Dandiya PC 1993 CNS and analgesic studies on *Nigella sativa*. Fitoterapia 54(5):407

32 El-Tahir KE, Ashour MM, Al-Harbi MM 1993 The cardiovascular actions of the volatile oil of the black seed (*Nigella sativa*) in rats: elucidation of the mechanism of action. General Pharmacology 24(5):1123

33 Agarwala IP, Achar MV, Tamankar BP 1971 Galactagogue action of *Nigella sativa*. Indian Journal of Medical Science 25(8):535

34 Steinmann A, Schatzle M, Agathos M, Breit R 1997 Allergic contact dermatitis from black cumin (*Nigella sativa*) oil after topical use. Contact Dermatitis 36(5):268

Ocimum sanctum L. (Lamiaceae)

English: Sacred basil, holy basil

Hindi: *Tulsi*

Sanskrit: *Surasa, vrinda*

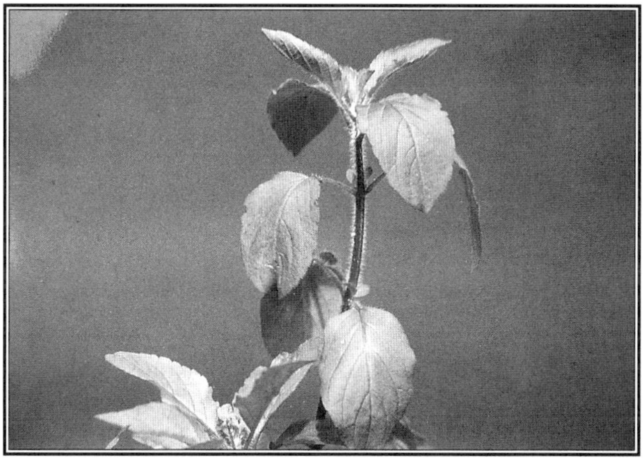

In Indian mythology the plant is considered to extirpate all sins and purify the body when touched. It is often grown outside dwellings and worshipped daily. It is said to daunt Yama, the god of death, but has a close affinity with Lord Krishna who is reputed to have grown the herb. If offered to Lord Krishna it is said to lead to salvation and is considered to have mystical powers of protection from death, disease and misfortune.

Habitat

The plant grows wild all over India and elsewhere in the tropics, ascending to a height of 1800 m, and is also widely cultivated.

Botanical description

An erect, annual herb or shrub, reaching a height of 0.5–1.5 m (Plate 40). The leaves are elliptical, oblong, acute or obtuse, pubescent on both sides. The flowers are very small, purplish or crimson, in long, close racemes. The fruits or nutlets are small, subglobose or broadly ellipsoid, pale brown or reddish with small markings.

Parts used

Leaves, seeds, root.

Traditional and modern use

The leaves are used as a demulcent, diaphoretic and expectorant in bronchitis, cough, cold and fever. It is an insecticide, anthelmintic and deodoriser and has also been used as a laxative, stimulant, antiinflammatory, cardiotonic and blood purifier in hepatic disorders. It can be used for indigestion, diminished appetite and all types of malaise. The oil is applied externally for chronic ulcers, inflammation and skin disorders.

Ethnoveterinary usage

The whole plant is used in glossitis, ulcers, maggots in wounds, anthrax, pneumonia, indigestion, tympanitis, pain in the abdomen, constipation, stoppage of urination, liver fluke, loss of appetite, stomach pain, dog bite, cold and cough, cannabis poisoning, opacity of cornea, swelling of lungs, tachycardia, sprains and sore eyes. The leaves are used in bleeding, coughs and cold, eye disease, udder infection and wound healing in ruminants.

Major chemical constituents

Essential oil

The leaf and flower contain an essential oil composed of eugenol, eugenal, carvacrol, methyl chavicol, linalool, caryophyllene, elemene and others.[1]

Fatty acids

Stearic, myristic, palmitic, oleic, linoleic and linolenic acids[2] and their methyl esters.

Triterpenes and sterols

Ursolic acid, campesterol, cholesterol, stigmasterol, β-sitosterol and others.[3]

Flavonoids and polyphenols

Vicenin-2, rosmarinic acid, galuteolin, cirsilineol, gallic acid, gallic acid methyl and ethyl esters, protocatechuic acid, vanillic acid, 4-hydroxybenzoic acid, vanillin, 4-hydroxybenzaldehyde, caffeic acid, chlorogenic acid and phenylpropane glucosides.[4]

Medicinal and pharmacological activities

Immunomodulatory activity: An ethanolic extract of the leaves of *Ocimum sanctum* was evaluated on the activities of the enzymes cytochrome P450, cytochrome B5 and aryl hydrocarbon hydroxylase in the liver and glutathione-S-transferase and reduced glutathione levels in the liver, lung and stomach of the mouse. Administration of the extract at a dose of 400 and 800 mg/kg for 15 days significantly increased the activities of these, all of which are important in the detoxification of both carcinogens and mutagens. An increase in extrahepatic glutathione-S-transferase and reduced glutathione levels in the liver, lung and stomach tissues was also observed[5] as well as stimulation of humoral immunological response, as indicated by an increase in antibody titre in both the Widal and sheep erythrocyte agglutination tests. An increase in cellular immunological response, represented by E-rosette formation and lymphocytosis, was seen with the methanolic extract (100 and 250 mg/kg) and an aqueous suspension (500 mg/kg) of *Ocimum sanctum* leaves in rats.[6] In an in vitro test, a significant inhibition of antigen-induced histamine release from peritoneal mast cells of sensitised rats was produced with an increase in anti-SRBC haemagglutination titre and IgE antibody titre. These results indicated that *O. sanctum* modulated the humoral immune responses by acting at various levels in the immune mechanism such as antibody production, release of mediators of hypersensitivity reactions and tissue response to the mediators in the target organs.[7]

Antistress activity: The plant extract exhibited antistress activity by improving SDH levels in albino rats.[8] It also showed a marked protective and inhibitory effect on stress-induced gastric ulcer in albino rats. Microscopical and histopathological findings, such as congestion, erosion, discrete and multiple haemorrhages, ulcers and perforation in the control group of rats served as a measure for scoring the intensity of the lesions.[9] An ethanolic extract of the leaves prevented changes in plasma levels of corticosterone induced by the exposure to both acute and chronic noise stress in rats.[10]

Antimicrobial activity: Spinach mosaic virus (SMV) was inhibited by an extract in a dose-dependent manner.[11]

Antiinflammatory activity: The fixed oil extracted from the leaves exhibited significant antiinflammatory activity against carrageenan and other mediator-induced paw oedema in rats. Using various inflammation models, it was inferred that the antiinflammatory activity was due to inhibition of both the cyclooxygenase and lipoxygenase pathways of arachidonic acid metabolism[12] and the active principle responsible was found to be linolenic acid.[13]

Antiasthmatic activity: A 50% hydroalcoholic extract and the volatile oil extracted from fresh leaves were evaluated against histamine- and acetylcholine-induced preconvulsive dyspnoea in pigs. Both the extract and the oil exhibited a significant dose-dependent antiasthmatic activity, with the percentage protection shown by 200 mg/kg of ethanol extract of fresh leaves equivalent to 0.5 ml of volatile oil. The volatile constituents of the fresh leaves were thought to be the main factor responsible for the activity.[14]

Anticarcinogenic activity: The essential oil showed a significant inhibition of benzo(a)pyrene-induced squamous cell carcinoma in the stomach of Swiss mice. The chemopreventive potential of the oil was studied by assessing its effect on the carcinogen detoxifying enzyme, glutathione-S-transferase, and 3,4-benzo(a)pyrene-induced neoplasia in Swiss mice.[15]

Hypoglycaemic and hypolipidaemic activity: *Ocimum sanctum* leaf powder at a level of 1% was fed to normal and diabetic rats for one month. A significant reduction in cholesterol and triglyceride levels in the liver, a reduction of total lipids in the kidney and a fall in total cholesterol and phospholipids in the heart were observed.[16]

Enhancement of bone marrow radioprotection: The radioprotective effect of a leaf extract of *Ocimum sanctum* in combination with WR-2721 was evaluated on bone marrow of adult Swiss mice. Mice were injected intraperitoneally with the extract (10 mg/kg daily for 5 consecutive days) or 100–400 mg/kg WR-2721 (single dose) or a combination of the two, and the whole body of the mouse exposed to γ-irradiation. A significant free radical scavenging activity in vitro was observed with the leaf extract and WR-2721, which was further enhanced by combining the two, and resulted in a higher bone marrow protection. Significant protection of chromosomes was obtained by a combination of leaf extract and WR-2721, with a reduction in the toxicity of the latter at higher doses, indicating that the combination may have promise for radioprotection in humans.[17]

Hypotensive activity: Administration of the leaf extract resulted in a fall of both diastolic and systolic pressure to normal levels, with no adverse side effects.[18]

Analgesic activity: The fixed oil showed significant analgesic activity in mice, using the acetic acid-induced writhing test, suggesting a possible mechanism related to the peripheral system.[19]

Safety profile

Few side effects, except for constipation, were reported for patients administered powdered leaves at 5–7 g/day for 3 months.[18] Large doses of leaf extract induced an antispermatogenic activity in animals.[20] The maximum tolerated dose of the 50% hydroalcoholic leaf extract was 1000 mg/kg body weight in albino rats.[21]

Dosage

Leaf infusion: 4–12 ml

Decoction: 28–56 ml

Seed powder: 1.5–2 g

Ayurvedic properties

Rasa: *Katu* (pungent), *tikta* (bitter)

Guna: *Laghu* (light), *ruksha* (dry)

Veerya: *Ushna* (hot)

Vipaka: *Katu* (pungent)

Dosha: Pacifies *kapha* and *vata*

Further reading

Bharatiya Vidya Bhavan's Swami Prakashananda Ayurveda Research Centre 1992 Selected medicinal plants of India. Chemexcil, Mumbai

Sairam TV 1999 Home remedies, vol II. Penguin India, New Delhi

References

1 Skaltsa-Diamantidis H, Tzakou O, Loukis A, Argyriadou N 1990 Analysis of essential oil of *Ocimum sanctum* L. New results. Plant Medicine and Phytotherapy 24(2):79

2 Singh S, Majumdar DK, Yadav MR 1996 Chemical and pharmacological studies on fixed oils of *Ocimum sanctum*. Indian Journal of Experimental Biology 34(12):1212

3 Skaltsa M, Couladi M, Philianos S, Singh M 1987 Phytochemical study of the leaves of *Ocimum sanctum*. Fitoterapia 58(4):286

4 Norr H, Wagner H 1992 New constituents from *Ocimum sanctum*. Planta Medica 58(6):547

5 Banerjee S, Prashar R, Kumar, Rao AR 1996 Modulatory influence of alcoholic extract of *Ocimum* leaves on carcinogen metabolizing enzyme activities and reduced glutathione levels in mouse. Nutrition and Cancer 25(2):205

6 Godhwani S, Godhwani JL, Vyas DS 1988 *Ocimum sanctum*. A preliminary study evaluating its immunoregulatory profile in albino rats. Journal of Ethnopharmacology 24:193

7 Mediratta PK, Dewan V, Bhattacharya SK, Gupta VS, Maiti PC, Sen P 1988 Effect of *Ocimum sanctum* Linn. on humoral immune responses. Indian Journal of Medical Research 87:384

8 Dadkar VN, Joshi AG, Jaguste VS, Billimoria FR, Dhar HL 1988 Antistress activity of *Ocimum sanctum* (Tulsi). Indian Drugs 25(5):172

9 Roy U, Mukhopadhyay S, Poddar MK, Mukherjee BP 1992 Evaluation of antistress activity of Indian medicinal plants, *Withania somnifera* and *Ocimum sanctum* with special reference to stress induced stomach ulcer in albino rats. Proceedings of an International Seminar on Traditional Medicine, Calcutta, 7–9 November

10 Sembulingam K, Sembulingam P, Namasivayam A 1997 Effect of *Ocimum sanctum* Linn. on noise induced changes in plasma corticosterone level. Indian Journal of Physiology and Pharmacology 41(2):139

11 Zaidi ZB, Gupta VP, Samad A, Naqui AQ 1988 Inhibition of Spinach mosaic virus by extracts of some medicinal plants. Current Science 57(3):151

12 Singh S, Majumdar DK, Rehan HM 1996 Evaluation of anti-inflammatory potential of fixed oil of *Ocimum sanctum* (Holy Basil) and its possible mechanism of action. Journal of Ethnopharmacology 46(3):195

13 Singh S, Majumdar DK 1997 Evaluation of anti-inflammatory activity of fatty acids of *Ocimum sanctum* fixed oil. Indian Journal of Experimental Biology 35(4):380

14 Singh S, Agrawal SS 1991 Anti-asthmatic and anti-inflammatory activity of *Ocimum sanctum*. International Journal of Pharmacognosy 29(4):306

15 Aruna K, Sivaramakrishnan VM 1996 Anticarcinogenic effects of the essential oils from cumin, poppy and basil. Phytotherapy Research 10:577

16 Rai V, Iyer U, Mani UV 1997 Effect of Tulsi (*Ocimum sanctum*) leaf powder supplementation on blood sugar levels, serum lipids and tissue lipids in diabetic rats. Plant Foods and Human Nutrition 50(1):9

17 Ganasoundari A, Devi PU, Rao BS 1998 Enhancement of bone marrow radioprotection and reduction of WR-2721 toxicity by *Ocimum sanctum*. Mutation Research 397(2):303

18 Subbulakshmi G, Sarvaiya SR 1991 Hypotensive effect of *Ocimum sanctum*. Bombay Hospital Journal 33(1):39

19 Singh S, Majumdar DK 1995 Analgesic activity of *Ocimum sanctum* and its possible mechanism of action. International Journal of Pharmacognosy 33(3):182

20 Seth SD, Johri N, Sundaram KR 1981 Antispermatogenic effect of *Ocimum sanctum*. Indian Journal of Experimental Biology 19:975

21 Dhar ML, Dhar MM, Dhawan BN, Mehrotra BN, Ray C 1968 Screening of Indian plants for biological activity: Part I. Indian Journal of Experimental Biology 6:242

Paederia foetida (Rubiaceae) (syn. *P. scandens* (Lour.) Merr; *P. tomentosa* Blume)

English: Chinese flower

Hindi: *Gandhaprasarini*

Sanskrit: *Prasarini*

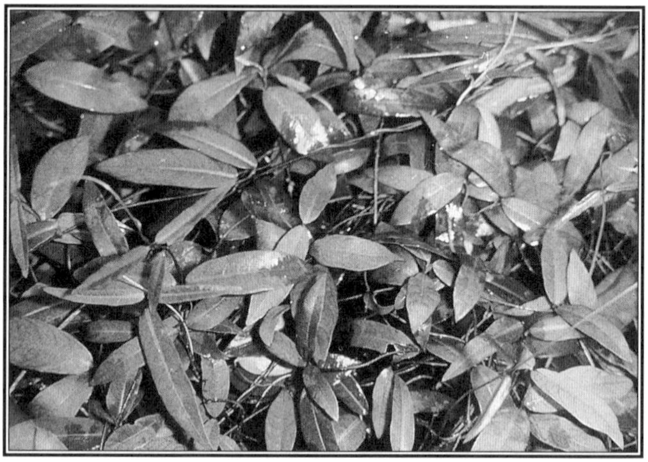

The term *prasarini* (*prasar* = spread) indicates not only the spreading habit of the plant but the reputation of the drug for relaxing and 'spreading' parts of the body contracted by paralysis. Because of this it is regarded as a specific remedy for rheumatic conditions associated with stiffness and contraction of the joints.

Habitat

Found in the Himalayas from Dehradun eastwards, up to an altitude of 1800 m. It is also found in Bihar, Orissa, Bengal and Assam.

Botanical description

An extensive climber (Plate 41), leaves ovate to lanceolate, entire, about 5 cm long and 2.5 cm broad, membranous with long petioles. Purple or violet flowers are found in scorpioid cymes. The fruits are compressed, ellipsoid, red or black in colour. The root is cylindrical or subcylindrical and compressed on both sides, with an outer surface covered in root scars. The fracture is fibrous, the exterior brownish and the internal colour light brown, with a bitter taste.

Parts used

Whole plant, leaves, roots.

Traditional and modern use

The main use of the plant is for arthritis and rheumatic disorders. The leaves, in the form of a poultice, are applied to the abdomen to relieve distension due to flatulence and in herpes infections. The roots are used as an emetic and the juice extracted from the roots is given in cases of inflammation of the spleen and for pains in the chest and liver. The fruits are used to prevent toothache. The whole plant shows tonic, astringent and antiphlogistic actions and has been used in tenesmus.

Ethnoveterinary usage

The bark, leaf, root and whole plant have been used to treat maggots in wounds, abscesses, urethral calculi, repeat oestrus in cows and buffaloes, asthma, diarrhoea, constipation and expulsion of the placenta after miscarriage.[1]

Major chemical constituents

Essential oil

The intense odour is due to methyl mercaptan. Linalool is the major component of the oil obtained from the stem, leaf and flower, together with α-terpineol and geraniol.[2] The leaf and stem also contain hentriacontane, hentriacontanol and ceryl alcohol, 2,3-dihydrobenzofuran, benzofuran and the sulphur-containing compounds dimethyl sulphide and dimethyl trisulphide.[3]

Iridoid glucosides

Asperuloside, paederoside and scandoside have been isolated from the leaf and stem.[4]

Triterpenoids and saponins

Ursolic acid, epifriedelinol, friedelin. The leaf and stem contain sitosterol, stigmasterol and campesterol.[4,5]

Quinones

Embelin has been isolated from the aerial parts.[4,5]

Alkaloids

α-Paederine and β-paederine have been isolated.[4,5]

Fatty acids

The leaf contains a mixture of fatty acids including non-ionic, capric, lauric, myristic, arachidic and palmitic acids.[6]

Carotene and vitamin C

The leaves are rich in carotene and vitamin C.[7]

Medicinal and pharmacological activities

Antiinflammatory activity: A 50% ethanolic extract of *P. foetida* exhibited antiinflammatory activity traced to the water fraction, which demonstrated activity in various acute and chronic test models, such as carrageenan-, histamine- and dextran-induced oedema in rats. The activity was dose dependent and showed a remarkable increase when the extract was administered intraperitoneally. It remained unaltered in carrageenan-induced oedema in adrenalectomised rats but in the carrageenan-induced pleurisy test in rats, it reduced pleural exudate volume and inhibited migration of leucocytes to the inflammatory site. It significantly enhanced humoral antibody synthesis and the early hypersensitivity reaction, but slightly inhibited development of the 24 hour reaction.[8] Another study reported that a butanol fraction of the leaves showed a significant antiinflammatory activity, producing a significant inhibition of granulation tissue formation in cotton pellet-implanted rats. It also decreased liver (but not serum) aspartate transaminase activity but did not affect adrenal weight and ascorbic acid content significantly. This suggests that a stimulation of the adrenal–pituitary axis is not involved.[9]

Antiarthritic activity: *Paederia foetida* extract was tested for its effect on osteoarthritis-like lesions induced in the knee joints of rabbits by ananase (the proteolytic enzyme from pineapple). It reduced the degradation changes in the articular cartilage induced by ananase and in vitro studies using ananase-treated chick embryonic bones showed that the plant (at a dose of 10 mg/ml of the medium) enhanced the growth of the chick bones cultivated in this medium.[10]

Anthelmintic activity: An aqueous extract administered orally was highly effective against Strongyloides, Trichostrongylus and Haemonchus spp. and moderately effective against Bunostomum and Monezia spp., when given at 2-day intervals in young calves.[11]

Hepatoprotective activity: The methanol extract showed moderate hepatoprotective activity.[12]

Antispasmodic activity: A 50% ethanolic extract of *Paederia foetida* exhibited antispasmodic activity on the isolated guinea pig ileum.[13]

Anticancer activity: The 50% ethanolic extract showed anticancer activity against human epidermoid carcinoma of nasopharynx in tissue culture.[13]

Safety profile

The LD_{50} of a 50% ethanolic extract of leaves was 1200 mg/kg in mice.[13] The water-soluble fraction was found to be non-toxic up to 2 g/kg (PO and IP) in rats and mice and it exerted no significant effect on gross general behaviour.

Dosage

Infusion: 12–24 ml

Decoction: 56–112 ml

Powder: 2–4 g

Ayurvedic properties

Rasa: *Tikta* (bitter)

Guna: *Guru* (heavy)

Veerya: *Ushna* (hot)

Vipaka: *Katu* (pungent)

Dosha: Balances *vata*

Further reading

Pandey GS (ed) 1998 Bhavprakash Nighantu. Chaukhambha Bharati Academy, Gokul Bhawan, Varanasi

Sivarajan VV, Balachandran I 1994 Ayurvedic drugs and their plant sources. Oxford and IBH Publishing, New Delhi

References

1 International Institute of Rural Reconstruction 1994 Ethnoveterinary medicine in Asia. An information kit on traditional animal health care practices. IIRR, Silang, Philippines

2 Wong KC, Tan GL 1994 Steam volatile constituents of the aerial parts of *Paederia foetida* L. Flavour and Fragrance Journal 9(1):25

3 Shukla YN, Lloyd HA, Morton JF, Kapadia GJ 1976 Iridoid glycosides and other constituents of *Paederia foetida*. Phytochemistry 15:1989

4 Ahmad MU, Islam MR, Huq E, Khan MW, Gupta S 1991 Chemical investigation of the aerial parts of *Paederia foetida* Linn. Journal of the Bangladesh Academy of Science 15(1):19

5 Desai HK, Gwad DH, Govindachari TR et al 1971 Chemical investigations of some Indian plants, VI. Indian Journal of Chemistry 9:611

6 De Subrata D, Bhavsar GC 1993 Fatty acid compositions of *Gymnosporia montana* and *Paederia foetida* leaves. Indian Journal of Pharmaceutical Science 55(3):110

7 Basu NM, Ray GK, De NK 1947 On the vitamin C and carotene content of several herbs and flowers used in the Ayurvedic system of medicine. Indian Chemistry Society Journal 24:358

8 Singh S, Bani S, Khajuria A et al 1994 Antiinflammatory activity of *Paederia foetida*. Fitoterapia 65(4):357

9 De S, Ravishankar B, Bhavsar GC 1994 Investigation of the anti-inflammatory effects of

Paederia foetida. Journal of Ethnopharmacology 43(1):31

10 Prasad GC, Singh RH 1969 Ananase-induced degenerative arthritis and the effect of an indigenous drug. Indian Journal of Medical Research 57:1095

11 Roychoudhary GK, Chakrabarty AK, Dutta B 1970 A preliminary observation on the effects of *Paederia foetida* on gastro-intestinal helminths in bovines. Indian Veterinary Journal 47(9):767

12 De S, Ravishankar B, Bhavsar GC 1993 Evaluation of *Paederia foetida* for hepatoprotective and anti-inflammatory activities. Indian Journal of Natural Products 9(1):7

13 Dhar ML, Dhar MM, Dhawan BN, Mehrotra BN Ray C 1968 Screening of Indian plants for biological activity: Part I. Indian Journal of Experimental Biology 6:242

Phyllanthus emblica L. (Euphorbiaceae) (syn. *Emblica officinalis* Gaertn.)

English: Emblic myrobalan, Indian gooseberry

Hindi: *Amla*

Sanskrit: *Amlaki*

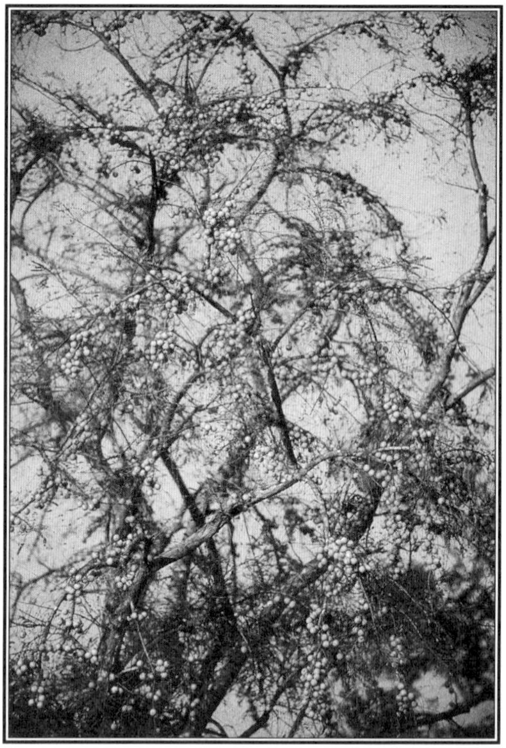

The fruits are held in high esteem and are associated with Kubera, the mythical Lord of Wealth. It is used widely in indigenous medicine and is an ingredient of *triphala*, an important *rasayana* drug thought to impart youthful vigour and strength. There are two varieties: the smaller, wild type and the larger cultivated one; both are used medicinally.

Habitat

Found wild and cultivated in all parts of India, especially the south, to an altitude of 1500 m.

Botanical description

A small or medium-sized deciduous tree with spreading branches, a crooked trunk and a smooth exfoliating bark (Plate 42). Leaves light green, digitate compound, subsessile, 10–15 mm long and 3–8 mm wide, closely set on the branchlets. Flowers are greenish-yellow in axillary fascicles. The fruits are fleshy, globose, shining yellowish-green when ripe, and contain three loculi each containing two trigonous seeds.

Parts used

Fruit, leaves, seed, root bark and flowers.

Traditional and modern use

The fruits are used as a general tonic, particularly in the winter, and for constipation, urinary problems, headache, anxiety, diabetes, vomiting and burning sensation. It is considered to improve memory and intelligence. A paste of the dried fruit powder is also applied to the hair and skin as a substitute for soap. The leaves are used in conjunctivitis and bronchitis and the powdered root bark mixed with honey and applied to mouth ulcers.

Ethnoveterinary usage

The fruits are used as food and the seeds applied to wounds in ruminants. All parts of the plant are used to cure cold and cough, burns, wounds, maggots in wounds, mastitis, haematuria, general poisoning and datura poisoning in particular, ringworm, sprained hoof, abscess, diarrhoea, bloody dysentery, *E. coli* bacillosis, indigestion, glossitis, tympanitis, lumbar fracture and stoppage of urine.

Major chemical constituents

Polyphenols

The fruit and most other parts of the plant contain gallic acid,[1] phyllemblin, phyllemblic acid, emblicol, ellagic acid, chebulagic acid, glucogallin, corilagin, 3,6-digalloyl glucose, putranjivin A, emblicanin A and B, punigluconin, pedunculagin and quercetin.

Organic acids

The fruit is a rich source of ascorbic acid.

Cytokinins

Zeatin, zeatin riboside and zeatin nucleotide have been isolated from the fruit.

Fatty acids

Arachidic and behenic acids have been isolated from the seed oil.[2]

Medicinal and pharmacological activities

Hypolipidaemic activity: The lipid-lowering and antiatherosclerotic actions of the fruit were evaluated in rabbits with hyperlipidaemia induced by an atherogenic diet which included cholesterol. Administration of the fresh juice of the fruit at a dose of 5 ml/kg per rabbit per day for 60 days lowered serum cholesterol, triglycerides, phospholipids and low-density lipoprotein levels by 82%, 66%, 77% and 90%, respectively. The lipid level of the tissues decreased significantly and regression of aortic plaques was observed. Increased amounts of cholesterol and phospholipids were excreted, suggesting the mode of absorption may have been affected.[3] A separate study revealed that *P. emblica* also reduces serum, aortic and hepatic cholesterol in rabbits.[4] In a clinical study the diet of normal and hypercholesterolaemic men aged 35–55 years was supplemented with raw *P. emblica* fruit for 28 days. Both groups showed a decrease in total serum cholesterol levels, which reverted almost to their initial values 2 weeks after withdrawal of the plant.[5] The ripe fruits are one of the chief constituents of a *siddha* preparation used for the prevention and reversal of atherosclerotic disease.[6]

Antiviral activity: A methanolic extract of the fruits showed significant inhibitory activity on HIV reverse transcriptase, with an IC_{50} of about 50 μg/ml. Putranjivin A, di-O-galloyl-β-D-glucose and digallic acid were also isolated from the fruit and shown to have antiviral activity. These exhibited a non-competitive mode of action with respect to the substrate, but competitive with respect to the template primer.[7]

Effect on experimentally induced cytotoxicity: Toxicity induced by lead nitrate, aluminium sulphate,[8] nickel chloride,[9] caesium chloride[10] and 3,4-benzo(a)pyrene[11] was reduced by administration of an extract of the fruit, which also reduced the clastogenic effects of all four compounds. A comparative study of *P. emblica* extract and synthetic ascorbic acid on their capability to modify adverse effects of environmental toxins showed that the extract afforded a more pronounced protective effect in counteracting the genotoxicity induced by both Al and Pb.[12,13] Similar results were found for the clastogenicity and carcinogenicity induced by nickel.[14] The more potent effect of the extract was attributed to a synergistic action between the naturally occurring compounds present.

Hepatoprotective activity: A 50% aqueous extract of *P. emblica* and quercetin (a flavonoid isolated from the same) for hepatoprotective action was assessed using country-made liquor (CML) and paracetamol-induced liver damage in albino rats and mice. The possible mechanism of action for their hepatoprotective activity was thought to be by decreasing glutathione depletion and prevention of stimulation of cytochrome P450. Since quercetin was more effective than the extract it was considered to be the active principle.[15] Toxic effects induced by lead nitrate and aluminium sulphate were also counteracted by the administration of *P. emblica* fruit extract and ascorbic acid in albino rats.[16]

Hypoglycaemic activity: A combined extract containing *P. emblica* and *Curcuma longa* produced a marked reduction in blood sugar levels in both normal fasting and alloxan-induced diabetic rats, with a good response in the glucose tolerance test.[17]

Activity against acute necrotising pancreatitis: An experiment was carried out in dogs with acute pancreatitis induced by injecting a mixture of trypsin, bile and blood into the duodenal opening of the pancreatic duct. Controls were normal and sham operated and the test group was pretreated with 28 mg of extract/kg per day given orally for 15 days before inducing pancreatitis. The rise in serum amylase was significant in the control pancreatitis group but not in the others and microscopical examination revealed that cell damage and inflammation in the *P. emblica*-treated group was lower than the untreated pancreatitis group.[18]

Immunomodulatory activity: An aqueous extract of the fruit enhanced natural killer cell activity and antibody-dependent cellular cytotoxicity in mice, resulting in an increase in lifespan of 35% in tumour-bearing mice. The drug's antitumour action may occur through its ability to augment natural cell-mediated cytotoxicity, since a functional NK cell or K cell population was an absolute requirement for activity.[19]

Protective effect in myocardial necrosis: An ethanolic extract of the fruits of *P. emblica* given orally at a dose of 1 g/kg for 2 consecutive days was found to protect against isoproterenol-induced myocardial necrosis.[20]

Antidyspepsia activity: *P. emblica* was found to be useful in the treatment of dyspepsia.[21]

Antioxidant and other activities: Phyllemblin showed a number of direct pharmacological actions including mild stimulation of isolated frog heart, mild cerebral depressant action, spasmolytic activity, potentiation of adrenaline and barbiturate sedation, in a similar manner to that of rutin. It was argued that rutin exerted its adrenergic action due to its antioxidant properties and it was concluded that phyllemblin, a powerful antioxidant, may be acting in the same manner.[22]

Antimicrobial activity: Phyllemblin was found to have activity against *Staph. aureus, E.coli, Staph. typhosa, C. albicans, Mycobacterium tuberculosis* and *Xanthomonas campestris*.[23]

Antiinflammatory and antipyretic activity: Extracts of the leaves inhibited polymorphonuclear leucocyte (PMN) and platelet activity, supporting their antiinflammatory and antipyretic action.[2]

Safety profile

The fruits are considered a food and no toxicity has been noted.

Dosage

Fresh fruit: As required

Infusion: 10–15 ml

Powder: 3–6 g

Ayurvedic properties

Rasa: Five *rasas* (except *lavana rasa*)

Guna: *Guru* (heavy), *ruksha* (dry)

Veerya: *Shita* (cold)

Vipaka: *Madhur* (sweet)

Dosha: Pacifies *tridosha*

Further reading

Bharatiya Vidya Bhavan's Swami Prakashananda Ayurveda Research Centre 1992 Selected medicinal plants of India. Chemexcil, Mumbai

Ministry of Health and Family Welfare 1989 Ayurvedic pharmacopoeia of India. Government of India, New Delhi

Sairam TV 1999 Home remedies, vol II. Penguin India, New Delhi

References

1 Basa SC, Srinivasulu C 1987 Constituents of leaves of *Phyllanthus emblica* Linn. Indian Journal of Natural Products 3(1):13

2 Ihantola-Vormisto A, Summanen J, Kankaanranta H, Vuorela H, Asmawi ZM, Moilanen E 1997 Anti-inflammatory activity of extracts from leaves of *Phyllanthus emblica*. Planta Medica 63(6):518

3 Mathur R, Sharma A, Dixit VP, Varma M 1996 Hypolipidaemic effect of fruit juice of *Emblica officinalis* in cholesterol-fed rabbits. Journal of Ethnopharmacology 50:61

4 Thakur CP 1985 *Emblica officinalis* reduces serum, aortic and hepatic cholesterol in rabbits. Experientia 41(3):423

5 Jacob A, Pandey M, Kapoor S, Saroja R 1988 Effect of the Indian Gooseberry (amla) on serum cholesterol levels in men aged 35–55 years. European Journal of Clinical Nutrition 42(11): 939

6 Shanmugasundaram KR, Seethapathy PG, Shanmugasundaram ER 1983 Anna Pavala Sindhooram – an antiatherosclerotic Indian drug. Journal of Ethnopharmacology 7(3):247

7 El-Mekkawy S, Meselhy MR, Kusumoto IT, Kadota S, Hattori M, Namba T 1995 Inhibitory effects of Egyptian folk medicines on human immunodeficiency virus (HIV) reverse transcriptase. Chemical and Pharmaceutical Bulletin 43(4):641

8 Dhir H, Roy AK, Sharma A, Talukder G 1990 Protection afforded by aqueous extracts of *Phyllanthus* species against cytotoxicity induced by lead and aluminium salts. Phytotherapy Research 4(5):172

9 Agarwal K, Dhir H, Sharma A, Talukder G 1992 The efficacy of two species of *Phyllanthus* in counteracting nickel clastogenicity. Fitoterapia 63(1):49

10 Ghosh A, Sharma A, Talukder G 1993 Comparison of the protection afforded by a crude extract of *Phyllanthus emblica* fruit and an equivalent amount of synthetic ascorbic acid against the cytotoxic effects of cesium chloride in mice. International Journal of Pharmacognosy 31(2):116

11 Nandi P, Talukdar G, Sharma A 1997 Dietary chemoprevention of clastogenic effects of 3,4-benzo(a)pyrene by *Emblica officinalis* Gaertn. fruit extract. British Journal of Cancer 76(10):1279

12 Dhir H, Roy AK, Sharma A 1993 Relative efficiency of *Phyllanthus emblica* fruit extract and ascorbic acid in modifying lead and aluminium induced sister-chromatid exchanges in mouse bone marrow. Environmental and Molecular Mutagenesis 21(3):229

13 Roy AK, Dhir H, Sharma A 1992 Modification of metal-induced micronuclei formation in mouse bone marrow erythrocytes by *Phyllanthus* fruit extract and ascorbic acid. Toxicology Letters 62(1):9–17

14 Dhir H, Agarwal K, Sharma A, Talukdar G 1991 Modifying role of *Phyllanthus emblica* and ascorbic acid against nickel clastogenicity in mice. Cancer Letters 59(1):9

15 Gulati RK, Agarwal S, Agrawal SS 1995 Hepatoprotective studies on *Phyllanthus emblica* Linn. and quercetin. Indian Journal of Experimental Biology 33(4):261

16 Roy AK, Dhir H, Sharma A, Talukder G 1991 *Phyllanthus emblica* fruit extract and ascorbic acid modify hepatotoxic and renotoxic effects of metals in mice. International Journal of Pharmacognosy 29(2):117

17 Singh AK, Chaudhary R, Manohar SJ 1991 Hypoglycaemic activity of *Curcuma longa* Linn., *Phyllanthus emblica* Linn. and their various extractive combinations on albino rats. Proc. Conf. Pharmacol. Symp. Herbal Drugs, New Delhi, 1–5 March 1991:33

18 Thorat SP, Rege NN, Naik AS et al 1995 *Emblica officinalis*: a novel therapy for acute pancreatitis – an experimental study. Hepatic, Pancreatic and Biliary Surgery 9(1):25

19 Suresh K, Vasudevan DM 1994 Augmentation of murine natural killer cell and antibody dependent cellular cytotoxicity activities by *Phyllanthus emblica*, a new immunomodulator. Journal of Ethnopharmacology 44(1):55

20 Tariq M, Hussain SJ, Asif M, Jahan M 1977 Protective effects of fruit extracts of *Emblica officinalis* Gaertn. and *Terminalia chebula* in experimental myocardial necrosis in rats. Indian Journal of Experimental Biology 15:485

21 Chawla YK, Dubey P, Singh R, Nundy S, Tandon BN 1982 Treatment of dyspepsia with Amalaki (*Emblica officinalis* Linn.) – an Ayurvedic drug. Indian Journal of Medical Research 76:S95

22 Rao MRR, Siddqui HH 1964 Pharmacological studies on *Emblica officinalis* Gaertn. Indian Journal of Experimental Biology 2:29

23 Khanna P, Nag TN 1973 Isolation, identification and screening of phyllemblin from *Emblica officinalis* Gaertn. tissue culture. Indian Journal of Pharmacy 35(1):23

Phyllanthus niruri L. (Euphorbiaceae)(syn. *P. amarus, P. sellowianus, P. fraternus* Webster)

English: Stone breaker, shatter stone

Hindi: *Bhuinanvalah*

Sanskrit: *Bhumyaamlaki, bahupatra*

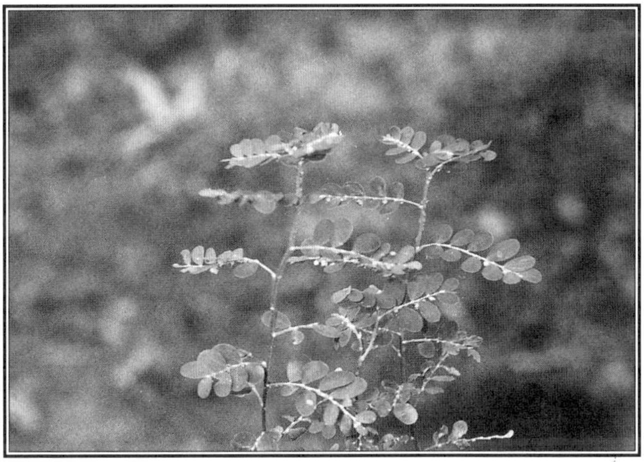

The herb has been used in Ayurveda for over 2000 years and has a wide range of traditional uses, both internally and externally. There is some botanical confusion between *P. niruri* and *P. amarus*, which is also referred to as Bhui-amla or Kheezanelli, and the Ayurvedic formulary of India accepts either. *P. sellowianus* is also closely related and often confused with these, so relevant information on all is given.

Habitat

It is a common weed indigenous to central and southern India but now found widely throughout the tropics in fields, gardens and on waste ground.

Botanical description

An erect annual herb reaching up to 60 cm in height (Plate 43). The leaves are small, green, closely arranged, with a short petiole and an obtuse or retuse apex. The flowers are numerous, inconspicuous, unisexual, monoecious, yellowish-green and borne in pairs in the axils of the leaves. The fruit is a globose capsule, slightly depressed at the top.

Parts used

Herb, leaf, roots.

Traditional and modern use

The plant is used mainly to treat all kinds of jaundice as a single remedy and as a choleretic and liver protectant, as well as for diabetes, dyspepsia, diarrhoea, inflammation, fever and frequent menstruation. In Brazil it is used for kidney and gall stones (hence the name 'stone breaker') and in the Bahamas as an aperient and laxative. It has also been used for urogenital conditions such as gonorrhoea and for worm infestation and viral diseases.[1]

Ethnoveterinary usage

The whole plant, root, leaves and latex are used in abscess of the neck, sprained hoof, haematuria, night blindness, colic, jaundice and stoppage of urination.

Major chemical constituents

Lignans

Phyllanthin, phyllanthinol, phyllanthinone, phyllnirurin, hypophyllanthin, hikokinin, nirurin, ninuretin, niranthin, nirphyllin, 4-hydroxysesamin, corylagin and others.

Flavonoids

Astragalin, fisetin glucoside, phyllocrysin, quercetin, quercitrin, isoquercitrin, rutin.

Phenols, polyphenols and tannins

Catechin, ellagic acid, eryiodictiol, gallic acid, geraniin, epicatechin, epigallocatechin, epigallocatechin-3-O-gallate, brevifolin (xanthoxylin), brevifolin carboxylic acid and others.

Triterpenes

Lupeol, sitosterol and others.

Alkaloids

Nor-securinine and 4-methoxysecurinine (phyllanthine) are present in the leaves.

Miscellaneous

Oestradiol, triacontanol, repandusinic acid, cymene, linalool, limonene and others.[1]

Medicinal and pharmacological activities

Diuretic activity: Nine mildly hypertensive patients, four of them with diabetes mellitus, were treated with a preparation of *P. niruri*. A significant increase in the 24-hour urine volume and serum Na levels was observed.[2]

Hypotensive activity: A significant reduction in systolic blood pressure in non-diabetic hypertensives and females was observed in the aforesaid study. Geraniin, one of the constituents, has been shown to inhibit angiotensin-converting enzyme (ACE).[3]

Hypoglycaemic activity: A significant reduction in blood glucose has been observed,[2] with no harmful side effects. Administration of ethanolic extract of the leaves of *P. niruri* orally at a dose of 250 mg/kg produced a marked decrease in the blood glucose level of alloxan-induced diabetic rats.[4] Two flavonoids, isolated from the water fraction of ethanolic extract of *P. fraternus*, exhibited hypoglycaemic action on oral administration in alloxan-treated albino rats.[5]

Antihepatotoxic activity: It has been shown in a small study that *P. niruri* extract, when administered to children with acute hepatitis, was able to normalise the liver function within 5 days.[6] The hexane extract elicited an in vitro hepatoprotective action in CCl_4-induced cytotoxicity, using primary cultured rat hepatocytes. Phyllanthin and hypophyllanthin exhibited significant inhibitory action in preventing CCl_4-produced hepatic lesions and triacontanal, along with those compounds, was effective in preventing galactosamine-induced cytotoxicity.[7] The ethanolic extract of the roots and leaves of *P. niruri* showed hepatoprotective effect in alcohol-induced liver cell damage in non-hepatectomised and partially hepatectomised rats. The root extract was found to be more active.[8]

Antimicrobial activity: The aqueous extract of *P. niruri* inhibited the human immunodeficiency virus type-1, reverse transcriptase (HIV-1-RT). The monosodium salt of repandusinic acid was identified as the active principle. The ID_{50} of this compound on HIV-1-RT and DNA polymerase-α (from HeLa cells) was 0.05 and 0.6 μM, respectively. The compound is a competitive inhibitor with respect to template-primer but non-competitive with respect to substrate.[9] The ethanolic and water extracts of *P. niruri* have been found to inhibit bacterial and fungal growth at concentrations of 100 and 400 μg/ml.[10] The aqueous extract inhibited endogenous DNA polymerase of hepatitis B virus and Woodchuck hepatitis virus (WHV) DNA, binding to the surface antigen of both viruses in vitro.[11]

Antimalarial activity: *P. niruri* extract produced an inhibition of *Plasmodium falciparum* growth (>60%) at a test concentration of 6 μg/ml.[12] The ethanolic, dichloromethane and lyophilised aqueous extracts have also been evaluated for antimalarial activity in vivo, in a 4-day assay against *P. berghei* in mice. At a dose of 200 mg/kg PO, both the ethanolic and dichloromethane extracts produced significant chemosuppression, reducing parasitaemia by 73% and 72% respectively, but the lyophilised aqueous extract was less active.[13]

Nematocidal activity: A decoction of bark at 1 mg/ml was active against *Toxocara canis*.[14]

Aldose reductase inhibitory activity: Ellagic acid, isolated from the 70% ethanolic extract of *P. niruri*, exhibited significant activity (six times more potent than quercitrin, a well-known inhibitor of aldose reductase). Brevifolin carboxylic acid was found to have a lesser order of activity.[15]

Antinociceptive activity: The hydroalcoholic extract of *P. niruri* exhibited a significant, dose-related inhibition of capsaicin-induced pain, with an ID_{50} of 6.1 mg/kg when given IP, and 35 mg/kg when given orally.[16]

Antiurolithiasis activity: The antispasmodic action of an alkaloid isolated from *P. sellowianus* was tested on isolated strips of guinea pig ileum, rat uterus and rat aorta. The alkaloid was more potent on ileum strips (comparable to papaverine) than the other tissues. Studies suggested a similar mode of action for both, a competitive antagonism of calcium entry into the cell. These results support its use for the treatment of kidney and bladder stones, since smooth muscle relaxation within the urinary or biliary tract would facilitate the passing of kidney or bladder calculi.[17]

Anticlastogenic and anticytotoxic activity: Oral administration of an aqueous extract of the leaves of *P. niruri* to mice resulted in a significant reduction in the cytotoxic action of lead nitrate and aluminium sulphate and a reduction in the clastogenic effects of both.[18] It also counteracted the clastogenic effects of nickel chloride in mouse bone marrow cells.[19]

Antioxidant activity: The plant has been shown to exhibit antioxidant action in rats.[20]

Safety profile

The herb is considered safe when given under clinical guidance. The maximum tolerated dose of the whole plant was 1000 mg/kg body weight in adult rats.[21]

Dosage

Decoction: 15 g

Infusion: 14–28 ml

Powder: 3–6 g

Ayurvedic properties

Rasa: *Tikta* (bitter), *kashaya* (astringent), *madhur* (sweet)

Guna: *Laghu* (light), *ruksha* (dry)

Veerya: *Shita* (cold)

Vipaka: *Katu* (pungent)

Dosha: Pacifies *kapha* and *pitta*

Further reading

Kapoor LD 1990 Handbook of Ayurvedic medicinal plants. CRC Press, Boca Raton

Ministry of Health and Family Welfare 1989 Ayurvedic pharmacopoeia of India. Government of India, New Delhi

Council of Scientific and Industrial Research 1985 The wealth of India. PID, New Delhi

References

1 Ross I 1999 Medicinal plants of the world, vol 1. Humana Press, Totowa, New Jersey

2 Srividya N, Periwal S 1995 Diuretic, hypotensive and hypoglycaemic effect of *Phyllanthus amarus*. Indian Journal of Experimental Biology 33(11):861

3 Ueno H, Horie Y, Nishi H, Shogawa M 1988 Chemical and pharmaceutical studies on medicinal plants in Paraguay. Geraniin, an angiotensin-converting enzyme inhibitor from 'Paraparai Mi', *Phyllanthus niruri*. Journal of Natural Products 51(2):357

4 Kumar NG, Nair AMC, Raghunandanan VR, Rajagopalan MK 1989 Hypoglycaemic effect of *Phyllanthus niruri* leaves in rabbits. Kerala Journal of Veterinary Science 20(1):77

5 Hukeri VI, Kalyani GA, Kakrani HK 1988 Hypoglycaemic activity of flavonoids of *Phyllanthus fraternus* in rats. Fitoterapia 59(1):68

6 Dixit SP, Achar MP 1983 Bhumyamlaki (*Phyllanthus niruri* L.) and jaundice in children. Journal of the Natural and Integrated Medicine Association 25:269

7 Kodakandla VS, Singh B, Thakur RS, Husain A, Kiso Y, Hikino H 1985 Antihepatotoxic principles of *Phyllanthus niruri* herb. Journal of Ethnopharmacology 14:41

8 Agrawal SS, Garg A, Agrawal S 1988 Screening of *Phyllanthus niruri* Linn. and *Ricinus communis* Linn. on alcohol-induced liver cell damage in non-hepatectomized and partially hepatectomized rats. Indian Journal of Pharmacology 18(4):211–214

9 Ogata T, Higuchi H, Mochida S et al 1992 HIV-1 reverse transcriptase inhibitor from *Phyllanthus niruri*. AIDS Research and Human Retroviruses 8(11):1937

10 Ramchandani M, Chungath JI 1988 Antibacterial, antifungal and antiviral studies on *Phyllanthus fraternus* Webster and *Jatropha glandulifera* Roxb. Indian Drugs 25(4):134

11 Venkateswaran PS, Millman I, Blumberg BS 1987 Effects of an extract from *Phyllanthus niruri* on hepatitis B and Woodchuck hepatitis viruses: in vitro and in vivo studies. Proceedings of the National Academy of Science of the USA 84:274

12 Tona L, Ngimbi NP, Tsakala M et al 1999 Antimalarial activity of 20 crude extracts from nine African medicinal plants used in Kinshasa, Congo. Journal of Ethnopharmacology 68(1–3):193

13 Tona L, Mesia K, Ngimbi NP et al 2001 *In vivo* antimalarial activity of *Cassia occidentalis, Morinda morindoides* and *Phyllanthus niruri*. Annals of Tropical Medicine and Parasitology 95(1):47

14 Kiuchi F, Hioki M, Nakamura N, Miyashita N, Tsuda Y, Kondo K 1989 Screening of crude drugs used in Sri Lanka for nematocidal activity on the larva of *Toxocara canis*. Shoyakugaku Zasshi 43(4):288

15 Shimizu M, Horie Y, Terashima S, Ueno H 1989 Studies on aldose reductase inhibitors from natural products II. Active components of a Paraguayan crude drug 'Paraparai Mi', *Phyllanthus niruri*. Chemical and Pharmaceutical Bulletin 37(9):2531

16 Santos AR, Filho VC, Yunes RA, Calixto JB 1995 Analysis of the mechanisms underlying the antinociceptive effect of the extracts of plants from the genus *Phyllanthus*. General Pharmacology 26(7):1499

17 Calixto JB, Yunes RA, Neto AS, Valle RM, Rae GA 1984 Antispasmodic effects of an alkaloid extracted from *Phyllanthus sellowianus*: a comparative study with papaverine. Brazilian Journal of Medical and Biological Research 17(3–4):313

18 Dhir H, Roy AK, Sharma A, Talukdar G 1990 Protection afforded by aqueous extracts of *Phyllanthus* species against cytotoxicity induced by lead and aluminium salts. Phytotherapy Research 4(5):172

19 Agarwal K, Dhir H, Sharma A, Talukdar G 1992 The efficacy of two species of *Phyllanthus* in counteracting nickel clastogenicity. Fitoterapia 63(1):49

20 Jhou G, Krishnamurthy S 1993 Some biochemical effects of *Phyllanthus niruri*, an Ayurvedic drug for hepatitis, in rats. Medical and Nutritional Research Communications 1(1):40

21 Dhar ML, Dhar MM, Dhawan BN, Mehrotra BN, Ray C 1968 Screening of Indian plants for biological activity: Part I. Indian Journal of Experimental Biology 6:232

Picrorrhiza kurroa Royle ex. Benth. (Scrophulariaceae)

English: Kutki, yellow gentian

Hindi: *Kutaki*

Sanskrit: *Katukarohini*

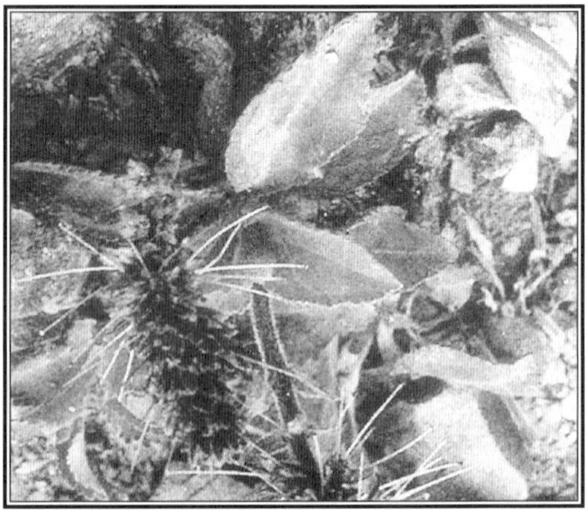

Kutki has long been known as a curative and preventive medicine and many complex preparations handed down from ancient Indian, Greek and Arabian physicians include it among their ingredients. In Indian mythology the herb is said to have been administered by Dhanwantary, the god of medicine himself, and because of this it is also known as *Dhanwantary grastya*.

Habitat

A perennial herb mainly confined to the alpine Himalayas, found between 2500 and 3600 m altitude.

Botanical description

A perennial, woody herb, with greyish-brown, cylindrical, irregularly curved rootstock (Plate 44). The leaves are spatulate, serrate, 5–10 cm long, with rounded tips and a narrowed base. The flowers are small, in spikes, with oblong or lanceolate bracts which are as long as the calyx and dark-violet in colour.

Parts used

Dried root, rhizome.

Traditional and modern use

The dried root and rhizomes are used as a hepatoprotective, antiasthmatic, immunomodulatory and antiinflammatory agent, particularly for liver disorders and jaundice, chest and digestive disorders, fever, dysentery and diarrhoea.[1,2]

Ethnoveterinary usage

Picrorrhiza kurroa is used in various diseases, including fever, in domestic animals. The roots are used as an appetite stimulant in swine.[3]

Major chemical constituents

Iridoid glycosides

Kutkoside, picroside-I, II, III, IV, V, veronicoside, specioside and pikuroside have been isolated from the roots.[4–7]

Cucurbitacin glycosides

Over 20 cucurbitacin glycosides have been reported.[8–12]

Phenolics

Phenolic compounds including apocynin,[13] androsin[4] and vanillic acid[14] and flavonoids have been reported.

Medicinal and pharmacological activities

Hepatoprotective activity: The hepatoprotective and therapeutic effect of *Picrorrhiza kurroa* roots have been shown in diverse models of liver injury. The crude extract, and the isolated active principles of the roots, have been shown to protect the liver from various types of drug-induced injury.[15] In a clinical study on patients with hepatitis and jaundice, kutki produced significantly reduced serum bilirubin levels, together with a more rapid clinical recovery from jaundice and without any untoward effects.[16] In a prospective double-blind controlled clinical trial of *Picrorrhiza kurroa* and *Berberis aristata* in patients with viral hepatitis, *P. kurroa* proved to be superior.[17] Isolated compounds from *Picrorrhiza kurroa* have also been shown to have hepatoprotective activity. Picroliv, a specific combination of iridoid glycosides from *P. kurroa*, has been reported to inhibit drug-induced hepatocarcinogenesis and to prevent the biochemical changes in Wistar rats administered with aflatoxin B1 and phenobarbitone experimentally.[18–21] A herbo-mineral preparation, *Arogyavardhini vati*, containing *P. kurroa* as the major ingredient, has been evaluated in two small clinical studies. Administration in a dose of 500 mg thrice daily for 3 weeks led to a significant improvement in clinical symptoms including appetite stimulation and a significant lowering of the serum transaminases (SGPT, SGOT) and serum bilirubin in the first week of the treatment. The medicine was well tolerated.[22]

Immunomodulatory activity: *Picrorrhiza kurroa* is considered to be one of the most promising immunomodulatory agents of herbal origin.[23] Various solvent extracts were screened for their influence on complement-mediated haemolysis and on the production of luminol-dependent chemiluminescense by activated human neutrophils. All exhibited dose-dependent inhibitory effects, the methanolic and aqueous extracts being the most potent.[24,25] In an experimental study in mice, the oral administration of Picroliv (a standardised fraction of iridoid glycosides) prior to immunisation with sheep red blood cells resulted in a significant increase in haemagglutinating antibody titre, plaque-forming cells and delayed hypersensitivity response to SRBC. Picroliv further enhanced the non-specific immune response characterised by an increase in the macrophage migration index.[25]

Antiasthmatic activity: *P. kurroa* has been studied extensively for its antiasthmatic activity.[26,27] A pilot study of 10 patients with acute bronchial asthma given a dose of 160 mg powder twice daily produced evidence of objective and subjective improvement.[28] In another study in 20 patients, the crude extract of *P. kurroa* roots reduced the frequency and severity of asthmatic attacks and the need for regular bronchodilators.[29] The activity has been attributed to compounds such as androsin and apocynin, which have been shown to inhibit allergen- and PAF-induced bronchoconstriction.[30,31] In another study, androsin produced an inhibition of ovalbumin- and PAF-induced bronchial reactions.[32] The antiallergic and antianaphylactic activity of Picroliv has also been investigated in vitro and in vivo. A dose of 25 mg/kg inhibited passive anaphylaxis in mice and rats and protected mast cells from degranulation, but bronchospasm induced by histamine could not be inhibited.[33]

Antiinflammatory activity: In a variety of test models, powdered roots, the alcohol extract and the active constituents kutkin, picroside-1 and kutkoside demonstrated antiinflammatory activity in adjuvant-induced and formaldehyde arthritis in rats and mice.[34]

Other activities: It has antioxidant,[35] anticholestatic[36–38] hypolipidaemic,[39] and laxative activity.[40]

Safety profile

No major untoward reactions have been reported when used within recommended doses, although in large doses the herb is reported to be laxative and mild gastric irritation may occur.

Dosage

Dried root powder: 1–1.5 g

Ayurvedic properties

Rasa: *Tikta* (bitter)

Guna: *Laghu* (light), *ruksha* (dry)

Veerya: *Shita* (cold)

Vipaka: *Katu* (pungent)

Dosha: Pacifies *kapha* and *pitta*

Further reading

Bharatiya Vidya Bhavan's Swami Prakashananda Ayurveda Research Centre 1992 Selected medicinal plants of India. Chemexcil, Mumbai

Kapoor LD 1990 Handbook of Ayurvedic medicinal plants. CRC Press, Boca Raton

Ministry of Health and Family Welfare 1989 Ayurvedic pharmacopoeia of India. Government of India, New Delhi

Pandey GS (ed) 1998 Bhavprakash Nighantu. Chaukhambha Bharati Academy, Gokul Bhawan, Varanasi

References

1 Mehrotra S, Rawat AKS, Usha S 1994 Ethnobiology of Kutki – *Picrorrhiza kurroa* Royle ex Benth. Proceedings of the 4th International Congress on Ethnobiology, NBRI, Lucknow, India

2 Dobriyal RM, Singh GS, Rao KS, Saxena KG 1997 Medicinal plants resource of Chhakinal Watershed in Northwestern Himalaya. Journal of Herbs, Spices and Medicinal Plants 5(1):15

3 International Institute of Rural Reconstruction 1994 Ethnoveterinary medicine in Asia. An information kit on traditional animal health care practices. IIRR, Silang, Philippines

4 Stuppner H, Wagner H 1989 Minor iridoid and phenol glycosides of *Picrorrhiza kurroa*. Planta Medica 55:467

5 Weinges K, Kloss P, Henkels WD 1972 Picroside II, ein neues 6-vanilloyl-cataphol aus *Picrorrhiza kurroa* Royle und Benth. Liebigs Annals of Chemistry 759:173

6 Singh B, Rastogi RP 1972 Chemical examination of *Picrorrhiza kurroa*. Part VI. Reinvestigation of Kutki. Indian Journal of Chemistry 10:29

7 Simons JM, T'Hart BA, Vai Ching I, Van Dijk T, Labadie RP 1989 Isolation of 5 low molecular compounds from a root extract of *Picrorrhiza kurroa* which affect the respiratory burst in activated human polymorphonuclear leucocytes. Planta Medica 55:113

8 Jia QH, Minter M, Minter D 1999 Pikuroside: a novel iridoid from *Picrorrhiza kurroa*. Journal of Natural Products 62:901

9 Stuppner H, Wagner H 1989 New cucurbitacin glycosides from *Picrorrhiza kurroa*. Planta Medica 55:559

10 Stuppner H, Muller EP, Wagner H 1991 Cucurbitacins from *Picrorrhiza kurroa*. Phytochemistry 30:305

11 Stuppner H, Muller EP 1991 Cucurbitacin with unusual side chains from *Picrorrhiza kurroa*. Phytochemistry 33:1139

12 Stuppner H, Kahling H, Seligmann O, Wagner H 1990 Minor cucurbitacin glycosides from *Picrorrhiza kurroa*. Phytochemistry 29:1633

13 Basu K, Dasgupta B, Bhattacharya SK, Devnath PK 1971 Chemistry and pharmacology of apocynin, isolated from *Picrorrhiza kurroa*. Current Science 22:603

14 Rastogi RP, Sharma VN, Siddiqui S 1950 Chemical examination of *Picrorrhiza kurroa* Benth Part-I. Indian Journal of Scientific Research 8B:173

15 Saraswat B, Visen PKS, Patnaik GK, Dhawan BN 1999 *Ex-vivo* and *in-vivo* investigations of Picroliv from *Picrorrhiza kurroa* in an alcohol intoxication model in rats. Indian Journal of Ethnopharmacology 66(3):263

16 Chaturvedi GN, Singh RH 1965 Treatment of jaundice with an indigenous drug, *Picrorrhiza kurroa*. A clinical and experimental study. Current Medical Practice 9:451

17 Singh DS, Gupta SS, Ansari SA, Singh RH 1991 A comparative study of Ayurvedic drugs *Picrorrhiza kurroa* (Kutaki) and *Berberis aristata* (Daruhardira) in acute viral hepatitis. Journal of Research and Education in Indian Medicine 4:1

18 Rajeshkumar NV, Kuttan R 2000 Inhibition of N-nitrosodiethylamine induced hepatocarcinogenesis by Picroliv. Journal of Experimental and Clinical Cancer Research 19(4):459

19 Rastogi R, Srivastava AK, Dhawan BN 1998 Prevention of phenobarbitone induced biochemical changes in liver and serum of rats by Picroliv. Acta Pharmaceutica 48(2):77

20 Rastogi R, Srivastava AK, Dhawan BN 1997 Effect of Picroliv on impaired hepatic mixed–function oxidase system in carbon tetrachloride intoxicated rats. Drug Development Research 41(1):44

21 Saraswat B, Visen PK, Patnaik GK, Dhawan BN 1997 Hepatoprotective effect of Picroliv against rifampicin induced toxicity. Drug Development Research 40(4):299

22 Antarkar DS, Vaidya AB, Doshi JC et al 1980 Double blind clinical trial of *Arogyavardhini*, an Ayurvedic drug, in acute viral hepatitis. Indian Journal of Medical Research 72:588

23 Agarwal SS, Singh VK 1999 Immunomodulators: a review of studies on Indian medicinal plants and synthetic peptides. Part I: medicinal plants. Journal of the Indian National Science Academy 65(3,4):179

24 Simsons JM, Hart LA, Labadie RP, Dijk HV, De Selva KTD 1991 Modulation of human complement activation and the human neutrophil oxidative burst by different root extracts of *Picrorrhiza kurroa*. Journal of Ethnopharmacology 34:61

25 Puri A, Saxena RP, Guru PYS, Kulshreshtha DK, Saxena KC, Dhawan BN 1992 Immunostimulant activity of Picroliv, the iridoid glycoside fraction of *Picrorrhiza kurroa*, and its protective action against *Leishmania donovani* infection in hamsters. Planta Medica 58:528

26 Kulkarni RD, Mahajani SS 1976 Studies of antiasthmatic potentials of *Picrorrhiza kurroa* in comparison with disodium chromoglycate. Aspects of Allergy and Applied Immunology 9:231

27 Rajaram D 1975 A preliminary clinical trial of *Picrorrhiza kurroa* in bronchial asthma. Indian Journal of Pharmacology 7:95

28 Shah BK, Kamat SR, Seth UK 1977 Preliminary report of use of *Picrorrhiza kurroa* root in bronchial asthma. Journal of Postgraduate Medicine 23(3):118

29 Yegnanarayana R, Dange SV, Vaidya SD, Bhalwani JH Study of *Picrorrhiza kurroa* in cases of bronchial asthma. Bombay Hospital Journal 24(2):15

30 Wagner H 1994 New potent anti-asthmatic constituents from higher plants. Second International Symposium on Innovations in Pharmaceutical Sciences and Technology, Ahmedabad, February 25–27

31 Stuppner H, Dorsch W, Wagner H, Gropp M, Kelper P 1991 Antiasthmatic effects of *Picrorrhiza kurroa*: inhibition of allergen and PAF induced bronchial obstruction in guinea pigs by androsin, apocynin and structurally related compounds. Planta Medica 57(2):A-60

32 Muller A, Antus S, Bittinger M et al 1993 Chemistry and pharmacology of the asthmatic

plants, *Galphamia glauca*, *Adhatoda vasica* and *Picrorrhiza kurroa*. Planta Medica 59:586

33 Baruah CC, Gupta PP, Nath A, Patnaik GK, Dhawan BN 1998 Anti-allergic and anti-anaphylactic activity of Picroliv, a standardized iridoid glycoside fraction of *Picrorrhiza kurroa*. Pharmacology Research 38(6):487

34 Singh GB, Bani S, Singh S et al 1993 Anti-inflammatory activity of the iridoids Kutkin, Picroside-I and kutkoside from *Picrorrhiza kurroa*. Phytotherapy Research 7:402

35 Chander R, Kapoor NK, Dhawan BN 1992 Picroliv, picroside-I, and Kutkoside from *Picrorrhiza kurroa* are scavengers of superoxide anions. Biochemistry and Pharmacology 44(1):180

36 Shukla B, Visen PKS, Patnaik GK, Dhawan BN 1992 Reversal of thioacetamide induced cholestasis by Picroliv in rodents. Phytotherapy Research 6(1):53

37 Visen PKS, Patnaik GK, Dhawan BN 1991 Cholerectic effect of Picroliv, the hepatoprotective principle of *Picrorrhiza kurroa*. Planta Medica 57(1):29

38 Saraswat B, Visen PKS, Patnaik GK, Dhawan BN 1993 Anticholestatic effect of Picroliv, active hepatoprotective principle of *Picrorrhiza kurroa*, against carbon tetrachloride induced cholestasis. Indian Journal of Experimental Biology 31:316

39 Khanna AK, Chander R, Kapoor NK, Dhawan BN 1994 Hypolipidemic activity of Picroliv in albino rats. Phytotherapy Research 8(7):403

40 Das PK, Raina MK 1967 Preliminary pharmacological studies on the roots of *Picrorrhiza kurroa*. Journal of Research in Indian Medicine 1(2):213

Piper longum L. (Piperaceae) (syn. *Piper latifolium* Hunter, *P. sarmentosum* Wall., *Chavica roxburghii* Miq, C.)

English: Long pepper

Hindi: *Pippali*

Sanskrit: *Pippali*

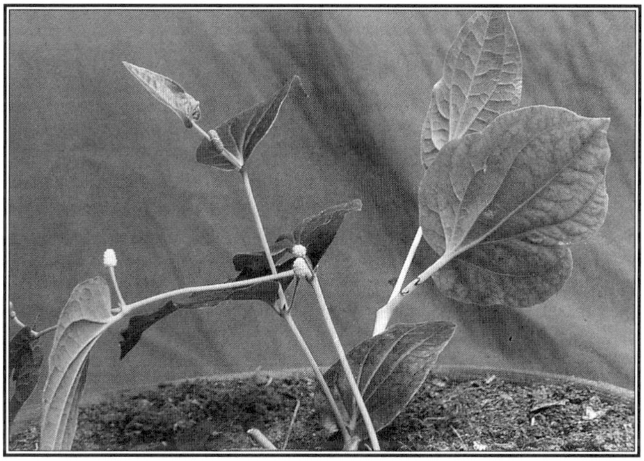

Long pepper has long been used in medicine and is an important culinary spice throughout the Indian subcontinent, Sri Lanka, Middle Eastern countries and the Americas. It became popular in Europe, northern and eastern Africa, where it was introduced by traders from India, and it is said that the Roman emperors valued it even more highly than black pepper.

Habitat

It is considered a native of South Asia and is found both wild as well as cultivated, throughout the hotter parts of India from central to the north-eastern Himalayas. The herb also grows wild in Malaysia, Singapore, Bhutan, Myanmar and elsewhere.

Botanical description

A slender, aromatic, perennial climber, with woody roots and numerous wide ovate, cordate leaves (Plate 45). The inflorescence is a cylindrical, pedunculate spike, the female flower is up to 2.5 cm long and 4–5 mm in diameter, the male flowers being larger and more slender. The fruits are small, ovoid berries, shiny blackish green, embedded in fleshy spikes.

Parts used

Immature spikes, roots.

Traditional and modern use

The dried fruit spikes are extensively used for flavouring a variety of foods. They are considered to have stimulant, carminative, laxative and stomachic properties. The berries are also given with honey for asthma, coughs and sore throats. The root is a stimulant and is also used in gout, rheumatism and lumbago. The whole plant is considered by tribal people in India to be useful in splenic disorders, cholera, dysentery, asthma, cough and bronchitis.

Ethnoveterinary usage

A decoction of the roots is given for swellings of the joints of cattle in the north-western Himalayan regions.

Major chemical constituents

Alkaloids and amides

The fruit contains a large number of alkaloids and related compounds, the most abundant of which is piperine, together with methyl piperine, pipernonaline, piperettine, asarinine, pellitorine, piperundecalidine, piperlongumine, piperlonguminine, retrofractamide A, pergumidiene, brachystamide-B, a dimer of desmethoxypiplartine, N-isobutyl-decadienamide, brachyamide-A, brachystine, pipercide, piperderidine, longamide, dehydropipernonaline piperidine and tetrahydropiperine. Piperine, piperlongumine, tetrahydropiperlongumine, trimethoxy cinnamyol-piperidine and piperlonguminine have been found in the root.[1-11]

Lignans

Sesamin, pulviatilol, fargesin and others have been isolated from the fruits.[2,3,5,12]

Esters

The fruits contain tridecyl-dihydro-p-coumarate, eicosanyl-(E)-p-coumarate and Z-12-octadecenoic-glycerol-monoester.[2,3,5,13]

Volatile oil

The essential oil of the fruit is a complex mixture, the three major components of which are (excluding the volatile piperine) caryophyllene and pentadecane (both about 17.8%) and bisaboline (11%). Others include thujine, terpinoline, zingiberine, p-cymene, p-methoxyacetophenone and dihydrocarveol.[2,3,5,14,15]

Medicinal and pharmacological activities

Immunomodulatory activity: Tests such as haemagglutination titre (HA), macrophage migration index (MMI) and phagocytic index (PI) in mice have demonstrated the immunostimulatory action of *Piper longum* fruits to be both specific and non-specific. The effect was more prominent at lower doses (225 mg/kg) and was marginally reduced when the dose was increased.[16] In another study, it was found to offer protection against externally induced stress.[17] A famous Ayurvedic preparation containing long pepper, *Pippali Rasayana*, was tested in mice infected with *Giardia lamblia* and found to produce significant activation of macrophages, as shown by an increased MMI and phagocytic activity.[18]

Stimulant effects: Isolated piperine showed a central stimulant action in frogs, mice, rats and dogs and increased the hypnotic response in mice. It antagonised respiratory depression induced by morphine or pentobarbitone in anaesthetised dogs[19] and a petroleum ether extract of the fruits antagonised morphine-induced respiratory depression in mice.[20] A comparative study conducted with piperine and nalorphine, for effects against morphine-induced respiratory depression and analgesia, found that both reversed respiratory depression but, unlike nalorphine, piperine did not antagonise morphine-induced analgesia in rats.[21]

Antiasthmatic activity: Studies have been carried out to validate the traditional claims of Ayurveda for antiasthmatic activity of *Piper* *longum*. An extract of the fruits in milk reduced passive cutaneous anaphylaxis in rats and protected guinea pigs against antigen-induced bronchospasm.[22,23]

Bio-availability enhancement: Piperine has been shown to enhance the bio-availability of structurally and therapeutically diverse drugs, possibly by modulating membrane dynamics, due to its easy partitioning and increasing permeability.[24] The effect of 'Trikatu', a compound Ayurvedic preparation containing *Piper longum* as one of the major ingredients, was tested in combination with other drugs. The study reported that 'Trikatu' increased their bio-availability either by promoting rapid absorption from the gastrointestinal tract or by protecting the drug from being metabolised during its first passage through the liver after being absorbed, or by combination of both mechanisms.[25]

Hepatoprotective activity: Piperine was evaluated and found to exert significant protection against tertiary butyl hydroperoxide and carbon tetrachloride-induced hepatotoxicity, by reducing both in vitro and in vivo lipid peroxidation.[26] A fruit extract was assessed in rodents for its hepatoprotective action against CCL_4-induced acute, chronic and reversible damage and chronic irreversible damage, using morphological, biochemical and histopathological assessment parameters. The extract improves the regeneration process by restricting fibrosis, but offered no protection against acute damage or against cirrhotic changes.[27]

Hypocholesterolaemic activity: Methyl piperine significantly inhibited the elevation of total serum cholesterol, and the total cholesterol to HDL-cholesterol ratio, in rats fed with a high cholesterol diet.[28] The unsaponifiable fraction of the oil of *Piper longum* also significantly decreased total serum cholesterol and hepatic cholesterol in hypercholesterolaemic mice.[29]

Antiinflammatory activity: A marked antiinflammatory activity of a decoction of *P. longum* fruits has been reported using carrageenan-induced rat oedema.[30]

Antiamoebic activity: The fruits were tested for their efficacy against *Entamoeba histolytica* in vitro and experimental caecal amoebiasis in vivo. Both the ethanolic extract and isolated piperine produced an improvement of 90% and 40% respectively, in rats with caecal amoebiasis.[31]

Antibacterial activity: The essential oil of *P. longum* showed antibacterial action against a number of bacterial strains[32,33] although a 50% ethanolic extract of the fruits did not show any effect.[34] Piperlonguminine was found to have potent activity against *Bacillus subtilis* while piperine was more effective against *Staphylococcus aureus*.[35]

Safety profile

Since it is so widely used in cooking and traditional medicine, it is generally assumed to be safe in moderate doses. However, as the fruits are reported to have contraceptive activity in experimental models, its use during pregnancy and lactation should be avoided.[36] Piperine may interfere with enzymatic drug biotransformations, resulting in the inhibition of hepatic arylhydrocarbon hydroxylase (AHH) and UDP-glucuronyltransferase, and alter the pharmacokinetic parameters of barbiturates and phenytoin. A single oral dose of 3 g/kg body weight in experimental animals, and chronic toxicity studies with 100 mg/kg body weight for 90 days, revealed no untoward effects.[34,37,38] Studies of isolated constituents in mice gave LD_{50} values for piperine, piperlongumine and piperlonguminine as 56.2 ± 3.0, 110.1 ± 7.8 and 115.3 ± 9.5 mg/kg body weight respectively.[39] In the evaluation of antifertility activity, long pepper at a dose of 1 g/kg body weight was found to be an effective contraceptive agent without toxic or teratogenic effects.[36]

Dosage

Powdered fruits and roots: 500 mg to 1 g

Ayurvedic properties

Rasa: *Katu* (pungent)

Guna: *Laghu* (light), *snigdha* (unctuous), *tikshna* (sharp)

Veerya: *Anushnashita* (slight cold)

Vipaka: *Madhur* (sweet)

Dosha: Pacifies *kapha* and *vata*

Further reading

Bharatiya Vidya Bhavan's Swami Prakashananda Ayurveda Research Centre 1992 Selected medicinal plants of India. Chemexcil, Mumbai

Ministry of Health and Family Welfare 1989 Ayurvedic pharmacopoeia of India, vol I. Government of India, New Delhi

Sairam TV 1998 Home remedies, vol I. Penguin India, New Delhi

References

1 Parmar VS, Jain SC, Gupta S et al 1998 Polyphenols and alkaloids from *Piper* species. Phytochemistry 49(4):1069

2 Tabuneng W, Bando H, Amiya T 1983 Studies on the constituents of the crude drug Piper Longi Fructus. Chemical and Pharmaceutical Bulletin 31(10):3562

3 Shankaracharya NB, Rao LJ, Naik JP, Nagalakshmi S 1997 Characterization of chemical constituents of Indian Long Peper (*Piper longum* L.). Journal of Food Science and Technology 34(1):73

4 Lee SE, Park BS, Kim KM et al 2001 Fungicidal activity of pipernonaline, a piperidine alkaloid derived from long pepper, *Piper longum* L., against phytopathogenic fungi. Crop Protection 20(6):523

5 Sharma RK, Rathore YKS, Kumar S 1983 Chemical examination of dried fruits of Pippali (*Piper longum* Linn). Journal of Scientific Research into Plant Medicines 4(4):63

6 Das B, Kashinathan A, Madhusudhan P 1998 One new and two rare alkamides from two samples of the fruits of *Piper longum*. Natural Product Science 4(1):23

7 Koul SK, Taneja SC, Agarwal VK, Dhar KL 1988 Minor amides of Piper species. Phytochemistry 27(11):3523

8 Zhang K, Chen C, Wang D, Wu Y 1996 A new amide dimer from *Piper longum*. Yunnan Zhiwu Yanjiu 18(3):353

9 Das B, Kashinathan A, Srinivas KVNS 1996 Alkamides and other constituents of *Piper longum*. Planta Medica 62(6):582

10 Shoji N, Umeyama A, Saito N, Takemoto T, Kajiwara A, Ohizumi Y 1986 Dehydropipernonaline, an amide possessing coronary vasodilating activity, isolated from *Piper longum* L. Journal of Pharmaceutical Sciences 75(12):1188

11 Madhusudhan P, Vandana KL 2001 Tetrahydropiperine, the first natural aryl pentanamide from *Piper longum*. Biochemistry, Systematics and Ecology 29(5):537

12 Atal CK, Girotra RN, Dhar KL 1966 Occurrence of sesamin in *Piper longum* Linn. Indian Journal of Chemistry 4:252

13 Das B, Kashinathan A, Madhusudhan P 1998 Long chain esters and alkamides from *Piper longum*. Bolletino Chimico Farmaceutico 137(8):319

14 Nigam SS, Radhakrishnan C 1968 Chemical examination of the essential oil derived from the berries of *Piper longum*. Bulletin of the National Institute of Science of India 37:189

15 Handa KL, Sharma ML, Nigam NC 1963 The essential oil of *Piper longum*, properties of the components and isolation of two monocyclic sesquiterpenes. Parfume Kosmetik 44(9):233

16 Tripathi DM, Gupta N, Lakshmi V, Saxena KC, Agarwal AK 1999 Antigiardial and immunostimulatory effect of *Piper longum* on giardiasis due to *Giardia lamblia*. Phytotherapy Research 13(7):561

17 Rege NN, Thatte UM, Dhanukar SA 1999 Adaptogenic properties of six rasayana herbs used in Ayurvedic medicines. Phytotherapy Research 13(4):275

18 Agarwal AK, Singh M, Gupta N et al 1994 Management of giardiasis by an immunomodulatory herbal drug 'Pippali Rasayana'. Journal of Ethnopharmacology 44(3):143

19 Singh N, Kulshreshta VK, Srivastava RK, Kohli RP 1973 Analeptic activity of some *Piper longum* alkaloids. Journal of Research into Indian Medicine 8(1):1

20 Dhanukar SA, Zha A, Karandikar SM 1981 Anti-allergic activity of *Piper longum*. Indian Journal of Pharmacology 13:122

21 Dhanukar SA, Karandikar SM, Desai SM 1984 Efficacy of *Piper longum* in childhood asthma. Indian Drugs 21:384

22 Kulshreshta VK, Srivastava RK, Singh N, Kohli RP 1969 A study of central stimulant effect of *Piper longum*. Indian Journal of Pharmacology 1(2):8

23 Kulshreshta VK, Singh N, Srivastava RK, Rastogi RK, Kohli RP 1971 Analysis of central stimulant activity of *Piper longum*. Journal of Research into Indian Medicine 6(1):17

24 Khajuria A, Zutshi U, Bedi KL 1998 Intestinal permeability characteristics of piperine, an active alkaloid from peppers and bioavailability enhancer. Indian Journal of Experimental Biology 36(1):46

25 Atal CK, Zutshi U, Rao PG 1981 Scientific evidence on the role of Ayurvedic herbals on bioavailability of drugs. Journal of Ethnopharmacology 4(2):229

26 Koul IB, Kapil A 1993 Evaluation of the hepatoprotective potential of piperine, an active principle of black and long peppers. Planta Medica 59(5):413

27 Rege N, Dhanukar S, Karandikar SM 1984 Hepatoprotective effects of *P. longum* against carbon tetrachloride induced liver damage. Indian Drugs 21:569

28 Li Y, Wang H, Wu E, Su W 1993 Effect of methyl piperate on rat serum cholesterol level and its mechanism of action. Zhonggacayao 24(1):27

29 Bao Z, Wu E 1992 Effects of unsaponifiable matter of *Piper longum* oil on cholesterol biosynthesis in experimental hypocholesterolaemic mice. Zhonggacayao 23(4):197

30 Sharma AK, Singh RH 1980 Screening of anti-inflammatory activity of certain indigenous drugs on carageenan induced hind paw oedema in rats. Indian Bulletin of Medical and Ethnobotanical Research 2:262

31 Ghosal S, Prasad K, Lakshmi V 1996 Anti-amoebic activity of *Piper longum* against *Entamoeba histolytica in vitro* and *in vivo*. Journal of Ethnopharmacology 50(3):167

32 Singh RH, Khosa KL, Upadhyaya BB 1974 Antibacterial activity of some Ayurvedic drugs. Journal of Research into Indian Medicine 9(2):65

33 Bhargava AK, Chauhan CS 1968 Antibacterial activity of some essential oils. Indian Journal of Pharmacy 30(6):150

34 Dhar ML, Dhar MM, Dhawan BN, Mehrotra BN, Ray C 1968 Screening of Indian plants for biological activity. Part I. Indian Journal of Experimental Biology 6:232

35 Reddy P, Srinivas J, Jamil K, Madhusudhan P, Anjani G, Das B 2001 Anti-bacterial activity of

isolates from *Piper longum* and *Taxus baccata*. Pharmaceutical Biology 39(3):236

36 Das PC, Sarkar AK, Thakur S 1987 Studies on animals of a herbo-mineral compound for long acting contraception. Fitoterapia 58(4):257

37 Atal CK, Dubey RK, Singh J 1984 Biochemical basis of enhanced drugs bio-availability by piperine: evidence that piperine is a potent inhibitor of monoxygenase system. Indian Journal of Pharmacology 16:52

38 Shah AH, Al-Shareef AH, Ageel AM, Qureshi S 1998 Toxicity studies in mice of common spices, *Cinnamomum zeylanicum* bark and *Piper longum* fruits. Plant Foods and Human Nutrition 52(3):231

39 Prasad BN, Chowdhury B 1967 Pharmacodynamics of extracts of *Piper longum* Linn., and its amides piperlongumine and piperine. Journal of Research into Indian Medicine 1(2):203

Piper nigrum L. (Piperaceae) (syn. *Piper tritoicum* Roxb., *Muldera multinervis* Miq.)

English: Black pepper

Hindi: *Golmirch, kalmirch*

Sanskrit: *Maricha*

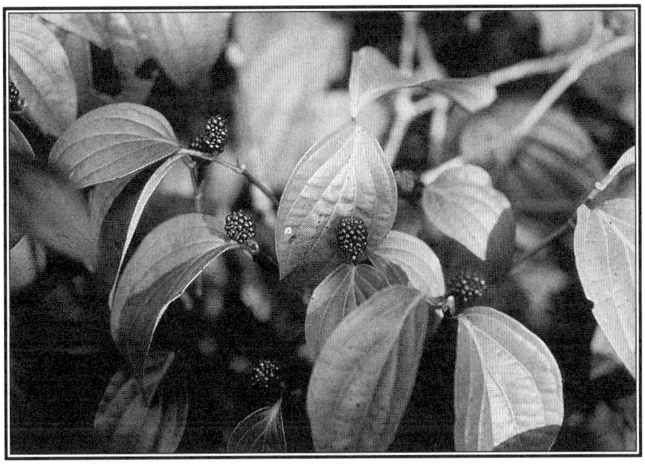

Originally from south-western India, *P. nigrum* is highly regarded as a condiment as well as a medicine, especially in Ayurveda and Unani. It is an important constituent of the Ayurvedic preparation *Trikatu*,[1] and historically was important to the Romans, Africans and Europeans. White pepper comes from the same plant but the fruits are ripe and peeled; it has a more pungent taste.

Habitat

The plant grows wild in tropical parts of India and is widely cultivated there and in many other countries including Sri Lanka, China and parts of Africa.

Botanical description

Pepper is a climbing perennial shrub cultivated on posts or wire and growing up to a height of 6 m (Plate 46). The branches are stout, trailing and rooting at the nodes. The glossy pale green leaves are entire, 8–18 cm in length and 5–10 cm in breadth, with an acute base, rounded or equally or unequally cordate. The flowers occur in minute spikes and are dioecious. The female bears two anthers and the male a single pistil. Fruiting spikes usually vary in length. Fruits are globular or oblong, 4–6 mm in diameter, and externally are bright red when ripe and blackish-brown when dried, with protruding reticulate wrinkles and a single seed. Seeds are white, hollow, globose with a thin testa and hard albumin. They are aromatic and strongly pungent.

Parts used

Dried unripe fruits, oleoresin and volatile oil.

Traditional and modern use

Black pepper is used particularly for stomach and digestive disorders and colds and bronchitis. It also finds use in conditions like neuralgia and scabies. External application helps to relieve pain due to cold and neuralgia, piles and various skin diseases. In Indian medicine it is used as an aromatic stimulant in cholera, weakness following fevers and vertigo, as an antiperiodic in malaria and for arthritic disease; *Trikatu* is used to enhance the bio-availability and efficacy of other medicines.[1] In Chinese medicine it is used to improve the appetite and in the treatment of cold, influenza, pains of the upper abdomen, diarrhoea and epilepsy.

Ethnoveterinary usage

The dried fruits are used to treat cold and cough in ruminants and to increase the flow of milk. It is administered to swine with retained placenta and given to poultry to treat fowl pox.[2] In Kerala it is used in combination with other drugs in the treatment of mastitis, fever, bloat, diarrhoea, helminthiasis, throat diseases and foot and mouth disease.[3]

Major chemical constituents

Volatile oil

The dried fruits contain 1.2–2.6% of volatile oil mainly composed of sabinene (15–25%), caryophyllene, α-pinene, β-pinene, β-ocimene, δ-guaiene, farnesol, δ-cadinol, guaiacol, 1-phellandrene, 1,8 cineole, p-cymene, carvone, citronellol, α-thujene, α-terpinene, bisabolene, dl-limonene, dihydrocarveol, camphene and piperonal.[4–7]

Alkaloids and amides

These are the main pungent principles and include piperine, piperylin, piperolein A and B, cumaperine, piperanine, piperamides, pipericide, guineensine and sarmentine. Other alkaloids include chavicine, piperidine and piperettine, methyl caffeic acid, piperidide, β-methyl pyrroline, and a series of vinyl homologues of piperine and their stereoisomers.[8,9]

Aminoacids

The dried fruits are rich in β-alanine, arginine, serine, threonine, histidine, lysine, cystine, asparagine and glutamic acid in combination with γ-aminobutyric acid and pipecolic acid.

Vitamins and minerals

Ascorbic acid, carotenes, thiamine, riboflavin and nicotinic acid are present and minerals including potassium, sodium, calcium, magnesium, iron, phosphorus, copper and zinc.[10]

Medicinal and pharmacological activities

Antimicrobial activity: Black pepper extracts inhibited aflatoxin production, via the β-glucuronidase reporter gene under the control of the aflatoxin biosynthesis gene promoter in the fungus *Aspergillus parasiticus*.[11] Using the agar diffusion method, both the ethanol and aqueous extracts of the dried fruits were found to have significant activity against a penicillin G-resistant strain of *Staphylococcus aureus*.[12] An extract was toxic to the culture of *Escherichia coli, Staphylococcus faecalis, Staph. aureus, Staph. albus, Corynebacterium diphtheriae, Salmonella dysenteriae and S. sonnei*.[13] The volatile oil also exhibited a high degree of antimicrobial activity against various types of organisms including animal pathogens, organisms involved in food poisoning and other spoilage bacteria and fungi.[4–7]

Effect on the gastrointestinal tract: An aqueous extract of black pepper perfused into pentobarbitone-anaesthetised rats increased acid secretion. This was mainly due to cholinergic activity but may involve other mechanisms also.[14] Piperine has the capability to increase absorption from the intestine by enhancing permeability of intestinal cells. This is thought to be due to stimulation of γ-glutamyl transpeptidase enzyme activity and increased lipid peroxidation.[15]

Melanocyte proliferating activity: An aqueous extract enhanced cell multiplication in a mouse melanocyte culture (melan-a), which was inhibited by protein kinase C, suggesting the involvement of PKC signalling.[16]

Thermogenic activity: Oxygen uptake by the perfused rat hind limb was increased by piperine, in association with vascular resistance which was blocked by glyceryl nitrate. This implies piperine may act as a thermogenic agent.[17]

Hepatic enzyme induction: Administration of black pepper to experimental animals resulted in a significant elevation of glutathione S-transferase (GST), cytochrome b5, cytochrome P450, acid-soluble sulfhydryl (-SH) content and malondialdehyde (MDA) levels in a dose-dependent manner. This shows it induces various detoxification enzymes, which suggests a possible role as a chemopreventive.[18] Piperine protected the liver against the toxic effects of tert-butyl hydroperoxide and carbon tetrachloride by a reduction in lipid peroxidation, prevention of enzymatic leakage of GPT and AP, and by the inhibition of GSH depletion and total thiols.[19]

Anticancer activity: Increased activities of β-glucuronidase in the distal colon, and levels of mucinase in the colon and faeces in experimental colon cancer, were brought down to almost normal by the ingestion of black pepper. This may prevent the hydrolysis of glucuronide conjugates, which liberate toxins, and the degradation of mucinase, which would prevent the hydrolysis of protective mucins in the colon.[20]

Antiinflammatory activity: Piperine exhibited activity by depressing both the acute inflammatory process and chronic granulative changes using carrageenan-induced rat paw oedema, cotton pellet and croton oil-induced granuloma pouch models. It was thought to act partially through the stimulation of the pituitary adrenal axis.[21]

Antioxidant effects: Pepper is rich in phenolic amides and possesses antioxidant effects that are more potent than α-tocopherol and equivalent to the synthetic antioxidants butylated hydroyanisole (BHA) and butylated hydroxytoluene (BHT).[9]

Anticonvulsant effects: In a recent study piperine and derivatives antagonised convulsions in animals induced by both physical and chemical methods.[22] In another experiment, convulsions produced by an intracerebroventricular injection of kainite was blocked by piperine, possibly due to activity at different aminoacid receptor subtypes.[23]

Safety profile

Pepper is widely used and considered safe at the usual therapeutic doses and as a flavouring. Use during pregnancy has not been properly evaluated and excessive intake is not encouraged in nursing mothers as metabolites are excreted into human milk. As it is known as an enzyme inducer it may reduce blood levels of concurrent medication if taken in large doses over a period of time.

Dosage

Dried fruit: 300–600 mg

Oleoresin: 15–20 mg

Ayurvedic properties

Rasa: *Katu* (pungent)

Guna: *Laghu* (light), *tikshna* (sharp)

Veerya: *Ushna* (hot)

Vipaka: *Katu* (pungent)

Dosha: Pacifies *vata* and *pitta*

Further reading

Chatterjee A, Prakashi SC 1995 Treatise on Indian medicinal plants, vol 4. PID, CSIR, New Delhi

Kapoor LD 1990 Handbook of Ayurvedic medicinal plants. CRC Press, Boca Raton

Rastogi RP, Mehrotra BN 1998 Compendium of Indian medicinal plants, vol 5. PID, New Delhi

Sivarajan VV, Balachandran I 1994 Ayurvedic drugs and their plant sources. Oxford and IBH Publishing, New Delhi

References

1 Johri RK, Zutshi U 1992 An Ayurvedic formulation 'Trikatu' and its constituents. Journal of Ethnopharmacology 37(2):85

2 International Institute of Rural Reconstruction 1994 Ethnoveterinary medicine in Asia. An information kit on traditional animal health care practices. IIRR, Silang, Philippines

3 Mathias E, Rangnekar DV, McCorkle CM 1988 Ethnoveterinary medicine: alternative for livestock development. Proceedings of an International Conference, BAIF Development Research Foundation, Pune, India

4 Dorman HJ, Deans SG 2000 Antimicrobial agents from plants: antibacterial activity of plant volatile oils. Journal of Applied Microbiology 88(2):308

5 Jain SR, Kar A 1971 Antibacterial activity of some essential oils and their combinations. Planta Medica 20:118

6 Rao CSS, Nigam SS 1976 Antimicrobial activity of some Indian essential oils. Indian Drugs 14:62

7 Jain SR, Jain MR 1972 Antifungal studies on some indigenous volatile oils and their combinations. Planta Medica 22:136

8 Williamson EM, Evans FJ 1988 Potter's new cyclopedia of botanical drugs and preparations. CW Daniel, Saffron Walden

9 Nakatani N, Inatani R, Ohta H, Nishioka A 1986 Chemical constituents of Peppers (*Piper* spp.) and application to food preservation: naturally occurring antioxidative compounds. Environmental Health Perspectives 67:135

10 Lavilla I, Filgueiras AV, Bendicho C 1999 Comparison of digestion of trace and minor metals in plant samples. Journal of Agricultural and Food Chemistry 47(12):5072

11 Annis SL, Velasquez L, Xu H, Hammerschmidt R, Linz J, Trail F 2000 Novel procedure for identification of compounds inhibitory to transcription of gene involved in mycotoxin biosynthesis. Journal of Agricultural and Food Chemistry 48(10):4656

12 Perez C, Anesini C 1994 Antibacterial activity of alimentary plants against *Staphylococcus aureus* growth. American Journal of Chinese Medicine 22(2):169

13 Subrahmanyan V, Sreenivasmurthy V, Krishnamurthy K, Swaminathan M, Studies on the antibacterial activity of spices. Indian Journal of Science and Industrial Research 16C:240

14 Vasudevan K, Vembar S, Veeraraghavan K, Haranath PS 2000 Influence of intragastric perfusion of aqueous spice extracts on acid secretion in anesthetized albino rats. Indian Journal of Gastroenterology 19(2):53

15 Johri RK, Thusu N, Khajuria A, Zutshi U 1992 Piperine-mediated changes in the permeability of rat intestinal epithelial cells. The status of gamma-glutamyl transpeptidase activity, uptake of amino acids and lipid peroxidation. Biochemistry and Pharmacology 1, 43(7):1401

16 Lin Z, Hoult JR, Bennett DC, Raman A 1999 Stimulation of mouse melanocyte proliferation by *Piper nigrum* fruit extract and its main alkaloids, Piperine. Planta Medica 65(7):600

17 Eldershaw TP, Colquhoun EQ, Bennett KL, Dora KA, Clark MG 1994 Resiniferatoxin and Piperine: capsaicin-like stimulators of oxygen uptake in the perfused rat hindlimb. Life Sciences 55(5):389

18 Singh A, Rao AR 1993 Evaluation of the modulatory influence of Black Pepper (*Piper nigrum* L.) on the detoxification system. Cancer Letters 72(1–2):5

19 Koul IB, Kapil A 1993 Evaluation of the liver protective potential of Piperine, an active principle of black and long peppers. Planta Medica 59(5):413

20 Nalini N, Sabitha K, Viswanathan P, Menon VP 1998 Influence of spices on the bacterial (enzyme) activity in experimental colon cancer. Journal of Ethnopharmacology 62(1):15

21 Mujumdar AM, Dhuley JN, Deshmukh VK, Raman PH, Naik SR 1990 Anti-inflammatory activity of Piperine. Japanese Journal of Medical Science and Biology 43(3):95

22 Pei YQ 1983 A review of pharmacology and clinical use of Piperine and its derivatives. Epilepsia 24(2):177

23 D'Hooge R, Pei YQ, Raes A, Lebrun P, Bogaert PP, de Deyn PP 1996 Anticonvulsant activity of Piperine on seizures induced by excitatory amino acid receptor agonists. Arzneimittelforschung 46(6):557

Plantago ovata Forsk. (Plantaginaceae)

English: Blond psyllium, ispaghula, spogel

Hindi: *Isapghul*

Sanskrit: *Ashwakarnabeez*

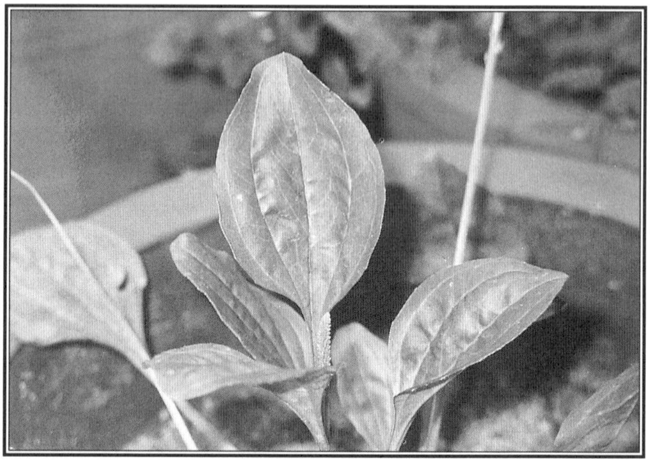

The plant is mentioned in ancient Arabic and Persian texts from as far back as the 10th century and from there was introduced to India where it is widely found. The name *isapghul* literally means 'horse's ear'.

Habitat

It is native to the Mediterranean regions of western Asia and widely cultivated in India, Pakistan, Russia, China and elsewhere on a commercial scale.

Botanical description

The plant is a softly hairy annual herb (Plate 47), with leaves that are narrowly linear or filiform up to 25 cm long, with an acute apex and an entire or faintly toothed margin. The flowers occur in cylindrical or oval spikes up to 4 cm long. The capsules are ellipsoid and up to 8 cm long, containing the seeds, which are ovoid or oblong, smooth and yellowish-brown with deep red husks.

Parts used

Seed and husks.

Traditional and modern use

The dried seeds and husk are used as a demulcent, emollient and laxative in the treatment of chronic constipation, amoebic and bacillary dysentery and diarrhoea due to irritant conditions of the gastrointestinal tract; in colds and coughs, bronchitis, rheumatism, kidney disorders and urethritis. They are also applied as a poultice.

Ethnoveterinary usage

The husked seed kernels are mixed with guar and used as cattle feed.[1]

Major chemical constituents

Polysaccharides

The main component of the mucilage of the seed is a large, linear, highly branched polymer comprising d-galactose, d-glucose, lignin, (1,2)-1-rhamnose, d-xylose, 1-arabinose, d-mannose with uronic acid side chains.

Others

Other parts of the plant contain monoterpene alkaloids such as boshniakine (indicaine) and boshniakinic acid (plantagonine), the iridoid aucubin and tannins.[2]

Medicinal and pharmacological activities

Laxative effects: The mucilage in the husk is responsible for this activity. It swells to a jelly-like mass with cold water, thereby increasing in volume, and this relieves constipation by stimulating intestinal peristalsis mechanically. The intraluminal pressure is decreased and colon transit therefore accelerated.[3–6] The toxins present in the gut are absorbed by the mucilage and are prevented from being absorbed in the system to some extent. The mucilage remains unaffected by the digestive enzymes and bacteria. Only a small part of the fibre is degraded by colon bacteria.[7]

Antihaemorrhoidal effects: In a placebo-controlled trial in 50 patients with bleeding internal haemorrhoids *P. ovata* was found to be helpful in alleviating symptoms. Parameters measured before and after the treatment included the degree of haemorrhoidal prolapse, the number of congested haemorrhoidal cushions and the amount of bleeding from the haemorrhoids. The average number of bleeding episodes decreased significantly over 15 days in the study group and in the last 10 days of treatment a further reduction was observed. The number of congested haemorrhoidal cushions also diminished after treatment. No differences were found in the control group. No modification of the degree of prolapse was observed after treatment. The addition of a preparation of *P. ovata* therefore improved most of the symptoms of internal bleeding haemorrhoids, although the effect was not immediate.[8]

Pharmacological activity: The ethanolic extract of the seeds exhibits cholinergic activity, lowering the blood pressure in anaesthetised animals.[2]

Protection of mucosa: A decrease in β-glucuronidase activity of colon bacteria has been observed, which inhibits cleavage of toxic compounds from their liver conjugates. The bacterial conversion of primary bile acids to the more toxic secondary ones was reduced in a study performed in rats.[9]

Antidiarrhoeal activity: The mucilage in *P. ovata* combines with the excess fluid in the intestines, thereby increasing the viscosity of the intestinal contents. Hence, transit time and defaecation frequency are normalised.[10]

Cholesterol-lowering activity: Levels of cholesterol in blood were lowered by *P. ovata* due to binding with bile acids and increasing their faecal excretion, thereby resulting in further synthesis of bile salts from cholesterol.[11]

Glucose-lowering activity: Levels of blood glucose are lowered by *P. ovata* due to delaying the intestinal absorption in the intestine.[12]

Safety profile

No harmful or deleterious effects during pregnancy or lactation have been reported. This is understandable as the constituents are not absorbed.[13] However, in rare cases hypersensitivity reactions may occur.

Dosage

Powdered seed and husk: 6–12 g daily

Ayurvedic properties

Rasa: *Madhur* (sweet)

Guna: *Guru* (heavy), *snigdha* (unctuous), *pichchhil* (sticky)

Veerya: *Shita* (cold)

Vipaka: *Madhur* (sweet)

Dosha: Pacifies *vata* and *kapha*

Further reading

Council of Scientific and Industrial Research 1995 The wealth of India. PID, New Delhi

References

1 Council of Scientific and Industrial Research 1995 The wealth of India: A dictionary of Indian raw materials and industrial products. PID, New Delhi

2 Williamson EM, Evans FJ 1988 Potter's new cyclopedia of botanical drugs and preparations. C W Daniels, Saffron Walden

3 Ligny G 1988 Therapie des colon irritabile: Knotrollierte Doppelblindstudie zur prufung der wirksamkeit einer hemizellulosehaltigen Arzneizubereitung. Therapeutikon 7:449

4 Sharma PK, Koul AK 1986 Mucilage in seeds of *Plantago ovata* and its wild allies. Journal of Ethnopharmacology 17:289

5 Read NW 1986 Dietary fibre and bowel transit. In: Vahouny GV, Kritchevsky D (eds). Dietary fiber. Basic and clinical aspects. Plenum Press, New York, 81

6 Stevens J, Van-Soest PJ, Robertson JB, Levitsky DA 1988 Comparison of the effects of psyllium and wheat bran on gastrointestinal transit time and stool characteristics. Journal of the American Dietetic Association 88:323

7 Kay RM, Strasberg SM 1978 Origin, chemistry, physiological effects and clinical importance of dietary fibre. Clinical and Investigative Medicine 1:9

8 Perez-Miranda M, Gomez-Cedenilla A, Leon-Colombo T, Pajares J, Mate-Jimenez J 1996 Effect of fiber supplements on internal bleeding hemorrhoids. Hepatogastroenterology 43(12):1504

9 Vahouny GB, Khalafi R, Satchithanandam S et al 1987 Dietary fibre supplementation and fecal bile acids, neutral steroids and divalent cations in rats. Journal of Nutrition 117:2009

10 Kovar F 1983 Was tun bei akuter, nicht bakteriell bedingter Diarrhoea. Arzneimittel und Praxis 35:1498

11 Leng-Peschlow E 1989 Cholesterol lowering effect of *Plantago ovata* seeds (abstract). Tenth International Symposium on Drugs Affecting Lipid Metabolism, Houston, Texas

12 Welsh JD, Manion CV, Griffiths WJ, Bird PC 1982 Effect of psyllium hydrophilic mucilloid on oral glucose tolerance and breath hydrogen in postgastrectomy patients. Digestive Diseases and Sciences 27:7

13 Lewis JH, Weingold AB 1985 The use of gastrointestinal drugs during pregnancy and lactation. American Journal of Gastroenterology 80:912

Plumbago zeylanica L. (Plumbaginaceae)

English: White leadwort

Hindi: *Chitra*

Sanskrit: *Chitraka*

Plumbago zeylanica is one of the oldest drugs known to Ayurvedic physicians. It is a component of several Indian preparations used as caustics or abortifacients.

Habitat

Found wild in the tropics and subtropics and widely cultivated as an ornamental plant.

Botanical description

A much-branched shrub with long and tuberous roots and a striate stem (Plate 48). The leaves are up to 8 cm long, simple, glabrous, alternate, ovate or oblong, with an entire or wavy margin, an acute apex and a short petiole. The flowers are white in terminal spikes, with a tubular calyx, a slender, glandular, hairy corolla tube, with five lobes and five stamens, a slender style and a stigma with five branches. The fruit is a membranous capsule enclosed within the persistent calyx. The dried roots occur as cylindrical pieces of varying length, less than 1.25 cm in width, reddish-brown in colour with a brittle, fairly thick, shrivelled, smooth or irregularly fissured bark. The roots have a short fracture, an acrid and biting taste and disagreeable odour.

Parts used

Roots, leaves.

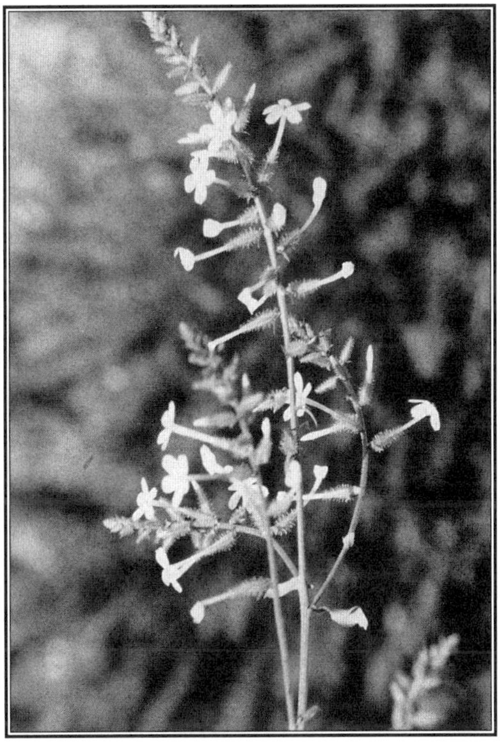

Traditional and modern use

The drug is an abortifacient and vesicant. It is also used in the treatment of rheumatism, dyspepsia, piles and diarrhoea and as a diuretic. It is used as a counterirritant and for skin diseases. The drug is apt to cause abortion and in Malaysia, eating the leaves is said to cause similar action. In Africa, a cold infusion of the root is used for influenza and black water fever. The powdered root is occasionally taken as a snuff to relieve headache.

Ethnoveterinary usage

The bark is used to stop bleeding in ruminants.[1] It is also used to cure baldness, cracked tail, worms in the eye, diarrhoea and boils.[2] In Java the root is used to expel worms from horses.[3]

Major chemical constituents

Naphthalene derivatives

The chief component is plumbagin, together with 3-chloroplumbagin, 3,3′-biplumbagin, 3′,6′-biplumbagin (chitranone), isozeylanicone, zeylanicone, elliptinone and droserone.[4,5]

Triterpenes

Lupeol and lupenyl acetate have been isolated from the root.[6]

Aminoacids

Aspartic acid, tryptophan, tyrosine, threonine, alanine, histidine, glycine, methionine and hydroxyproline were isolated from the aerial parts.[7]

Medicinal and pharmacological activities

Anticancer activity: Plumbagin has been reported as having anticancer activity against fibrosarcoma induced by methyl cholanthrene and P388 lymphocytic leukaemia, but not against L1210 lymphoid leukaemia in mice. It is thought to be an inhibitor of mitosis.[8] It has also been evaluated against Dalton's ascitic lymphoma, where an inhibition of tumour growth and a significant enhancement of mean survival time were observed for treated mice compared to the control group. Peritoneal cell counts were also enhanced. Plumbagin-treated groups were able to reverse the changes in various haematological parameters which are a consequence of tumour inoculation.[9] Studies have shown that plumbagin, when administered orally at a dose of 4 mg/kg body weight, caused tumour regression in rats with 3-methyl-4-dimethyl aminoazobenzene (3MeDAB)-induced hepatoma. It reduced levels of glycolytic enzymes such as hexokinase, phosphoglucoisomerase and aldolase levels, which are increased in hepatoma-bearing rats, and increased levels of gluconeogenic enzymes such as glucose-6-phosphatase and fructose-1,6-diphosphatase which are decreased in tumour hosts.[10]

Antifertility activity: In rats, treatment during the first week of pregnancy abolished certain uterine proteins resulting in both pre-implantationary loss and abortion of the foetus.[11] Uterine endopeptidases (cathepsin D, remin and chymotrypsin) were studied after the root powder had induced these effects and cathepsin D and renin activities were found to be decreased whilst chymotrypsin activity was increased. The results indicated that cathepsin D and renin may play a role in maintenance of pregnancy and chymotrypsin may be involved in postabortive involution.[12] Plumbagin, at a dose of 1 and 2 mg/100 g body weight, prevented implantation and induced abortion in albino rats without any teratogenic effects, and produced a significant inhibitory effect on copper acetate-induced ovulation in rabbits.[13]

Antiinflammatory activity: A phosphate buffered saline extract of the roots of *P. zeylanica* stabilised red blood cells subjected to both heat- and hypotonic-induced lyses. A biphasic response and a reduction in the enzymatic activities of alkaline and acid phosphatases were observed and adenosine triphosphate activity was stimulated in liver homogenates of formaldehyde-induced arthritic rats.[14]

Antimicrobial activity: A chloroform extract from *P. zeylanica* showed significant activity against penicillin- and non-penicillin resistant strains of *Neisseria gonorrhoeae*.[15] It also showed antibacterial activity against *Bacillus mycoides*, *B. pumilus*, *B. subtilis*, *Salmonella typhi*, *Staphylococcus aureus* and others.[16] Eye drops containing 50 µg/ml of plumbagin demonstrated significant antibacterial, antiviral and antichlamydial effects in eye diseases with few side effects.[17] Aqueous, hexane and alcoholic extracts of the plant were found to show interesting antibacterial activity. The alcoholic extract was the most active and showed no toxicity when assayed using fresh sheep erythrocytes.[18]

Antibiotic resistance modification: Plumbagin has been studied for its effect on the development of antibiotic resistance using sensitive strains of *Escherichia coli* and *Staphylococcus aureus*. When the organisms were inoculated into the antibiotic (streptomycin/rifampicin) medium, some growth was observed due to development of resistance. However, it was completely prevented when plumbagin was added to the medium and this was attributed to prevention of antibiotic resistance.[19]

Antioxidant activity: At a concentration of 1 mM, plumbagin prevented peroxidation in liver and heart homogenates. By a comparison with menadione (which has one hydroxyl group less) it was suggested that plumbagin may prevent NADPH and ascorbate-induced microsomal lipid peroxidation by forming hydroquinones. These may trap free radical species involved in catalysing lipid peroxidation.[20]

Immunomodulatory activity: The effect of plumbagin was studied on peritoneal macrophages of BALB/c mice, evaluated by bactericidal activity, hydrogen peroxide production and superoxide anion release. The bactericidal activity in vivo of plumbagin-treated mouse macrophages was estimated using *Staphylococcus aureus* and in low doses plumbagin caused a constant increase in bactericidal activity. It was also seen to exert a similar response on oxygen radical release, showing a correlation between oxygen radical release and bactericidal activity. Plumbagin appeared to augment macrophage bactericidal activity at low concentrations by potentiating oxygen radical release, whereas at higher concentrations it had an inhibitory effect.[21]

Hypolipidaemic activity: When administered to hyperlipidaemic rabbits, plumbagin reduced serum cholesterol and LDL cholesterol by 53–86% and 61–91% respectively. It also lowered the cholesterol/phospholipid ratio and elevated HDL cholesterol significantly. Furthermore, plumbagin treatment prevented the accumulation of cholesterol and triglycerides in the liver and aorta and caused regression of atheromatous plaques of the thoracic and abdominal aorta. The animals treated with plumbagin excreted more faecal cholesterol and phospholipids.[22]

Uterine stimulant activity: The juice extracted from the root was found to have potent activity when tested on rat uterus in vitro, as well as on isolated human myometrial strips. This ecbolic effect was not blocked by either atropine sulphate or pentolinium bitartrate.[23]

Anticoagulant activity: Plumbagin significantly increased prothrombin time, GPT, total protein and alkaline phosphatase levels in liver tissue and decreased GPT levels in serum. The anti-vitamin K activity was thought to be associated with the hydroxyl group attached to the naphthoquinone ring of the compound.[24]

Digestive effects: The roots of *Plumbago zeylanica* were found to stimulate the proliferation of coliform bacteria in mice and act as an intestinal flora normaliser. This supports claims that the plant is a digestive stimulant.[25]

Safety profile

The LD_{50} of plumbagin is approximately 10 mg/kg body weight (oral and IP) in mice and a 50% alcoholic extract of the root or whole plant has an LD_{50} of 500 mg/kg body weight when given IP.[26] In view of the documented abortifacient activity, it should be avoided at all stages of pregnancy.

Dosage

Powdered root: 1–2 g

Ayurvedic properties

Rasa: *Katu* (pungent)

Guna: *Laghu* (light), *ruksha* (dry), *tikshna* (sharp)

Veerya: *Ushna* (hot)

Vipaka: *Katu* (pungent)

Dosha: Pacifies *kapha*

Further reading

Ministry of Health and Family Welfare 1989 Ayurvedic pharmacopoeia of India. Government of India, New Delhi

Pandey GS (ed) 1998 Bhavprakash Nighantu. Chaukhambha Bharati Academy, Gokul Bhawan, Varanasi

Sivarajan VV, Balachandran I 1994 Ayurvedic drugs and their plant sources. Oxford and IBH Publishing, New Delhi

References

1. International Institute of Rural Reconstruction 1994 Ethnoveterinary medicine in Asia. An information kit on traditional animal health care practices. IIRR, Silang, Philippines
2. Jha MK 1992 Folk veterinary medicine of Bihar – a research project. NDDB, Anand, Gujrat
3. Watt JM, Breyer-Brandwijk MG 1962 The medicinal and poisonous plants of east and southern Africa, 2nd edn. AJ & S Livingstone, Edinburgh
4. Sidhu GS, Sankaran AVB 1971 A new biplumbagin and 3-chloroplumbagin from *Plumbago zeylanica*. Tetrahedron Letters 26:2385
5. Sankaram AVB, Srinivasarao A, Sidhu GS 1976 Chitranone, a new binaphthoquinone from *Plumbago zeylanica*. Phytochemistry 15:237
6. Dinda B, Saha S 1990 Chemical constituents of *Plumbago zeylanica* aerial parts and *Thevetia nerifolia* roots. Journal of the Indian Chemical Society 67:88
7. Dinda B, Saha S 1987 Free amino acids of *Plumbago zeylanica*. Journal of the Indian Chemical Society 64(4):261
8. Krishnaswamy M, Purushothaman KK 1980 Plumbagin: a study of its anticancer, antibacterial and antifungal properties. Indian Journal of Experimental Biology 18:876
9. Kavimani S, Ilango R, Madheswaran M, Jayakar B, Gupta M, Majumdar UK 1996 Antitumor activity of plumbagin against Dalton's ascitic lymphoma. Indian Journal of Pharmaceutical Science 58(5):194
10. Parimala R, Sachdanandam P 1993 Effect of plumbagin on some glucose metabolizing enzymes studied in rats in experimental

hepatoma. Molecular and Cellular Biochemistry 125(1):59

11 Devarshi P, Patil S, Kanase A 1991 Effect of *Plumbago zeylanica* root powder induced preimplantationary loss and abortion on uterine luminal proteins in albino rats. Indian Journal of Experimental Biology 29(6):521

12 Devarshi P, Patil S, Kanase A 1992 Studies on uterine endopeptidases in albino rats after *Plumbago zeylanica* root powder induced preimplantationary loss and abortion. Indian Journal of Comparative Animal Physiology 10(1):32

13 Premakumari P, Rathinam K, Santhakumari G 1977 Antifertility activity of plumbagin. Indian Journal of Medical Research 65:829

14 Oyedapo OO 1996 Studies on the bioactivity of the root extract of *Plumbago zeylanica*. International Journal of Pharmacognosy 34(5):365

15 Gundidza M, Manwa G 1990 Activity of chloroform extract from *Plumbago zeylanica* against *Neisseria gonorrhoeae*. Fitoterapia 61(1):47

16 Mukharya D, Dahia MS 1977 Antimicrobial activity of some plant extracts. Indian Drugs 14:160

17 Zeng Y, Deng YM, Yao MY 1997 Pharmacological study of plumbagin and its use in eye drops. Chinese Pharmaceutical Journal 8(4):161

18 Ahmed I, Mehmood Z, Mohammad F 1998 Screening of some Indian medicinal plants for their antimicrobial properties. Journal of Ethnopharmacology 62(2):183

19 Durga R, Sridhar P, Polasa H 1990 Effects of plumbagin on antibiotic resistance in bacteria. Indian Journal of Medical Research 91(A):18

20 Sankar R, Devamanoharan PS, Ragupathi G, Shyamala Devi CS 1987 Anti-lipid peroxidative efficacy of plumbagin and menadione: an *in vitro* study. Current Science 56(17):890

21 Abdul KM, Ramchender RP 1995 Modulatory effect of plumbagin (5-hydroxy-2-methyl-1, 4-naphthoquinone) on macrophage functions in BALB/c mice I. Potentiation of macrophage bactericidal activity. Immunopharmacology 30:231

22 Sharma I, Gusain D, Dixit VP 1991 Hypolipidaemic and antiatherosclerotic effects of plumbagin in rabbits. Indian Journal of Physiology and Pharmacology 35(1):10

23 Tewari PV, Prasad DN, Das PK 1966 Preliminary studies on uterine activity of some Indian medicinal plants. Journal of Research in Indian Medicine 1(1):68

24 Santhakumari G, Rathinam K, Seshadri C 1978 Anticoagulant activity of plumbagin. Indian Journal of Experimental Biology 16:485

25 Iyengar MA, Pendse GS 1966 *Plumbago zeylanica* L. (Chitrak) – a gastrointestinal flora normalizer. Planta Medica 14:337

26 Bhakuni DS, Dhar ML, Dhar MM, Dhawan BN, Mehrotra BN 1969 Screening of Indian plants for biological activity: Part II. Indian Journal of Experimental Biology 7:258

Polygonum aviculare L. (Polygonaceae)

English: Prostrate knotweed, wireweed, knotgrass

Hindi: *Machoti, anjawar*

Sanskrit: *Nasomali*

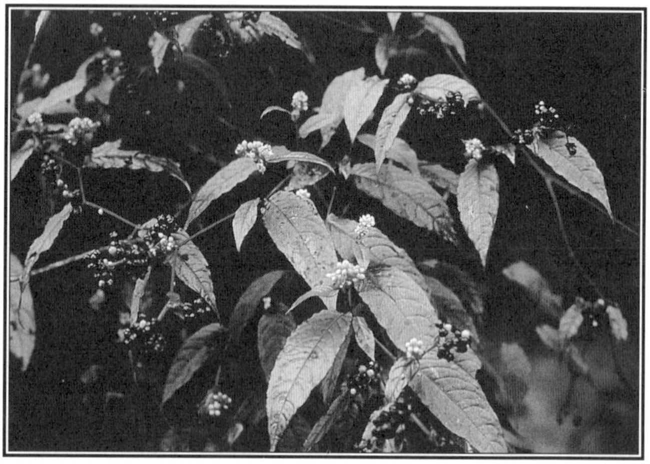

The generic name comes from the Latin word *aviculus*, a diminutive of '*avis*' meaning 'bird', because a large number of small birds feed on the seeds. The plant is used as a fodder for sheep and goats and also yields a dye rather like indigo.

Habitat

It is native to Europe, Russia and parts of Asia up to an altitude of 3600 m.

Botanical description

It is an annual herb with both erect and prostrate branches, reaching about 60 cm high and with tough fibrous roots (Plate 49). The leaves are narrowly lanceolate or elliptical, up to 1 cm long with lanceolate stipules. The flowers are green, edged with white or red, and present in axillary clusters. The nutlets are ovoid and minutely edged.

Parts used

Whole plant, leaves.

Traditional and modern use

A decoction of the herb is given in dysentery, diarrhoea, bronchitis, diabetes, jaundice and malaria. It is particularly useful for bleeding disorders including menorrhagia, haematuria and bleeding piles and has been used as an anodyne, antiseptic, diuretic, vermifuge and tonic. It is less often used for eczema, gonorrhoea and vaginitis.

Ethnoveterinary usage

Leaves are used in cuts, bruises and sores. It is also used in urinary complaints, problems of polyurea, diarrhoea and dysentery.

Major chemical constituents

Flavonoids and anthocyanins

Avicularin, catechin, delphinidin, hyperin, myricetin, quercetin, quercitrin, quercetin-3-arabinoside, rutin, astragalin are present.[1]

Polyphenolics and anthraquinones

Oxymethyl anthraquinone, polygonic acid, salicylic acid, tannic acid, fuglanin, betmidin and a lignan glycoside have been isolated.[1]

Medicinal and pharmacological activities

Antifibrotic activity: The antifibrotic effect of a methanolic extract has been studied. Liver fibrosis was induced by a bile duct ligation and scission (BDL/S) operation. In BDL/S rats, the levels of aspartate transaminase (AST), alanine transaminase (ALT), alkaline phosphatase (ALP), total bilirubin in serum and hydroxyproline content in liver were dramatically increased. Rats treated with extract showed reduction in all the liver enzymes and the liver hydroxyproline content of the treated group was reduced to 40% that of the BDL/S control group. The morphological characteristics of fibrotic liver were also improved in the extract-treated BDL/S group.[2]

Antimicrobial activity: An aqueous extract showed antifungal activity in vitro. Dermatophytes were inoculated on Sabouraud's dextrose agar medium containing different concentrations of the extract. After 2 weeks, growth of some strains of *Trichophyton rubrum*, *T. mentagrophytes* and *Microsporum canis* were completely inhibited by the extract and a moderate inhibitory effect was observed for other strains.[3] The efficacy of *P. aviculare* extract was tested against gingivitis using 60 male dentistry students between the ages of 18 and 25 years, over a period of 2 weeks. These students used the extract (1 mg/ml) as an oral rinse twice daily and the O'Leary Plaque Index and the Loe and Silness Gingivitis Index were recorded at baseline (day 0) in all the subjects. The antibacterial and antiinflammatory effects of the extract were evaluated and the results showed that the extract in the oral rinse significantly decreased gingivitis from day 0 to day 14. However, a significant increase in dental plaque was observed during the same period although the consistency of this plaque permitted its mechanical flushing easily.[4]

Antiinflammatory activity: *Polygonum aviculare* was found to inhibit prostaglandin biosynthesis and platelet-activating factor (PAF) induced in vitro.[5]

Hepatoprotective and lipid peroxidation activity: A crude fraction consisting primarily of flavonoid glucosides inhibited the lipid peroxidation of rat liver in vitro. It decreased liver enzymes including GOT and GPT, and the thiobarbituric acid value compared to the control, suggesting strong protective action against hepatotoxicity induced by carbon tetrachloride.[6]

Hypotensive and anticoagulant activity: Extracts of the aerial parts were hypotensive in dogs, cats and rabbits and showed anticoagulant activity in sheep blood.[7]

Safety profile

The LD_{50} of a 50% ethanolic extract of aerial parts was 500 mg/kg (IP in rats).[7] Overdosage has been observed in farm animals. Six horses died and one was slaughtered after grazing on farms cultivating *P. aviculare*. The animals showed recumbency, hyperaesthesia and circulatory collapse. However, the plant accumulates nitrites and this may have caused the toxicity.[8]

Dosage

Powdered herb (or equivalent extract): 4 g twice daily

Ayurvedic properties

Rasa: *Tikta* (bitter), *katu* (pungent)

Guna: *Laghu* (light)

Veerya: *Ushna* (hot)

Vipaka: *Katu* (pungent)

Dosha: Pacifies *kapha* and *vata*

Further reading

Duke JA 1992 Handbook of phytochemical constituents of GRAS herbs and other economic plants. CRC Press, Boca Raton

References

1 Kim HJ, Woo ER, Park H 1994 A novel lignan and flavonoids from *Polygonum aviculare*. Journal of Natural Products 57(5):581

2 Nan JX, Park EJ, Kim HJ, Ko G, Sohn DH 2000 Antifibrotic effects of the methanol extract of *Polygonum aviculare* in fibrotic rats induced by bile duct ligation and scission. Biological and Pharmaceutical Bulletin 23(2):240

3 Kim HS, Cho KH 1980 A study of antifungal activity with *Polygonum aviculare*. Korean Journal of Mycology 8(1):1

4 Gonzalez Begne M, Yslas N, Reyes E, Quiroz V, Santana J, Jimenez G 2001 Clinical effect of a Mexican 'sanguinaria' extract (*Polygonum aviculare* L.) on gingivitis. Journal of Ethnopharmacology 74(1):45–51

5 Tunon H, Olavsdotter C, Bohlin L 1995 Evaluation of anti-inflammatory activity of some Swedish medicinal plants. Inhibition of prostaglandin biosynthesis and PAF-induced exocytosis. Journal of Ethnopharmacology 48(2):61

6 Lee CG, Kim NJ, Hong ND, Kwon CH 1994 Anti-lipid peroxidation and liver protective effects of *Polygonum aviculare* L. Korean Journal of Pharmacognosy 25(1):59–69

7 Sharma ML, Chandokhe N, Ray Ghatak BJ et al 1978 Pharmacological screening of Indian medicinal plants. Indian Journal of Experimental Biology 16:228

8 Knight PR 1979 Suspected nitrite toxicity in horses associated with the ingestion of wireweed (*Polygonum aviculare*). Australian Veterinary Practitioner 9(3):175

Punica granatum L. (Punicaceae)

English: Pomegranate

Hindi: *Anar*

Sanskrit: *Dadim*

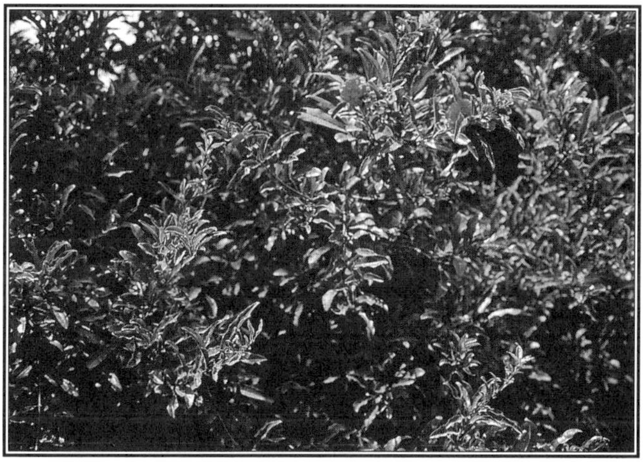

Pomegranate is mentioned in the ancient literature, including Ayurvedic texts and the Ebers papyrus from 1500BC. It has been depicted in many illustrations dating from the time of the Egyptians. 'Punica' is derived from the Latin *malum punicum* meaning 'apple of Carthage' or 'an apple with many seeds'. For this reason the pomegranate became a symbol of fertility and was consumed by childless women.

Habitat

It is thought to have originated from Iran and grows in the Mediterranean region and North Africa, Egypt and parts of Asia including India. It is cultivated for its fruit or as an ornamental tree.

Botanical description

A small, dense tree or shrub, 5–10 m high, with slender branches often tipped with a spine (Plate 50). The leaves are pale green, shiny, simple, ovate or lanceolate, with an acute or marginate apex. The flowers are orange-red in colour. The fruits are large, leathery skinned, globose berries, with a yellowish-red external surface or rind, containing numerous seeds and a juicy red pulp.

Parts used

Whole fruit, rind, leaf and root.

Traditional and modern use

Pomegranate is used as a vermifuge, anodyne, astringent, bactericide, refrigerant, stimulant, stomachic, styptic, hair dye and even as a poison. It can be used in asthma, bronchitis, cough, cardiac problems, dysentery, diarrhoea, colic, dyspepsia, fever, inflammation and bleeding disorders including metrorrhagia, menorrhagia, and piles and for leucorrhoea and dysmenorrhoea.

Ethnoveterinary usage

The bark, root and fruit are used mainly for intestinal worms in poultry and ruminants. The fruit and leaves are used to treat eye diseases in swine and ruminants and the leaves and stem for diarrhoea in swine.[1]

Major chemical constituents

Anthocyanins and flavonoids

The rind and seeds contain glycosides of malvidin and petunidin and pelargonidin 3,5-diglucoside was found to be the main pigment of the flowers. Leaf extracts have yielded apigenin-4′-O-β-glucopyranoside, luteolin-4′-O-β-glucopyranoside, luteolin-3′-O-β-glucopyranoside, luteolin-3′-O-β-xylopyranoside and isoquercetin.[2]

Alkaloids

Punicalin, punicalagin, granatin B, gallagyldilactone, casuarinine, pedunculagin and tellimagrandin I were isolated from the pericarp. The fruits also contain punicalagin, punicalin and granatin B. The bark contains iso-pelletierine, pseudo-pelletierine, methyl iso-pelletierine and pelletierine.[3]

Tannins

Gallic acid, granatin A, corilagin and ellagic acid have been isolated from the pericarp. The fruit contains an ellagitannin and ellagic acid.[4]

Triterpenes and phytosterols

Sitosterol, friedelin, ursolic acid, maslinic acid and asiatic acid are present.[4]

Medicinal and pharmacological activities

Anthelmintic activity: A clinical study of natural nematodiasis in calves below 6 months of age gave a successful treatment rate of 78.2%.[4] The ethanolic extract of the rind showed in vitro anthelmintic action against human *Ascaris lumbricoides*.[5] An aqueous extract was more potent than piperazine citrate against roundworm[6] and activity was seen in infections of pups with *Taenia hydatigena* and chickens naturally infected with helminths.[7,8] The pelletierine alkaloids paralyse tapeworms and laxatives may be used to expel them.

Antimicrobial activity: An extract of *P. granatum* rind possessed strong in vitro antimicrobial activity against *Staphylococcus aureus*, *Escherichia coli*, *Pseudomonas aeruginosa* and *Candida albicans*.[9] The hot water and other extracts of *P. granatum* fruit pericarp showed antibacterial action against organisms such as *Salmonella typhi* and *Vibrio cholerae*.[10–12]

Antiamoebic activity: Aqueous extracts of the rind and flowers of *P. granatum* showed encouraging in vitro activity against *Entamoeba histolytica*. Complete inhibition of the organism was observed when treated with rind extract at a dose of 1 g/kg body weight and flower extract at 2.5 g/kg.[13] The root extract showed a higher inhibition of *Entamoeba histolytica* than *E. invadens*. Alkaloids from the root, at a concentration of 1 mg/ml, had no amoebicidal effect but the tannins (at a concentration of 10 μg/ml for *E. histolytica* and 100 μg/ml for *E. invadens*) produced an inhibition of 100%.[14]

Antiviral activity: Tannins from the pericarp of *P. granatum* were effective against genital herpes virus (HSV-2). They inhibited replication of the virus, blocked its absorption into cells and had a strong virucidal effect.[15]

Antidiabetic activity: A rind extract administered at a dose of 2.5 g/kg body weight exhibited hypoglycaemic action in mildly diabetic albino rats.[16] Oral administration of an aqueous-ethanolic extract of the male flowers at a dose of 400 mg/kg produced a significant blood glucose lowering effect in normal, glucose-fed hyperglycaemic and alloxan-induced diabetic rats.[17]

Antiimplantation activity: Aqueous and methanolic extracts of *P. granatum* inhibited pregnancy in 70–90% of albino rats.[18]

Antimutagenic activity: Aqueous extracts consisting primarily of ascorbic and citric acids of pomegranate showed varying activity against the mutagenicity of direct-acting and S-9 dependent mutagens.[19]

Safety profile

The fruits, eaten as a food, are regarded as safe. The LD_{50} of a 50% ethanolic extract of the whole plant (excluding roots) was found to be 250 mg/kg, given IP to adult rats.[20] The tannin fraction has shown hepatotoxic effects.[4]

Dosage

Fruit powder: 4–8 g
Flower powder: 4–5 g
Root and bark powder: 1.5–3 g
Bark decoction: 100–200 ml

Ayurvedic properties

Rasa: *Madhur* (sweet), *kashaya* (astringent), *amla* (sour)

Guna: *Laghu* (light), *snigdha* (unctuous)

Veerya: *Anushna* (tepid)

Vipaka: *Madhur* (sweet)

Dosha: Pacifies *tridosha*

Further reading

Ross I 1999 Medicinal plants of the world, vol 1. Humana Press, Totowa, New Jersey

Sairam TV 1998 Home remedies, vol 1. Penguin India, New Delhi

References

1 International Institute of Rural Reconstruction 1994 Ethnoveterinary medicine in Asia. An information kit on traditional animal health care practices. Part I, general information. IIRR, Silang, Philippines

2 Nawwar MAM, Hussein SAM, Merfort I 1994 Leaf phenolics of *Punica granatum*. Phytochemistry 37(4):1175

3 Ross I 1999 Medicinal plants of the world, vol 1. Humana Press, Totowa, New Jersey

4 Pradhan KD, Thakur DK, Sudhan NA 1992 Therapeutic efficacy of *Punica granatum* and *Cucurbita maxima* against clinical cases of nematodiasis in calves. Indian Journal of Indigenous Medicines 9(1/2):53

5 Raj RK 1975 Screening of indigenous plants for anthelmintic action against human *Ascaris lumbricoides*: Part II. Indian Journal of Physiology and Pharmacology 19(1)

6 Hukkeri VI, Kalyani GA, Hatapaki BC, Manvi FV 1993 In vitro anthelmintic activity of aqueous extract of rind of *Punica granatum*. Fitoterapia 61(1):69

7 Pandey BB 1978 Developmental studies of some tapeworms with special reference to haematological, biochemical observations and therapeutics. Veterinary Research Bulletin 1(1):89

8 Matta SC, Ahluwalia SS 1979 Efficacy of two indigenous drugs – Helminta P and Sonex – against some common helminths of poultry. Indian Veterinary Journal 56(7):616

9 Navarro V, Villarreal ML, Rojas G, Lozoya X 1996 Antimicrobial evaluation of some plants used in Mexican traditional medicine for the treatment of infectious diseases. Journal of Ethnopharmacology 53(3):143

10 Perez C, Anesini C 1994 In vitro antibacterial activity of Argentine folk medicinal plants against

Salmonella typhi. Journal of Ethnopharmacology 44(1):41

11 Guevara JM, Chumpitaz J, Valencia E 1994 The *in vitro* action of plants on *Vibrio cholerae*. Revista Gastroenterologia de Peru 14(1):27

12 Prashanth D, Asha MK, Amit A 2001 Antibacterial activity of *Punica granatum*. Fitoterapia 72(2):171

13 Naqvi SAH, Siddiqui TO, Hamdard ME, Hameed A Antiamoebic activity of rind and flowers of *Punica granatum* Linn. Journal of Science of the Islam Republic of Iran 4(1):1

14 Segura JJ, Morales-Ramos LH, Verde-Star J, Guerra D 1990 Growth inhibition of *Entamoeba histolytica* and *E. invadens* produced by pomegranate roots. Archives of Investigative Medicine (Mex) 21(3):235

15 Zhang J, Zhan B, Yao X, Gao Y, Shong J 1995 Antiviral activity of tannin from the pericarp of *Punica granatum* L. against genital *Herpes* virus *in vitro*. Chung Kuo Chung Yao Tsa Chih 20(9):556

16 Zafar R, Singh J 1990 Antidiabetic activity of *Punica granatum* Linn. Science and Culture 56(7):303

17 Jafri MA, Aslam M, Javed K, Singh S 2000 Effect of *Punica granatum* Linn. (flowers) on blood glucose level in normal and alloxan-induced diabetic rats. Journal of Ethnopharmacology 70(3):309

18 Prakash AO, Saxena V, Shukla S et al 1985 Anti-implantation activity of some indigenous plants in rats. Acta Europaea Fertilitas 16(6):441

19 Saroj B, Grover IS 1992 Antimutagenic effect of pomegranate (*Punica granatum* var *anardana*) fruit extracts on direct acting and S-9 dependent mutagens in *Salmonella typhimurium*. Journal of Plant Science and Research 8(1–4):14

20 Dhawan BN, Patnaik GK, Rastogi RP, Singh KK, Tandon JS 1977 Screening of Indian plants for biological activity: PartVI. Indian Journal of Experimental Biology 15:208

Ricinus communis L. (Euphorbiaceae)

English: Castor bean, castor oil plant

Hindi: *Endi*

Sanskrit: *Eranda*

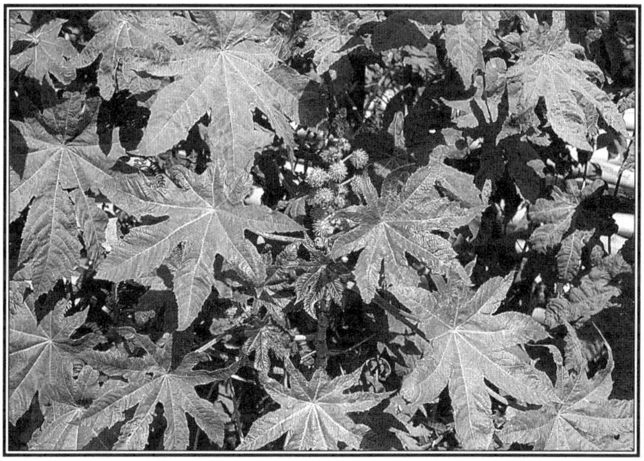

The plant has been cultivated for over 6000 years and was a source of oil for lamps and cosmetics in ancient Egypt. The toxicity of the plant has been well publicised as a result of a political assassination in London that was carried out using an umbrella tipped with the plant's main toxin, ricin. Greek physicians of the first century AD regarded the oil as suitable only for external application, a view which persisted until the 18th century, when it was listed in many pharmacopoeias as a purgative. The generic name is from the Latin *ricinus*, meaning 'tick', because the mottled seeds of the plant are similar in shape to these insects. The Egyptian Ebers papyrus of *c*. 1500 BC lists the plant.

Habitat

The castor oil plant is probably native to eastern Africa, but it is cultivated in hot climates around the world, especially India and other parts of southern Asia. It is also widely naturalised.

Botanical description

A tall, glaucus, branched shrub, reaching up to 4 m in height (Plate 51). The stem is erect and hollow, greyish-green when young and becoming brownish-red when older. The leaves are petioled, green and occasionally frosted blue or red, and arranged in a spiral. The blade is peltate, usually divided into palmate, ovate-oblong or lanceolate lobes up to 60 cm in diameter. The ribs are palmate and the margins irregularly serrate. The inflorescences are terminal panicles, 15–50 cm long, with the female flowers in the upper section of the inflorescence. The perianth is divided into five lobes and the style has three red, doubly split stigma branches. The male flowers bear numerous, heavily branched stamens with up to 1000 separate bursting anthers. The fruit capsule is soft and prickly or smooth and grooved, 1–2.5 cm in diameter. The capsule bursts open when ripe, showing the large, brightly speckled seeds. Castor oil is fatty oil obtained from the seeds.

Parts used

Oil, leaves, seeds and root.

Traditional and modern use

Castor oil is used internally in folk medicine for acute constipation, intestinal inflammation, for removal of worms, rheumatism and as a form of birth control. The extracts of the seeds are also used for this purpose. The oil is used externally for inflammatory skin disorders, furuncles, carbuncles, abscesses, inflammation of the middle ear and headaches. In Chinese medicine oil is used to treat sore throat, facial paralysis, dry stool, furuncles, ulcers and festering inflammation of the skin. The leaves are used as an emmenagogue, antiinflammatory and febrifuge and the root has been used to treat liver diseases and various forms of inflammation. Castor oil is used as a lubricant in hard candy production, as a component of protective coatings in tablets and as a flavour component.

Ethnoveterinary usage

It is used as feed after detoxification.

Major chemical constituents

Phytosterols

Brassicasterol, campesterol, β-sitosterol, β-amyrin, lupeol and derivatives are present in the aerial parts.[1,2]

Flavonoids, coumarins and phenolic acids

Epicatechin, corilagin, ellagic, gallic, chlorogenic and neo-chlorogenic acids, hyperoside, kaempferol, quercetin, isoquercetin and rutin, 6,7-dihydroxy-8-methoxy coumarin and 6,8-dihydroxy-3,4-dimethoxy coumarin[3–6] are all present in the aerial parts.

Alkaloid

Ricinine is present in the seed.[7]

Proteins

Ricin-A, B, C, D and E, and α-, β- and γ-ricin[8–10] have been found in the seed.

Fatty acids

Ricinoleic acid is the main component of the oil, together with linoleic, palmitic, oleic and stearic acids.[11,12]

Medicinal and pharmacological activities

Lipolytic activity: Ricin showed lipolytic activity on neutral lipids both in emulsions and in a membrane-like model. The activity was found to be proportional to ricin and substrate concentrations and to be pH and galactose dependent. These data support the idea that a lipolytic step may be involved in the process of cell poisoning by ricin.[13]

Antibacterial activity: Various types of extracts exhibit antibacterial activity, including an ethanolic extract of an in vitro callus culture of *Ricinus communis* which showed activity against six bacterial strains.[14] The methanol extract of the root was active against *Staphylococcus aureus* and produced weak activity against *Shigella boydii*.[15] The ethanol extract of the dried leaf was active against *Bacillus subtilis* as well as *Staphylococcus aureus* and an acetone extract against *Serratia marcescens, Shigella flexneri, Escherichia coli, Pseudomonas aeruginosa, Salmonella typhi* and others. The water extract was active on *E. coli, P. aeruginosa, S. typhi, Sh. flexneri, Sarcina lutea* and *Staph. aureus*.[16]

Anthelmintic activity: Potent anthelmintic

activity was observed from a tissue culture of the plant against *Mesocestoides corti* and *Taenis crassiceps*.[14]

Immunomodulating activity: Peptides from the seeds have been used in the preparation of immunomodulating drugs controlling the production of tumour necrosis factor (TNF).[17]

Central nervous system (CNS) stimulant: An extract of the pericarp of the castor bean showed typical CNS stimulant effects when administered to mice. The animals became exophthalmic, presented tremors and clonic seizures, and died a few minutes after receiving high doses of the extract. At lower doses, the extract improved memory consolidation and showed some neuroleptic-like properties, including a decrease in exploratory behaviour and catalepsy. Similar properties were also observed using ricinine, a neutral alkaloid isolated from the extract. The therapeutic index of ricinine is of the order of 200 and it may therefore be a promising cognition-enhancing drug.[18]

Laxative effects: Castor oil has been used since ancient times as a laxative, the active principle being ricinoleic acid. This hydroxylated, long-chain fatty acid has multiple effects on the intestinal mucosa, resulting in fluid secretion. Mucosal effects were considered to be due to enteritis or interference with cellular metabolism but more recent studies have revealed that castor oil increases mucosal permeability, associated with release of eicosanoids, platelet-activating factor, other autacoids and nitric oxide. In addition, ricinoleic acid disrupts normal intestinal motility. The combination of these effects on the mucosa and smooth muscle of the gut is thought to account for its laxative action.[19] Castor oil decreases fluid absorption and increases secretion in the small intestine and colon and decreases activity of the circular smooth muscle, which is believed to produce an increase in intestinal transit. The mechanism by which it produces the effect on the gut may involve inhibition of Na+ and K+-ATPase, activation of adenylate cyclase, stimulation of prostaglandins and nitric oxide biosynthesis. Castor oil changes the intestinal permeability and causes histological abnormalities, but these alterations are not essential for the laxative effect. Platelet-activating factor (PAF) is most likely one of the mediators of castor oil-induced damage, while nitric oxide has a protective role possibly by reducing PAF biosynthesis.[20] Other properties may be due to the presence of lectins which interfere with bacterial adhesion.[21]

Antiinflammatory activity: The petroleum ether extract exhibited significant antiinflammatory activity against induced rat paw arthritis and was safe up to a dose of 1 g/kg PO. A water extract of the root bark showed analgesic activity when administered to rats, using the tail flick response to radiant heat.[22,23]

Hepatoprotective activity: The alcoholic extract of the leaf showed activity against galactosamine- and paracetamol-induced hepatotoxicity in rats. N-demethylricinine, isolated from the butanol fraction, was found to be the active compound. It restored the altered levels of several enzymatic and non-enzymatic parameters in the serum and liver and in hepatocytes isolated from paracetamol-treated rats, the compound reversed the biochemical changes produced by galactosamine. It was also found to possess significant choleretic and anticholestatic effects.[24,25] An ethanol:water (1:1) extract of the root was active on hepatocytes against carbon tetrachloride-induced hepatotoxicity and PGE-induced paw oedema.[28]

Abortifacient and contraceptive activity: The oil showed abortifacient activity when taken orally by pregnant women.[26] Extracts of the seed have been tested in women and found to produce long-term contraception.[27]

Anticonvulsant activity: The ethanol extract of the fresh root, administered to mice at variable dosage levels, was active against phenmetrazole-induced convulsions.[28]

Diuretic effects: Ethanol extracts of the seed and an aqueous extract of the aerial parts produced diuresis when administered intragastrically to rats.[29,30]

Antifilarial and nematocidal activity: Methanol extract of the dried leaf was effective against *Onchocerca volvulus*.[31] Castor leaves alone, or in combination with different levels of N, P and K-enhanced plant growth fertilisers, reduced the nematode population.[32]

Antiamoebic activity: Ethanol:water (1:1) extracts of the root and stem in broth culture were active against *Entamoeba histolytica*.[33]

Antischistosomal activity: The seed oil, when administered intragastrically to mice at a dose of 0.3 ml/day for 7 days, showed activity against *Schistosoma mansonii*.[34]

Antioxidant effects: *Ricinus communis* extract produced an inhibition of aryl hydrocarbon hydroxylase (AHH) activity and H_2O_2 production by lindane-induced mouse hepatic microsomes, indicating the antioxidant activity of the plant.[35] The methanol extract of the seed also demonstrated strong antioxidant activity.[36]

Safety profile

The seeds are highly toxic and ornamental use increases the likelihood of poisoning, since they may have been drilled, rupturing the seed coat and exposing the contents. If swallowed without chewing, poisoning is less likely because the impermeable seed coat remains intact. The oil is used more commonly and as the protein ricin is denatured during processing, therapeutic dosages of castor oil are reasonably safe. The oil should be used only occasionally and is contraindicated in intestinal obstruction, acute inflammatory intestinal diseases, appendicitis, abdominal pain of unknown origin, during pregnancy and lactation. The drug should not be administered to children under 12 years of age.

Dosage

Oil: 14–28 ml

Leaf paste: 9–15 g

Root paste: 3–6 g

Ayurvedic properties

Rasa: *Madhur* (sweet), *katu* (pungent), *kashaya* (astringent)

Guna: *Guru* (heavy), *snigdha* (unctuous), *tishna* (sharp), *sukshma* (subtle)

Veerya: *Ushna* (hot)

Vipaka: *Madhur* (sweet)

Dosha: Pacifies *kapha* and *vata*

Further reading

Bown D 1995 Encyclopaedia of herbs and their uses. Dorling Kindersley, London

Chevallier A 1996 The encyclopedia of medicinal plants. Dorling Kindersley, London

Ministry of Health and Family Welfare 1989 Ayurvedic pharmacopoeia of India, vol III. Government of India, New Delhi

Ross I 2000 Medicinal plants of the world, vol 2. Humana Press, Totowa, New Jersey

References

1 Khafagy SM, Mahmoud YA, Abdel Salam NA, Mahmoud ZF 1983 Crystalline principles from the leaves of *Ricinus communis* L. Journal of Drug Research (Egypt) 14(1/2):189

2 Thompson MJ, Bowers WS 1968 Lupeol and 30-norlupan-3-beta-ol-20-one from the coating of the castor bean (*Ricinus communis* L.). Phytochemistry 7:845

3 Khafagy SM, Mahmoud ZF, Salam NAE 1979 Coumarins and flavonoids of *Ricinus communis* growing in Egypt. Planta Medica 37:191

4 Kang SS, Cordell GA, Soejarto DD, Fong HHS 1985 Alkaloids and flavonoids from *Ricinus communis*. Journal of Natural Products 48(1):155

5 Khafagy SM, Abdel Salam NA, Mohamed YA, Mahmoud ZF 1983 Determination of the flavonoidal content of *Ricinus communis* L. and *Euphorbia terraina* L. Journal of Drug Research (Egypt) 14(1/2):183

6 Kang SS, Cordell GA, Soejarto DD, Fong HHS 1985 Alkaloids and flavonoids from *Ricinus communis*. Journal of Natural Products 48(1):155

7 Pahuja DN, Gavnekar SV, Shah DH, Jathar VS, Kulkarni PR, Ganatra RD 1979 Goitrogenic principle from castor seeds. Biochemical Pharmacology 28:641

8 Lin JY, Liu SY 1986 Studies on the antitumor lectins isolated from the seeds of *Ricinus communis* (castor bean). Toxicon 24(8):757

9 Funatsu G, Funatsu M 1977 Separation of the two constituent polypeptide chains of ricin-D. Agricultural and Biological Chemistry 41:1217

10 Funatsu G, Mise T, Matsuda H, Funatsu M 1978 Isolation and characterization of two constituent polypeptide chains of Ricin E. Agricultural and Biological Chemistry 42:851

11 Borodulina AA, Bukhatchenko SL 1980 Chemical composition of castor seeds. Kleschevina 92

12 Donaldson RP 1977 Accumulation of free ricinoleic acid in germinating castor bean endosperm. Plant Physiology 59:1064

13 Lombard S, Helmy ME, Pieroni G 2001 Lipolytic activity of ricin from *Ricinus sanguineus* and *Ricinus communis* on neutral lipids. Biochemistry Journal 358(3):773

14 Khafagy SM, Ishrak K 1999 Screening cultures of some Sinai medicinal plants for their antibiotic activity. Egyptian Journal of Microbiology 34(4):613

15 Chhabra SC, Uiso FC 1991 Antibacterial activity of some Tanzanian plants used in traditional medicine. Fitoterapia 62(6):499

16 Verpoorte R, Dihal PP 1987 Medicinal plants of Surinam-IV. Antimicrobial activity of some medicinal plants. Journal of Ethnopharmacology 21(3):315

17 Brieva DA, Garcia VV, Guerrero A, Pivel RJ, Gimenez GG, Matji TJ 2000 Glycoconjugates obtained from *Candida utilis* cells and *Ricinus communis* seeds for immunomodulation. Industrial Farmaceutica Cantabria SA, Spain. PCT International Patent Application WO 2000050087

18 Ferraz AC, Angelucci M, Da Costa ML, Batista IR, De Oliveira BH, Da Cunha C 1999 Pharmacological evaluation of ricinine, a central nervous system stimulant isolated from *Ricinus communis*. Pharmacology, Biochemistry and Behaviour 63(3):367

19 Gaginella TS, Capasso F, Mascolo N, Perilli S 1998 Castor oil: new lessons from an ancient oil. Phytotherapy Research 12:S128

20 Izzo AA 1996 Castor oil: an update on mechanism of action. Phytotherapy Research 10:S109

21 Coutino-Rodriguez R, Hernandez-Cruz P 2001 Lectins in fruits having gastrointestinal activity: their participation in the hemagglutinating property of *Escherichia coli* 0157:H7. Archives of Medical Research 32(4):251

22 Yangf LL, Yen KY, Kiso Y, Kikino H 1987 Antihepatotoxic actions of Formosan plant drugs. Journal of Ethnopharmacology 19(1):103

23 Banerjee S, Bandhyopadhyay SK, Mukherjee PK, Mukherjee A, Sikdar S 1991 Further studies on the anti-inflammatory activities of *Ricinus communis* in albino rat. Indian Journal of Pharmacology 23(3):149

24 Visen PKS, Shukla B, Patnaik GK et al 1992 Hepatoprotective activity of *Ricinus communis* leaves. International Journal of Pharmacognosy 30(4):241

25 Tripathi SC, Patnaik GK, Shukla B, Visen PKS, Srimal RC, Dhawan BN 1991 Hepatoprotective activity of N-demethylricinine, the active principle of *Ricinus communis* L. Proceedings of the 24th Indian Pharmacological Society Conference, Ahmedabad, Gujrat, India, December 29–31

26 Mathieu A, Sichel MS 1931 Further observations on the use of castor oil, quinine, and pituitary extract in the induction of labor. An analysis based on the study of 320 consecutive cases from private practice. Surgery, Gynecology and Obstetrics 53:676

27 Okwuasaba FK, Das SC, Isichei CO et al 1997 Pharmacological studies on the antifertility effects of RICOM-1013-J from *Ricinus communis* var *minor* and preliminary clinical studies on women volunteers. Phytotherapy Research 11(8):547

28 Adesina SK 1982 Studies on some plants used as anticonvulsants in Amerindian and African traditional medicine. Fitoterapia 53:147

29 Abraham Z, Bhakuni SD, Garg HS, Goel AK, Mehrotra BN, Patnaik GK 1986 Screening of Indian plants for biological activity. Part-XII. Indian Journal of Experimental Biology 24:48

30 Tanira MOM, Ageel AM, Al-Said MS 1989 A study of some Saudi medicinal plants used as diuretics in traditional medicine. Fitoterapia 60(5):443

31 Titanii VPK, Ayafor JF, Mulufi JP, Mbacham WF 1987 *In vitro* killing of *Onchocerca volvulus* (Filaroidea) adults and microfilariaeby selected Cameroonian medicinal plant extracts. Fitoterapia 58(5):338

32 Zaki FA, Bhatti DS 1991 Effect of castor *Ricinus communis* leaves in combination with different fertilizer doses in *Meloidogyne javanica* infecting tomato. Indian Journal of Nematology 19(2):171

33 Dhar ML, Dhar MM, Dhawan BN, Mehrotra BN, Ray C 1968 Screening of Indian plants for biological activity: Part I. Indian Journal of Experimental Biology 6:232

34 Salafsky B, Fusco AC, Li LH, Mueller J, Ellenberger B 1989 *Schistosoma mansoni*: experimental chemoprophylaxis in mice using oral anti-penetration agents. Experimental Parasitology 69(3):263

35 Awney HA, Amara AA, El-Masry MH, Baghdadi HH 1997 Effect of 12 plant extracts on hepatic microsomal benzo(a)pyrene hydroxylation and hydrogen peroxide production in mice treated with lindane. Environmental and Nutritional Interactions 1(3–4):129

36 Kim SY, Kim JH, Kim SK, Oh MJ, Jung MY 1994 Antioxidant activities of selected oriental herb extracts. Journal of the American Oil and Chemical Society 71(6):633

Rubia cordifolia L. (Rubiaceae) (syn. *R. munjista* Roxb., *R. secunda* Moon, *R. mungisth* Desv.)

English: Indian madder, dyer's madder

Hindi: *Manjit, majeeth*

Sanskrit: *Manjista, chitravalli*

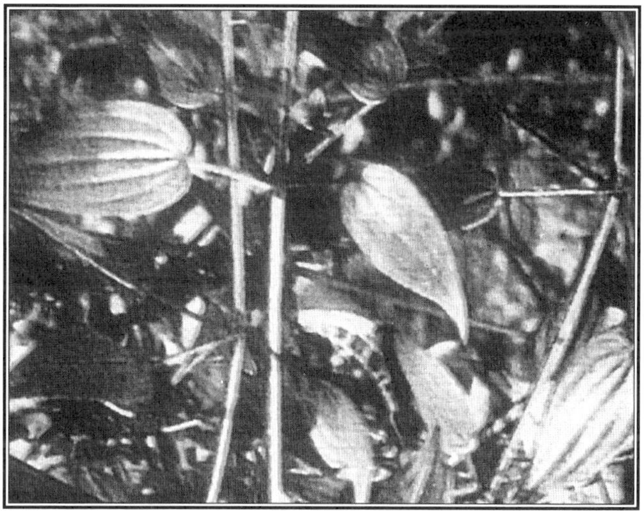

Madder has been used in many Asian countries as a dye, for imparting shades of red, scarlet, brown and mauve to cotton and woollen fabrics. In India and neighbouring countries, madder also has a long history in skin care and treatment and it has been used internally in disorders of the urinary tract.

Habitat

A perennial climber, growing throughout India, where it is common throughout the lower hills of the Indian Himalayas in the north and the Western Ghats in the South, and Japan, Indonesia and Sri Lanka in moist temperate and tropical forests, up to an altitude of 3500 m.

Botanical description

A prickly climber, usually growing over other bushes or trees (Plate 52). The rootstocks are perennial, the roots very long, twisted and cylindrical with a thin, red-coloured bark. The stem is quadrangular, leaves cordate to ovate-lanceolate, in whorls of 2–8 but more usually four. Flowers small, white or greenish in terminal panicles or cymes. Fruits globose, dark purplish or black.

Parts used

Dried roots and stem.

Traditional and modern use

The root is widely used as a tonic and also credited with astringent, deobstruent and antiinflammatory properties. A decoction is used in paralysis, jaundice, dropsy and infections or obstructions of the urinary passage and the plant is given in inflammatory conditions of the chest and in rheumatism. It has been used in tuberculosis and intestinal ulcer and is recommended by Ayurvedic physicians as a blood purifier for skin diseases and to improve the complexion.

Ethnoveterinary usage

Rubia cordifolia is used in the treatment of liver fluke, dysentery, maggots, wounds and intestinal worms in animals.[1]

Major chemical constituents

Quinones

These are mainly anthraquinone glycosides and include 1-hydroxy 2-methoxy anthraquinone, 1,4-dihydroxy-2-methyl-5-methoxy anthraquinone, 1,3-dimethoxy 2-carboxy anthraquinone and rubiadin.[2]

Iridoids

6-Methoxygeniposidic acid is found along with manjistin, garancin and alizarin.[3]

Triterpenoids

Oleananes such as rubiprasin A, B and C along with arborane triterpenoids including rubiarbonol A, B, C, D, E and F have been isolated.[4,5]

Medicinal and pharmacological activities

Antioxidant activity: The antioxidant properties have been well established. The herb significantly inhibited $FeSO_4$-induced lipid peroxidation and glutathione depletion.[6,7] The activity was ascribed to the quinone rubiadin.[8]

Antiinflammatory activity: *Rubia cordifolia* inhibited the lipoxygenase enzyme pathway[9] and the production of cumene hydroperoxides. The lipoxygenase pathway catalyses the production of various inflammatory mediators such as the leukotrienes which are involved in asthma, arthritis and other inflammatory disorders.

Antiplatelet activity: Platelet-activating factor (PAF) is a phospholipid involved in thrombosis, allergy and nervous disorders. *Rubia cordifolia* extract inhibited the aggregation of rabbit platelets in a dose-dependent manner, measured in a binding assay using ^{3}H-labelled PAF.[10]

Anticancer activity: The cyclic hexapeptides and quinones of Rubia exhibited a significant anticancer activity against various proliferating cells. The hexapeptides showed potent antitumour activity by binding to eukaryotic 80S ribosomes, resulting in inhibition of aminoacyl-tRNA binding and peptidyl-tRNA translocation, thus leading to the stoppage of protein synthesis.[11–14]

Hepatoprotective activity: Protection against different liver toxins has been established.[15,16] It has been found to be effective against acute and chronic hepatitis caused by the hepatitis B virus (HBV) by interfering with the secretion of hepatitis B surface antigen (HBsAg) in human hepatoma cells (Hep 3B). The quinone derivatives are thought to be the active components.[17]

Others: The plant has activity against allergies,[18] bacterial infection,[19] excessive bleeding[20] and diabetic ulcer.[21]

Safety profile

No adverse effects have been reported at recommended doses and the herb is usually categorised as GRAS (generally recognised as safe).

Dosage

Powdered root: 1–3 g

Decoction: 56–112 ml

Ayurvedic properties

Rasa: *Kashaya* (astringent), *tikta* (bitter), *madhur* (sweet)

Guna: *Guru* (heavy), *ruksha* (dry)

Veerya: *Ushna* (hot)

Vipaka: *Katu* (pungent)

Dosha: Pacifies *kapha* and *pitta*

Further reading

Bharatiya Vidya Bhavan's Swami Prakashananda Ayurveda Research Centre 1992 Selected medicinal plants of India. Chemexcil, Mumbai

Duke JA 1992 Handbook of phytochemical constituents of GRAS herbs and other economic plants. CRC Press, Boca Raton

Kapoor LD 1990 Handbook of Ayurvedic medicinal plants. CRC Press, Boca Raton

Ministry of Health and Family Welfare 2001 Ayurvedic pharmacopoeia of India, vol 3. Government of India, New Delhi

References

1 Jha MK 1992 The folk veterinary system of Bihar – a research survey. NDDB, Anand, Gujrat

2 Dosseh C, Tessier AM 1981 Nouvelles quinones des racines de *Rubia cordifolia* L. III. Planta Medica 43:360

3 Wu LJ, Wang SX, Hua HM et al 1991 6-Methoxygeniposidic acid, an iridoid glycoside from *Rubia cordifolia*. Phytochemistry 30(5):1710

4 Itokawa H, Qiao YF, Takeya K, Iitaka Y 1989 New triterpenoids from *Rubia cordifolia* var. *pratensis* (Rubiaceae). Chemical and Pharmaceutical Bulletin 37(6):1670

5 Itokawa H, Qiao YF, Takeya K, Iitaka Y 1990 Arborane type triterpenoids from *Rubia cordifolia* var. *pratensis*, and *R. oncotricha*. Chemical and Pharmaceutical Bulletin 38(5):1435

6 Tripathi YB, Sharma M 1999 The interaction of *Rubia cordifolia* with iron redox status: a mechanistic aspect in free radical reactions. Phytomedicine 6(1):51

7 Tripathi YB, Shukla S, Sharma M, Shukla VK 1995 Antioxidant property of *Rubia cordifolia* extract and its comparison with Vitamin E and parabenzoquinone. Phytotherapy Research 9(6):440

8 Tripathi YB, Sharma M, Manickam M 1997 Rubiadin, a new antioxidant from *Rubia cordifolia*. Indian Journal of Biochemistry and Biophysics 34(3):302

9 Tripathi YB, Sharma M, Shukla S, Tripathi P, Thyagaraju K, Reddanna P 1995 *Rubia cordifolia* inhibits potato-lipoxygenase. Indian Journal of Experimental Biology 33:109

10 Tripathi YB, Pandey S, Shukla SD 1993 Anti-platelet activating factor property of *Rubia cordifolia* Linn. Indian Journal of Experimental Biology 31:533

11 Tripathi YB, Shukla SD 1998 *Rubia cordifolia* extract inhibits cell proliferation in A- 431 cells. Phytotherapy Research 12(6):454

12 Morita H, Yamamiya T, Takeya K et al 1993 Conformational recognition of RA-XII by 80S ribosomes: a differential line broadening study in ^{1}H NMR spectroscopy. Chemical and Pharmaceutical Bulletin 41(4):781

13 Morita H, Yamamiya T, Takeya K, Itokawa H 1992 New anti-tumor bicyclic hexapeptides, RA-IX, XII, XIII and XIV from *Rubia cordifolia*. Chemical and Pharmaceutical Bulletin 40(5):1352

14 Itokawa H, Ibraheim ZZ, Ya-Fang Q, Takeya K 1993 Anthraquinones, naphthohydroquinones and naphthohydroquinone dimers from *Rubia cordifolia* and their cytotoxic activity. Chemical and Pharmaceutical Bulletin 41(10):1869

15 Gilani AH, Janbaz KH 1995 Effect of *Rubia cordifolia* extract on acetaminophen and CCl_4-induced hepatotoxicity. Phytotherapy Research 9(5):372

16 Pandey S, Sharma M, Chaturvedi P, Tripathi YB 1994 Protective effect of *Rubia cordifolia* on lipid peroxide formation in isolated rat liver homogenate. Indian Journal of Experimental Biology 32(3):180

17 Ho LK, Don MJ, Chen HC, Yeh SF, Chen JM 1996 Inhibition of hepatitis B surface antigen

secretion on human hepatoma cell components from *Rubia cordifolia*. Journal of Natural Products 59:330

18 Gupta PP, Srimal RC, Tandon JS 1993 Antiallergenic activity of some traditional Indian medicinal plants. International Journal of Pharmacognosy 31(1):15

19 Qiao YF, Wang SX, Wu LJ, Li X, Zhu TR 1990 Studies on antibacterial constituents from the roots of *Rubia cordifolia* L. Acta Pharmaceutica Sinica 25:834

20 Kosuge T, Yokota M, Yoshida M, Ochiali A 1981 Studies on antihemorrhagic principles in crude drugs for hemostatics. Part I. Hemostatic activities of the crude drugs for hemostatics. Yakugaku-Zasshi 101(6):501

21 Ojha JK, Dwivedi KN, Chaurasiya AK 1994 Effect of *Rubia cordifolia* plant extract on non-healing diabetic foot ulcer. Proceedings of a National Seminar on Traditional Medicinal Plants in Skin Care. November 25–26, CIMAP, Lucknow

Salmalia malabarica Schott. (Malvaceae) (syn. *Bombax malabaricum* DC.)

English: Silk cotton tree

Hindi: *Semul*

Sanskrit: *Rakta-pushpa*

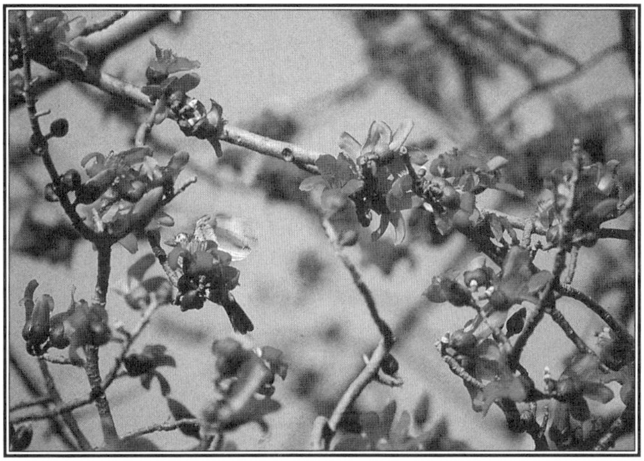

The long silky seed hairs ('cotton') have been used as a source of kapok.

Habitat

It is found all over India and other parts of tropical Asia up to an altitude of 1500 m.

Botanical description

A tall deciduous tree up to 40 m in height, with horizontally spread branches (Plate 53). The bark is ash coloured or silvery grey, leaves large and digitate with lanceolate leaflets. The flowers are bright crimson or yellow to orange, bunched at the tip of branches, the fruits oblong-ovoid capsules with many seeds.

Parts used

Seeds, leaves, fruit, roots, flowers and gum exuded by the stem bark (known as 'mocharus').

Traditional and modern use

The gum is used mainly in the treatment of acute dysentery, haemoptysis of pulmonary tuberculosis, influenza and menorrhagia. It acts as an astringent, diuretic, expectorant, tonic, emetic, stimulant, alterative, antiinflammatory, styptic and demulcent. It has also been used in bladder disorders, calculus, catarrh, cystitis, gonorrhoea and skin troubles such as sores and wounds. The seeds are used in chicken pox, gonorrhoea, chronic cystitis and catarrhal affections.

Ethnoveterinary usage

Applied to wounds and sores.

Major chemical constituents

Tannins

The gum contains 8.9% mineral matter and a large proportion of catechol tannin, along with tannic, gallic and catechutannic acids.

Aminoacids

The gum yielded DL-valine and indicamine.

Fatty acids

The seeds contain linoleic acid, myristic acid, oleic acid, palmitic acid and stearic acid.

Iridoids

Aucubin was isolated from the gum.[1]

Medicinal and pharmacological activities

Oxytocic activity: An aqueous extract of seeds exhibits oxytocic action on rat uteri and guinea pig and rabbit uterine strips.[2]

Cardiac activity: An aqueous extract of the seeds acts as a direct and indirect stimulant to the frog heart in situ.[3]

Safety profile

The maximum tolerated doses of the stem bark and flowers are 50 and 250 mg/kg body weight (IP in adult albino rats).[4]

Dosage

Root powder: 6–12 g

Infusion of flower: 12–20 g

Fruit powder: 1–3 g

Gum: 1–3 g

Ayurvedic properties

Rasa: *Madhur* (sweet), *shita* (cold)

Guna: *Guru* (heavy), *ruksha* (dry)

Veerya: *Shita* (cold)

Vipaka: *Madhur* (sweet)

Dosha: Pacifies *pitta* and *vata*

Further reading

Kapoor LD 1990 Handbook of Ayurvedic medicinal plants. CRC Press, Boca Raton

References

1 Council of Scientific and Industrial Research 1972 The wealth of India. A dictionary of Indian raw materials and industrial products. PID, CSIR, New Delhi

2 Misra MB, Mishra SS, Misra RK 1968 Pharmacology of *Bombax malabaricum* D.C. Indian Journal of Pharmacy 30:165

3 Misra MB, Mishra SS 1966 Studies in indigenous uterotonic drugs (a preliminary note). Indian Journal of Physiology and Pharmacology 10:59

4 Dhar ML, Dhar MM, Dhawan BN, Mehrotra BN, Ray C 1968 Screening of Indian plants for biological activity: Part I. Indian Journal of Experimental Biology 6:232

Semecarpus anacardium L. f. (Umbelliferae, Apiaceae)

English: Marking-nut tree

Hindi: *Bhilawa*

Sanskrit: *Bhallataka*

Semecarpus has long been used in Ayurveda. The tree produces sap which dries to a black resin and this has been mixed with lime or alum and used as a dye or marking ink (hence the name). Trade in the bhilawa nut is ancient and this fruit is considered to be the 'golden acorn' of Galen and Avicenna.

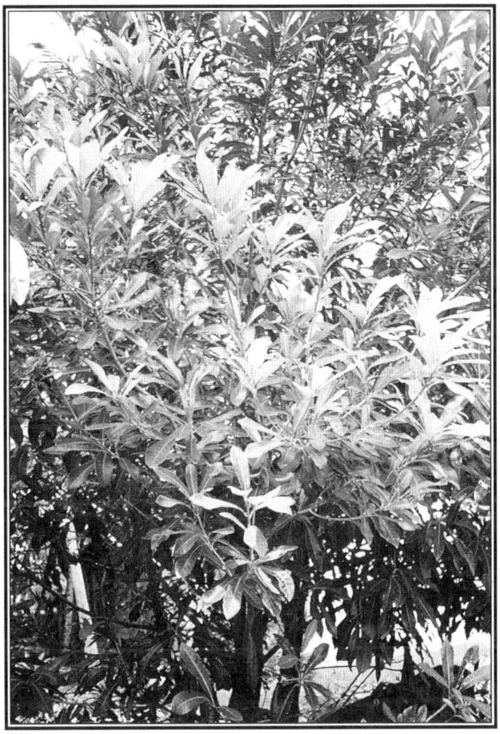

Habitat

The tree is distributed throughout the hotter parts of India and in the deciduous forests of the Malaysian archipelago and northern Australia.

Botanical description

A medium-sized deciduous tree, reaching up to a height of 12–15 m (Plate 54). The bark is dark brown and rough, the leaves large, ovate and simple up to 60 cm long and 30 cm wide. The flowers are small, dioecious, dull greenish-yellow; the fruits are drupes about 2.5 cm long, obliquely ovoid, smooth and shining, black when ripe, on a fleshy orange receptacle in terminal panicles.[4]

Parts used

Fruit, gum and oil.

Traditional and modern use

The resinous juice is applied to heel cracks. In traditional medicine, it is highly valued for the treatment of tumours and malignant growths. The fruit is reported to be caustic, astringent, alterative, antirheumatic, carminative, counterirritant, rubefacient and vesicant. It is also used in anorexia, cough, asthma, indigestion, enlargement of the spleen, alopecia, ulcers, corns, leprosy, leucoderma, rheumatism, piles and for various nervous diseases.

Ethnoveterinary usage

The crushed seeds are applied to cuts, bruises and scratches to stop bleeding. The oil is applied to cracks and fissures in the tails and hooves of animals. Bhilawa fruits are cooked in mustard oil and then applied to sores to kill maggots.[1]

Major chemical constituents

Phenolic compounds

The seed contains anacardoside and other derivatives of anacardic acids, including 'bhilawanol', which is a mixture of 1,2-dihydroxy-3-(pentadecenyl-8′) benzene and 1,2-dihydroxy-3-(pentadecadienyl-8′,11′) -benzene.[2,3]

Flavonoids

Semecarpetin, semecarpuflavone, nallaflavone, galluflavanone, jeediflavanone, tetrahydroarmentoflavone and tetrahydrobustaflavone have all been isolated.[4–9]

Fixed oil

The oil from the nut contains palmitic, stearic, oleic, linoleic and arachidic acids.[10]

Medicinal and pharmacological activities

Antineoplastic activity: *Semecarpus anacardium* nut milk extract, 'Serankottai nei', was tested against experimental mammary carcinoma in rats and treatment resulted in a significant reduction in the activity of aspartate and alanine aminotransferases and a sharp increase in lactate dehydrogenase, γ-glutamyl transpeptidase, alkaline phosphatase and 5′-nucleotidase. The activity of these enzymes returned almost to normal control levels.[11] 1,2-Dihydroxy-3-pentadeca-7′,10′-dienylbenzene and 1,2-dihydroxy-3-pentadec-8′-enylbenzene, isolated from *S. anacardium*, showed antitumour activity in vitro in the Eagles 9KB nasopharyngeal carcinoma cell culture system, but not against P388 leukaemia in mice at doses of 80 mg/kg.[12] When the effect of the nut milk extract on the host detoxification system in aflatoxin B1-induced hepatocellular carcinoma was studied in male albino rats, oral administration (200 mg/kg body weight per day for 14 days) was found to be effective in inducing phase I and phase II biotransformation enzymes. It was suggested that the anticarcinogenic effect is mediated through the induction of these enzymes.[13] The antioxidant defence system plays a critical role in carcinogenesis and is severely altered in aflatoxin B1-induced hepatocellular carcinoma. Non-enzymic antioxidant levels were analysed in rats to assess the antitumour activity and administration of nut extract produced a marked increase in antioxidant levels and a dramatic elevation in cytochrome P450 content. The observed anticancer properties may be due to its ability to induce the in vivo antioxidant system.[14] A marked increase in lipid peroxide levels and a concomitant decrease in enzymic antioxidant levels was observed in carcinoma-induced rats, whilst drug treatment reversed conditions to near normal levels.[15] The extract also stabilised lysosomal membranes in experimental hepatocellular carcinoma, which may have benefits in treating such disorders where the membranes are abnormally fragile.[16]

Immunomodulatory activity: The immunomodulatory activity of the nut milk extract was studied in rats bearing aflatoxin B1-induced hepatocellular carcinoma. Immunomodulatory activity was assessed measuring serum Ig levels. Reduced IgG, and elevated IgA and IgM, in the hepatocellular carcinoma condition were returned to near normal levels in rats treated with 200 mg/kg extract.[17]

Antiarthritic activity: The nut extract was shown to have antiarthritic activity[18] and its effect was studied on carbohydrate metabolic changes associated with adjuvant arthritis in albino rats. The drug was administered at a dose level of 150 mg/kg for 14 days to arthritic animals, 14 days after the day of adjuvant induction. The decreased activity of glycolytic enzymes, and the concomitant increase in that of gluconeogenic enzymes, which had developed during the arthritic condition, reverted back to near normal in drug-treated animals. Carbohydrate metabolism, which had been affected during arthritic condition, became normalised with the drug.[19] The nut milk extract also decreased lipid peroxide levels in both plasma and tissues and brought the altered antioxidant defence components back to near normal levels.[20] It also stabilised lysosomes obtained from liver and kidney of adjuvant-induced arthritic animals.[21]

Antimicrobial activity: Anacardic acid possessed antibacterial and antifungal activity against *Staphylococcus aureus*, *Escherichia coli* and *Candida albicans*.[22] It also had antiamoebic effects in rats inoculated with *Entamoeba histolytica*, reducing the degree of infection compared to untreated animals.[23]

Anthelmintic activity: Anacardic acid was lethal to earthworms.[24]

Hypocholesterolaemic activity: Administration of *S. anacardium* nut shell extract to cholesterol-fed rabbits resulted in a significant reduction in serum cholesterol levels and LDL cholesterol. It also prevented accumulation of cholesterol and triglycerides in the liver, heart muscle and aorta.[25]

Safety profile

The drug should be used with care, preferably under the direction of a qualified practitioner, since the anacardic acids are allergenic. The maximum tolerated dose of a 50% alcoholic extract of the fruit when given intraperitoneally to mice was found to be 250 mg/kg body weight.[26]

Dosage

Oil: 1–2 drops

Fruit: 0.5–1.5 g

Ayurvedic properties

Guna: *Laghu* (light), *snigdha* (unctuous), *tikshna* (sharp)

Rasa: *Madhur* (sweet), *kasaya* (astringent)

Veerya: *Ushna* (hot)

Vipaka: *Madhur* (sweet)

Dosha: Pacifies *vata*

Further reading

Bharatiya Vidya Bhavan's Swami Prakashananda Ayurveda Research Centre 1992 Selected medicinal plants of India. Chemexcil, Mumbai

Kapoor LD 1990 Handbook of Ayurvedic medicinal plants. CRC Press, Boca Raton

Ministry of Health and Family Welfare 1999 Ayurvedic pharmacopoeia of India, vol 2. Government of India, New Delhi

Nadkarni AK 1976 Indian materia medica. Popular Prakashan PVT Ltd, Bombay

Sairam TV 1999 Home remedies, vol II. Penguin India, New Delhi

Sivarajan VV, Balachandran 1994 Ayurvedic drugs and their plant sources. Oxford and IBH Publishing, New Delhi

References

1 Jha MK 1992 The folk veterinary system of Bihar – a research survey. NDDB, Anand, Gujrat

2 Gil RR, Lin L-Z, Cordell GA et al 1995 Anacardoside from the seeds of *Semecarpus anacardium*. Phytochemistry 39(2):405

3 Govindachari TR, Joshi BS, Kamat VN, Viswanathan N 1971 Phenolic constituents of *Semecarpus anacardium*. Indian Journal of Chemistry 9(10):1044

4 Murthy SSN 1988 Naturally occurring biflavonoid derivatives. Part 10. Semecarpetin, a biflavanone from *Semecarpus anacardium*. Phytochemistry 27(9):3020

5 Murthy SSN 1986 Semecarpuflavone – a new biflavone from *Semecarpus anacardium* Linn. Proceedings of the Indian Academy of Sciences, Chemical Sciences 97(1):63

6 Murthy SSN 1987 Naturally occurring biflavonoid derivatives IX. New dimeric flavanone from *Semecarpus anacardium* Linn. Proceedings of the Indian National Academy of Science 53(5):632

7 Murthy SSN 1985 Naturally occurring biflavonoid derivatives: Part VII – galluflavanone, a new biflavonoid from *Semecarpus anacardium* Linn. Indian Journal of Chemistry 24B(4):398

8 Murthy SSN 1985 Naturally occurring biflavonoid derivatives: Part VI – jeediflavanone, a biflavonoid from *Semecarpus anacardium*. Phytochemistry 24(5):1065

9 Ishratullah K, Ansari WH, Rahman W, Okigawa M, Kawano N 1977 Biflavonoids from *Semecarpus anacardium* Linn. (Anacardiaceae). Indian Journal of Chemistry 15B(7):615

10 Agarwala KL, Absar N 1993 Chemical investigations on the kernel oil of marking nut (*Semecarpus anacardium* Linn). Journal of the Bangladesh Chemistry Society 6(1):83

11 Sujatha V, Sachdanandam P 2000 Effect of *Semecarpus anacardium* Linn. nut extract on experimental mammary carcinoma in Sprague-Dawley rats with reference to tumor marker enzymes. Pharmacy and Pharmacology Communications 6(8):375

12 Hembree JA, Chang CJ, McLaughlin JL, Peck G, Cassady JM 1978 The anticancer activity of *Semecarpus anacardium* I. 9KB active pentadecylcatechols. Lloydia 41(5):491

13 Premalatha B, Sachdanandam P 2000 Potency of *Semecarpus anacardium* Linn. nut milk extract against aflatoxin B1-induced hepatocarcinogenesis: reflection on microsomal biotransformation enzymes. Pharmacological Research 42(2):161

14 Premalatha B, Sachdanandam P 1999 *Semecarpus anacardium* L. nut extract administration induces the *in vivo* antioxidant defense system in aflatoxin B1-mediated hepatocellular carcinoma. Journal of Ethnopharmacology 66(2):131

15 Premalatha B, Muthulakshmi V, Vijayalakshmi T, Sachdanandam P 1997 *Semecarpus anacardium* nut extract induced changes in enzymic antioxidants studied in aflatoxin B1 caused hepatocellular carcinoma bearing Wistar rats. International Journal of Pharmacognosy 35(3):161

16 Premalatha B, Sachdanandam P 2000 Stabilization of lysosomal membranes and cell membrane glycoprotein profile by *Semecarpus anacardium* Linn. nut milk extract in experimental hepatocellular carcinoma. Phytotherapy Research 14 (5):352

17 Premalatha B, Sachdanandam P 1998 Immunomodulatory activity of *Semecarpus anacardium* Linn. nut milk extract in aflatoxin B1-induced hepatocellular carcinoma in rats. Pharm. Pharmacol. Commun 4(10):507

18 Vijayalakshmi T, Muthulakshmi V, Sachdanandam P 1996 Effect of the milk extract of *Semecarpus anacardium* nut on adjuvant arthritis – a dose-dependent study in Wistar albino rats. General Pharmacology 27(7):1223

19 Vijayalakshmi T, Narayanan P, Jayaprakash, Sachdanandam P 1998 Changes in glucose metabolizing enzymes in adjuvant arthritis and its treatment with a Siddha drug: Serankottai nei. Indian Journal of Pharmacology 30(2):89

20 Vijayalakshmi T, Muthulakshmi V, Sachdanandam P 1997 Salubrious effect of *Semecarpus anacardium* against lipid peroxidative changes in adjuvant arthritis studied in rats.

Molecular and Cellular Biochemistry 175(1&2):65

21 Vijayalakshmi T, Muthulakshmi V, Sachdanandam P 1997 Effect of milk extract of *Semecarpus anacardium* nuts on glycohydrolases and lysosomal stability in adjuvant arthritis in rats. Journal of Ethnopharmacology 58(1):1

22 Chattopadhyaya MK, Khare RL 1970 Antimicrobial activity of anacardic acid and its metallic complexes. Indian Journal of Pharmacology 32(2):46

23 Dutta D, Khare RL 1971 Antiamebic activity of anacardic acid and its sodium salt. Indian Journal of Pharmacology 33(6):112

24 Chattopadhyaya MK, Khare RL 1969 Isolation of anacardic acid from *Semecarpus anacardium* and study of its anthelmintic activity. Indian Journal of Pharmacology 31(4):104

25 Sharma A, Mathur R, Dixit VP 1995 Hypocholesterolemic activity of nut shell extract of *Semecarpus anacardium* (Bhilawa) in cholesterol fed rabbits. Indian Journal of Experimental Biology 33(6):444

26 Dhar ML, Dhar MM, Dhawan BN, Mehrotra BN, Ray C 1968 Screening of Indian medicinal plants for biological activity: Part I. Indian Journal of Experimental Biology 6:232

Solanum nigrum L. (Solanaceae) (syn. *Solanum americanum* Mill.)

English: Garden or black nightshade

Hindi: *Makoi*

Sanskrit: *Kakamachi*

Black nightshade is considered to be a *rasayana* and is used as a food. The fruits resemble small tomatoes and are made into a spicy sauce in southern India and the young leaves are steamed and eaten like spinach.

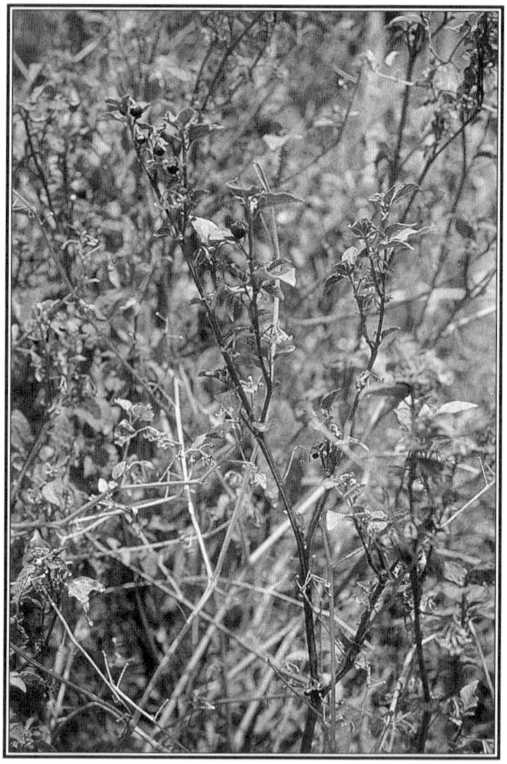

Habitat

The plant is found throughout the drier areas of India and other parts of Asia and Africa on wasteland and roadsides and in gardens.

Botanical description

A glabrous, dense, erect annual herb reaching up to 45 cm (Plate 55). The leaves are ovate-lanceolate, with an acute apex, thin and may be lobed or toothed. The flowers are typically solanaceous, small and violet, borne in lateral, umbellate cymes. The fruits are smooth, shiny berries, green when unripe and becoming red to purplish-black on ripening, containing numerous small, yellow discoid seeds.

Parts used

Whole plant, fruit.

Traditional and modern use

A decoction is taken internally for hepatitis and other disorders of the liver and for inflammation of the spleen, digestive system and uterus. It is used in the form of a gargle as an antiseptic and antiinflammatory for conditions of the pharynx and larynx. The leaves are made into a poultice and applied to burns, wounds and skin affections.

Ethnoveterinary usage

The whole plant, leaves, berries and young shoots are used to treat blindness, fever, skin diseases, diarrhoea and stoppage of urine.[1]

Major chemical constituents

Steroidal glycoalkaloids

Solanine, solamargine, solasonine, α- and β-solanigrine, which are based on the aglycone solasodine, are found in the unripe fruit.[2]

Steroidal saponins

Diosgenin, trigogenin and nigrumnins I and II have also been isolated.[3,4]

Medicinal and pharmacological activities

Hepatoprotective activity: Administration of the fruit powder in water reduced elevated levels of SGPT and SGOT in carbon tetrachloride-treated rats. This protective action was also observed with paracetamol-induced hepatotoxicity and depleted hepatic glutathione was restored. The petroleum ether and 50% ethanolic extracts brought about a moderate reversal of hepatotoxin-induced changes in serum and liver enzyme concentrations, but the effect of the extracts was less marked than that of the crude fruit powder. Diarrhoea, lethargy and pyloric obstruction were noted as side effects and higher doses of the alcoholic and petroleum ether extracts caused mortality.[5] The aerial parts of *S. nigrum* increased the in vitro demethylation of aflatoxin B_1 and aflatoxin G_1 and the concentration of some drug-metabolising enzymes.[6]

Antiulcerogenic activity: Powdered aerial parts of *S. nigrum* and the methanolic extract were shown to decrease the ulcer index significantly in aspirin-induced gastric ulcers. The activity may be due to the inhibition of acid and pepsin secretion.[7]

Antiinflammatory activity: The plant showed activity in both acute and chronic models of inflammation.[8]

Molluscicidal activity: All parts of the plant exhibit molluscicidal activity against *Biomphalaria alexandrina* and other snail species, which are intermediate hosts of the parasites causing human schistosomiasis or fascioliasis.[9]

Safety profile

The presence of the steroidal alkaloids, especially in the unripe fruit, can lead to toxicity and solanine is known to be teratogenic. Symptoms include gastrointestinal problems which can then lead to cyanosis, shock and even paralysis. The maximum tolerated dose of the 50% ethanolic extract of whole plant was found to be 1000 mg/kg in adult albino rats.[10]

Dosage

Infusion: 15–25 ml

Fruit powder: 1–2 g

Decoction: 28–56 ml

Ayurvedic properties

Rasa: *Tikta* (bitter)

Guna: *Laghu* (light), *snigdha* (unctuous)

Veerya: *Ushna* (hot)

Vipaka: *Katu* (pungent)

Dosha: Pacifies *kapha*

Further reading

Kapoor LD 1990 Handbook of Ayurvedic medicinal plants. CRC Press, Boca Raton

Nadkarni AK 1976 Indian materia medica. Popular Prakashan PVT Ltd, Bombay

Pandey GS (ed) 1998 Bhavprakash Nighantu. Chaukhambha Bharati Academy, Gokul Bhawan, Varanasi

References

1 Jha MK 1992 Folk veterinary medicine of Bihar – a research project. NDDB, Anand, Gujrat

2 Varshney IP, Duke NK 1970 Chemical investigation of *Solanum nigrum*. Journal of the Indian Chemical Society 47(7):717

3 Varshney IP, Sharma SC 1965 Saponins of *Solanum nigrum* berries. Phytochemistry 4(6):967

4 Ikeda T, Tsumagari H, Nohara T 2000 Steroidal oligoglycosides from *Solanum nigrum*. Chemical and Pharmaceutical Bulletin 48(7):1062

5 Nadeem M, Dandiya PC, Pasha KV et al 1997 Hepatoprotective activity of *Solanum nigrum*. Fitoterapia 68(3):245

6 Domngang F 1985 Detoxification des aflatoxins par o-demethylase chez les rats consommant les legue feuilles. *S. nigrum* et *Amaranthus hybridus*. Annales Faculte des Sciences. Biologie et Biochemie 81

7 Akhtar MS, Munir M 1989 Evaluation of the gastric antiulcerogenic effects of *Solanum nigrum*, *Brassica oleracea* and *Ocimum basilicum* in rats. Journal of Ethnopharmacology 27(1–2):163

8 Reddy KRK, Tehara SS, Goud PV, Alikhan MM 1990 Comparison of the anti-inflammatory activity of *Eclipta alba* (Bhangra) and *Solanum nigrum* (Mako Khushk) in rats. Journal of Research and Education in Indian Medicine 9(4):43

9 Kloos H, McCullough FS 1988 Plants with recognized molluscicidal activity. In: Mott K (ed) Plant molluscicides. John Wiley and Sons, Chichester

10 Dhar ML, Dhar MM, Dhawan BN, Mehrotra BN, Ray C 1968 Screening of Indian plants for biological activities. Part I. Indian Journal of Experimental Biology 6:232

Solanum xanthocarpum Schrad (Solanaceae) (syn. *Solanum surattense* Burm.f.)

English: Yellow-berried nightshade

Hindi: *Choti katheri, kateli*

Sanskrit: *Kantkari, laghu kantkari*

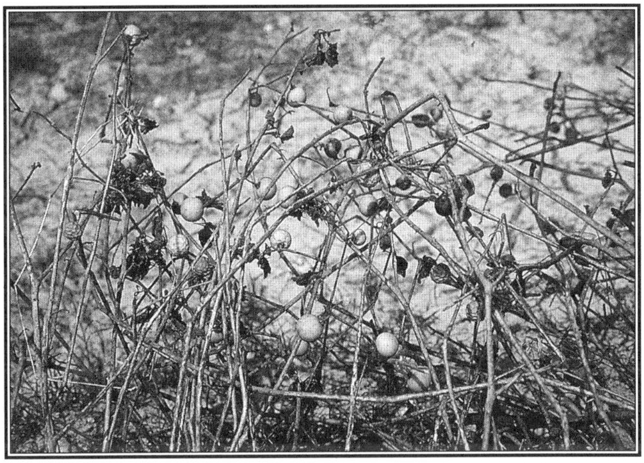

Kateli has long been known for its medicinal value and is reputed to facilitate conception.

Habitat

A common perennial herb growing in dry plains and low hills throughout India, Sri Lanka and other parts of Asia.

Botanical description

A spiny, diffuse, much-branched, perennial herb reaching up to 3 m (Plate 56). The leaves are bright green, ovate and lobed, with purplish hairs on both surfaces and yellow sharp spines. Flowers purple, in lateral cymes. Berries globose, up to 1.5 cm in diameter, green with whitish patches when young, yellow and glabrous with green or white veins.

Parts used

Whole plant.

Traditional and modern use

The root is used in fever, cough, asthma and inflammation and as a diuretic and antiemetic. It is often used in combination with other drugs; for example, a decoction prepared with chiretta and ginger is prescribed as a febrifuge, with black pepper to treat rheumatism and with *Tinospora cordifolia* as a tonic in fever and cough. The powdered fruit with honey relieves chronic cough in children. Juice extracted from the fruits is used to treat sore throats and the vapours of the burning seeds have been used to relieve toothache.

Ethnoveterinary usage

The leaves mixed with neem oil are given to cattle for chronic cough.

Major chemical constituents

Alkaloids

Solasodine is the main constituent isolated from the berries of the plant, together with solanine in the unripe fruits and solacarpidin.[1–3]

Sterols

Carpesterol, β-sitosterol and norcarpesterol.[4–7]

Polyphenols

Chlorogenic, isochlorogenic, neochlorogenic and caffeic acids and the flavonoids quercitrin and apigenin glycosides are present in the fruits.[1,2]

Medicinal and pharmacological activities

Antifertility activity: This has been demonstrated in various species. The crude alcoholic extract of the seeds showed spermicidal activity on rat epididymal spermatozoa which was 100% effective after 60 days of treatment at a dose of 100 mg/kg.[8] Androgen deprivation was also observed after administration of the extract and a decrease in spermatids was found in rhesus monkeys. It reduced the number of immature and mature Leydig cells, along with a decrease in testicular protein, sialic acid and glycogen contents.[9,10] Administration of solasodine lead to testicular lesions, causing a reduction of spermatozoa in the epididymis. The total protein, sialic acid and glycogen contents of the testis and epididymis were also reduced significantly and the testicular cholesterol content was elevated.[11,12]

Antiasthmatic and respiratory activity: A whole plant extract of *S. xanthocarpum* produced a significant improvement in certain parameters of pulmonary functions in asthmatic subjects.[13] Clinically the herb has also proved to be useful in treating individuals with cough and bronchial asthma.[14]

Insecticidal activity: Antifeedant and insecticidal effects have been noted.[15,16]

Other activities: Hepatoprotective, hypertensive, antihistaminic and antimicrobial activities have been described.[17–21]

Safety profile

No health hazards or side effects have been observed with the proper administration of usual doses, but in view of the toxicity of the alkaloids, excessive use should be avoided. The plant should not be taken by pregnant women.

Dosage

Decoction: 56–112 ml

Powder: 1–2 g

Ayurvedic properties

Rasa: *Katu* (pungent), *tikta* (bitter)

Guna: *Laghu* (light), *tikshna* (sharp), *rukshna* (dry)

Veerya: *Ushna* (hot)

Vipaka: *Katu* (pungent)

Dosha: Pacifies *kapha* and *vata*

Further reading

Chopra RN, Chopra IC, Handa KL, Kapoor LD 1994 Indigenous drugs of India. Academic Publishers, Calcutta

Chopra RN, Chopra IC, Verma BS 1969 Supplement to glossary of Indian medicinal plants. PID, CSIR, New Delhi

Kapoor LD 1990 Handbook of Ayurvedic medicinal plants. CRC Press, Boca Raton

Ministry of Health and Family Welfare 1989 Ayurvedic pharmacopoeia of India, vol 2. Government of India, New Delhi

Nadkarni AK 1976 Indian materia medica. Popular Prakashan PVT Ltd, Bombay

Rastogi RP, Mehrotra BN 1998 Compendium of Indian medicinal plants, vol 5. PID, New Delhi

References

1 Gupta SS, Verma SC, Singh C, Khandelwal P, Gupta NK 1967 Chemical and pharmacological studies on *Solanum xanthocarpum* (Kantakari). Indian Journal of Medical Research 55(7):723

2 Tupkari SV, Saoji AN, Deshmukh VK 1972 Phytochemical study of *Solanum xanthocarpum*. Planta Medica 22(2):184

3 Menon VP, Jolly IC 1996 Microbial conversion and formation studies on the secondary metabolites of *Solanum xanthocarpum* (Schrad and Wendle). Indian Journal of Pharmaceutical Science 58(1):37

4 Kusano G, Beisler JA, Sato Y 1973 Steroidal constituents of *Solanum xanthocarpum*. Phytochemistry 12(2):397

5 Beisler JA, Sato Y 1971 The chemistry of carpesterol, a novel sterol from *Solanum xanthocarpum*. Journal of Organic Chemistry 36(25):39–46

6 Sate Y, Latham HG 1953 The isolation of diosgenin from *Solanum xanthocarpum*. Journal of the American Chemistry Society 60–67

7 Heble MR, Narayanaswami S, Chadha MS 1967 Diosgenin and beta-sitosterol: isolation from *Solanum xanthocarpum* tissue cultures. Science 161(846):1145

8 Mali PC, Chaturvedi M 1996 Antispermatogenic activity of *Solanum xanthocarpum* (50 percent EtOH-extract) in rats. Journal of Phytologic Research 9(1):13

9 Dixit VP, Gupta RS, Gupta S 1989 Antifertility plant products: testicular cell population dynamics following solasodine (C27H43O2N) administration in rhesus monkey (*Macaca mulatta*). Andrologia 21(6):542

10 Rao MV 1988 Effects of alcoholic extract of *Solanum xanthocarpum* seeds in adult male rats. Indian Journal of Experimental Biology 26(2):95

11 Kanwar U, Batla A 1988 Effect of solasodine on morphology, motility and glycolytic enzymes of buffalo bull spermatozoa. Indian Journal of Experimental Biology 26(12):941

12 Dixit VP, Gupta RS 1982 Antispermatogenic/antiandrogenic properties of solasodine (C27H43O2N) obtained from *Solanum xanthocarpum* berries on the male genital tract of dog. A histophysiological approach. International Journal of Andrology 5(3):295

13 Govindan S, Viswanathan S, Vijayasekaran V, Alagappan R 1999 A pilot study on the clinical efficacy of *Solanum xanthocarpum* and *Solanum trilobatum* in bronchial asthma. Journal of Ethnopharmacology 66(2):205

14 Bector NP, Puri AS 1971 *Solanum xanthocarpum* (Kantakari) in chronic bronchitis, bronchial asthma and non-specific unproductive cough (an experimental and clinical co-relation). Journal of the Association of Physicians of India 19(10):741

15 Verma GS, Pandey UK 1987 Insect antifeedant property of some indigenous plant products. Zeitschrift Fuer Angewandte Zoologie 74(1):113

16 Verma RR, Srivastava PM 1988 Effect of plant origin insecticides against the fourth instar caterpillars of *Spilosoma rhodophila* Walk. Journal of Entomological Research 12(2):179

17 Ansari MS, Gupta RC, Prasad S 1971 Pharmacological studies on *Solanum surattense* Burm. (Kantakari). Journal of Research in Indian Medicine 6(2):143

18 Khan FZ, Saeed MA 1993 Biological studies of indigenous medicinal plants: III. Phytochemical and antimicrobial studies on the non-alkaloidal constituents of some solanaceous fruits. Journal of the Faculty of Pharmacy, Gazi University 10(2):105

19 Chatterjee S 1999 Bronchodilatory and anti-allergic effect of PulmoFlex-A proprietary herbal formulation. Indian Journal of Physiology and Pharmacology 43(4):486

20 Gupta SS, Gupta NK 1967 Effect of *Solanum xanthocarpum* and *Clerodendron serratum* on histamine release from tissues. Indian Journal of Medical Science 21(12):795

21 Kapur V, Pillai KK 1994 Hepatoprotective activity of "Jigrine" on liver damage caused by alcohol-carbon tetrachloride and paracetamol in rats. Indian Journal of Pharmacology 26(1):35

Swertia chirata Buch-Ham (Gentianaceae)

English: Chiretta
Hindi: *Kirat, chirayita*
Sanskrit: *Kirata-tikta, bhunimba*

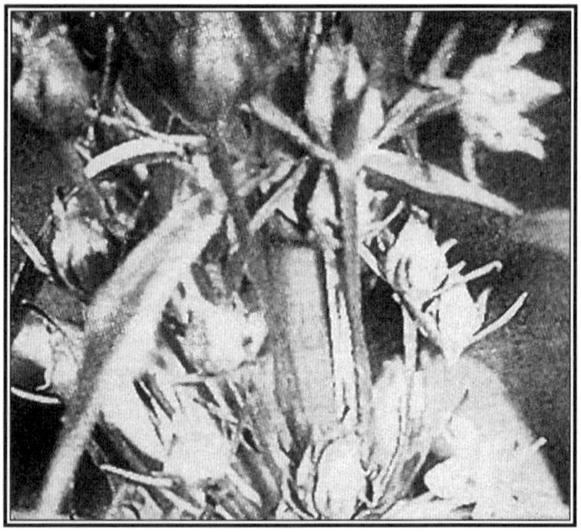

Chirata is an ancient Ayurvedic drug, sometimes known as 'Nepali Neem' because it is common in the forests of Nepal. The name is sometimes used for other gentian-like plants sold in Indian bazaars. It was introduced into Europe in 1839 and is still widely used there.

Habitat

It is found in the temperate Himalayas from Kashmir to Bhutan up to a height of 1200–1500 m.

Botanical description

An erect or prostrate herb, much branched, with lanceolate leaves (Plate 57). The flowers are greenish-yellow with a purplish tinge, in large panicles. The fruits are egg-shaped capsules containing a large number of seeds.

Parts used

Whole plant.

Traditional and modern use

The drug is used to stimulate the appetite and relieve acidity, biliousness and nausea and is highly valued as a tonic in debility and convalescence and for liver disorders. It is also an alterative, laxative, vermifuge and sedative and has been used in asthma, cough, bronchitis and malaria.

Ethnoveterinary usage

The whole plant is used to treat fever in swine and ruminants and to stimulate the appetite in swine.[1]

Major chemical constituents

Iridoids

Amarogenin, amarogentin, amaroswerin, chiratin, chiratanin, chiratogenin, decussatin, enicoflavine, gentianine, gentiocrucin, gentiopicrin, isobellidifolin, swertiamarin, sweroside, swerchirin, swertianin and swertinin.[2–4]

Xanthones

1,3,7,8-Tetrahydroxyxanthone, 1,8-dihydroxy-3,7-dimethoxyxanthone, 1-hydroxy-3,5,8-trimethoxyxanthone and mangiferin.[2]

Triterpenes

The plant yields β-amyrin and lupeol.[2]

Medicinal and pharmacological activities

Hepatoprotective activity: The methanol extract has been evaluated for antihepatotoxic activity using paracetamol and galactosamine models. It was found to be active at a dose of 100 mg/kg and on fractionating the activity was found to reside mainly in the chloroform fraction which was most active at a dose level of 25 mg/kg. These two hepatotoxins induce hepatotoxicity by different mechanisms, suggesting a broad and non-specific protection of the liver for *Swertia chirata*.[5] The liver-protecting activity was also ascertained in carbon tetrachloride-induced liver damage in albino rats over 16 days. Simultaneous administration of *S. chirata* at a dose of 50 mg/kg produced an improvement in both biochemical and histopathological parameters and again the chloroform extract was the most active.[6,7]

Leishmanicidal activity: Amarogentin, isolated from the methanolic extract of *S. chirata*, exhibited potent inhibitory action against type I DNA topoisomerase from *Leishmania donovani*. The mechanism of action is thought to be by preventing binary complex formation.[2]

The activity of amarogentin, in the form of liposomes and niosomes, was also examined in a hamster model of experimental leishmaniasis. The liposomal, and particularly the niosomal, forms were found to be more effective than the free amarogentin. Blood pathology, histological staining of tissues and specific enzyme levels related to normal liver function revealed no toxicity.[8]

Antiulcer activity: An ethanolic extract of *S. chirata* markedly reduced the intensity of gastric ulcers induced by indomethacin and necrotising agents in rats. Ethanol-induced gastric wall mucus depletion and restoration of the non-protein sulfhydryl (NP-SH) content in the glandular stomachs was also achieved by pretreating the rats with the extract. It also showed anticholinergic activity by inhibiting acetylcholine-induced contraction of guinea pig ileum.[9]

CNS depressant activity: An ethanolic extract (excluding mangiferin) of *S. chirata* reversed mangiferin-induced CNS stimulation effects in albino mice and rats. Swertiamarin and mangiferin, both present in the same plant, antagonised each other in vivo.[4]

Hypoglycaemic activity: Significant blood sugar lowering effects of the 95% ethanolic extract were observed in fed, fasted and glucose-loaded albino rats. The hypoglycaemic activity of tolbutamide was increased in healthy albino rats by giving *S. chirata* extract orally.[10]

Antiinflammatory activity: The ethanolic extract of *S. chirata* exhibited significant antiinflammatory activity when tested in acute, subacute and chronic models of inflammation.[11]

Antimicrobial activity: Antimicrobial activity has been demonstrated by *S. chirata*.[12]

Safety profile

The drug normally produced no problems at recommended doses. The maximum tolerated dose of the 50% ethanolic extract of the whole plant was 1000 mg/kg IP in adult rats.[13]

Dosage

Whole plant: 0.5–2 g

Liquid extract or tincture 1:1: 2–5 ml

Ayurvedic properties

Rasa: *Tikta* (bitter)

Guna: *Laghu* (light), *ruksha* (dry)

Veerya: *Ushna* (hot)

Vipaka: *Katu* (pungent)

Dosha: Balances *tridosha*

Further reading

Ministry of Health and Family Welfare 1989 Ayurvedic pharmacopoeia of India, vol 1. Government of India, New Delhi

Sairam TV 2000 Home remedies, vol III. Penguin India, New Delhi

References

1 International Institute of Rural Reconstruction 1994 Ethnoveterinary medicine in Asia. An information kit on traditional animal health care practices. Part I, general information. IIRR, Silang, Philippines

2 Ray S, Majumdar HK, Chakravarty AK, Mukhopadhyay S, Gill RR, Cordell GA 1996 Amarogentin, a naturally occurring secoiridoid glycoside and a newly recognised inhibitor of topoisomerase I from *Leishmania donovani*. Journal of Natural Products 59(1):27

3 Prasad S, Nayar KC, Bhattacharya IC 1960 Pharmacognostical studies on chirata and its substitutes and adulterants, Part I; *Swertia chirata* Ham. Indian Journal of Scientific and Industrial Research 19c:119

4 Bhattacharya SK, Reddy PK, Ghosal S, Singh AK, Sharma PV 1976 Chemical constituents of Gentianaceae XIX: CNS-depressant effects of swertiamarin. Journal of Pharmaceutical Science 65(10):1547

5 Karan M, Vasisht K, Handa SS 1999 Antihepatotoxic activity of *Swertia chirata* on paracetamol and galactosamine induced hepatotoxicity in rats. Phytotherapy Research 13(2):95

6 Mukherjee S, Sur A, Maiti BR 1997 Hepatoprotective effect of *S. chirata* on rat. Indian Journal of Experimental Biology 35(4):384

7 Karan M, Vasisht K, Handa SS 1999 Antihepatotoxic activity of *Swertia chirata* on carbon tetrachloride induced hepatotoxicity in rats. Phytotherapy Research 13(1):24

8 Medda S, Mukhopadhyay S, Basu MK 1999 Evaluation of the in-vivo activity and toxicity of amarogentin, an antileishmanial agent, in both liposomal and niosomal forms. Journal of Antimicrobial Chemotherapy 44(6):791

9 Rafatullah S, Tariq M, Mossa JS, al-Yahya MA, al-Said MS, Ageel AM 1993 Protective effect of *S. chirata* against indomethacin and other ulcerogenic agent-induced gastric ulcers. Drugs under Experimental and Clinical Research 19(2):69

10 Mukherjee B, Mukherjee SK 1987 Blood sugar lowering activity of *Swertia chirata* (Buch-Ham) extract. International Journal of Crude Drug Research 25(2):97

11 Das PC, Mandal S, Chatterjee A, Islam CN, Patra BB, Dutta MK 1995 Anti-inflammatory activity of *Mangifera indica* L. and *Swertia chirata* Buch-Ham. Proceedings of an International Conference on Progress in Medicinal Aromatic Plant Research, Calcutta, India, 30 December 1994–1 January 1995

12 Leslie ER,Chungath JI 1988 Studies on *Swertia chirata*. Indian Drugs 25(4):143

13 Dhar ML, Dhar MM, Dhawan BN, Mehrotra BN, Ray C 1968 Screening of Indian plants for biological activity: Part I. Indian Journal of Experimental Biology 6:232

Symplocos racemosa Roxb. (Symplocaceae)

English: Symplocos

Hindi: *Lodh*

Sanskrit: *Lodhra*

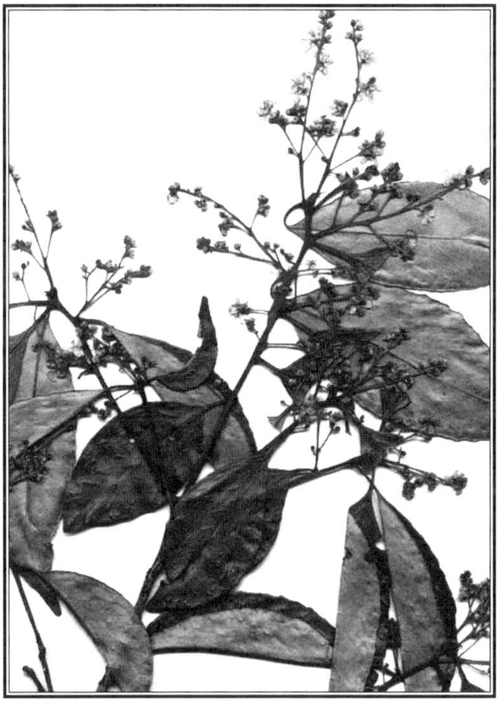

The name *Lodhra* comes from its reputed remedy as a cure for ophthalmia. It is an ingredient of many *rasayanas*. A yellow dye is extracted from the leaves which, in combination with other plants, is used for dyeing silk.

Habitat

It is found commonly in the plains and hills of northern India and other Asian countries, up to a height of 1400 m.

Botanical description

It is a small evergreen tree reaching a height of 6–8.5 m (Plate 58). The leaves are leathery, orbicular and dark green in colour. The flowers are white or cream, in axillary, simple or compound racemes. The fruit is a purplish black drupe containing 1–3 seeds.

Parts used

Bark, root.

Traditional and modern use

The bark is astringent and therefore used to treat diarrhoea and dysentery and also liver complaints and dropsy. It is used as a tonic, antioxytocic, amoebicide and in conjunctivitis and ophthalmia. A decoction of bark is used to treat bleeding gums, menorrhagia and other uterine disorders.

Ethnoveterinary usage

Bark is used in stomach troubles, sores and eye diseases.

Major chemical constituents

Triterpenes

Betulin, betulinic acid, acetyloleanolic acid, oleanolic acid and others have been isolated.[1]

Flavonoids and anthocyanins

3-Monoglucofuranoside of 7-O-methyl leucopelargonidin glucosides, symposide.[2]

Tannins

Ellagic acid has also been reported from the bark.[3]

Alkaloids

The bark has yielded loturine, loturidine and colloturine.[3]

Medicinal and pharmacological activities

Antimicrobial activity: A crystalline fraction obtained from the ethanolic extract of the bark of *S. racemosa* exhibited the inhibition of the growth of Staphylococci, *Escherichia coli* and other dysenteric organisms.[4]

Antifibrinolytic activity: Symposide showed antifibrinolytic activity.[2]

Antispasmodic activity: The alcoholic extract reduced the frequency and intensity of contractions in vitro in both pregnant and non-pregnant uteri. Antagonisation of acetylcholine-induced contractions and prolongation of the quiescent period were also observed.[2]

Safety profile

The LD_{50} of the 50% ethanolic extract of the whole plant (excluding roots) was found to be 750 mg/kg in adult male albino rats.[5]

Dosage

Powder: 1–3 g

Decoction: 56–112 ml

Ayurvedic properties

Rasa: *Kashaya* (astringent)

Guna: *Laghu* (light), *ruksha* (dry)

Veerya: *Ushna* (hot)

Vipaka: *Katu* (pungent)

Dosha: Balances *kapha* and *pitta*

Further reading

Kapoor LD 1990 Handbook of Ayurvedic medicinal plants. CRC Press, Boca Raton

References

1 Ali M, Bhutani KK, Srivastava TN 1990 Triterpenoids from *Symplocos racemosa* bark. Phytochemistry 29(11):3601

2 Dhaon R, Jain GK, Sarin JPS, Khanna NM 1989 Symposide – a new anti-fibrinolytic glycoside from *Symplocos racemosa* Roxb. Indian Journal of Chemistry 28B(11):982

3 De Silva LB, De Silva ULL, Mahendran M 1979 The chemical constituents of *Symplocos racemosa*. Journal of the National Science Council for Sri Lanka 7(1):1

4 Sirsi M 1964 Pharmacology of *Symplocos racemosa* Roxb. Indian Journal of Pharmacy 26(5):129

5 Dhawan BN, Patnaik GK, Rastogi RP, Singh KK, Tandon JS 1977 Screening of Indian plants for biological activities. Indian Journal of Experimental Biology 15:208

Syzygium cumini L. Skeels (Myrtaceae) (syn. *Eugenia jambolana* Lam., *E. cumini* Druce, *Myrtus cuminii* L.)

English: Java plum, jambul, Indian blackberry

Hindi: *Jamun*

Sanskrit: *Jambu*

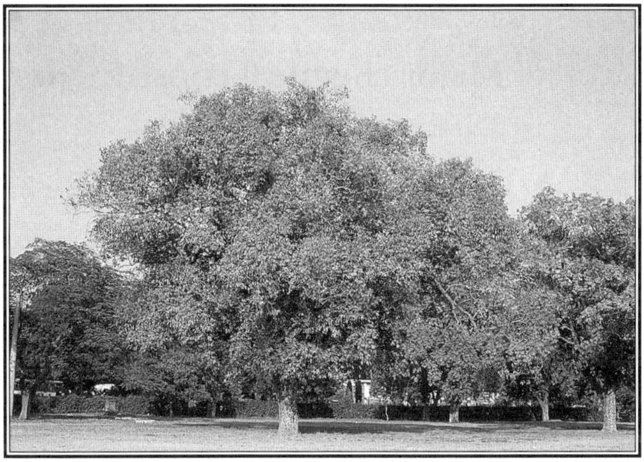

Jamun has a rich history of use in India and it is known to have been cultivated in England by the herbalist Miller during the 1700s. Almost all the parts of the tree are used in folk medicine. The plant is associated with the Lord Krishna and the elephant-headed Ganesh in Hindu mythology and it is sacred to Buddhists also. The ripe fruits are eaten throughout India and a wine is made from the fruits in Goa.

Habitat

It is indigenous to India and Indonesia, but is naturalised in Thailand, the Philippines and Madagascar and cultivated widely throughout Africa, the Caribbean and tropical America. It grows commonly along streams and in damp places and in evergreen forests. The tree is planted as an ornamental in gardens and at roadsides.

Botanical description

A moderate-sized evergreen tree with a dense canopy attaining a height of up to 50 m (Plate 59). The bark is brown to greyish, smooth and exfoliating in hard woody scales. The leaves are lanceolate, oblong or broadly ovate and elliptic, smooth, shiny and coriaceous with visible glands dotted over the surface and an aromatic scent. The flowers are greenish white and the fruits black and plum-like, with a juicy pink pulp, containing a single oblong seed.

Parts used

Bark, fruit, seed and leaves.

Traditional and modern use

Almost all the parts of the tree are used in folk medicine. The fruits are used as an astringent and to treat diarrhoea and are eaten to relieve the symptoms of diabetes. The bark and seeds are also popular antidiabetic agents in many parts of India. Extracts of the bark are given as an astringent for chronic diarrhoea in adults and in children are mixed with goats' milk. The bark is also used for mouth freshening and to treat disorders of the gums and teeth.

Ethnoveterinary usage

The bark is used to staunch bleeding in ruminants.[1]

Major chemical constituents

Triterpenes and sterols

Betulinic acid, friedelin, friedelanol, β-sitosterol, daucosterol and a β-sitosterol glucoside have been found in the bark.[2–4]

Flavonoids

Quercetin has been isolated from the pulp and kaempferol, myricetin, quercetin and astragalin from the bark.[2]

Fatty acids

Lauric acid, myristic acid, palmitic acid, stearic acid, oleic acid, linoleic acid, malvalic acid, sterculic acid and vernolic acid in the seeds.[5,6]

Phenolics

Gallic, ellagic, caffeic and ferulic acids and derivatives, guaicol, resorcinol dimethyl ether and corilaginin are found in the seeds and gallic acid in the bark.[2,18]

Monoterpenoids

β-Pinene, γ-terpinene, terpinolene, borbeneol, β-phellanderene, α-terpineol and eugenol are present in the seeds.[2]

Carbohydrates

Glucose, galactose, mannose and fructose are the principal sugars in the ripe fruit pulp and 3,6,hexahydroxy diphenoyl glucose, 4,6,hexahydroxy-diphenoyl glucose, 1-galloyl glucose, 3-galloyl-glucose and 6-galloyl-glucose occur in the seeds.[2]

Minerals and vitamins

Calcium, iron, potassium, vitamin A, thiamin, riboflavin, nicotinic acid and ascorbic acid are present in the fruit pulp.[2]

Medicinal and pharmacological activities

Hypoglycaemic activity: A number of scientific studies in animals have substantiated the role of *jambul* in the management of diabetes.[7] Antihyperglycaemic effects of the aqueous and alcoholic extracts and the lyophilised seed powder were evaluated in diabetic animals. Although all produced a reduction in blood glucose levels, the lyophilised powder was the most potent.[8] In combination with *Momordia charantia* (qv), the effect of different doses of aqueous and alcoholic extracts was studied on metabolic parameters including body weight, serum glucose, insulin and triglyceride levels. Fructose feeding for 15 days increased serum glucose and insulin levels markedly, and triglyceride levels marginally, but treatment with 400 mg per day of the aqueous extracts prevented hyperglycaemia and hyperinsulinaemia.[9] The seeds have also been found to be active in rats at doses of 170–510 mg/animal/day for 15 days.[10] In rabbits, a hot water extract equivalent to 50 g of dried fruit pulp, when administered by gastric intubation, was active in reducing blood glucose levels.[11]

In human volunteers, the ethanol (95%) and hot water extracts of dried seeds at variable doses levels were found to have potent hypoglycaemic activity when given both orally and intravenously.[12] The seeds themselves, at a dose of 4–24 g/person, were found to have a hypoglycaemic effect in a trial of 28 diabetic patients.[13] A decoction of the aerial parts, also in human adults, was reported to have hypoglycaemic effects; however, this was associated with oliguria and pain, which resolved within one week.[2]

Diuretic activity: The leaf extract when administered by gastric intubation at a concentration of 2.5% was found to have a diuretic effect in experimental rats. Animals were divided into two categories and the first category was given water while the second category was given 2.5% extract. The results showed urinary excretion of 59% for controls and 68% for the extract group. No changes in sodium and potassium levels were found.[2]

Antiinflammatory activity: The antiinflammatory activity of orally administered hexane, dichloromethane, ethylacetate and methanol extracts was investigated in rats. All inhibited both the acute and chronic phases of experimental inflammation in a dose-dependent manner. The ethyl acetate and methanol extracts were the most active and were comparable to phenylbutazone; however, in a chronic model, the methanolic extract was found to be more potent.[14] The chloroform extract of the seeds, when administered intraperitoneally to rats at a dose of 100 mg/kg, was found to have potent effects in reducing carageenan-induced paw oedema.[15] In a separate study, the hydroalcoholic extract of the aerial parts, given at a dose of 0.375 mg/kg orally, had no effect.[16]

Antidiarrhoeal activity: The ethanol extract was evaluated for activity against different experimental models of diarrhoea in rats. It produced significant inhibition of castor oil-induced diarrhoea and PGE_2-induced entero-pooling and a significant reduction in gastrointestinal motility in charcoal meal tests.[17]

Antiplaque activity: Aqueous, methanolic and methanol-water (1:1) extracts of the bark were able to suppress plaque formation in vitro. All were active against *Streptococcus mutans* at 260, 120 and 380 μg per ml respectively.[18]

Safety profile

The use of the leaves, fruit, seeds and bark is prevalent throughout the Indian subcontinent and no harmful effects have been reported.

Dosage

Seed: 2 g per day

Bark: 3–6 g per day

Leaves: Extract equivalent to 15–20 g dried leaves per day

Ayurvedic properties

Rasa: *Kashaya* (astringent), *madhur* (sweet)

Guna: *Laghu* (light), *ruksha* (dry)

Veerya: *Shita* (cold)

Vipaka: *Madhur* (sweet)

Dosha: Pacifies *kapha* and *pitta*

Further reading

Husain A, Virmani OP, Popli SP et al 1992 Dictionary of Indian medicinal plants. CIMAP, Lucknow

Kapoor LD 2001 Handbook of Ayurvedic medicinal plants. CRC Press, Boca Raton

Ross I 1999 Medicinal plants of the world, vol 1. Humana Press, Totowa, New Jersey

Sairam TV 1999 Home remedies, vol 2. Penguin India, New Delhi

References

1 International Institute of Rural Reconstruction 1994 Ethnoveterinary medicine in Asia: an information kit on traditional animal health care practices, part 1. IIRR, Silang, Philippines

2 Ross I 1999 Medicinal plants of the world. Humana Press, Totowa, New Jersey

3 Sengupta P, Das PB 1965 Terpenoids and related compounds IV. Triterpenoids from the stem-bark of *Eugenia jambolana*. Journal of the Indian Chemical Society 42(4):255

4 Bhargava KK, Dayal RS, Seshadri TR 1974 Chemical components of *Eugenia jambolana* stem bark. Current Science 43(20):645

5 Mahmood JD, Mirajkar AM, Hosamani KM, Mulla GMM 1988 Epoxy and cyclopropenoid fatty acids in *Syzygium cumini* seed oil. Journal of Science in Food and Agriculture 43(1):91

6 Bhatia IS, Bajaj KL 1975 Thin layer chromatography of the phenolic constituents of *Eugenia jambolana* seeds. Journal of the Institute of Chemistry 47(4):127

7 Grover JK, Vats V, Rathi SS, Dawar R 2001 Traditional Indian anti-diabetic plants attenuate progression of renal damage in streptozotocin induced diabetic mice. Journal of Ethnopharmacology 76(3):233

8 Grover JK, Vats V, Rathi SS 2000 Anti-hyperglycemic effect of *Eugenia jambolana* and *Tinospora cordifolia* in experimental diabetes and their effects on key metabolic enzymes involved in carbohydrate metabolism. Journal of Ethnopharmacology 73(3):461

9 Vikrant V, Grover JK, Tandon N, Rathi SS, Gupta N 2001 Treatment with extracts of *Momordica charantia* and *Eugenia jambolana* prevents hyperglycemia and hyperinsulinemia in fructose fed rats. Journal of Ethnopharmacology 76(2):139

10 Bansal RN, Ahmead, Kidwai JR 1981 Effect of oral administration of *Eugenia jambolana* seeds and chloropropamide on blood glucose level and pancreatic cathepsin B in rats. Indian Journal of Biochemistry and Biophysics 18:377

11 Jain SR, Sharma SN 1967 Hypoglycemic drugs of Indian indigenous origin. Planta Medica 15(4):439

12 Bhatt HV, Gupta OP, Gupta PS 1983 Hypoglycemia induced by *Syzygium cumini* Linn. seeds in diabetes mellitus. Asian Medical Journal 26(7):489

13 Khan AH, Burney A 1962 A preliminary study of the hypoglycemic properties of indigenous plants. Pakistan Journal of Medical Research 2:100

14 Slowing K, Carretero E, Villar A 1994 Anti-inflammatory activity of leaf extracts of *Eugenia jambos* in rats. Journal of Ethnopharmacology 43(1):9

15 Mahapatra PK, Chakraborthy D, Chaudhuri AKN 1986 Anti-inflammatory and antipyretic activities of *Syzygium cumini*. Planta Medica 6:540

16 Dhawan BN, Patnaik GK, Rastogi RP, Singh KK, Tandon JS 1977 Screening of Indian plants for biological activity. Indian Journal of Experimental Biology 15:208

17 Mukherjee PK, Saha K, Murugesan T, Mandal SC, Pal M, Saha BP 1989 Screening for anti-diarrheal profile of some plant extract of specific region of West Bengal, India. Journal of Ethnopharmacology 60(1):85

18 Namba TM, Tsunezuka NK, Dissanayake UP, Saito K, Hattori M 1985 Studies on dental caries prevention by traditional medicines (Part VII). Screening of Ayurvedic medicines for antiplaque action. Shoyakugaku Zasshi 39(2):146

Tamarindus indica L. (Leguminosae)

English: Tamarind

Hindi: *Imli*

Sanskrit: *Tintiri, amlika*

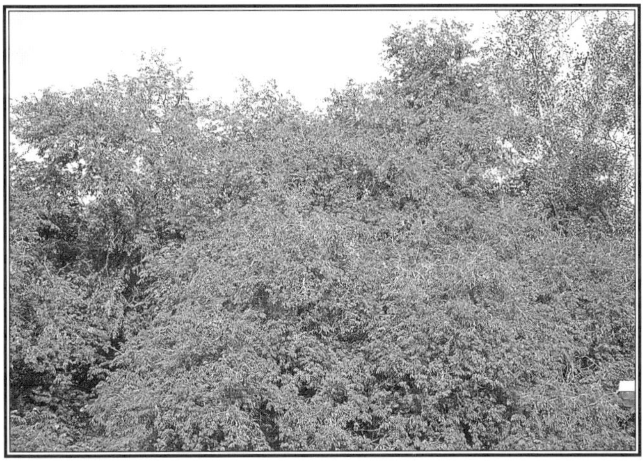

Tamarind has been cultivated in India for centuries and was taken by the Spanish conquistadores to the West Indies and Mexico in the 17th century. It is now widely grown in the tropics as an ornamental to provide shade as well as for the fruit. The name tamarindus comes from the Arabic *Tamar-Hindi*, meaning 'date of India', and refers to the date-like pulp inside the pods. According to folklore the sailors used to eat tamarind fruit as a complement to their otherwise starchy diet, in the belief that eating it would prevent scurvy.

Habitat

The tree is native to tropical Africa and is now naturalised and widely cultivated throughout India as well as other tropical countries, including the Caribbean, south east Asia and China, where it is found on roadsides and in gardens.

Botanical description

A large tree up to 30 m high, with spreading branches (Plate 60). The bark is brownish-grey, peeling off in flakes. Leaves are even-pinnate, consisting of 10–18 pairs of small leaflets, rather close together. Petioles and rachis up to 12 cm long; leaflets oblong, up to 30 by 10 mm; opposite, pink or reddish when young, membranous, glabrous, with an obtuse apex and unequal base. The inflorescence is a terminal raceme, yellowish orange to pale green, consisting of a narrow turbinate calyx tube with four imbricate segments. There are three unequal petals, the upper cordate about 1 cm long, and two lateral petals, narrowed towards the base. There are three fertile stamens, the base conical; ovary linear, about 7 mm long, pubescent, on a stalk adnate to the calyx tube. Pods are oblong, slightly curved, up to 15 cm long and reddish brown. The seed is glossy, dark brown, embedded in a thick, sticky aromatic and acid brown pulp.

Parts used

Fruits, fruit pulp, seeds, leaves, flowers and bark.

Traditional and modern use

The fruits are eaten fresh and made into a refreshing drink and the pulp is an important ingredient of Indian cuisine. Fresh and dried fruits are used as a sour flavouring agent in curries, fish, chutneys and sauces. They are sweet and sour, cooling, carminative, digestive, laxative and antiscorbutic. The bark, leaves and seeds are astringent. The tender leaves and flowers are cooling and antibilious and are used in constipation, colic, cough, dyspepsia, fever, flatulence and urinary infection. The fruit pulp or the leaves may be used in the form of a poultice for external application to inflammatory swellings to relieve pain, and a poultice of the flowers is useful in inflammatory affections of the conjunctiva. The ripe pulp of the fruit is considered as an effective laxative in habitual constipation and enters into many Ayurvedic preparations, where it may be given for loss of appetite and nausea and vomiting in pregnancy. An infusion of the leaves is used as a gargle for aphthous ulcers and sore throats and for washing indolent ulcers. In other parts of the world the plant is equally regarded: in Nigeria, leaf extracts are used in guinea worm infection;[1] in Fiji, the fruit and leaves are taken orally for piles[2] and in Tanzania, a decoction of dried leaves is given for malaria.[3] In Guatemala the dried fruit is taken as a febrifuge, for urinary tract infections and infections of the skin and mucosa,[4] including ringworm and other fungal diseases.[5] The bark is used as a tonic and febrifuge and the ash obtained by heating it with salt in an earthen pot is mixed with water and taken orally for colic and as a gargle or mouth wash.[6] In the Canary Islands the dried fruit is eaten as a choleretic.[7] Tamarind seed xyloglucan (TSX) is used as a thickener, stabiliser, gelling agent and starch modifier for food, textile and toiletry use.

Ethnoveterinary usage

The bark is used to treat intestinal parasites in swine. Fruits and leaves are given to ruminants for fever, internal parasites, bloat and as an appetiser, to pigs for coughs and colds, and to both for constipation. The leaves have been used to treat fractures.[8]

Major chemical constituents

Cardenolides and bufadienolides

Uzarigenin-3-O-β-D-xylopyranosyl-α-L-rhamnopyranoside[9] and scilliphaeosidin 3-O-β-D-glucopyranosyl-L-rhamnopyranoside[10] have been isolated from the seed.

Phytosterols and triterpenes

β-Sitosterol, campesterol, stigmasterol and β-amyrin occur in the seed.

Polysaccharides and sugars

Arabinose, ribose, xylose, mannose, fructose, galactose, glucose, inositol, sucrose, maltose, raffinose,[11] xyloglucan[12] and polyose (a polysaccharide gum)[13] are present in the seed and pectin,[14] glucose, mannose, maltose and arabinose in the fruit.

Flavones and flavonols

Apigenin, vitexin, isovitexin, orientin and others occur in the leaf.[15]

Organic and aminoacids

Aspartic, glutamic, tartaric, citric, oxalic and succinic acids, serine, methionine, phenylalanine and others are present in the fruit and seeds and glyoxalic, oxaloacetic, oxalosuccinic and α-oxoglutaric acid in the leaf and seed.[16,17]

Vitamins

L-ascorbic acid, tocopherol, carotenes in the fruit.[18]

Minerals

Calcium, phosphorus, magnesium, potassium, sodium, copper, iron, zinc, manganese[19,20] in the fruit.

Fatty acids

Palmitic, oleic acid, linoleic, arachidic, behenic, lignoceric, linolenic, and decosatetraenoic acid are present in the seed.[21,22]

Monoterpenoids and other volatiles

2-Acetyl furan, benzaldehyde, phenyl acetaldehyde, dibutyl phthalate,[23] furfural,[24] linalool, linalool oxides, geraniol, α-terpineol, tamarindineal (5-hydroxy-2-oxo-hexa-3,5-dienal)[25] and others have been found in the fruit.

Medicinal and pharmacological activities

Immunomodulatory activity: A polysaccharide isolated from *Tamarindus indica* showed phagocytic enhancement, leucocyte migration inhibition and inhibition of lymphocyte proliferation.[26] A biologically active xyloglucan oligosaccharide, obtained by treatment of tamarind xyloglucan with a fungal b-glucanase, was found to be useful for the prevention and/or treatment of immunological damage to skin exposed to UV irradiation. This was due to prevention of the suppression of delayed hypersensitivity and a reduction in the amount of interleukin-10 produced by keratinocytes in the skin.[27] Tamarind xyloglucans were immunoprotective at low (picogram) doses and prevented suppression of immune responses to alloantigen in mice exposed to 30 kJ/m^2 UVB radiation.[28]

Antioxidant activity: 2-Hydroxy-3′,4′-dihydroxyacetophenone, methyl 3,4-dihydroxybenzoate and 3,4-dihydroxyphenyl acetate were isolated from the ethyl acetate extract of the seed coat and demonstrated strong antioxidative activity in the linoleic acid autoxidation system as measured by the thiocyanate and thiobarbituric acid methods.[29]

Antiinflammatory activity: Aqueous, ethanol and chloroform extracts demonstrated antiinflammatory activity in mice (ear oedema induced by arachidonic acid) and rats (subplantar oedema induced by carrageenan) after topical or intraperitoneal administration, respectively.[30]

***Hypolipidaemic activity*:** Tamarind xyloglucan has a β-1,4-glucan backbone, so is not digested by human digestive enzymes and acts as a dietary fibre. Both intact and hydrolysed xyloglucan reduced plasma and liver lipids in rats fed a high-cholesterol diet and significantly reduced adipose tissue weight.[31] In another study, high-fat diets containing 5% w/w of xyloglucan or cellulose were given to the test or control groups of rats for 4 weeks. Blood total cholesterol, plasma triglyceride and lipoprotein levels of the test groups were reduced, indicating the beneficial effect of xyloglucan supplementation. Blood GOT and GPT levels of the test groups were also lower than those of the control group.[32]

Hypoglycaemic activity: The effect of oligosaccharides obtained from tamarind xyloglucan on absorption of 3-O-methyl-D-glucose was studied using everted sacs from rat small intestine. Among the oligosaccharides tested, octasaccharide and nonasaccharide, which contain D-galactose residues at their non-reducing terminals, inhibited absorption of 3-O-methyl-D-glucose and inhibition was concentration dependent. The results indicate that the octasaccharide and nonasaccharide may not only serve as a soluble dietary fibre of low molecular weight but also lower the blood sugar level.[33]

Antibacterial activity: An acetone extract of the fruit showed antibacterial activity against *Salmonella typhimurium* on agar plates. The 70% alcoholic extract was active on *Bacillus cereus*, *B. megatherium*, *Escherichia coli*, *Pseudomonas aeruginosa*, *Salmonella typhimurium*, *Staphylococcus alba* and *Staph. aureus*.[34] The methanol extract of the dried stem bark was active on *Sarcina lutea*.[35]

Antifungal activity: The ethanol (95%) extract of the fruit was active against *Trichophyton mentagrophytes* and *T. rubrum*.[36] An aqueous alcoholic extract was also active against *Aspergillus fumigatus*, *A. niger*, *Penicillium digitatum* and *Rhizophus nigricans*.[37]

Molluscicidal activity: Water and methanol extracts of the fruit pulp were found to have molluscicidal activity against *Bulinus truncatus*. The LC_{50}s were 400 ppm and 300 ppm respectively.[38]

Antiviral activity: Tamarind gum (glyloid) and three sulphate derivatives (GP4311, GP4327 and GP4324) were evaluated for their inhibitory effect on Rubella virus (RV) infection of Vero cells. Glyloid sulphate 4324 had the highest inhibitory effect on RV antigen synthesis. The results indicated that the polysaccharides blocked a step in virus replication subsequent to virus attachment, such as internalisation and/or uncoating.[39] Glyloid sulphate 4323 and glyloid sulphate 4327 were also found to inhibit rabies virus infection in chicken embryo-related cells by interfering with the virus adsorption process, in a dose-dependent manner. The effective concentration was far below the cytotoxicity threshold.[40]

Effect on fluoride toxicity: The effect of tamarind ingestion on fluoride retention was studied in dogs. The urinary excretion of fluoride was significantly higher in dogs supplemented with fluoride and tamarind in comparison with the fluoride-only supplemented group and the control group, indicating the beneficial effect of tamarind ingestion on fluoride retention and toxicity.[41]

Ophthalmic delivery system: Tamarind seed polysaccharide (TS-P) has been used as an ophthalmic delivery system for ocular administration of hydrophilic and hydrophobic antibiotics.[42] TS-P has high viscosity and mucoadhesive properties, which make it suitable for addition to ophthalmic solutions to prolong the residence time on the cornea. The effect of a preparation containing TS-P on intraocular pressure (IOP) was evaluated in rabbits. Administration into the conjunctival sac of 0.5% timolol, or 0.5% timolol with 1% and 2% TS-P, had no effect on normal IOP but significantly reduced betamethasone-induced ocular hypertension over 20 days. Timolol in conjunction with TS-P had a longer duration of action.[43]

Bioavailability enhancement: The influence of tamarind fruit extract, incorporated into a traditional meal, on the bioavailability of aspirin tablets 600 mg dose was studied. There was an increase in plasma levels of aspirin and salicylic acid when the meal containing the extract was administered with the aspirin, compared to when it was taken in the fasting state or with the meal but without the fruit extract.[44]

Safety profile

No health hazards or side effects are known in conjunction with therapeutic dosages. A 90-day repeated dose toxicity study of flavonoid tamarind pigments cocoa brown (TRSP(B)) and roasted seed pigments was conducted in Sprague-Dawley SPF rats. During the entire period of administration, there were changes in clinical signs, body weight, food consumption, ophthalmological, urinalysis, haematological, blood chemistry or pathological parameters.[45] An ethanol/water (1:1) extract of the flowers, when administered orally to mice, gave a maximum tolerated dose of 1.0 g/kg.[46]

Dosage

Fruits: 1–3 g

Seed powder: 1–2 g

Ayurvedic properties

Rasa: *Amla* (sour)

Guna: *Guru* (heavy), *ruksha* (dry)

Veerya: *Ushna* (hot)

Vipaka: *Amla* (sour)

Dosha: Pacifies *vata;* increases *kapha* and *pitta*

Further reading

Bown D 1995 Encyclopaedia of herbs and their uses. Dorling Kindersley, London

Chevallier A 1996 The encyclopedia of medicinal plants. Dorling Kindersley, London

Duke JA 1992 Handbook of phytochemical constituents of GRAS herbs and other economic plants. CRC Press, London

Ross I 1999 Medicinal plants of the world, vol 1. Humana Press, Totowa, New Jersey

References

1 Fabiyi JP, Kela SL, Tal KM, Istifanus WA 1993 Traditional therapy of dracunculiasis in the state of Bauchi – Nigeria. Dakar Medicine 38(2):193

2 Singh YN 1986 Traditional medicine in Fiji. Some herbal folk cures used by Fiji Indians. Journal of Ethnopharmacology 15(1):57

3 Gessler MC, Nkunyak MHH, Mwasumbi LB, Heinrich M, Tanner M 1994 Screening of Tanzanian medicinal plants for antimalarial activity. Acta Tropica 56(1):65

4 Caceres A, Giron LM, Alvarado SR, Torres MF 1987 Screening of antimicrobial activity of plants popularly used in Guatemala for the treatment of dermatomucosal diseases. Journal of Ethnopharmacology 20(3):223

5 Caceres A, Lopez BR, Giron MA, Logemann H 1991 Plants used in Guatemala for the treatment of dermatophytic infections. I. Screening for antimycotic activity of 44 plant extracts. Journal of Ethnopharmacology 31(3):263

6 Khan MA, Khan T, Ahmad Z 1994 Barks used as source of medicine in Madhya Pradesh, India. Fitoterapia 65(5):444

7 Darias V, Brando L, Rabanal R et al 1989 New contribution to the ethnopharmacological study of the Canary Islands. Journal of Ethnopharmacology 25(1):77

8 International Institute of Rural Reconstruction 1994 Ethnoveterinary medicine in Asia: an information kit on traditional animal health care practices. 4 vols. IIRR, Silang, Philippines

9 Yadava RN, Yadav S 1999 A new cardenolide uzarigenin-3-O-β-D-xylopyranosyl (1→2)-α-L-rhamnopyranoside. Journal of Asian Natural Products Research 1(4):245–249

10 Yadava RN, Yadav S, Vardhan D 1999 A new

bufadienolide from the seeds of *Tamarindus indica* (Linn). Res. J. Chem. Environ. 3(2):55–56

11 Sone Y, Sato K 1994 Measurement of oligosaccharides derived from tamarind xyloglucan by competitive ELISA assay. Bio. Sci. Biotech. Biotech. Bio. Chem. 58:2295–2296

12 Yamada H 2001 Application of xyloglucan (functional property and application). Cellular Communication 8(1):30–33

13 Khanna M, Dwivedi AK, Singh S 1999 Polyose from seeds of *Tamarindus indica* of unique property and immense pharmaceutical use. Trends in Carbohydrate Chemistry 4:79–81

14 Kulkarni MG, Kulkarni SS, Nene SN, Thakar MJ, Gaikwad BG 1999 Process for the recovery of tartaric acid and other products from tamarind pulp. US Patent No. 5994533

15 Bhatia VK, Gupta SR, Seshadri TR 1966 C-glycosides of tamarind leaves. Phytochemistry 5(1):177–181

16 De Lumen B, Beeker R, Reyes PS 1986 Legumes and a cereal with high methionine/cysteine content. Journal of Agricultural and Food Chemistry 34:361–364

17 Shankaracharya NB 1998 Tamarind – chemistry, technology and uses – a critical appraisal. Journal of Food Science and Technology 35(3):193–208

18 Schmandke H, Olivarez GO 1969 The carotene, L-ascorbic acid, dehydroascorbic acid and tocopherol content of Cuban vegetable products; Nahrung 13:523–530

19 Ishola MM, Agbaji EB, Agbaji AS 1990 A chemical study of *Tamarindus indica* fruits grown in Nigeria. J. Sci. Food Agric. 51:141–143

20 Marangoni A, Alli I, Kermasha S 1988 Composition and properties of seeds of the tree legume *Tamarindus indica*. Journal of Food Science 53(5):1452–1455

21 Andriamanantena RW, Artaud J, Gaydou EM, Iatrides MC, Chevalier JL 1983 Fatty acid and sterol composition of Malagasy tamarind kernel oils. JACOS 60(7):1318–1321

22 Sivarama Reddy G, Jaganmohan Rao S, Achyutaramayya D, Azeemoddin G, Tirumala Rao SD 1979 Extraction, characteristics and fatty acid composition of tamarind kernel oil. Journal of the Oil Technology Association of India 11:91–93

23 Lee PL, Swords G, Hunter GLK 1975 Volatile constituents of tamarind. Journal of Agricultural and Food Chemistry 23:1195–1199

24 Zhang Y, Ho CT, Khurana AL 1990 Volatile flavour components of tamarind (*Tamarindus indica* L.). Journal of Essential Oil Research 2(4):197–198

25 Imbabi ES, Ibrahim KE, Ahmed BM, Abulfutuh IM, Hulbert P 1992 Chemical characterization of tamarind bitter principle, tamarindineal. Fitoterapia 63(6):537–538

26 Sreelekha TT, Vijayakumar T, Ankanthil R, Vijayan KK, Nair MK 1993 Immunomodulatory effects of a polysaccharide from *Tamarindus indica*. Anti-cancer Drugs 4(2):209–212

27 Strickland F, Pelley R, Albersheim P, Darvill A, Pauly M, Eberhard S 2001 Inhibition of UV-induced immune suppression and interleukin-10 production by cytoprotective tamarind oligosaccharides. US Patent No. 6251878

28 Strickland FM, Darvill A, Albersheim P, Eberhard S, Pauly M, Pelley RP 1999 Inhibition of UV-induced immune suppression and interleukin-10 production by plant oligosaccharides and polysaccharides. Photochemistry and Photobiology 69(2):141–147

29 Tsuda T, Watanabe M, Ohshima K, Yamamoto A, Kawakishi S, Osawa T 1994 Antioxidative components isolated from the seed of tamarind (*Tamarindus indica* L.). Journal of Agricultural and Food Chemistry 42(12):2671–2674

30 Rimbau V, Cerdan C, Vila R, Iglesias J 1999 Antiinflammatory activity of some extracts from plants used in the traditional medicine of north-African countries (II). Phytotherapy Research 13(2):128–132

31 Yamatoya K, Shirakawa M, Baba O 2000 Effects of xyloglucan on lipid metabolism: hydrocolloids Fourth International Conference on Hydrocolloids, Osaka City University, 1998:405–410

32 Baba O, Suzuki J, Shirakawa M, Yamatoya K 1997 Lipid increase inhibitors containing xyloglucan. Japanese Patent No. 09224608

33 Sone Y, Makino C, Misaki A 1992 Inhibitory effect of oligosaccharides derived from plant xyloglucan on intestinal glucose absorption in rat. Journal of Nutritional Science and Vitaminology 38(4):391–395

34 Ross SA, Megalla SE, Bishay DW, Awad AH 1980 Studies for determining antibiotic substances in some Egyptian plants. Part 1. Screening for antimicrobial activity. Fitoterapia 51:303–308

35 Laurens A, Mboup S, Tignokpa M, Sylla O, Masquelier J 1985 Antimicrobial activity of some medicinal species of Dakar markets. Pharmazie 40(7):482–485

36 Ray PG, Majumdar SK 1976 Antimicrobial activity of some Indian plants. Economic Botany 30:317–320

37 Guerin JC, Reveillere HP 1984 Antifungal activity of plant extract used in therapy I. Study of 41 plant extracts against 9 fungal species. Annales Pharmaceutiques Francaises 42(6):553–559

38 Imbabi ES, Abu-al-Futuh IM 1992 Investigation of the molluscicidal activity of *Tamarindus indica*. Indian Journal of Pharmacy 30(2):157–160

39 Mastromarino P, Petruzziello R, Macchia S, Rieti S, Nicoletti R, Orsi N 1997 Antiviral activity of natural and semisynthetic polysaccharides on the early steps of rubella virus infection. Journal of Antimicrobial Chemotherapy 39(3):339–345

40 Pietropaolo V, Seganti L, Marchetti M, Sinibaldi L, Orsi N, Nicoletti R 1993 Effect of natural and semisynthetic polymers on rabies virus infection in CER cells. Research in Virology 144(2):151–158

41 Khandare AL, Kumar PU, Lakshmaiah N 2000 Beneficial effect of tamarind ingestion on fluoride toxicity in dogs. Fluoride 33(1):33–38

42 Ghelardi E, Tavanti A, Celandroni F et al 2000 Effect of a novel mucoadhesive polysaccharide obtained from tamarind seeds on the intraocular penetration of gentamicin and ofloxacin in rabbits. Journal of Antimicrobial Chemotherapy 46(5):831–834

43 D'Amico M, Filippo C, Lampa E et al 1999 Effects of timolol and timolol with tamarind seed polysaccharide on intraocular pressure in rabbits. Pharm. Pharmacol. Commun 5(5):361–364

44 Mustapha A, Yakasai IA, Aguye IA 1996 Effect of *Tamarindus indica* on the bioavailability of aspirin in healthy human volunteers. European Journal of Drug Metabolism and Pharmacokinetics 21(3):223–226

45 Mochizuki M, Katsumata T, Hatayama K et al 1998 A 90-day oral (dietary) toxicity study of tamarind pigments cocoa brown TRSP(B) in rats. Nippon Shokuhin Kagaku Gakkaishi 5(2):140–145

46 Dhar ML, Dhar MM, Dhawan BN, Mehrotra BN, Ray C 1968 Screening of Indian plants for biological activity. Part I. Indian Journal of Experimental Biology 6:232–247

Terminalia arjuna (Roxb.) Wight & Arn (Combretaceae) (syn. *Terminalia cuneata* Roth.)

English: Arjun myrobalan

Hindi: *Arjun*

Sanskrit: *Arjuna, kakubha*

Arjuna has a prominent place in Indian mythology; it is considered sacred and is mentioned in ancient folklore. In Ayurveda it is thought necessary to maintain basic health and has a reputation as a heart medicine; it is also an important ingredient in many classical herbal formulae.

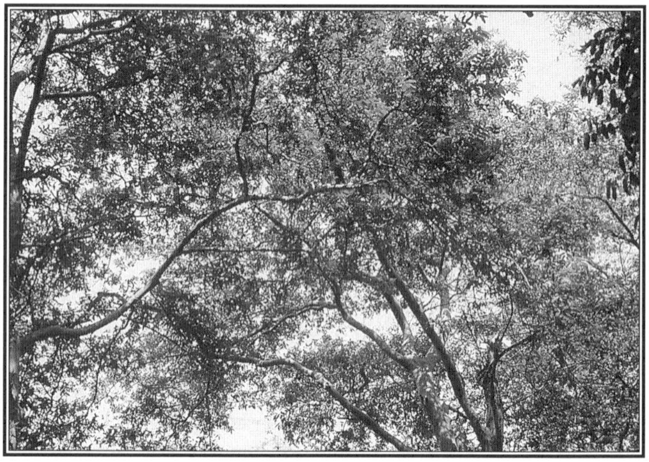

Habitat

Arjuna is common in the plains of India, along riversides, streams, ravines and dry watercourses. It is also cultivated for decoration and shade in avenues and gardens.

Botanical description

A large evergreen tree with spreading crown, buttressed trunk and drooping branches (Plate 61). The bark is smooth, pinkish grey, exfoliating in large, thin irregular sheets. The leaves are subopposite, elliptical, coriaceous, up to 15 cm long, with a pair of oil glands visible on the lower surface near the petiole. The flowers are cup-shaped, in panicled spikes. The fruits are 2–5 cm long, glabrous and ovoid-oblong in shape, bearing 5–7 wings.

Parts used

Bark and fruit.

Traditional and modern use

Terminalia arjuna is traditionally used for heart problems. The bark is considered to be a cardiotonic and used in the treatment of cardiovascular diseases such as angina, myocardial infarction, hypertension, congestive heart failure, coronary artery diseases and hypercholesterolaemia. It is also used to treat hepatic, urogenital and venereal diseases.[1] It has been reported as useful for fractured bones, bacterial and viral infections, colic, piles, dysentery and dyspepsia and as an antidote in cases of poisoning. The powdered bark mixed with honey is recommended for bilious disorders, diarrhoea, dysentery and haemorrhage. A decoction is used topically as an astringent for treating ulcers, sores and wounds.

Ethnoveterinary usage

An extract of the bark is used to staunch bleeding in animals, especially goats and sheep.[2]

Major chemical constituents

Triterpenoids

Arjunosides I–IV, arjunine, arjunetin, arjunctine, friedelin and arjungenin, oleanolic acid, arjunic acid, arjunolic acid and various other saponin glycosides have been isolated.[3,4]

Flavonoids and polyphenols

Arjunolone, arjunone, catechol, gallocatechol, epicatechol and epigallocatechol are present.

Medicinal and pharmacological activities

Cardiovascular activity: An experimental study, using an ischaemic reperfusion injury model, showed that *Terminalia arjuna* bark powder produced an increase in superoxide dismutase, catalase and glutathione levels and demonstrated the protective effect of the drug against oxidative stress.[5] Other experiments have confirmed the direct positive inotropic effects on heart muscle[6] and the hypotensive activity.[7,8] *T. arjuna* was found to be effective in relieving stable anginal pain[9] and shown to lower systolic blood pressure and frequency of angina attacks without any evidence of renal or hepatic impairment.[10] When given to patients with refractory chronic congestive heart failure over a period of 12 weeks, the bark extract was effective in the management of the disease as judged by an improvement in various parameters.[11] In ventricular arrhythmia a dose of 500 mg three times a day was reported to be effective.[12]

Hypolipidaemic activity: Studies have been conducted in animals using the administration of a cholesterol-rich diet to induce experimental arteriosclerosis.[13] Parameters such as total cholesterol, LD lipoprotein, HD lipoprotein and triglyceride were measured before and after treatment and, together with histopathological tests, these showed a significant decrease in LDL and total cholesterol levels after administration of *T. arjuna*. The action appears to be mediated through the inhibition of hepatic cholesterol biosynthesis, increased faecal bile acid secretion and enhanced catabolism.[14–16] A recent trial has confirmed these effects in humans.[17]

Hepatoprotective activity: Ayurvedic preparations Nagarjunabhram and Somesvararasam, containing arjuna bark as the main ingredient, are used in hepatic complaints. Recent studies have indicated that the bark might act through the inhibition of hepatitis B virus surface antigen secretion.[18]

Antineoplastic activity: Gallic acid, ethyl gallate and the flavone luteolin were found to be useful in retarding the growth of cancer cells.[19]

Antimutagenic activity: Ellagic acid and other extracts isolated from *Terminalia arjuna* were antimutagenic to various strains of *Salmonella typhimurium* against directly or indirectly acting mutagens.[20–22]

Antibacterial and antiviral activity: The bark has been reported as having significant antibacterial activity against *Escherichia*,

Klebsiella, *Proteus* and *Pseudomonas* species[23] as well as against human immunodeficiency virus. The bark inhibited HIV type I protease enzyme activity by more than 70% at a concentration of 0.2 mg/ml.[24]

Safety profile

T. arjuna is well tolerated when used within the recommended doses.

Dosage

Powder: 1–3 g

Juice: 12–24 ml

Decoction: 60–120 ml

Ayurvedic properties

Rasa: *Kashaya* (astringent)

Guna: *Laghu* (light), *ruksha* (dry)

Veerya: *Shita* (cold)

Vipaka: *Katu* (pungent)

Dosha: Pacifies *kapha* and *pitta*

Further reading

Bharatiya Vidya Bhavan's Swami Prakashananda Ayurveda Research Centre 1992 Selected medicinal plants of India. Chemexcil, Mumbai

Kapoor LD 1990 Handbook of Ayurvedic medicinal plants. CRC Press, Boca Raton

Rastogi RP, Mehrotra BN 1993 Compendium of Indian medicinal plants, vol 3. PID, New Delhi

References

1 Kumar DS, Prabhakar YS 1987 On the ethnomedical significance of the Arjuna tree, *Terminalia arjuna* (Roxb.) Wight & Arnot. Journal of Ethnopharmacology 20(2):173

2 International Institute of Rural Reconstruction 1994 Ethnoveterinary medicine in Asia. An information kit on traditional animal health care practices. IIRR, Silang, Philippines

3 Dwivedi S, Udupa N 1989 *Terminalia arjuna*: pharmacognosy, phytochemistry, pharmacology and clinical use: a review. Fitoterapia 60:413

4 Honda T, Murae T, Tsuyuki T, Takahashi T, Sawai M 1998 Arjugenin, arjunglycoside I and arjunglycoside II. A new triterpene and new triterpene glucosides from *Terminalia arjuna*. Bulletin of the Chemistry Society of Japan 49:3213

5 Gauthaman K, Maulik M, Kumar R, Manchanda SC, Dinda AK, Maulik SK 2001 Effect of chronic treatment with bark of *Terminalia arjuna*: a study on the isolated ischemic-reperfused rat heart. Journal of Ethnopharmacology 75(2–3):197

6 Radhakrishnan R, Wadsworth RM, Gray AI 1993 *Terminalia arjuna*, an Ayurvedic cardiotonic, increases contractile force of rat isolated atria. Phytotherapy Research 7(3):266

7 Singh N, Kapur KK, Singh SP, Shanker K, Sinha JN, Kohil RP 1982 Mechanism of cardiovascular action of *Terminalia arjuna*. Planta Medica 45:102

8 Takahashi S, Tanaka H, Hano Y, Ito K, Nomura T, Shigenobu K 1997 Hypotensive effects in rats of hydrophilic extract from *Terminalia arjuna* containing tannin-related compounds. Phytotherapy Research 11:424

9 Dwivedi S, Jauhari R 1997 Beneficial effects of *Terminalia arjuna* in coronary artery disease. Indian Heart Journal 49(5):507

10 Kumar PU, Adhikari P, Pereira P, Bhat P 1999 Safety and efficacy of Hartone in stable angina pectoris – an open comparative trial. Journal of the Association of Physicians of India 47(7):685

11 Bharani A, Ganguly A, Bhargava KD 1995 Salutary effect of *T. arjuna* in patients with severe refractory heart failure. International Journal of Cardiology 49:191

12 Dwivedi S, Avasthi R, Mahajan S 1994 Case report: role of *Terminalia arjuna* in ventricular tachyarrhythmias. Indian Practitioner 57(6):523

13 Tiwari AK, Gode JD, Dubey GP 1990 Effect of *Terminalia arjuna* on lipid profiles of rabbits fed hypercholesterolemic diet. International Journal of Crude Drug Research 28(1):43

14 Pathak SR, Upadhyaya L, Singh RH, Dubey GP, Udupa KN 1989 Effect of *Terminalia arjuna* W.& A. on autacoidal and lipid profiles of rabbits. Indian Drugs 27(4):221

15 Ram A, Lauria P, Gupta R, Kumar P, Sharma VN 1997 Hypocholesterolaemic effects of *Terminalia arjuna* tree bark. Journal of Ethnopharmacology 55(3):165

16 Shaila HP, Udupa SL 1997 Hypolipidemic effects of *Terminalia arjuna* in cholesterol fed rabbits. Fitoterapia 57(5):405

17 Gupta R, Singhal S, Goyle A, Sharma VN 2001 Antioxidant and hypocholesterolaemic effects of *Terminalia arjuna* tree-bark powder: a randomized placebo-controlled trial. Journal of the Association of Physicians of India 49:231

18 Goto W, Kusumoto I, Kadota S, Namba T, Kurokawa M, Shiraki K 1996 Suppression of hepatitis B virus surface antigen secretion by traditional plant medicines. Phytotherapy Research 10(6):504

19 Pettit GR, Hoard MS, Doubek DL et al 1996 Antineoplastic agents 338. The cancer cell growth inhibitory constituents of *Terminalia arjuna* (Combretaceae). Journal of Ethnopharmacology 53(2):57

20 Kaur S, Grover IS, Kumar S 1997 Antimutagenic potential of ellagic acid isolated from *Terminalia arjuna*. Indian Journal of Experimental Biology 35(5):478

21 Kaur S, Grover IS, Kumar S 2001 Antimutagenic potential of extracts isolated from *Terminalia arjuna*. Journal of Environmental Pathology, Toxicology and Oncology 20(1):9

22 Jain AK, Shimoi K, Nakamura Y, Tomita I, Kada T 1987 Preliminary study on the desmutagenic and antimutagenic effects of some natural products. Current Science 56(24):1266

23 Perumal SR, Ignacimuthu S, Sen A 1998 Screening of 34 Indian medicinal plants for antibacterial properties. Journal of Ethnopharmacology 62(2):173

24 Ines KT, Takeshi NH, Kida MH, Masao HT, Namba KS 1995 Screening of various plant extracts used in Ayurvedic medicine for inhibitory effects on human immunodeficiency virus type I (HIV-I) protease. Phytotherapy Research 9:180

Terminalia belerica (Gaertn.) Roxb. (Combretaceae) (syn. *Myrobalanus bellirica* Gaertn.)

English: Beleric myrobalan

Hindi: *Bhaira, bahera*

Sanskrit: *Vibitaki, vibeekaka, bibhitaki*

Terminalia belerica has deep roots in Indian mythology as well as in Ayurveda. It is part of a compound *rasayana* preparation of three myrobalan fruits, known as *Triphala* (or *trifla*), which is important in both Indian and Tibetan traditional medicine. The name *Vibheekaki* indicates that regular use keeps a person healthy and free from disease. The fixed oil from the seeds is used for cooking.

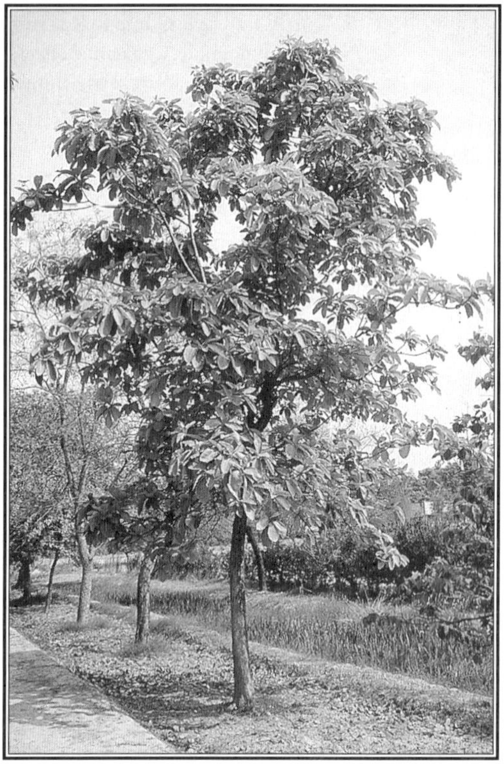

Habitat

The tree is found commonly throughout the forests of India, Sri Lanka and other Asian countries, in different climatic conditions apart from very arid zones, up to an altitude of about 1200 m. It is also cultivated in gardens, parks and at roadsides.

Botanical description

A large deciduous tree reaching up to 29 m (Plate 62). The trunk and stems are straight with a characteristic blue-grey, cracked bark. The leaves are broadly elliptical, about 10–25 cm in length and 5–8 cm in width, coriaceous, alternate and mainly directed toward the apex of the branches. The flowers are in axillary spikes, pale greenish-yellow with an unpleasant odour. The fruits are globular, grey, hairy and about 1–2 cm in diameter.

Parts used

Fruit.

Traditional and modern use

The fruit is used extensively by many ethnic groups of India and neighbouring countries to treat a variety of ailments and is considered to be a tonic, hepatoprotective, antiviral, purgative, hypolipidaemic, astringent and antidiarrhoeal. It is also reputed to improve immunity and bodily resistance to infectious disease and is therefore used for coughs, sore throats, and eye and skin diseases such as conjunctivitis and leprosy. The preparation *Triphala* is widely prescribed for liver disorders and gastrointestinal problems.

Ethnoveterinary usage

The seeds are generally used to treat wounds of ruminants.[1]

Major chemical constituents

Triterpenoids

Belleric acid, the glycoside saponins bellericoside and bellericanin, and sterols such as β-sitosterol have been isolated from the fruit.[2]

Polyphenols

Phyllembin, ellagic acid, gallic acid, ethyl gallate, chebulagic acid and hexahydroxydiphenic acid ester[3,4] are present.

Fixed oil

A fixed oil is extracted from the seed.

Medicinal and pharmacological activities

Antioxidant activity: Free radical-induced cellular damage is involved in several pathological conditions such as cancer, rheumatism, liver injury, ischaemic heart disease and ageing. *Triphala*, which contains *T. belerica*, showed scavenging activity against mitochondrial lipid peroxidation. The phenolic compounds present were credited for the antioxidant activity.[5]

Cardiovascular activity: In vivo and in vitro studies have shown cardiovascular activity, including negative inotropic and chronotropic activity as well as hypotensive effects. This was attributed to cholinergic activity.[6,7]

Hypolipidaemic activity: When *T. belerica* was given to animals in which arteriosclerosis had been induced by feeding a cholesterol-rich diet, significant decreases in the cholesterol level of the liver and aorta were observed.[8–10]

Antimicrobial activity: Antibacterial activity was shown against a wide range of bacterial organisms.[11] *Sukshma Triphala* was active against *Clostridium tetani*[12] and several viruses such as the vesicular stomatitis virus and a rotavirus.[13,14]

Hepatoprotective activity: The fruit is hepatoprotective and this is thought to be due at least in part to the presence of gallic acid.[15] When administered orally it showed a good protective effect against carbon tetrachloride-induced hepatotoxicity as shown by an improvement in serum transaminase and bilirubin levels and a significant inhibition of microsomal lipid peroxidation and a reduction in triglyceride levels in the liver.[16] This supports the traditional use of *T. belerica* in the treatment of liver disease.

Antiulcer activity: The fruit was effective in reducing the total acidity and peptic activity and increasing the mucin content, which suggests a role in ulcer management.[17] *Triphala Churna* was found to be effective in ulcers induced by pylorus ligation, aspirin and prednisolone.[18] A documented case of healing a leg ulcer and generation of new tissue growth showed its potential use in the management of other types of ulcer.[19]

Antiobesity effects: *Triphala Guggulu* is an antiobesity agent, reducing weight, skinfold thickness and circumference of hips and waist in obese subjects. Clinical studies also revealed the preparation to be safe.[20–22]

Use in eye disorders: Myopia and hypermetropia were controlled by *Triphala Gritha*, an ancient Ayurvedic recipe which contains the fruit of belleric myrobalan as one of the main ingredients.[23] Also *Sukshma Triphala* has been recommended for the management of *anjananamika* (stye) of eye disease.[24]

Antimutagenicity: This effect was attributed to the polyphenols present in the fruit.[25]

Hypoglycaemic activity: The preparation *Triphala* showed hypoglycaemic activity.[26]

Antiinflammatory effects: Classical combinations containing *T. belerica* have been found to be useful in the treatment of rheumatic diseases.[27,28]

Safety profile

T. belerica is a safe and well-tolerated herb when used at recommended doses and in the form of *Triphala*. The fixed oil is purgative in large doses.[29]

Dosage

Powder: 1–3 g

Ayurvedic properties

Rasa: *Kashaya* (astringent), *madhur* (sweet)

Guna: *Laghu* (light), *ruksha* (dry)

Veerya: *Ushna* (hot)

Vipaka: *Madhur* (sweet)

Dosha: Pacifies *tridosha*

Further reading

Bharatiya Vidya Bhavan's Swami Prakashanandra Ayurveda Research Centre 1992 Selected medicinal plants of India. Chemexcil, Mumbai

Kapoor LD 1990 Handbook of Ayurvedic medicinal plants. CRC Press, Boca Raton

Khare CP 2000 Indian herbal therapies. Vishv Vijay PVT Ltd, New Delhi

References

1 International Institute of Rural Reconstruction 1994 Ethnoveterinary medicine in Asia. An information kit on traditional animal health care practices. IIRR, Silang, Philippines

2 Nandy AK, Podder G, Sahu NP, Mahato SB 1989 Triterpenoids and their glycosides from *Terminalia belerica*. Phytochemistry 28(10):2769

3 Ali M, Bhutani KK 1991 Occurrence of hexahydroxydiphenic acid ester in *Terminalia belerica* fruits. Indian Journal of Natural Products 7(1):16

4 Row LR, Murty PS 1970 Chemical examination of *Terminalia belerica* Roxb. Indian Journal of Chemistry 8:1047–1048

5 Vani T, Rajani M, Sarkar S, Shishoo CJ 1997 Antioxidant properties of the Ayurvedic formulation Triphala and its constituents. International Journal of Pharmacognosy 35(5):313

6 Srivastava RD, Swivedi S, Sreenivasan KK, Chandrashekhar CN 1992 Cardiovascular effects of *Terminalia* species of plants. Indian Drugs 29(4):144

7 Sharma JN, Rajpal MN, Rao TS, Gupta SK 1988 Some pharmacological investigations on the alcoholic extract of Triphala alone and in combination with petroleum ether extract of oleogum resin of *Commiphora mukul*. Indian Drugs 25(6):220

8 Shaila HP, Udupa SL, Udupa AL 1998 Hypolipidemic activity of three indigenous drugs in experimentally induced atherosclerosis. International Journal of Cardiology 67(2):119

9 Shaila HP, Udupa AL, Udupa SL 1995 Preventive actions of *Terminalia belerica* in experimentally

induced atherosclerosis. International Journal of Cardiology 4(2):101

10 Thakur CP, Thakur B, Singh S, Sinha PK, Sinha SK 1998 The Ayurvedic medicines Haritaki, Amla, and Behera reduce cholesterol-induced atherosclerosis in rabbits. International Journal of Cardiology 21(2):167

11 Ahmad I, Mehmood Z, Mohammad F 1998 Screening of some Indian medicinal plants for their antibacterial properties. Journal of Ethnopharmacology 62(2):183

12 Kulkarni GG, Ravetkar SD, Kulkarni PH 1995 Antibacterial properties of Ayurvedic preparations '*Bhallatakasava*' and '*Sukshma Triphala*'. Deerghayu International 11(42):3

13 Bopegamage SA, Petrovicova A 1995 Antiviral effect of selected Ayurvedic preparations on vesicular stomatitis virus. In Kulkarn PH (ed) Biorhythm. Ayurved Acad. Pune, p20

14 Bopegamage SA, Petrovicova A, Nossik NN, Lavrukina LA 1995 Compilation of the *in-vitro* and *in-vivo* antiviral activities of some Ayurvedic products. In Kulkarn PH (ed) Biorhythm. Ayurved Acad. Pune, p24

15 Anand K, Singh B, Saxena AK, Chandan BK, Gupta VN, Bhardwaj VN 1997 3,4,5-Trihydroxy benzoic acid (gallic acid), the hepatoprotective principle in the fruits of *Terminalia belerica*: bioassay guided activity. Pharmacological Research 36(4):315

16 Anand KK, Singh B, Saxena AK, Chandan BK, Gupta VN 1994 Hepatoprotective studies of a fraction from the fruits of *Terminalia belerica* Roxb. on experimental liver injury in rodents. Phytotherapy Research 8(5):287

17 Satyanaryanana S, Savitir M, Visweswaram D 1994 Anti-gastric ulcer activity of brucine and Triphala. Indian Journal of Pharmaceutical Science 56(4):165

18 Elango K, Suresh B, Kumar EP et al 1995 Pharmacological validation of certain Siddha drugs for their antiulcer and anti-inflammatory activity. International Seminar on Recent Trends in Pharmaceutical Science, Ootacamund, February

19 Kumar K, Junius M 1995 A spectacular case history of Pyoderma gangrenosum at the Ayurvedic Health Care Centre of South Australia. In Kulkarn PH (ed) Biorhythm. Ayurved Acad. Pune, p1

20 Paranjpe P, Patki P, Patwardhan B 1990 Ayurvedic treatment of obesity: a randomized double-blind, placebo-controlled clinical trial. Journal of Ethnopharmacology 29(1):1

21 Kulkarni PH, Paranjpe P 1990 Clinical assessment of Ayurvedic anti-obesity drugs. A double blind placebo controlled trial. Journal of Natural and Integrated Medicine 32(1):7

22 Kulkarni PH 1996 Clinical study of effect of Sukshma (subtle) *Triphala Guggulu* (TC.3x) in obesity. Med. Aromat. Plant Abs. 18(5):512

23 Sripathi P, Tarpanam R 1995 Boon to Drusti Lopa (refractive errors). Proc. Seminar on Research in Ayurveda and Siddha, CCRAS, New Delhi, p25, March

24 Sudrik UV 1995 Management of *Anjananamika* in amavastha with Swedana and Sookshma Triphala. Med. Aromat. Plant Abs. 18(5):514

25 Padam SK, Grover IS, Singh M 1996 Antimutagenic effects of polyphenols isolated from *Terminalia belerica* (Myrobalan) in *Salmonella typhimurium*. Indian Journal of Experimental Biology 43(2):98

26 Ghosh D, Uma R, Thejomoorthy P, Veluchamy G 1990 Hypoglycemic and toxicity studies of Triphala – a Siddha drug. Journal of Research in Ayurveda and Siddha 11(1–4):78

27 Pandey VK, Sharma AK 1986 Evaluation of Vatahari Guggulu and Nadivaspa-Sweda in the management of rheumatic diseases. Rheumatism 22(1):1

28 Ghosh D, Thejomoorthy P, Veluchamy G 1989 Anti-inflammatory, anti-arthritic and analgesic activities of Triphala. Journal of Research in Ayurveda and Siddha 10 (3–4):168

29 Dhar HL, Miglani BD, Dhawan D 1969 Studies on purgative action of an oil obtained from *Terminalia belerica*. Indian Journal of Medical Research 57(1):103

Terminalia chebula Retz. (Combretaceae)

English: Myrobalan, inknut

Hindi: *Hara*

Sanskrit: *Haritaki*

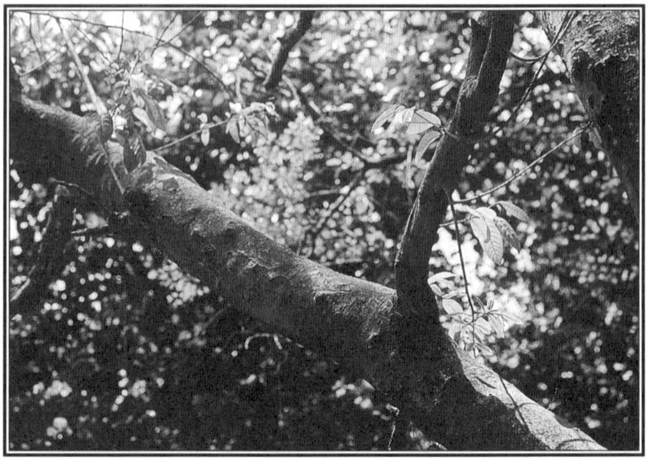

The chebulic myrobalan is of great importance in Ayurvedic medicine. It is known as *haritaki* in Sanskrit because it is sacred to Shiva (Hara). It is an ingredient of *Triphala*, or 'three fruits', a *rasayana* which also contains *T. belerica* (*Bibhitaki*) and *Phyllanthus emblica* (*Amalaki*). The plant was first mentioned in Chinese medicine in 1061 and it is also used in Tibetan medicine, where it is referred to as the 'king of medicines'. It has been known as *Abhay* as it is thought to promote fearlessness.

Habitat

It is found in the sub-Himalayan tract of India and in Myanmar, Sri Lanka and other Asian countries, up to an altitude of 1500 m.

Botanical description

A large deciduous tree reaching up to 30 m in height with a trunk girth of up to 2.5 m (Plate 63). The bark is dark brown, often longitudinally cracked, exfoliating in woody scales. The leaves are glabrous, opposite, ovate or elliptic and up to 20 cm long with an acute apex. The flowers are yellowish-white, in terminal spikes, with an unpleasant odour. The fruit is an ellipsoidal, pendulous drupe, up to 5 cm long, yellow to orange-brown in colour, sometimes tinged with red or black and hard when ripe. The seeds are hard and pale yellow.

Parts used

Fruits, leaves and stem.

Traditional and modern use

The fruits are used as an aperient, astringent, cardiotonic, carminative, fungicide, laxative, tonic, demulcent, purgative, alterative, febrifuge, antiasthmatic and antidysenteric. It is thought to strengthen the brain and enrich the blood. It is also used in bronchitis, burns, conjunctivitis, cough, dysurea, inflammation, leucorrhoea, measles, metritis, prolapse, ulcer, splenomegaly and cancer.

Ethnoveterinary usage

The fruits are used in bloat and as an appetite stimulant and the seeds are used to treat wounds in ruminants.[1]

Major chemical constituents

Triterpenoid glycosides

Chebulosides I and II, arjunin, arjunglucoside, 2α-hydroxyursolic acid and 2α-hydroxymicromiric acid have been reported.[2,3]

Tannins and polyphenols

Chebulinic acid, chebulin, punicalagin, punicalin, terflavins A, B, C and D, maslinic acid, gallic acid, synergic acid, terchebulin I, 1,2,3,4,6-penta-O-galloyl-β-D-glucopyranose and others have been isolated.[2]

Medicinal and pharmacological activities

Cardiotonic activity: Extracts prepared from the fruit rind of *T. chebula*, when tested on normal as well as hypodynamic isolated frog hearts, increased the force of contraction and cardiac output without changing the heart rate.[4]

Antianaphylactic activity: The water-soluble fraction was studied on systemic and local anaphylaxis and found to be effective. Systemic and passive cutaneous anaphylaxis was inhibited and serum histamine levels were reduced in a dose-dependent manner. The fraction also significantly inhibited histamine release from rat peritoneal mast cells, indicating that it may possess antianaphylactic action.[5]

Antimutagenic activity: The antimutagenicity of an aqueous extract of dry fruits of *T. chebula* was determined for two direct-acting mutagens, sodium azide and 4-nitro-O-phenylenediamine (NPD). Strains TA100, TA1535, TA97a and TA98 of *Salmonella typhimurium* and the S9-dependent mutagen 2-aminofluorene (2-AF) were used. The extract reduced NPD as well as 2-AF induced histidine revertants, but did not have any perceptible effect against sodium azide in TA100 and TA1535 strains. Preincubation studies showed an enhanced inhibitory effect.[6]

Antitumour activity: Gallic acid, 1,2,3,4,6-penta-O-galloyl-β-D-glucopyranose, chebulagic acid and chebulinic acid, isolated from the methanol fraction of *T. chebula* fruits, exhibited moderate cytotoxicity against cultured human tumour cell lines.[7]

Antibacterial activity: Gallic acid and its ethyl ester exhibited strong antimicrobial activity against methicillin-resistant strains of *Staphylococcus aureus* (MRSA).[8] In another study, an extract of *T. chebula* showed a potent wide-spectrum antibacterial activity against human pathogenic Gram-positive and Gram-negative bacteria.[9]

Antiviral activity: The fruit extract, when orally administered in combination with aciclovir, exhibited a strong anti-HSV-I activity by reducing virus in brain and skin more strongly than aciclovir alone.[10] The extract also showed a significant inhibitory activity on HIV-1 reverse transcriptase.[11]

Immunomodulatory activity: The crude extract of a formula containing *T. chebula, Tinospora cordifolia, Berberis aristata* and *Zingiber officinale* showed a significant enhancement in humoral immunity measured by haemagglutination titre and cell-mediated immune response, exhibited by inhibition of leucocyte migration.[12]

Antiamoebic activity: Antiamoebic effects of an ethanolic extract of the formulation above

(*T. chebula, Tinospora cordifolia, Berberis aristata, Zingiber officinale*) against experimental caecal amoebiasis in rats (*Entamoeba histolytica*) showed an effective cure rate compared with controls.[13]

Antioxidant activity: An ethanolic extract of the leaves significantly inhibited lipid peroxidation in mouse liver, lung homogenate and mitochondria, by effectively scavenging oxygen free radicals and inhibiting H_2O_2-induced red cell haemolysis. It also produced a significant inhibition in the chemiluminescence of human leucocytes induced by tissue plasminogen activator (TPA, 20 ng/ml). The extract also prevented DNA breaks in human leucocytes induced by TPA and cigarette smoke condensates.[14]

Safety profile

No adverse effects of *T. chebula* have been reported in the literature. The maximum tolerated doses of the 50% ethanolic extract of the stem bark and fruit were found to be 25 mg/kg body weight and 100 mg/kg body weight respectively, in adult albino rats.[15]

Dosage

Powder: 1–6 g (higher doses are laxative)

Decoction: 56–112 ml

Ayurvedic properties

Rasa: All *rasas* (except *lavana*)

Guna: *Laghu* (light), *ruksha* (dry)

Veerya: *Ushna* (hot)

Vipaka: *Madhur* (sweet)

Dosha: Pacifies *tridosha*

Further reading

Bharatiya Vidya Bhavan's Swami Prakashanandra Ayurveda Research Centre 1992 Selected medicinal plants of India. Chemexcil, Mumbai

Sairam TV 1999 Home remedies, vol II. Penguin India, New Delhi

References

1 International Institute of Rural Reconstruction 1994 Ethnoveterinary medicine in Asia. An information kit on traditional animal health care practices. Part I, general information. IIRR, Silang, Philippines

2 Singh C 1990 2alpha-Hydroxymicromeric acid, a pentacyclic triterpene from *Terminalia chebula*. Phytochemistry 29(7):2348

3 Kundu AP, Mahato SB 1993 Triterpenoids and their glycosides from *Terminalia chebula*. Phytochemistry 32(4):999

4 Reddy VRC, Rammana Kumari SV, Reddy BM, Anzeem MA, Prabhakar MC, Appa Rao AVN 1990 Cardiotonic activity of the fruits of *Terminalia chebula*. Fitoterapia 61(6):517

5 Shin TY, Jeong HJ, Kim DK et al 2001 Inhibitory action of water soluble fraction of *Terminalia chebula* on systemic and local anaphylaxis. Journal of Ethnopharmacology 4(2):133

6 Grover IS, Saroj B 1992 Antimutagenic activity of *T. chebula* (myrobalan) in *Salmonella typhimurium*. Indian Journal of Experimental Biology 30(4):399

7 Lee SH, Ryu SY, Choi SU et al 1995 Hydrolysable tannins and related compound having cytotoxic activity from the fruits of *Terminalia chebula*. Archives of Pharmacological Research 18(2):118

8 Sato Y, Oketani H, Singyouchi K et al 1997 Extraction and purification of effective antimicrobial constituents of *Terminalia chebula* Retz. against methicillin-resistant *Staphylococcus aureus*. Biological and Pharmaceutical Bulletin 20(4):401

9 Phadke SA, Kulkarni SD 1989 Screening of *in vitro* antibacterial activity of *Terminalia chebula, Eclipta alba* and *Ocimum sanctum*. Indian Journal of Medical Sciences 43(5):113

10 Kurokawa M, Nagasaka K, Hirabayashi T et al

1995 Efficacy of traditional herbal medicines in combination with acyclovir against herpes simplex virus type I infection *in vitro* and *in vivo*. Antiviral Research 27(1–2):19

11 El-Mekkawy S, Meselhy MR, Kusumoto IT, Kadota S, Hattori M, Namba T 1995 Inhibitory effects of Egyptian folk medicines on human immunodeficiency virus (HIV) reverse transcriptase. Chemical and Pharmaceutical Bulletin 43(4):641

12 Sohni YR, Bhatt RM 1996 Activity of a crude extract formulation in experimental hepatic amoebiasis and in immunomodulation studies. Journal of Ethnopharmacology 54(2–3):119

13 Sohni YR, Bhatt RM 1995 The antiamoebic effects of crude drug formulation of herbal extracts against *Entamoeba histolytica in vitro* and *in vivo*. Journal of Ethnopharmacology 45(1):43

14 Fu N, Quan L, Huang L, Zhang R, Chen Y 1992 Antioxidant action of extract of *Terminalia chebula* and its preventive effect on DNA breaks in human white cells induced by TPA. Chinese Traditional Herbal Drugs 23(1):26

15 Dhar ML, Dhar MM, Dhawan BN, Mehrotra BN, Ray C 1968 Screening of Indian plants for biological activity. Part I. Indian Journal of Experimental Biology 6:232

Tinospora cordifolia (Willd.) Miers. (Menispermaceae) (syn. *T. glabra* (N. Burm) Merr., *Menispermum cordifolium* Willd.)

English: Gulancha tinospora
Hindi: *Guruchi*
Sanskrit: *Guluchi, amrita*

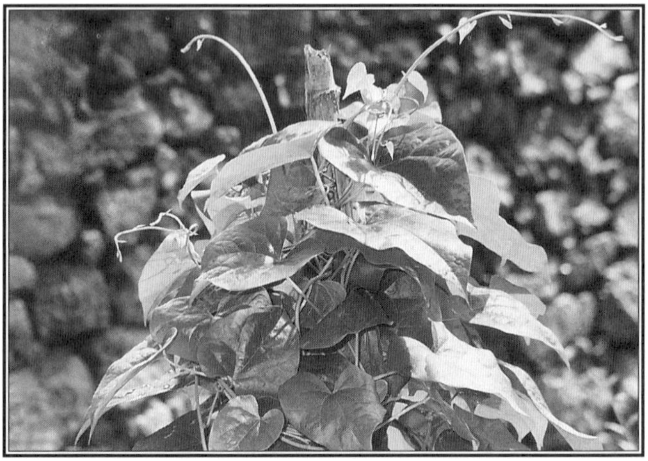

The term *amrita* refers to a heavenly elixir which was reputed to protect the celestial people from senescence and keep them eternally young.

Habitat

The plant grows throughout India from Kumaon to Kanyakumari.

Botanical description

Large, glabrous twiner with terete stem with long filiform, fleshy, aerial roots (Plate 64). The stem has a loose greyish bark when mature. The leaves are simple, alternate, long petioled and possess a characteristic heart shape, giving the name *cordifolia* to the plant. Flowers are green, unisexual, in dioecious spikes. The fruits are ovoid, glossy, red drupes, containing curved seeds.

Parts used

Stem, root and leaves.

Traditional and modern use

A decoction of leaves is used for the treatment of gout. The root is a powerful emetic and is used for visceral obstructions. Water extract is used in leprosy. It is used as a bactericide, emetic, tonic, stimulant, diuretic, aphrodisiac, sedative, stomachic and in asthma, erysipelas, fever, gout, inflammation, jaundice, leprosy, rheumatism, sores, tuberculosis, tumours, liver disorders and malaria.

Ethnoveterinary usage

The whole plant is used in scabies in swine. The vine is used as an appetiser and for internal parasites in ruminants and for diarrhoea in poultry.[1] It is also used in stomach trouble. Stem, root and whole plant are used in sprain, abscess, tumour, wound, broken horn, cracked tail, anthrax, as a galactagogue and in the treatment of pneumonia, asthma, cough, swelling of lungs colic, constipation, tetanus, pox and compound fracture.

Major chemical constituents

Diterpenes

Columbin, chasmanthin, palmarin, tinosporone, tinosporic acid, tinosporol, tinosporaside, cordifolisides A, B, C, D and E, cordioside, syringin and cordiol have all been isolated from the plant.[2]

Alkaloids

Berberine and related alkaloids have been reported, although this has been disputed.[3]

Medicinal and pharmacological activities

Antiallergic activity: An aqueous extract of *T. cordifolia* decreased bronchospasm in guinea pigs, decreased capillary permeability in mice and reduced the number of disrupted mast cells in rats.[4]

Anticancer activity: A formulation containing *Tinospora cordifolia, Asparagus racemosus, Withania somnifera* and *Picrorrhiza kurroa* markedly inhibited the suppression of chemotactic activity and production of interleukin-1 and tumour necrosis factor induced by the carcinogen ochratoxin in mouse macrophages.[5]

Antineoplastic activity: Aqueous, methanolic and dichloromethane extracts of *T. cordifolia* showed dose-dependent increases in lethality to HeLa cells in vitro. The most potent activity was found in the dichloromethane extract.[6]

Antioxidant activity: An extract of *T. cordifolia* reduced the toxicity induced by free radicals and inhibited lipid peroxidation and the generation of superoxide and hydroxyl radicals in vitro. It reduced the toxic side effects of cyclophosphamide in mice, as shown by the total white blood cell count, bone marrow cellularity and esterase-positive cells. It also partially reduced elevated lipid peroxides in serum and liver, as well as alkaline phosphatase and glutamine pyruvate transaminase.[7]

Antistress activity: An ethanolic extract of the roots of *T. cordifolia* normalised stress-induced biochemical changes in norepinephrine, dopamine, 5-hydroxytryptamine and 5-hydroxyindoleacetic acid levels in experimental rat models.[8]

Antiulcer activity: An ethanolic extract of the roots of *T. cordifolia*, in combination with *Centella asiatica*, afforded significant protective action against restraint stress-induced ulcer formation. The activity was comparable to diazepam in rats.[9]

Immunomodulatory activity: Syringin and cordiol, isolated from *T. cordifolia*, inhibited the in vitro immunohaemolysis of antibody-coated sheep erythrocytes by guinea pig serum. This was found to be due to inhibition of C3-convertase in the classic complement pathway. Humoral and cell-mediated immunity were also dose dependently enhanced and an increase in IgG antibody in serum was observed. Cordioside, cordiofolioside and cordiol also activated macrophages significantly.[2] In order to elucidate the mode of action, colony-forming units of the granulocyte-macrophage series (CFU-GM) in mouse serum were treated with *T. cordifolia*. The extract induced a significant ($p<0.01$) increase in the number of CFU-GM, indicating that activation of macrophages by *T. cordifolia* had occurred, leading to an increase in leucocytosis and enhanced neutrophil functions.[10] The protective effects were also studied in *Escherichia coli*-induced peritonitis and compared with gentamicin. Pretreatment of mice with *T. cordifolia* or gentamicin reduced the mortality rate of those injected with 1×10^8 *E. coli*, from 100% in the control to 17.8% and 11.1% respectively. This was associated with a significantly improved bacterial clearance and improved phagocytic and intracellular bactericidal capacities of neutrophils in the *T. cordifolia*-treated groups. Gentamicin cleared bacteria rapidly, although polymorph phagocytosis remained depressed.[11] In obstructive jaundice, phagocytic and microbicidal activity of polymorphonuclear cells (PMN) tend to be lower than normal. In a model of cholestasis using rats, a depression in the activity of PMN and peritoneal macrophages was observed and the rats showed an increased susceptibility to *E. coli* infection. Treating the animals with a water extract of *T. cordifolia* improved cellular immune functions and mortality following *E. coli* infection was significantly reduced. The study showed that cholestasis resulted in immunosuppression and suggests a role for immunomodulation in the management of obstructive jaundice.[12]

Hepatoprotective activity: A study in goats showed an improvement in clinical and haematobiochemical parameters of the liver, suggesting a protective action for *T. cordifolia*.[13]

Hypoglycaemic activity: The aqueous, alcoholic and chloroform extracts of the leaves of *T. cordifolia* exerted a significant hypoglycaemic effect in normal and alloxan-treated rabbits at doses of 50, 100, 150 and 200 mg/kg body weight.[14] Oral administration of an aqueous root extract to alloxan diabetic rats caused a significant reduction in blood glucose and brain lipids, an increase in body weight, haemoglobin and hepatic hexokinase levels, and a lowering of hepatic glucose-6-phosphatase, serum acid phosphatase, alkaline phosphatase and lactate dehydrogenase.[15]

Safety profile

Safe with appropriate clinical guidance. However, excessive doses of berberine inhibit vitamin B assimilation and can cause nausea. The maximum tolerated doses of 50% ethanolic extracts of the stem and whole plant were 250 and 500 mg/kg in adult rats.[16]

Dosage

Powder: 1–3 g

Extract: 1–2 g

Decoction: 56–112 ml

Ayurvedic properties

Rasa: *Tikta* (bitter), *kashaya* (astringent)

Guna: *Guru* (heavy), *snigdha* (unctuous)

Veerya: *Ushna* (hot)

Vipaka: *Madhur* (sweet)

Dosha: Pacifies *tridosha*

Further reading

Bharatiya Vidya Bhavan's Swami Prakashananda Ayurveda Research Centre 1992 Selected medicinal plants of India. Chemexcil, Mumbai

Ministry of Health and Family Welfare 1989 Ayurvedic pharmacopoeia of India, vol 1. Government of India, New Delhi

Sairam TV 1999 Home remedies, vol II. Penguin India, New Delhi

Sivarajan VV, Balachandran I 1994 Ayurvedic drugs and their plant sources. Oxford and IBH Publishing, New Delhi

References

1 International Institute of Rural Reconstruction 1994 Ethnoveterinary medicine in Asia. An information kit on traditional animal health care practices. Part I, general information. IIRR, Silang, Philippines

2 Kapil A, Sharma S 1997 Immunopotentiating compounds: *Tinospora cordifolia*. Journal of Ethnopharmacology 58:89

3 Bisset NG, Nwaiwa J 1983 Quaternary alkaloids of *Tinospora* species. Planta Medica 48:225

4 Nayampalli SS, Desai NK, Ainapure SS 1988 Antiallergic properties of *Tinospora cordifolia* in animal models. Indian Journal of Pharmacology 18(4):250

5 Dhuley JN 1997 Effect of some Indian herbs on macrophage functions in ochratoxin A treated mice. Journal of Ethnopharmacology 58(1):15

6 Jagetia GC, Nayak V, Vidyasagar MS 1998 Evaluation of the antineoplastic activity of guduchi (*Tinospora cordifolia*) in cultured HeLa cells. Cancer Letters 127(1–2):71

7 Mathew S, Kuttan G 1997 Antioxidant activity of *Tinospora cordifolia* and its usefulness in the amelioration of cyclophosphamide induced toxicity. Journal of Experimental and Clinical Cancer Research 16(4):407

8 Sarma DNK, Khosa RL, Chansauria JPN, Ray AK 1995 Effect of *Tinospora cordifolia* on brain neurotransmitters in stressed rats. Fitoterapia 66(5):421

9 Sarma DNK, Khosa RL, Chansauria JPN, Sahai M 1995 Antiulcer activity of *Tinospora cordifolia* Miers and *Centella asiatica* Linn. extracts. Phytotherapy Research 9(8):589

10 Thatte UM, Rao SG, Dahanukar SA 1994 *Tinospora cordifolia* induces colony stimulating activity in serum. Journal of Postgraduate Medicine 40(4):202

11 Thatte UM, Kulkarni MR, Dahanukar SA 1992 Immunotherapeutic modification of *Escherichia coli* peritonitis and bacteremia by *Tinospora cordifolia*. Journal of Postgraduate Medicine 38(1):13

12 Rege NN, Nazareth HM, Bapat RD, Dahanukar SA 1989 Modulation of immunosuppression in obstructive jaundice by *Tinospora cordifolia*. Indian Journal of Medical Research 90:478

13 Peer F, Sharma MC 1989 Therapeutic evaluation of *Tinospora cordifolia* in carbon tetrachloride induced hepatopathy in goats. Indian Journal of Veterinary Medicine 9(2):154

14 Wadood N, Wadood A, Shah SAW 1992 Effect of *Tinospora cordifolia* on blood glucose and total lipid levels of normal and alloxan-diabetic rabbits. Planta Medica 58(2):131

15 Stanley P, Prince M, Menon VP 2000 Hypoglycaemic and other related actions of *Tinospora cordifolia* roots in alloxan-induced diabetic rats. Journal of Ethnopharmacology 70(1):9

16 Dhar ML, Dhar MM, Dhawan BN, Mehrotra BN, Ray C 1968 Screening of Indian plants for biological activity: Part I. Indian Journal of Experimental Biology 6:232

Trachyspermum ammi L. Sprague (Umbelliferae)(syn. *Carum copticum* Benth. Hook; *Sison ammi* L.)

English: Ajowan, omum, bishop's weed

Hindi: *Ajwain*

Sanskrit: *Yavanika, agnivardhana*

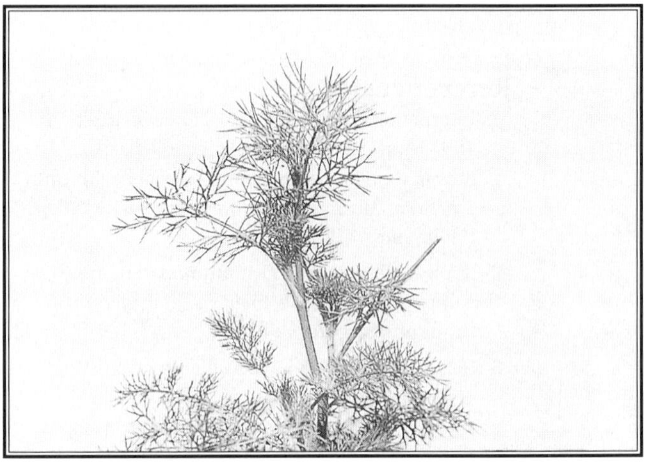

The name *agnivardhana* implies stimulation of the digestive fire or *agni*. It has been employed medicinally since ancient times and was described by the seer Charaka as useful in urticaria and as an antiflatulent and anticolic drug. Ajowan, with its characteristic aromatic smell and pungent taste, is widely used as a spice in curries, pickles, biscuits, confectionery and beverages. The crushed seeds are also dried for use in scented powders and pot pourri.

Habitat

The herb originated in the Mediterranean region and is now cultivated in Iraq, Iran, Afghanistan and Pakistan. Commercial ajowan is mainly produced in India and grown throughout the country, mainly in the plains but also at higher altitudes. Under irrigation, it is grown extensively as a garden crop or in small fields. The plant also grows in Africa, China and other countries of central Asia.

Botanical description

An erect, glabrous or minutely pubescent, branched annual up to 30–90 cm tall (Plate 65). Stems striate; leaves rather distant, 2–3 pinnately divided, segments linear, ultimate segments 1–2.5 cm long. The flowers are white and small, occurring in terminal or lateral pedunculate, compound umbels. Fruits ovoid, muricate, cremocarps, 2–3 mm long, greyish brown; mericarps compressed, with distinct ridges and tubercular surface. The essential oil obtained from the seed is a yellowish-orange or reddish liquid with a herbaceous-spicy medicinal odour, much like thyme.

Parts used

Seed, oil.

Traditional and modern use

The seeds are carminative, stimulant and antispasmodic and are given in colic and diarrhoea. For the relief of flatulence and dyspepsia, they may be eaten with betel leaves or rock salt and a mixture of the seeds and buttermilk is a commonly used expectorant. They are considered efficacious in sore throats, bronchitis and for habitual drunkenness and as a stimulating decongestant for the respiratory and digestive tracts. Internally the seeds are given for colds, coughs, influenza, asthma, arthritis and rheumatism and are a component of many important Ayurvedic formulations. Crude crystals from the oil, known as *Ajwain-ka-phool*, are used in stomach ache. In Unani medicine ajowan is used as a liver tonic, an antiinflammatory agent and for paralysis. The tincture, essential oil and extracted thymol have been used in Indian medicine to treat cholera. The distilled oil in water, sometimes known as 'omum water', is used as an antiseptic, to aid digestion and applied externally for relief of rheumatic and neuralgic pains. A paste of the seeds may be applied topically to relieve colic pains and a hot dry fomentation of the seeds is a household remedy for asthma. For relief of migraine and delirium the seeds are sometimes smoked or taken as snuff.

Ethnoveterinary usage

The seeds are used in stoppage of rumination and chewing the cud, pox, fever, mastitis, tympanitis, haematuria, ascites and indigestion.[1]

Major chemical constituents

Monoterpenoids

The essential oil contains thymol as the major component, with p-cymene, dipentene, α-pinene, β-pinene, γ-terpinene, camphene, myrcene, δ-3-carene, limonene, carvacrol and others.[2,3]

Glycosides

The seed contains 6-O-β-D-glucopyranosyloxythymol.[4]

Fatty acids

Fixed oil extracted from the seeds was found to contain resin acids, palmitic acid, petroselenic acid, oleic acid and linoleic acid.[5]

Vitamins and trace elements

The fruit contains riboflavin, thiamin, nicotinic acid, carotene, calcium, chromium, cobalt, copper, iodine, iron, manganese, phosphorus and zinc.[6]

Medicinal and pharmacological activities

Antiplatelet activity: An ether extract of *Trachyspermum ammi* inhibited platelet aggregation induced by arachidonic acid (AA), epinephrine and collagen. It reduced thromboxane B2 formation from added arachidonate in intact platelet preparations and also after stimulation with Ca^{2+} ionophore A23187. A direct action on cyclooxygenase was indicated as there was no effect on the release of AA from labelled platelets. An increased formation of lipoxygenase-derived products from exogenous AA in treated platelets was also observed, apparently due to the redirection of AA metabolism from the cyclooxygenase to the lipoxygenase pathway.[7]

Hypotensive activity: In anaesthetised rats, thymol (1–10 mg/kg) produced a dose-dependent fall in blood pressure and heart rate. These effects were not blocked by atropine (1 mg/kg) and thymol did not modify the presser response of norepinephrine, eliminating the possibility of cholinergic stimulation or adrenergic blockade. In spontaneously beating atria, thymol caused a decrease in force and rate of atrial contractions which remained unaltered in the presence of atropine. In rabbit aorta, thymol caused relaxation of norepinephrine- and potassium-induced contractions in a concentration-dependent manner. These relaxant effects remained unchanged after the removal of the endothelium. Moreover, atropine, propranolol, indomethacin and glibenclamide did not alter vasorelaxation, suggesting that thymol exhibits calcium channel blocking activity, which may explain the hypotensive and bradycardiac effects.[8]

Inhibition of the hepatitis C virus: The methanol extract of *Trachyspermum ammi* showed inhibitory effects on hepatitis C virus protease, using in vitro assay methods. It showed 90% inhibition at 100 μg/ml.[9]

Insecticidal activity: The oil of *Trachyspermum spp*. exhibited significant larvicidal activity against *Aedes aegypti* and *Culex quinquefasciatus*. It also produced significant metamorphic inhibition against *Dysdercus koenigii*, oviposition deterrence against *Phthorimaea operculella* and antifeedant effects against *Spodoptera litura* and *Achoea janata*.[10]

Molluscicidal activity: The effects of sublethal treatment with *Trachyspermum ammi* in combination with piperonyl butoxide (PBO) on the reproduction of the snail *Lymnaea acuminata* were studied. The combination of its active molluscicidal component (thymol) with PBO caused a significant reduction in fecundity, rate of hatching and survival of young snails.[11] In vivo exposure of *Lymnaea acuminata* to thymol indicated that it significantly altered acetylcholinesterase, lactic dehydrogenase, succinic dehydrogenase and cytooxidase activity in the nervous tissue of snails. However, in vitro exposure produced an effect only on acetylcholinesterase and lactic dehydrogenase. Thymol affected all known neurotransmission mechanisms in the snail via a complex interaction, which may account for its toxicity to snails.[12]

Antifungal activity: The essential oil demonstrated toxicity to *Aspergillus niger* and *Curvularia ovoidea*, two common storage fungi, inhibiting the mycelial growth of both test fungi completely at a minimum inhibitory concentration (MIC) of 500 ppm, at which level it was fungicidal. The oil also showed a broad fungitoxic spectrum.[13] Toxicity to the mycelial growth of *Macrophomina phaseolina* was also seen in vitro, at an MIC of 200 ppm. At this concentration the oil was fungistatic, but not phytotoxic, to germinating French beans (*Phaseolus vulgaris*). The oil was thermostable and more efficacious than some synthetic fungicides, including Benlate, Ceresan, copper oxychloride, Dithan M-45 and Thiovit. Thymol was also isolated as the main fungitoxic factor.[14] In another study *Trachyspermum ammi* oil inhibited growth of *Aspergillus flavus* and *A. niger* completely at an MIC of 800 ppm. At this concentration it was fungicidal in 50 seconds and the effect persisted for at least 365 days of storage. Peanuts, the seeds of *Arachis hypogea*, could be protected from fungal deterioration during storage by treating with the oil at 5000 ppm. Thymol and p-cymene isolated from the oil showed antifungal properties at 1000 ppm.[15] The oil was more active than some synthetic fungicides to *Helminthosporium oryzae* and was also toxic to various human pathogens.[16]

Antibacterial activity: The oil was shown to be antibacterial to *Salmonella typhosa*, *Micrococcus pyogenes* var. *aureus* and *E. coli*.[17] Thymol is well known as an antiseptic.

Spermicidal activity: Oil of ajowan showed spermicidal activity on human spermatozoa in vitro.[18]

Safety profile

The undiluted oil is a mucous membrane and dermal irritant. Due to the high thymol content it should be avoided in pregnancy. The acute oral LD_{50} of thymol is reported as 0.98 g/kg in the rat and 0.88 g in the guinea pig.[19]

Dosage

Powder: 3–6 g

Extract: 125 mg

Ayurvedic properties

Rasa: *Katu* (pungent), *tikta* (bitter)

Guna: *Laghu* (light), *ruksha* (dry), *tikshna* (sharp)

Veerya: *Ushna* (hot)

Vipaka: *Katu* (pungent)

Dosha: Promotes *pitta*, pacifies *vata* and *kapha*

Further reading

Bown D 1995 Encyclopaedia of herbs and their uses. Dorling Kindersley, London

Bharatiya Vidya Bhavan's Swami Prakashananda Ayurveda Research Centre 1992 Selected medicinal plants of India. Chemexcil, Mumbai

Kapoor LD 1990 Handbook of Ayurvedic medicinal plants. CRC Press, Boca Raton

Ministry of Health and Family Welfare 1989 Ayurvedic pharmacopoeia of India, vol III. Government of India, New Delhi

Sairam TV 1998 Home remedies, vol I. Penguin India, New Delhi

Thakur RS, Puri HS, Husain A 1989 Major medicinal plants of India. CIMAP, Lucknow

References

1 Jha MK 1992 The folk veterinary system of Bihar – a research survey. NDDB, Anand, Gujrat

2 Nigam IC, Skakum W, Levi L 1963 Determination of trace constituents of oil of ajowan. Perfume and Essential Oil Research 54:25

3 Nagalakshmi S, Shankaracharya NB, Naik JP, Jagan Mohan Rao L 2000 Studies on chemical and technological aspects of ajowan (*Trachyspermum ammi* syn. *Carum copticum*) seeds. Journal of Food Science and Technology 37(3):277

4 Garg SN, Kumar S 1998 A new glucoside from *Trachyspermum ammi*. Fitoterapia 69(6):511

5 Farooq MO, Osman SM, Ahmad MS 1953 The fixed oil from the seeds of *Carum copticum*. Journal of the Science of Food and Agriculture 4:132

6 Duke JA 1992 Handbook of phytochemical constituents of GRAS herbs and other economic plants. CRC Press, Boca Raton

7 Srivastava KC 1988 Extract of a spice – Omum (*Trachyspermum ammi*) – shows antiaggregatory effects and alters arachidonic acid metabolism in human platelets. Prostaglandins, Leukotrienes and Essential Fatty Acids 33(1):1

8 Aftab K, Atta-Ur-Rahman, Usmanghani K 1995 Blood pressure lowering action of active principle from *Trachyspermum ammi* (L.) Sprague. Phytomedicine 2(1):35

9 Hussein G, Miyashiro H, Nakamura N, Hattori M, Kakiuchi N, Shimotohno K 2000 Inhibitory effects of Sudanese medicinal plant extracts on hepatitis C virus (HCV) protease. Phytotherapy Research 14(7):510

10 Tare V 2001 Bioactivity of some medicinal plants against chosen insect pests/vectors. Journal of Medicinal and Aromatic Plant Sciences 23:120

11 Singh K, Singh DK 2000 Effect of different combinations of MGK-264 or piperonyl butoxide with plant-derived molluscicides on snail reproduction. Archives of Environmental Contamination and Toxicology 38(2):182

12 Singh VK, Singh S, Singh DK 1999 Effect of active molluscicidal component of spices on different enzyme activities and biogenic amine levels in the nervous tissue of *Lymnaea acuminata*. Phytotherapy Research 13(8):649

13 Singh J, Tripathi NN 1999 Inhibition of storage fungi of blackgram (*Vigna mungo* L.) by some essential oils. Flavour and Fragrance Journal 14(1):1

14 Dwivedi SK, Singh KP 1998 Fungi toxicity of some higher plant products against *Macrophomina phaseolina* (Tassi) Goid. Flavour and Fragrance Journal 13(6):397

15 Tripathi SC, Singh SP, Dube S 1986 Studies on antifungal properties of essential oil of *Trachyspermum ammi* (L.) Sprague. Journal of Phytopathology 116(2):113

16 Singh AK, Dikshit A, Sharma ML, Dixit SN 1980 Fungitoxic activity of some essential oils. Economic Botany 34(2):186

17 Council of Scientific and Industrial Research 1976 The wealth of India: a dictionary of Indian raw materials and industrial products. PID, CSIR, New Delhi

18 Buch JG, Dikshit RK, Mansuri SM 1988 Effect of certain volatile oils on ejaculated human spermatozoa. Indian Journal of Medical Research 87:361

19 Jenner PM 1964 Food flavouring and compounds of related structure-I. Acute oral toxicity. Food and Cosmetics Toxicology 2:327

Tribulus terrestris L. (Zygophyllaceae)

English: Caltrops
Hindi: *Gokhru*
Sanskrit: *Gokshura*

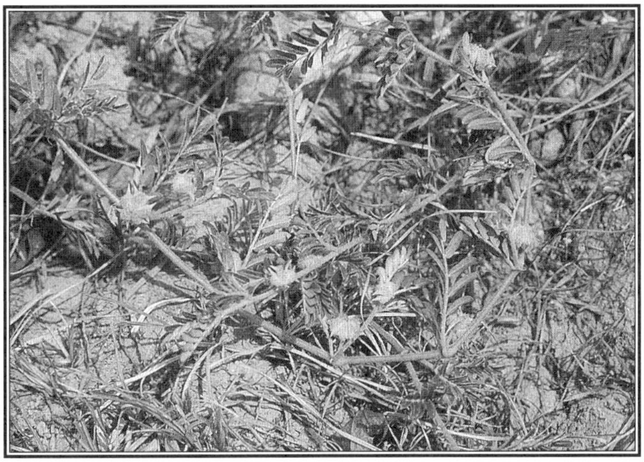

The name *gokhru* derives from the appearance of the fruit, which resembles the cloven hoof of a cow. It is a component of several Ayurvedic preparations and is used worldwide for many different applications.

Habitat

The plant grows throughout India, China, Vietnam, parts of Europe and South Africa on wasteland.

Botanical description

It is a thorny, perennial, trailing plant, up to 90 cm in length (Plate 66). The leaves are composed of 5–8 pairs of leaflets, subequal and oblong. Flowers are solitary and pale yellow in colour and the fruits are globose, each with two pairs of spines, one pair longer than the other, with five woody cocci each containing several seeds. The roots are cylindrical, 10–15 cm long, light brown and faintly aromatic.

Parts used

Fruit, root.

Traditional and modern use

The fruits are used for many purposes, including as an aperient, aperitif, astringent, antiinflammatory, emmenagogue, stomachic, tonic, diuretic, alterative, galactagogue and aphrodisiac. They are used in bladder disorders as a diuretic and to treat urinary calculi and for hepatitis, rheumatism and skin complaints including psoriasis, leprosy and scabies. The seeds are astringent and diuretic and are sometimes given to women to aid fecundity.

Ethnoveterinary usage

The fruits and whole plant are used in bloody dysentery, urinary disorders in ruminants and rheumatism.[1]

Major chemical constituents

Phytosterols and saponins

The fruits yielded protodioscin, the terrestrosins A–E, desgalactotigonin, F-gitonin, desglucolanatigonin, gitonin and other tigogenin and furostanol glycosides together with β-sitosterol, spirosta-3,5-diene and stigmasterol. The flowers also contain steroidal sapogenins based on diosgenin, hecogenin and ruscogenin.[2,3]

Flavonoids

Kaempferol and quercetin are present in the flowers.[4]

Lignans

Tribulusamides A and B have been isolated.[2,4]

Medicinal and pharmacological activities

Antiurolithitic activity: An ethanolic extract of *Tribulus terrestris* provided a strong, dose-dependent protection against calculus formation induced by glass bead implantation in albino rats. The activity was traced to the aqueous methanolic fraction.[5] The litholytic effect was also studied in rats where hyperoxalurea had been induced and maintained by hydroxypyroline and sodium glycolate. Oral administration of an aqueous extract caused urinary oxalate excretion to reverse to normal within 21 days of administration and it remained so until 15 days after withdrawal of the extract and sodium glycolate.[6] Another study confirmed these effects of *Tribulus terrestris* extract and a possible mechanism was proposed: inhibition of the enzyme glycolic acid oxidase (GAO) which catalyses the conversion of glycolate to glyoxylate. GAO activity results in the oxidation of glycolic acid to glyoxylate, which is a potentially toxic metabolite, and finally to oxalate. The aqueous extract of *Tribulus terrestris* has also been shown to have a high potassium content which may be responsible for the diuretic effect.[7]

Nephroprotective activity: The renal damage produced by gentamicin was decreased when given simultaneously with *Tribulus terrestris* extract to rats.[8]

Antimicrobial activity: Extracts of the fruit and leaf of *Tribulus terrestris* were active against *Escherichia coli* and *Staphylococcus aureus*.[9,10]

Cardiac stimulant activity: A semipurified aqueous fraction had a potent stimulant effect on isolated heart muscle. An increase in the force of contraction, together with a negative chronotropic effect, was noted.[11] Saponins isolated from *Tribulus terrestris* resulted in dilation of the coronary artery and improved coronary circulation in patients suffering from coronary heart disease.[12]

Fertility potentiating activity: Furostanol biglycosides isolated from the alcoholic extract stimulated spermatogenesis and Sertoli cell activity in rats. Terrestrioside-F increased libido and sexual response in male rats, and potentiated oestrus and increased fertility in female rats.[13]

Management of sexual dysfunction: Protodioscin is thought to improve sexual desire and enhance erection via the conversion of protodioscin to DHEA (dehydroepiandrosterone). However, the plant does not consistently produce protodioscin.[14] A study was conducted to investigate the effect of *Tribulus terrestris* extract on isolated corpus cavernosum tissue of rabbits to determine the mechanism by which protodioscin exerts its effects. The extract was administered orally, once daily, for a period of 8 weeks, in varying doses. The rabbits were then sacrificed and their penile tissue isolated to evaluate responses to pharmacological agents and electrical field stimulation. The relaxant responses to acetylcholine, nitroglycerin and EFS compared to their control values, and the lack of effect on the contractile response to noradrenaline and histamine, indicated that protodioscin has proerectile activity, which may account for its claims as an aphrodisiac. This may be due to an increase in nitric oxide release from the endothelium and nitrergic neurons.[15]

Cytotoxicity: An ethanolic extract was tested on FL-cells using the neutral red assay and was found to be active.[16]

Safety profile

The maximum tolerated dose of a 50% ethanolic extract of fruit was 100 mg/kg in rats.[17]

Dosage

Infusion: 4–8 ml

Decoction: 56–112 ml

Powder: 0.5–1 g

Ayurvedic properties

Rasa: *Madhur* (sweet)

Guna: *Guru* (heavy), *snigdha* (unctuous)

Veerya: *Shita* (cold)

Vipaka: *Madhur* (sweet)

Dosha: Pacifies *vata* and *pitta*

Further reading

Bharatiya Vidya Bhavan's Swami Prakashananda Ayurveda Research Centre 1992 Selected medicinal plants of India. Chemexcil, Mumbai

Ministry of Health and Family Welfare 1989 Ayurvedic pharmacopoeia of India, vol 1. Government of India, New Delhi

Sairam TV 1999 Home remedies, vol II. Penguin India, New Delhi

References

1 International Institute of Rural Reconstruction 1994 Ethnoveterinary medicine in Asia. An information kit on traditional animal health care practices. Part I, general information. IIRR, Silang, Philippines

2 Bedir E, Khan IA 2000 New steroidal glycosides from the fruits of *Tribulus terrestris*. Journal of Natural Products 63(12):1699

3 Yan W, Ohtani K, Kasai R, Yamasaki K 1996 Steroidal saponins from fruits of *Tribulus terrestris*. Phytochemistry 42(5):1417

4 Zafar R, Aeri V 1992 Constituents of *Tribulus terrestris* flowers. Fitoterapia 63(1):90

5 Anand R, Patnaik GK, Kulshreshtha DK, Dhawan BN 1994 Activity of certain fractions of *Tribulus terrestris* fruits against experimentally induced urolithiasis in rats. Indian Journal of Experimental Biology 32(8):548

6 Sangeeta D, Sidhu H, Thind SK, Nath R, Vaidyanathan S 1993 Therapeutic response of *Tribulus terrestris* (Gokhru) aqueous extract on hyperoxaluria in male adult rats. Phytotherapy Research 7(2):116

7 Sangeeta D, Sidhu H, Thind SK, Nath R 1994 Effect of *Tribulus terrestris* on oxalate metabolism in rats. Journal of Ethnopharmacology 44(2):61

8 Nagarkatti DS, Rege NN, Mittal BV, Uchil DA, Desai NK, Dhanukar SA 1994 Nephroprotection by *Tribulus terrestris*. Update Ayurveda, Bombay

9 Singh RH 1974 Antibacterial activity of some Ayurvedic drugs. Journal of Research in Indian Medicine 9(2):66

10 George M, Venkataraman PR, Pandalai KM 1947 Investigations on plant antibiotics II. Journal of Science and Industrial Research 6B(3):42

11 Seth SD, Jagdeesh G 1976 Cardiac action of *T. terrestris* L. Indian Journal of Medical Research 64(12):1821

12 Bowen W, Long'en M, Tongku L 1990 Clinical observation on 406 cases of angina pectoris of coronary heart disease treated with saponin of *Tribulus terrestris*. Chinese Journal of Integrated Traditional and Western Medicine 10(2):85

13 Kumar P, Despande PJ, Singh LM 1980 Studies on urolithylitic action of indigenous drugs. J. Science Res. and Plant Med. (India) 1:9

14 Adimoelja A 2000 Phytochemicals and the breakthrough of traditional herbs in the management of sexual dysfunctions. International Journal of Andrology 23(suppl 2):82

15 Adaikan PG, Gauthaman K, Prasad RN, Ng SC 2000 Proerectile pharmacological effects of *Tribulus terrestris* extract on the rabbit corpus cavernosum. Annals of the Academy of Medicine of Singapore 29(1):22

16 Ali NA, Julich WD, Kusnick C, Lindequist U 2001 Screening of Yemeni medicinal plants for antibacterial and cytotoxic activities. Journal of Ethnopharmacology 74(2):173

17 Dhar ML, Dhar MM, Dhawan BN, Mehrotra BN, Ray C 1968 Screening of Indian plants for biological activity: Part I. Indian Journal of Experimental Biology 6:245

Trigonella foenum-graecum L. (Fabaceae)

English: Fenugreek, bird's foot

Hindi: *Methi*

Sanskrit: *Methika*

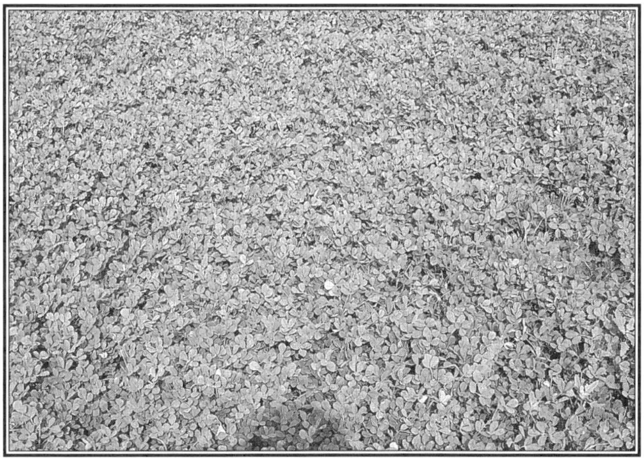

Fenugreek has been in use as a food and flavouring since time immemorial. The specific name *foenum-graecum* means 'Greek hay', since it was used there at one time to improve the nutritional quality of low-grade fodder. The herb is still used in parts of Europe to improve the palatability of poor hay. Both the seeds and leaves are well regarded for their medicinal value and were held in high esteem in India, Egypt, Greece and Italy in the time of the Romans.

Habitat

Indigenous to eastern Europe, the herb is now grown widely as a field crop for its leaves and seeds, and cultivated mainly in southern France, Turkey, northern Africa, India and China. It is naturalised throughout the Mediterranean region, India, China and Africa, as far south as Ethiopia.

Botanical description

A robust, erect, aromatic annual herb reaching up to 60 cm in height (Plate 67). The leaves are compound, up to 5 cm in length, with long pedicels. Leaflets are lanceolate or obovate, about 2.5 cm long, with slightly toothed margins. The flowers are axillary, occurring singly or in pairs, sessile, yellow in colour. The fruits are typically leguminous pods 5–8 cm long, narrow and with a persistent 'beak', enclosing 10–20 golden yellow seeds, which possess a characteristic savoury aroma.

Parts used

Dried seeds, leaves.

Traditional and modern use

Young plants and aromatic leaves are often eaten as a vegetable and the seeds are widely used as a condiment in curries. A poultice made of the herb can be applied locally to relieve swelling and the leaves are also made into paste and applied over burns or to the scalp to prevent premature greying of the hair. Internally, the leaves may be taken for indigestion and bilious disorders and a decoction of the whole herb is given for leucorrhoea. The seeds are given to breastfeeding mothers to increase the flow of milk. Various traditional Indian preparations are made from the seeds, together with other herbal ingredients, for example in the treatment of dyspepsia and to regulate blood sugar. After roasting, the seeds are powdered and given in dysentery and in the central Himalayas they are given to children with worm infestations.

Ethnoveterinary usage

The seeds are mixed with cottonseed and given to cattle to enhance milk production and utilised in the manufacture of nutritional supplements for horses and cattle. In rural areas of Bihar, they are applied over swellings and wounds in cattle. The seeds are also given to ruminants and poultry with diarrhoea and are considered useful in ruminants after calving.[1,2]

Major chemical constituents

Saponins

The sapogenins diosgenin, hederagin, tigogenin, neotigogenin, yuccagenin, gitogenin, smilagenin, sarsasapogenin and yamogenin have been isolated from the seed, together with their glycosides such as foenugraecin, trigoneosides Ia, Ib, IIa, IIIa, IIIb, IVa, Va, Vb, VI, VIIb and VIIIb, trigofoenosides A, B, C, and D, and fenugrin B.[3–8]

Coumarins

3,4,7, Trimethyl coumarin, 4, methyl coumarin and trigocoumarin.[9,10]

Flavonoids

Isoorientin, isovitexin, orientin, saponaretin, vicenin-l, kaempferol, quercetin, lilyn, vitexin, tricin, tricin-7-O-D-glucopyranoside, naringenin and luteolin have been reported in the stems and seeds.[11,12]

Alkaloids and aminoacids

Trigonelline, choline 4-hydroxyisoleucine, lysine, tryptophan, histidine, arginine, cystine and tyrosine are present.[13]

Carbohydrates

Sucrose, glucose, fructose, myoinositol, galactose, raffinose, verbascose, digalactosylmyoinositol, galactomannan, xylose and arabinose.[14]

Others

Calcium, iron, potassium, ascorbic acid, nicotinic acid, thiamin, riboflavin, biotin, β-carotene, fixed oil and traces of essential oil.[13,14,15]

Medicinal and Pharmacological activities

Antidiabetic activity: The seeds of *Trigonella foenum-graecum* have been extensively studied for antidiabetic properties in animals as well as in human clinical studies.[13] Creatine kinase levels were decreased compared to control subjects in the tissues of rats induced with experimental diabetes after administration of fenugreek. The seeds alone, and in combination with vanadate, produced a normalisation of glucose-6-phosphatase and fructose-1, 6-bisphosphatase in the liver and kidney of diabetic rats, with a combination of both showing the most potent lowering effect. Fenugreek seeds have also been reported to normalise the activity of glyoxalase I in the diabetic liver of experimental rats.[16,17,18] At a dose of 2 and 8 g/kg in normal and alloxan-induced diabetic rats it produced a significant, dose-dependent fall in blood glucose levels[19] and both doses showed marked hypoglycaemic effects in normal mice.[20] The hypoglycaemic activity of the seeds and various extracts was studied in experimental rabbits and the glucose tolerance test showed a significant hypoglycaemic activity in the alkaloid-rich fraction.[21] Antidiabetic properties have also been reported by various other workers.[22–24]

The traditional use has also been validated clinically. Studies on human volunteers support the use of fenugreek seeds in diabetes, especially in non-insulin dependent diabetes mellitus (NIDDM). In a controlled clinical trial, the effect of three preparations of the seeds (raw, boiled and germinated) was seen in six healthy and six diabetic patients taking raw and germinated seeds. Raw and germinated seeds significantly reduced postprandial glucose levels in all subjects; however, boiled seeds did not produce any such effects.[25] A trial conducted on 21 NIDDM patients showed that whole seeds of fenugreek lowered postprandial blood glucose levels. This effect was seen with a single dose (15 g) taken with the test meal, although no significant changes in insulin levels were noted.[26] In another study, defatted seeds, when given to 15 NIDDM patients for 10 days, resulted in a significant decrease in fasting blood glucose levels and a reduction in urinary glucose excretion by 64%. This suggests an effect of dietary fibre in intestinal absorption and an improvement in peripheral insulin activity, as possible mechanisms of action for the improvements in diabetic parameters.[27] As well as an improvement in biochemical parameters, fenugreek seeds suppressed some of the clinical symptoms of diabetes such as polyuria, polydypsia, weakness and weight loss.[28]

Hypocholesterolaemic activity: A number of experimental studies have shown hypocholesterolaemic effect in rats.[29] Fenugreek seeds have been shown to prevent the elevation of cholesterol in rats when given with a hypercholesterolaemic diet.[30] Steroidal saponins isolated from fenugreek seeds administered to rats with food (at a daily dose of 12.5 g per 300 g body weight) significantly reduced plasma cholesterol in both normal and diabetic rats.[31] One study suggests that the fraction producing the hypoglycaemic effect is also responsible for its hypocholesterolaemic effect.[32]

Antiinflammatory activity: Fenugreek seeds were screened for antiinflammatory activity against experimentally induced inflammation in albino rats. Ether, alcohol and aqueous extracts were tested in acute, subacute and chronic models of inflammation and the activity compared with that of sodium salicylate. Antiinflammatory activity was exhibited by all three extracts but the ether extract was the most potent and comparable to sodium salicylate.[33]

Antimicrobial activity: *Trigonella foenum-graecum* was screened against 26 common pathogens and demonstrated a broad-spectrum antibacterial activity.[34] The fatty oil and unsaponifiable matter of fenugreek seeds were evaluated against six bacterial and six fungal strains and the study concluded that the unsaponifiable matter was more active than the oil.[35]

Antioxidant activity: Several studies have suggested that the seeds may be useful as an antioxidant agent for preserving foods. In one study, the antioxidant potential was compared to the synthetic antioxidants butylated hydroxyanisole and butylated hydroxytoluene[37] and antioxidant activity of seeds was reported in pork patties prepared from both fresh and previously frozen meat.[38] A freeze-dried extract of fenugreek was reported to be antioxidant in a carotene and linoleic acid emulsion, with an activity comparable to standard commercial antioxidants.[39]

Safety profile

Since fenugreek has been used in both human and animal nutrition for so long without any untoward effects, it is considered safe. Systematic studies of the toxicity of the seeds, given to rats for 90 days at an equivalent dose of 2–4 times the therapeutic dose recommended in humans, did not produce any toxic effects on normal liver function tests and no changes in haematological parameters.[40] Furthermore, administration of seeds at 25 g/day in human diabetic subjects for 24 weeks produced no clinical changes in hepatic or renal function or haematological abnormalities.[26] However, it should be used with caution in individuals undergoing hypoglycaemic therapy as it may potentiate the action of other hypoglycaemic agents.

Dosage

Powdered seeds: 6 g per day

Ayurvedic properties

Rasa: *Katu* (pungent)

Guna: *Laghu* (light), *snigdha* (unctuous)

Veerya: *Ushna* (hot)

Vipaka: *Katu* (pungent)

Dosha: Pacifies *vata* and *kapha*

Further reading

Duke JA 1985 Handbook of medicinal plants. CRC Press, London

Sairam TV 1999 Home remedies, vol 1. Penguin India, Bombay

References

1 Jha MK 1992 The folk veterinary system of Bihar – a research survey. NDDB, Anand, Gujrat

2 International Institute of Rural Reconstruction 1994 Ethnoveterinary medicine in Asia: an information kit on traditional animal health care practices, part 1. IIRR, Silang, Philippines

3 Taylor WG, Elder JL, Chang PR, Richards KW 2000 Microdetermination of diosgenin from Fenugreek (*Trigonella foenum-graecum*) seeds. Journal of Agricultural and Food Chemistry 48(11):5206

4 Yoshikawa M, Murakami T, Komatsu H, Yamahara J, Matsuda H 1998 Medicinal foodstuffs VIII. Fenugreek seed. (2) Structures of six new furostanol saponins trigoneosides IVa, Va, Vb, VI, VIIb, VIIIb, from the seeds of Indian *Trigonella foenum-graecum* L. Heterocycles 47(1):397

5 Gupta RK, Jain DC, Thakur RS 1984 Plant saponins part 6: furostanol glycosides from *Trigonella foenum-graecum* seeds. Phytochemistry 23(11):2605

6 Gupta RK, Jain DC, Thakur RS 1985 Furostanol glycosides from *Trigonella foenum-graecum* seeds. Phytochemistry 24(10):2399

7 Gupta RK, Jain DC, Thakur RS 1986 Plant saponins. Part 10. Two furostanol saponins from *Trigonella foenum-graecum*. Phytochemistry 25(9):2205

8 Gupta RK, Jain DC, Thakur RS 1986 Minor steroidal sapogenins from Fenugreek seeds *Trigonella foenum-graecum*. Journal of Natural Products 49(6):1153

9 Khurana SK, Krishnamurthy V, Parmar VS, Sandeya R, Chawla HL 1982 3,4,7, trimethyl coumarin from *Trigonella foenum-graecum*. Phytochemistry 21(8):2154

10 Raj K, Kapil RS, Bhaumik HL, Mahesh VK 1999 Biosynthesis of 4-methylcoumarin. Indian Journal of Chemistry 38B(7):759

11 Han Y, Nishibe S, Noguchi Y, Jin Z 2001 Flavonol glycosides from stems of *Trigonella foenum-graecum*. Phytochemistry 58(4):577

12 Sood AR, Boutard B, Chandenson M, Chopin J, Lebreton P 1976 A new flavone C-glycoside from *Trigonella foenum-graecum*. Phytochemistry 15(2):351

13 Al-habbori M, Raman A 1998 Anti-diabetic and hypocholesterolemic effects of fenugreek. Phytotherapy Research 12(4):233

14 Aboutabl EA, Goneid MH, Soilman SN, Selim AA 1999 Analysis of certain plant polysaccharides and study of their antihyperlipidemic activity. Journal of Pharmaceutical Sciences 24:187

15 Leonard SW, Harn K, Leklem JE 2001 Vitamin B-6 content of spices. Journal of Food Composition and Analysis 14(2):163

16 Genet S, Kale RK, Baquer NZ 1999 Effects of vanadate, insulin and Fenugreek (*Trigonella foenum-graecum*) on creatine kinase levels in tissues of diabetic rats. Indian Journal of Experimental Biology 37(2):200

17 Gupta D, Raju J, Baquer NZ 1999 Modulation of some gluconeogenic enzyme activities in diabetic rat liver and kidney. Indian Journal of Experimental Biology 37(2):196

18 Raju J, Gupta D, Rao AR, Baquer NZ 1999 Effect of anti-diabetic compounds on glyoxalase I activity in experimental diabetic rat liver. Indian Journal of Experimental Biology 37(2):193

19 Khosla P, Gupta DD, Nagpal RK 1995 Effect of *Trigonella foenum-graecum* on blood glucose in normal and diabetic rats. Indian Journal of Physiology and Pharmacology 39(2):173

20 Zia T, Hasnain SN, Hasan SK 2001 Evaluation of the oral hypoglycemic effect of *Trigonella foenum-graecum* L. (Methi) in normal mice. Journal of Ethnopharmacology 75(2–3):191

21 Jain SC, Lohiya NK, Kapoor A 1987 *Trigonella foenum-graecum* Linn. – a hypoglycemic agent. Indian Journal of Pharmaceutical Science May–June:113

22 Ravikumar P, Anuradha CV 1999 The effect of Fenugreek seeds on blood lipid peroxidation and antioxidants in diabetic rats. Phytotherapy Research 13(3):197

23 Ali L, Azad Khan AK, Hassan Z et al 1995 Characterization of the hypoglycemic effects of *Trigonella foenum-graecum* seeds. Planta Medica 61(4):358

24 Vetrichelven T, Kavimani S, Gupta JK, Narasimhan CL 1988 Effect of rifampicin on *Trigonella foenum-graecum*-induced hypoglycemia in rats. Indian Journal of Pharmaceutical Science 60(4):244

25 Neeraja A, Rajyalakshmi P 1996 Hypoglycemic effect of processed Fenugreek seeds in humans. Journal of Food Science and Technology 33(5):427

26 Sharma RD, Sarkar A, Hazra DK 1996 Use of fenugreek seed powder in the management of non-insulin dependent diabetes mellitus. Nutrition Research 16(8):1331

27 Sharma RD, Raghuram TC 1990 Hypoglycemic effect of fenugreek seeds on non-insulin dependent diabetic subjects. Nutrition Research 10:731

28 Sharma RD 1986 Effect of fenugreek seeds and leaves on blood glucose and serum insulin responses in human subjects. Nutrition Research 6:1353

29 Singhal PC, Gupta RK, Joshi LD 1982 Hypocholesterolaemic effect of *Trigonella foenum-graecum* (Methi). Current Science 51:136

30 Stark A, Madar Z 1993 The effect of ethanol extract derived from fenugreek (*T. foenum-graecum*) on bile acid absorption and cholesterol levels in rats. British Journal of Nutrition 69:277

31 Petit PR, Sauvarie YD, Hillaire BDM et al 1995 Steroidal saponins from fenugreek seeds, extraction, purification and pharmacological investigation on feeding behavior and plasma cholesterol. Steroids 60(10):674

32 Puri D, Prabhu KM, Murthy PS 1994 Hypocholesterolaemic effect of the hypoglycemic principle of fenugreek (*Trigonella foenum-graecum*) seeds. Indian Journal of Clinical Biochemistry 9(1):13

33 Khare AK, Srivastava MC, Tewari JP, Puri JN, Singh S, Ansri NA 1982 Experimental evaluation of anti-inflammatory activity of Methi seeds. Indian Drugs February:191

34 Omoloso AD, Vagi JK 2001 Broad-spectrum antibacterial activity of *Allium cepa, Allium roseum, Trigonella foenum-graecum* and *Curcuma domestica*. Natural Product Science 7(1):13

35 Rathee PS, Mishra SH, Kaushal R 1980 Antimicrobial activity of fatty oil and unsaponifiable matter of *Trigonella foenum-graecum* Linn. Indian Drugs 17(5):136

36 McCarthy TL, Kerry JP, Kerry JF, Lynch PB, Buckley DJ 2001 Evaluation of the anti-oxidant potential of natural food/plant extracts as compared with synthetic antioxidants and vitamin E in raw and cooked pork patties. Meat Science 58(1):45

37 McCarthy TL, Kerry JP, Kerry JF, Lynch PB, Buckley DJ 2001 Assessment of the antioxidant potential of natural food and plant extracts in fresh and previously frozen pork patties. Meat Science 57(2):177

38 Mansour EH, Khalil AH 2000 Evaluation of antioxidant activity of some plant extracts and their application to ground beef patties. Food Chemistry 69(2):135

39 Rao UP, Sesikeran B, Rao SP 1996 Short term nutritional and safety evaluation of fenugreek. Nutrition Research 16:1495

40 Sharma RD, Sarkar A, Hazar DK, Mishra B, Singh JB, Maheshwari BB 1996 Toxicological evaluation of fenugreek seeds: a long term feeding experiment in diabetic patients. Phytotherapy Research 10:519

Withania somnifera L. Dunal (Solanaceae)

English: Winter cherry

Hindi: *Asagandh*

Sanskrit: *Ashwagandha*

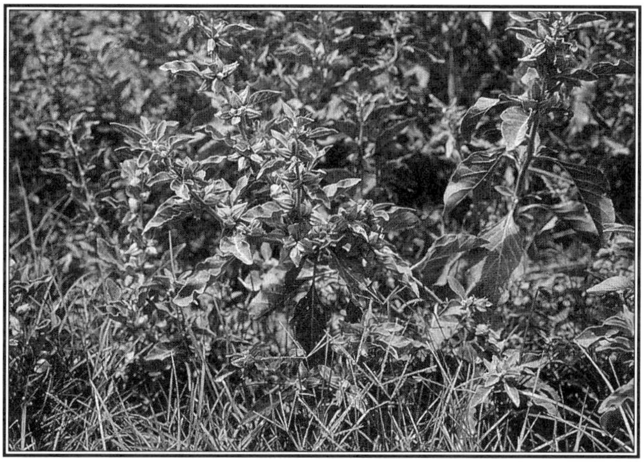

Withania somnifera holds a place in Ayurveda similar to that of ginseng in Chinese medicine. It is reputed to be capable of imparting long life, youthful vigour and intellectual prowess and is an ingredient of many traditional preparations. It has been used in parts of Africa and is now used increasingly elsewhere, including the USA and Europe. The name *ashwagandha* comes from the smell of horses, which the root emits, and the botanical suffix *somnifera* from the use of the plant as a sedative.

Habitat

It is indigenous to India, other Asian countries and parts of Africa and found widely on waste land. It is also cultivated widely for medicinal purposes.

Botanical description

It is an erect, greyish, tomentose undershrub (Plate 68). Leaves are simple, ovate, glabrous and those in the floral region smaller and opposite. The flowers are inconspicuous, greenish or yellow, in axillary or umbellate cymes. Berries are small, globose, orange red when mature, containing seeds which are yellow and reniform.

Parts used

Root, leaf, whole plant.

Traditional and modern use

It is known best as a rejuvenative herb, particularly for males, as it strengthens the muscles, bone marrow and semen. The plant is used as an abortifacient, anodyne, antiasthmatic, bactericide, contraceptive, diuretic, sedative, tonic and antiinflammatory and in cold, dropsy, anaemia, fever, hypertension and lumbago. The fresh fruits are used as an antiasthmatic, sedative and emetic; the dried fruits as a carminative, depurative and in dyspepsia. The leaves are used as a febrifuge and tonic.

Ethnoveterinary usage

The plant is used in cough, dropsy, rheumatism, scabies and sores. The roots are used to promote milk flow in ruminants.

Major chemical constituents

Steroid lactones

Withanolides A–Y, dehydrowithanolide-R, withasomniferin-A, withasomidienone, withasomniferols A–C, withaferin A, 27-deoxy-14α-hydroxywithaferin A, withanone, witha-2,24-dienolide and other derivatives have been isolated from the root and leaf.[1]

Phytosterols

Sitoindosides VII–X (acylsteryl-glucosides), β-sitosterol.[1]

Alkaloids

Ashwagandhine, ashwaghandhinine, cuscohygrine, anahygrine, tropine, pseudotropine, anaferine, dl-isopelletierine, withasomine, visamine, somniferine, somniferinine, withanine, withaninine, pseudowithaninine and solasodine have been isolated.[1,2]

Medicinal and pharmacological activities

Memory enhancement: The sitoindosides VII–X and withaferin A, isolated from the aqueous extract of the root, were investigated for nootropic activity in an experimental model of Alzheimer's disease. The syndrome was induced by ibotenic acid and cognitive deficits were assessed by the attenuation of a learned active avoidance task and a decrease in acetylcholine concentration, choline acetyltransferase activity and muscarinic cholinergic receptor (MCR) binding. The active principles of *Withania somnifera* were able to reverse various cognitive deficits and cholinotoxic effects after 2 weeks of treatment.[3]

Adaptogenic and antistress activity: An extract of the roots of *Withania somnifera* and equimolecular combination of sitoindosides (VII, VIII and withaferin A) was assessed using a diverse spectrum of stress-inducing paradigms. It exhibited significant activity in widely different stress situations including attenuation of pentylenetetrazol (PTZ)-induced defaecation and urination in a novel environment; reduction in the duration of immobility in the forced swimming-induced immobility test in mice; decreased incidence and severity of restraint stress gastric ulcers in rats; inhibition of time-dependent restraint stress-induced autoanalgesia in rats; and inhibition of the restraint stress effect on the thermic response of morphine in rats.[4] Antistress drugs (adaptogens) appear to have a corticosteroid-sparing effect and are able to protect the organism from unfavourable stress conditions. One of their features is the capacity to depress the central nervous system (CNS). A 50% ethanolic extract of *Withania somnifera* was evaluated on mouse CNS after injecting a single dose of pentobarbitol. The results demonstrated that the recovery of the righting reflex was sex and dose dependent and the extract had a close synergy with pentobarbitol in depressing the mouse CNS response.[5] A withadienolide derivative and solasodine also showed significant antistress activity in albino mice and rats and augmented learning acquisition and memory retention in both young and old rats.[6]

Immunomodulatory activity: *Withania somnifera* exhibited non-specific immunostimulatory activity in various models including oxazolone-induced erythema, the carbon clearance test and *Escherichia coli*-induced sepsis. The activity of the root extract was studied in three models of mice. Myelosuppression was induced by cyclophosphamide, azathioprine or prednisolone and haematological and serological tests were done to assess the immunomodulatory activity. A significant increase in haemoglobin concentration, red blood cell count, white blood cell count, platelet count and body weight resulting in the prevention of myelosuppression induced by the compounds was observed in all the three animal models used.[7] In another study, the immunomodulatory activity of sitoindosides IX and X was studied in rats and mice. A statistically significant mobilisation and activation of peritoneal macrophages, phagocytosis and increased activity of the lysosomal enzymes secreted by the activated macrophages were observed.[8]

Inhibition of morphine tolerance in mice: Treatment with a root extract inhibited the development of tolerance to the analgesic effect of morphine and inhibited withdrawal 'jumps' (a sign of opiate dependence).[9] *Withania somnifera* has a wide spectrum of psychotropic and antistress effects and because it is non-analgesic per se, it may have a potential role in treating opiate withdrawal syndrome.

Antihypertensive activity: An extract induced a significant decrease in the arterial and diastolic blood pressure in normotensive pentobarbitol anaesthetised dogs.[10]

Antiinflammatory activity: *Withania somnifera* extract exhibited significant antiinflammatory activity against carrageenan-induced paw oedema in rats, as well as a number of other experimental models.[11]

Antiviral activity: An extract showed a dose-dependent inhibition of spinach mosaic virus.[12]

Hepatoprotective activity: Administration of a herbal preparation containing extracts of *Piper longum* and *Withania somnifera* produced marked histopathological improvements in hepatotoxicity induced by antitubercular drugs, indicating that it may have potential as an adjuvant to antitubercular therapy.[13]

Antimicrobial activity: Withaferin A and 3-β-hydroxy-2,3,-dihydrowithanolide F exhibited antibacterial activity with no major toxicity observed.[14]

Antioxidant activity: The sitoindosides VII–X and withaferin A were studied on rat brain concentrations of superoxide dismutase (SOD), catalase (CAT) and glutathione peroxide (GPX). The efficacy was compared with the effects induced by deprenyl, a known antioxidant. The compounds produced a dose-related increase in SOD, CAT and GPX activity in the frontal cortex and striatum and may explain many of the reported effects of the plant.[15]

Antitumour activity: An ethanolic extract of the dried roots of *Withania somnifera* showed significant antitumour activity and radiosensitising effects in experimental tumours in vivo, without any noticeable toxicity.[16,17] Administration of a 75% methanolic extract significantly increased the total white blood cell count in mice and reduced the leucopenia induced by a sublethal dose of γ radiation.[18]

Safety profile

A daily dose of 100 mg/kg body weight (=1/12 LD_{50}) for 30 days in rats did not lead to any deaths or changes in peripheral blood constituents.[19] The maximum tolerated dose of a 50% ethanolic extract of the whole plant was 1000 mg/kg in rats and the LD_{50} of a 50% ethanolic extract of the roots was 1000 mg/kg.[20]

Dosage

Powder: 3–6 g

Ayurvedic properties

Rasa: *Tikta* (bitter), *katu* (pungent)

Guna: *Laghu* (light), *snigdha* (unctuous)

Veerya: *Ushna* (hot)

Vipaka: *Madhur* (sweet)

Dosha: Balances *kapha* and *vata*

Further reading

Kapoor LD 1990 Handbook of Ayurvedic medicinal plants. CRC Press, Boca Raton

Ministry of Health and Family Welfare 1989 Ayurvedic pharmacopoeia of India, vol 1. Government of India, New Delhi

References

1 Upton R (ed) 2000 Ashwagandha root. In: American herbal pharmacopoeia and therapeutic compendium. American Herbal Pharmacopoeia, Santa Cruz, California

2 Sharma K, Dandiya PC 1991 *Withania somnifera* Dunal – present status (review). Indian Drugs 29(6):24

3 Bhattacharya SK, Kumar A, Ghosal S 1995 Effects of glycowithanolides from *Withania somnifera* on an animal model of Alzheimer's disease and perturbed central cholinergic markers of cognition in rats. Phytotherapy Research 9(2):110

4 Bhattacharya SK, Goel RJ, Kaur R, Ghosal S 1987 Antistress activity of sitoindosides VII and VIII. New acylsterylglucosides from *Withania somnifera*. Phytotherapy Research 1(1):32

5 Ahumada F, Trincado MA, Arellano JA, Hancke J, Wikman G 1991 Effect of certain adaptogenic plant extracts on drug-induced narcosis in female and male mice. Phytotherapy Research 5(1):29

6 Bahr V, Hansel R 1982 Immunomodulating properties of 5,20α(R)-dihydroxy-6α,7α-epoxy-1-oxo-(5α)-witha-2,24-dienolide and solasodine. Planta Medica 44:32

7 Ziauddin M, Phansalkar N, Patki P, Diwanay S, Patwardhan B 1996 Studies on the immunomodulatory effects of Ashwagandha. Journal of Ethnopharmacology 50:69

8 Ghosal S, Jawahar L, Srivastava R et al 1989 Immunomodulatory and CNS effects of sitoindosides IX and X, two new glycowithanolides from *Withania somnifera*. Phytotherapy Research 3(5):201

9 Kulkarni SK, Ninan I 1997 Inhibition of morphine tolerance and dependence by *Withania somnifera* in mice. Journal of Ethnopharmacology 57:213

10 Ahumada F, Aspee F, Wikman G, Hancke J 1991 *Withania somnifera* extract. Its effect on arterial blood pressure in anaesthetized dogs. Phytotherapy Research 5(3):111

11 Agarwal R, Diwanay S, Patki P, Patwardhan B 1999 Studies on immunomodulatory activity of *Withania Somnifera* (ashwagandha) extracts in experimental immune inflammation. Journal of Ethnopharmacology 67:27

12 Zaidi ZB, Gupta VP, Samad A, Naqui AQ 1988 Inhibition of spinach mosaic virus by extract of some medicinal plants. Current Science 57(3):151

13 Chhajed S, Baghel MS, Ravishankar B 1991 Evaluation of hepatoprotective effect of *Piper longum* (Pippali) and *Withania somnifera* (Ashwagandha) in hepatotoxicity induced by antitubercular drugs in mice. Journal of Research Education in Indian Medicine 10(3):9

14 Budhiraja RD, Sudhir S 1987 Review of biological activity of withanolides. Journal of Scientific Indian Research 46(11):488

15 Bhattacharya SK, Satyan KS, Ghosal S 1997 Antioxidant activity of glycowithanolides from *Withania somnifera*. Indian Journal of Experimental Biology 35(3):236

16 Devi PU 1996 *Withania somnifera* Dunal (ashwagandha): potential plant source of a

promising drug for cancer chemotherapy and radiosensitization. Indian Journal of Experimental Biology 34(10):927

17 Sharad AC, Solomon FE, Devi PU, Udupa N, Srinivasan KK 1996 Antitumor and radiosensitizing effects of withaferin A on mouse Ehrlich ascites carcinoma *in vivo*. Acta Oncologia 35(1):95

18 Kuttan G 1996 Use of *Withania somnifera* Dunal as an adjuvant during radiation therapy. Indian Journal of Experimental Biology 34(9):854

19 Sharada AC, Emerson Soloman F, Uma Devi P 1993 Toxicity of *Withania somnifera* root extract in rat and mice. International Journal of Pharmacognosy 31(3):205

20 Bhakuni DS, Dhar ML, Dhar MM, Dhawan BN, Mehrotra BN 1969 Screening of Indian plants for biological activity: Part II. Indian Journal of Experimental Biology 7:260

Woodfordia fruticosa Kurz (Lythraceae)(syn. *Woodfordia floribunda* Salisb)

English: Fire-flame bush, shiranjitea

Hindi: *Dhai*

Sanskrit: *Dhataki*

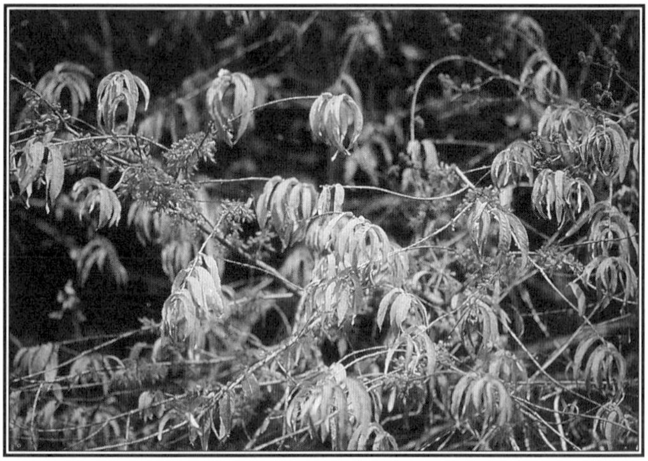

The flowers are flame coloured, hence the name, and yield a red dye used to colour fabric. It has been used medicinally for centuries.

Habitat

It is found commonly throughout India, Sri Lanka and other Asian countries and is widely cultivated as an ornamental shrub.

Botanical description

A much-branched, leafy shrub with fluted stems and long, spreading branches (Plate 69). It usually reaches about 3 m in height or, more rarely, up to 7 m. The smooth, reddish-brown bark peels off in thin fibrous strips. Leaves lanceolate, oblong or ovate-lanceolate; flowers numerous, brilliant red in dense axillary paniculate-cymose clusters. The capsules are ellipsoid and membranous, containing the minute, brown, smooth seeds.

Parts used

Flowers.

Traditional and modern use

The flowers are stimulant and astringent and an infusion of the flowers and leaves is used as a herbal tea. The flowers are added to prepared liquids to make many of the *aristas* and *asavas* by alcoholic fermentation, before the pots are sealed and stored. Powdered dried flowers in curdled milk are used in the treatment of dysentery, diarrhoea and internal haemorrhages and, with honey, are given for leucorrhoea and menorrhagia. Externally, the powder is sprinkled over foul ulcers and wounds to diminish discharge and promote granulation, and used in lotions for the same purpose. Dried flowers are useful in disorders of the mucous membranes, haemorrhoids and disorders of the liver.

Ethnoveterinary usage

Flower and root used in the treatment of rheumatism, dysentery, foot and mouth disease, lumbar and rib fracture.[1]

Major chemical constituents

Tannins

The flowers contain the hydrolysable tannins

oenothein A and B, woodfordins A–I and isoschimawalin A.[2,3,4]

Flavones and anthocyanins

The flowers contain pelargonidin-3,5, diglucoside, cyanidin-3,5, diglucoside and the leaves contain numerous quercetin and myricetin glycosides.[5]

Phytosterols and hydrocarbons

The flowers contain octacosanol and β-sitosterol.[6]

Anthraquinone

Chrysphanol-8-O-β-D-glucopyranoside has been isolated from the flowers.[6]

Medicinal and pharmacological activities

Antiinflammatory and antipyretic activity: A water extract of the flowers exhibited antiinflammatory activity against cotton pellet-induced granuloma in rats. Tissue granuloma formation was prevented but no effect on adrenal ascorbic acid was observed. The ethanolic extract also showed significant antiinflammatory and antipyretic activity, at a dose of 500 mg/kg.[7]

Antitumour activity: Woodfordin C, isolated from the dried flowers of *Woodfordia fruticosa*, prolonged the lifespan of mice inoculated with sarcoma 180 cells by 160%. One of the five mice survived to the 60th day at a dose of 10 mg/kg.[8] The in vitro and in vivo antitumour activity of woodfordin C compared favourably with the topoisomerase-II inhibitors adriamycin and etoposide. Woodfordin C strongly inhibited intracellular DNA synthesis but not RNA and protein synthesis and showed remarkable activity against PC-1 cells although only moderate activity against MKN45 and KB cells. Furthermore, woodfordin C had in vivo inhibitory activity against the growth of inoculated colon 38 cells, suggesting that the mechanism by which woodfordin C exhibits antitumour activity may be through inhibition of topoisomerase-II.[9]

Antiviral activity: Methanolic and aqueous extracts of the flowers and leaves inhibited avian myeloblastosis virus reverse transcriptase (RT). No cytotoxicity was observed in the extracts even at concentrations where there was over 90% inhibition of RT activity.[10]

Immunomodulatory activity: The contribution of *Woodfordia fruticosa* flowers to the immunomodulatory activity of the Ayurvedic drug *Nimba arishta* was investigated and the preparation was found to inhibit both human complement activity and chemiluminescence generated by zymosan-stimulated human polymorphonuclear leucocytes. It was established that the increased biological activity was not due to microbial interference, but to immunoactive constituents released from the Woodfordia flowers.[11]

Safety profile

The 50% ethanolic extract of the whole plant had a maximum tolerated dose of 100 mg/kg body weight in rats.[12]

Dosage

Powder: 3–6 g

Ayurvedic properties

Rasa: *Kashaya* (astringent), *katu* (pungent)
Guna: *Laghu* (light)
Veerya: *Shita* (cold)
Vipaka: *Katu* (pungent)
Dosha: Pacifies *pitta* and *kapha*

Further reading

Khory RN, Katrak NN 1980 Materia medica of India and their therapeutics. Neeraj Publishers, New Delhi

Pandey GS (ed) 1998 Bhavprakash Nighantu. Chaukhambha Bharati Academy, Gokul Bhawan, Varanasi

References

1 Jha MK 1992 Folk veterinary medicine of Bihar – a research survey. NDDB, Anand, Gujrat

2 Yoshida T, Chou T, Nitta A, Okuda T 1992 Tannins and related polyphenols of lythraceous plants III. Hydrolyzable tannin oligomers with macrocyclic structures, and accompanying tannins from *Woodfordia fruticosa* Kurz. Chemical and Pharmaceutical Bulletin 40(8):2023

3 Yoshida T, Chou T, Matsuda M et al 1991 Woodfordin D and oenothein A, trimeric hydrolyzable tannins of macro-ring structure with antitumor activity. Chemical and Pharmaceutical Bulletin 39(5):1157

4 Yoshida T, Chou T, Nitta A, Okuda T 1989 Woodfordins A, B and C, dimeric hydrolysable tannins from *Woodfordia fruticosa* flowers. Heterocycles 29(8):2267

5 Kadota S, Takamori Y, Nyein NK, Kikuchi T, Tanaka K, Ekimoto H 1990 Constituents of the leaves of *Woodfordia fruticosa* Kurz. I. Isolation, structure, and proton and carbon-13 nuclear magnetic resonance signal assignments of woodfruticosin (woodfordin C), an inhibitor of deoxyribonucleic acid topoisomerase II. Chemical and Pharmaceutical Bulletin 38(10):2687

6 Chauhan JS, Srivastava SK, Srivastava SD 1979 Phytochemical investigation of the flowers of *Woodfordia fruticosa*. Planta Medica 36(2):183

7 Alam M, Susan T, Joy S, Ali SU, Kundu AB 1990 Antiinflammatory activity of *Plectranthus urticifolius* Hook F. and *Woodfordia fruticosa* Kurz. in albino rats. Indian Drugs 27(11):559

8 Yoshida T, Chou T, Nitta A, Miyammoto K, Koshiura R, Okuda T 1990 Woodfordin C, a macro-ring hydrolyzable tannin dimer with antitumor activity, and accompanying dimers from *Woodfordia fruticosa* flowers. Chemical and Pharmaceutical Bulletin 38(5):1211

9 Kuramochi-Motegi A, Kuramochi H, Kobayashi F et al 1992 Woodfruticosin (woodfordin C), a new inhibitor of DNA topoisomerase II. Experimental antitumor activity. Biochemical Pharmacology 44(10):1961

10 Kusumoto IT, Shimada I, Kakiuchi N, Hattori M, Namba T, Supriyatna S 1992 Inhibitory effects of Indonesian plant extracts on reverse transcriptase of an RNA tumour virus (I). Phytotherapy Research 6:241

11 Kroes BH, Van den Berg AJJ, Abeysekara AM, De Silva KTD, Labadie RP 1993 Fermentation in traditional medicine: the impact of *Woodfordia fruticosa* flowers on the immunomodulatory activity, and the alcohol and sugar contents of Nimba arishta. Journal of Ethnopharmacology 40(2):117

12 Dhar ML, Dhar MM, Dhawan BN, Mehrotra BN, Ray C 1968 Screening of Indian plants for biological activity: Part I. Indian Journal of Experimental Biology 6:246

Zingiber officinale Rosc. (Zingiberaceae)

English: Ginger

Hindi: *Adrak* (fresh), *sonth* (dried)

Sanskrit: *Viswabhesaja, ardhrakam*

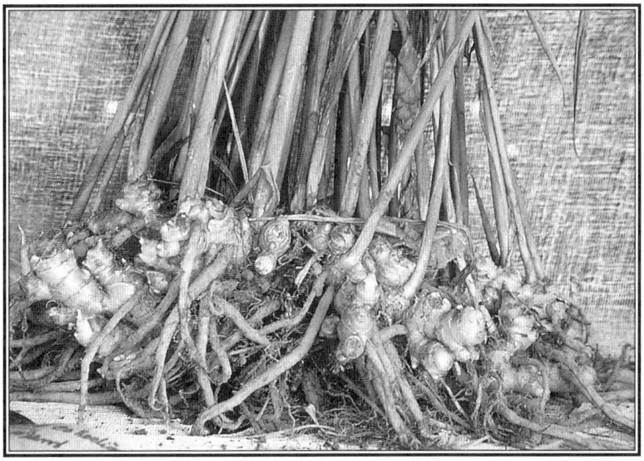

Ginger has been known for centuries as a culinary spice and medicinal plant all over the world, and is used even more today. Arabic physicians knew it as *Zanzabil* and it was widely used by the Greeks and Romans.

Habitat

The plant is widely cultivated in warm, moist areas of India, China, Sri Lanka, Nigeria, Jamaica and many south-east Asian countries.

Botanical description

It is a perennial herb with a stout, horizontal, tuberous, jointed, rootstock (Plate 70). The leaves are lanceolate, subsessile and glabrous, with a prominent midrib. The rhizome is thick and fleshy, laterally compressed, bearing short, ovate, oblique branches on the upper surface each having at its apex a depressed scar. Externally it is buff coloured with longitudinal striations. The flowers are yellowish-green, solitary, in oblong cylindrical spikes. The calyx is gamosepalous with three teeth at the apex and the corolla tube is cylindrical and three-lobed, greenish, subequal and lanceolate. The fruits are oblong capsules containing globose seeds.

Parts used

Rhizomes, leaves.

Traditional and modern use

The rhizome is used specifically for the treatment of rheumatism and inflammation. It is considered to be carminative, diuretic and aphrodisiac. It promotes digestive power, cleanses the throat and tongue, dispels flatulence and colic, suppresses vomiting and coughs, improves dyspnoea, anorexia, fever, constipation, swelling and dysurea. Ginger is valuable in many painful affections of the stomach and bowels and for cold, cough, asthma, dyspepsia and indigestion.

Ethnoveterinary usage

The rhizome is used in coughs and colds, eye diseases, retained placenta, bloat, diarrhoea and sprains in poultry, ruminants and swine. The leaves and rhizome are used as a preventive for mastitis and to treat wounds, haemorrhagic septicaemia, pneumonia, asthma, coughs, swelling of the nasal mucous membranes, stomach pain, tympanitis, constipation, dysentery, loss of appetite, lumbar fracture and stoppage of urination.

Major chemical constituents

Phenolic compounds

The pungent components are a series of gingerols, gingerdiols and gingerdiones and their dehydration products, the shogaols.[1]

Essential oil

Major constituents of the essential oil are the monoterpenes β-phellandrene, perillaldehyde, neral and geranial and the sesquiterpenes α-zingiberene, β-santalol, β-bisabolene, α-curcumene, zingiberol, nerolidol, β-eudesmol, farnesol, elemol and zingerone.[1]

Medicinal and pharmacological activities

Antiemetic activity: Ginger was found to be superior to dimenhydrinate in preventing motion sickness and the gingerols and shogaols were identified as the main antiemetic principles.[2] Studies suggest that the action of ginger modulated vestibular impulses to the autonomic centres of the central nervous system.[3] In a study of 30 pregnant women, in a double-blind randomised cross-over trial, it was observed that powdered root ginger was superior to placebo in reducing the symptoms of hyperemesis gravidarum (morning sickness).[4]

Antiulcer activity: β-Sesquiphellandrene, β-bisabolene, curcumene, 6-gingesulphonic acid and 6-shogaol were identified as antiulcer active principles from the dried rhizome when tested against hydrochloric acid or ethanol-induced gastric lesions in rats.[5,6] 6-Gingesulphonic acid was found to be the most potent compound.[7]

Antihepatotoxic activity: Protection by the gingerols and shogaols against carbon tetrachloride- and galactosamine-induced toxicity was observed in cultured rat hepatocytes.[8]

Antiinflammatory activity: An ethanolic extract of the rhizome reduced carrageenan-induced paw swelling and yeast-induced fever in rats, but was ineffective in suppressing the writhing induced by acetic acid. The essential oil inhibited chronic adjuvant arthritis in rats.[9]

Antiplatelet activity: An aqueous extract of ginger inhibited platelet aggregation induced by ADP, epinephrine, collagen and arachidonic acid in vitro and inhibited prostacyclin synthesis in rat aorta. It is thought to act by inhibiting thromboxane synthesis;[10] 6-gingerol acts in a similar manner.[11]

Antipyretic activity: Oral administration of ginger extract reduced fever in rats by 38% as compared to aspirin (where 44% reduction was observed), as did 6-shogaol and 6-gingerol.[10] Ginger is also used for the treatment of migraine headaches and a mechanism of action via the inhibition of prostaglandin and thromboxane synthesis was proposed.[12] However, in contrast to feverfew (*Tanacetum parthenium*), ginger did not inhibit serotonin release from bovine platelets.[13]

Cardiovascular activity: Ginger decreased serum and hepatic cholesterol and inhibited cholesterol biosynthesis levels in cholesterol-fed rats.[14] It also stimulated bile acid biosynthesis from cholesterol.[15] Ginger had a positive inotropic effect on isolated guinea pig atria[16] and 6-shogaol showed pressor response.[17]

Hypolipidaemic activity: An ethanolic extract of ginger reduced hyperlipidaemia induced by an atherogenic diet. A reduction in the levels of serum and total cholesterol, serum triglycerides and phospholipids and an increased coagulation time were observed when compared with the control group. The extract of ginger was comparable to gemfibrozil.[18]

Antioxidant activity: The pungent principles, including gingerol[19] and zingerone,[20] demonstrated in vitro effects in scavenging the superoxide and hydroxyl radicals[21] and inhibiting lipid peroxidation.[22]

Immunomodulatory activity: Humoral immunity was enhanced, as shown by humoral antibody titre, and cell-mediated response was also stimulated in leucocyte migration inhibition tests.[23]

Thermogenic activity: Studies suggest that the pungent principles of ginger stimulate thermoregulatory receptors. Zingerone induced catecholamine secretion from the adrenal medulla in vivo and thus induced a warming action.[24] 6-Gingerol was one of the more potent compounds isolated.[25]

Antiviral activity: β-Sesquiphellandrene exhibited significant antirhinoviral activity against rhinovirus B in vitro.[26]

Nematocidal activity: 6-Shogaol and 6-gingerol were lethal to *Anisakis* larvae at doses of 62.5 and 250 µg/ml. A synergistic effect appeared to exist between the two compounds.[27]

Insect repellent activity: The essential oil was found to be highly repellent to the cockroach, *Periplaneta americana*, and the agricultural pest *Bruchus pisorum*.[28]

Molluscicidal activity: Gingerol and shogaol exhibited potent molluscicidal activity against *Biomphalaria glabrata*. At a concentration of 5 ppm gingerol completely abolished the infectivity of *Schistosoma mansoni* miracidia and cercariae in the snail host and in mice.[29]

Safety profile

It is generally considered as safe (GRAS). Pregnancy has been considered to be a contraindication (although there is no evidence to support this and it has been demonstrated to be helpful in allaying nausea of pregnancy) as it could potentially induce uterine contractions.[1]

Dosage

Infusion: 7–20 ml

Powder: 1–2 g

Ayurvedic properties

Rasa: *Katu* (pungent), *tikta* (bitter)

Guna: *Laghu* (light), *snigdha* (unctuous)

Veerya: *Shita* (cold)

Vipaka: *Katu* (pungent)

Dosha: Pacifies *kapha* and *vata*

Further reading

Kapoor LD 1990 Handbook of Ayurvedic medicinal plants. CRC Press, Boca Raton

Ministry of Health and Family Welfare 1989 Ayurvedic pharmacopoeia of India, vol 1. Government of India, New Delhi

Pandey GS (ed) 1998 Bhavprakash Nighantu. Chaukhambha Bharati Academy, Gokul Bhawan, Varanasi

References

1 Newall CA, Anderson LA, Phillipson JD 1996 Ginger. In: Herbal medicines: a guide for health-care professionals. Pharmaceutical Press, London

2 Kawai T, Kinoshita K, Koyama K, Takahashi K 1994 Anti-emetic principles of *Magnolia obovata* bark and *Zingiber officinale* rhizome. Planta Medica 60:17

3 Grontved A, Hentzer E 1986 Vertigo-reducing effect of ginger root: a controlled clinical study. Journal of Oto-rhino-laryngology 48(5):282

4 Fischer-Rasmussen W, Kjaer SK, Dahl C, Asping U 1991 Ginger treatment of hyperemesis gravidarum. European Journal of Obstetrics, Gynaecology and Reproductive Biology 38(1):19

5 Yoshikawa M, Hatakeyama S, Taniguchi K, Matsuda H, Yamahara J 1992 6-Gingesulfonic acid, a new anti-ulcer principle, and gingerglycolipids A, B and C, three new monoacylgalactosylglycerols from Zingiberis rhizoma originating in Taiwan. Chemical and Pharmaceutical Bulletin 40(8):2239

6 Yamahara J, Hatakeyama S, Taniguchi K, Kawamura M, Yoshikawa M 1992 Stomachic principles in ginger. II. Pungent and anti-ulcer effects of low polar constituents isolated from ginger, the dried rhizoma of *Zingiber officinale* Roscoe cultivated in Taiwan. The absolute stereostructure of a new diarylheptanoid. Yakugaku Zasshi 112(9):645

7 Yoshikawa M, Yamaguchi S, Kunimi K et al 1994 Stomachic principles in ginger. III. An antiulcer principle, 6-gingesulfonic acid, and three monoacyldigalactosylglycerols, gingerglycolipids A, B and C, from Zingiberis rhizoma originating in Taiwan. Chemical and Pharmaceutical Bulletin (Tokyo) 42(6):1226

8 Hikino H, Kiso Y, Kato N et al 1985 Antihepatotoxic actions of gingerols and diarylhepanoids. Journal of Ethnopharmacology 14:31

9 Mascolo N, Jain R, Jain SC, Capasso F 1987 Ethnopharmacologic investigation of ginger (*Zingiber officinale*). Journal of Ethnopharmacology 27(1–2):129

10 Srivastava KC 1984 Effects of aqueous extracts of onion, garlic and ginger on platelet aggregation and metabolism of arachidonic acid in the blood vascular system: *in vitro* study. Prostaglandins, Leukotrienes and Medicine 13(2):227

11 Guh JH, Ko FN, Jong TT, Teng CM 1995 Antiplatelet effect of gingerol isolated from *Zingiber officinale*. Journal of Pharmacy and Pharmacology 47(4):329

12 Mustafa T, Srivastava KC 1990 Ginger (*Zingiber officinale*) in migraine headache. Journal of Ethnopharmacology 29:267

13 Marles RJ, Kaminski J, Arnason T 1992 A bioassay for inhibition of serotonin release from bovine platelets. Journal of Natural Products 55:1044

14 Tanabe M, Chen YD, Saito K, Kano Y 1993 Cholesterol biosynthesis inhibitory component from *Zingiber officinale* Roscoe. Chemical and Pharmaceutical Bulletin 41(4):710

15 Srinivasan K, Sambaiah K 1991 Effect of spices on cholesterol 7-α-hydroxylase activity and on serum and hepatic cholesterol levels in the rat. International Journal for Vitamin and Nutrition Research 61(4):364

16 Shoji N, Iwasa A, Takemoto T, Ishida Y, Ohizume Y 1982 Cardiotonic principles of ginger (*Zingiber officinale* Roscoe). Journal of Pharmaceutical Science 71(10):1174

17 Suekawa M, Aburada M, Hosoya E 1986 Pharmacological studies on ginger. II Pressor action of (6)-shogaol in anaesthetised rats. Journal of Pharmacobio-dynamics 9(10):842

18 Bhandari U, Grover JK, Sharma JN 1995 Effect of *Zingiber officinale* (ginger) on lipid metabolism in albino rabbits. Proc. International Seminar on Recent Trends in Pharmaceutical Sciences, Ootacamund, February 18–21

19 Aeschbach R, Loliger J, Scott BC et al 1994 Antioxidant actions of thymol, carvacrol, 6-gingerol, zingerone and hydroxytyrosol. Food Chemistry and Toxicology 32(1):31

20 Krishnakantha TP, Lokesh BR 1993 Scavenging of superoxide anions by spice principles. Indian Journal of Biochemistry and Biophysics 30(2):133

21 Cao ZF, Chen ZG, Guo P 1993 Scavenging effects of gingerone superoxide anion and hydroxyl radical. Chung-kuo Yao Tsa Chih 18(12):750

22 Zhou Y, Xu R 1992 Antioxidative effect of Chinese drugs. Chung-kuo Yao Tsa Chih 17(6):368

23 Sohni YR, Bhatt RM 1996 Activity of a crude extract formulation in experimental hepatic amoebiasis and in immunomodulation studies. Journal of Ethnopharmacology 54(2–3):119

24 Kawada T, Sakabe S, Watanabe T, Yamamoto M, Iwai K 1988 Some pungent principles of spices cause the adrenal medulla to secrete catecholamine in anaesthetised rats. Proccedings of the Society for Experimental Biology and Medicine 188(2):229

25 Eldershaw TP, Colquhoun EQ, Dora KA, Peng ZC, Clark MG 1992 Pungent principles of ginger (*Zingiber officinale*) are thermogenic in the perfused rat hindlimb. International Journal of Obesity and Related Metabolic Disorders 16(10):755

26 Denyer CV, Jackson P, Loakes DM, Ellis MR, Young DA 1994 Isolation of antirhinoviral sesquiterpenes from ginger (*Zingiber officinale*). Journal of Natural Products 57(5):658

27 Goto C, Kasuya S, Koga K, Ohtomo H, Kagei N 1990 Lethal efficacy of extract from *Zingiber officinale* (traditional Chinese medicine) or (6)-shogaol and (6)-gingerol in *Anisakis* larvae *in vitro*. Parasitology Research 76(8):653

28 Garg SC, Jain R 1991 The essential oil of *Zingiber officinale* Rosc. – a potential insect repellent. Journal of Economic Botany and Phytochemistry 2(1–4):21

29 Adewunmi CO, Oguntimein BO, Furu P 1990 Molluscicidal and antischistosomal activities of *Zingiber officinale*. Planta Medica 56(4):374

Therapeutic guide to plants, according to clinical applications

Gastrointestinal and hepatobiliary systems

Antispasmodics: all types of digestive complaints

- *Acorus calamus*
- *Bacopa monniera*
- *Cedrus deodara*
- *Centella asiatica*
- *Curcuma longa*
- *Gardenia gummifera*
- *Paederia foetida*
- *Phyllanthus niruri*
- *Plumbago zeylanica*
- *Symplocos racemosa*

Antiemetics: motion and pregnancy sickness

- *Cyperus rotundus*
- *Zingiber officinale*

Antidiarrhoeals: including dysentery

- *Abrus precatorius*
- *Aegle marmelos*
- *Andrographis paniculata*
- *Berberis aristata*
- *Caesalpinia bonducella*
- *Euphorbia hirta*
- *Holarrhena antidysenterica*
- *Piper longum*
- *Plantago ovata*
- *Punica granatum*
- *Syzygium cumini*

Bulk laxative

- *Plantago ovata*

Stimulant laxative

- *Ricinus communis* (oil)

Antiulcer agents

- *Acorus calamus*
- *Aegle marmelos*
- *Asparagus racemosus*
- *Azadirachta indica*
- *Carica papaya*
- *Centella asiatica*
- *Curcuma longa*
- *Cyperus rotundus*
- *Ficus religiosa*
- *Glycyrrhiza glabra*
- *Ocimum sanctum*
- *Solanum nigrum*
- *Swertia chirata*
- *Terminalia belerica*
- *Tinospora cordifolia*
- *Withania somnifera*
- *Zingiber officinale*

Antiobesity agents

- *Commiphora mukul*
- *Cyperus rotundus*
- *Tamarindus indica*
- *Terminalia belerica*

Liver protectants: cirrhosis and hepatitis

- *Acacia catechu*
- *Allium sativum*
- *Andrographis paniculata*
- *Azadirachta indica*
- *Berberis aristata*
- *Boerhaavia diffusa*
- *Curcuma longa*
- *Eclipta alba*

- *Fumaria indica*
- *Glycyrrhiza glabra*
- *Gymnema sylvestre*
- *Mangifera indica*
- *Momordica charantia*
- *Nigella sativa*
- *Paederia foetida*
- *Phyllanthus emblica*
- *Phyllanthus niruri*
- *Picrorrhiza kurroa*
- *Piper longum*
- *Polygonum aviculare*
- *Ricinus communis*
- *Rubia cordifolia*
- *Solanum nigrum*
- *Swertia chirata*
- *Terminalia arjuna*
- *Terminalia belerica*
- *Tinospora cordifolia*
- *Withania somnifera*
- *Zingiber officinale*

Cholagogues and choleretics

- *Adhatoda vasica*
- *Curcuma longa*

Cardiovascular system

Cardiotonics and cardioprotectants

- *Terminalia arjuna*
- *Terminalia chebula*
- *Tribulus terrestris*

Antihypertensives

- *Allium sativum*
- *Andrographis paniculata*
- *Azadirachta indica*
- *Carica papaya*
- *Cyperus rotundus*
- *Eclipta alba*
- *Fumaria indica*
- *Leptadenia reticulata*
- *Ocimum sanctum*
- *Phyllanthus niruri*
- *Polygonum aviculare*
- *Terminalia belerica*
- *Trachyspermum ammi*

Diuretics: hypertension and oedema

- *Boerhaavia diffusa*
- *Eucalyptus globulus*
- *Gymnema sylvestre*
- *Phyllanthus niruri*
- *Ricinus communis*
- *Syzygium cumini*
- *Tribulus terrestris*

Antifibrinolytics and anticoagulants

- *Boerhaavia diffusa*
- *Commiphora mukul*
- *Plumbago zeylanica*
- *Polygonum aviculare*

Antiplatelet and antithrombotic agents

- *Abrus precatorius*
- *Allium sativum*
- *Andrographis paniculata*
- *Berberis aristata*
- *Rubia cordifolia*
- *Zingiber officinale*

Calcium channel antagonist

- *Boerhaavia diffusa*

Antiatherosclerotics: hyperlipidaemia and hypercholesterolaemia

- *Allium sativum*
- *Andrographis paniculata*
- *Azadirachta indica*

- *Boswellia serrata*
- *Caesalpinia bonducella*
- *Carica papaya*
- *Commiphora mukul*
- *Curcuma longa*
- *Ficus religiosa*
- *Gymnema sylvestre*
- *Ocimum sanctum*
- *Phyllanthus emblica*
- *Piper longum*
- *Plantago ovata*
- *Semecarpus anacardium*
- *Tamarindus indica*
- *Terminalia arjuna*
- *Terminalia belerica*
- *Trigonella foenum-graecum*
- *Zingiber officinale*

Respiratory system

Antiasthmatics and broncholytics

- *Adhatoda vasica*
- *Bacopa monniera*
- *Boswellia serrata*
- *Curcuma longa*
- *Euphorbia hirta*
- *Ficus religiosa*
- *Ocimum sanctum*
- *Picrorrhiza kurroa*
- *Piper longum*
- *Solanum xanthocarpum*

Antitussive

- *Asparagus racemosus*

Central nervous system

Analgesics: all kinds of pain

- *Acorus calamus*
- *Azadirachta indica*
- *Bacopa monniera*
- *Boswellia serrata*
- *Eclipta alba*
- *Embelia ribes*
- *Fumaria indica*
- *Mucuna pruriens*
- *Nigella sativa*
- *Ocimum sanctum*
- *Phyllanthus niruri*
- *Ricinus communis*

Antipyretics: all types of fevers

- *Abrus precatorius*
- *Acacia catechu*
- *Acorus calamus*
- *Aegle marmelos*
- *Azadirachta indica*
- *Berberis aristata*
- *Boerhaavia diffusa*
- *Boswellia serrata*
- *Caesalpinia bonducella*
- *Cedrus deodara*
- *Commiphora mukul*
- *Crataeva nurvala*
- *Curcuma longa*
- *Cyperus rotundus*
- *Eclipta alba*
- *Eucalyptus globulus*
- *Euphorbia hirta*
- *Fumaria indica*
- *Glycyrrhiza glabra*
- *Mangifera indica*
- *Mucuna pruriens*
- *Nigella sativa*
- *Paederia foetida*
- *Phyllanthus emblica*
- *Picrorrhiza kurroa*
- *Piper longum*
- *Piper nigrum*
- *Plumbago zeylanica*
- *Polygonum aviculare*
- *Ricinus communis*

- *Rubia cordifolia*
- *Solanum nigrum*
- *Swertia chirata*
- *Syzygium cumini*
- *Tamarindus indica*
- *Trigonella foenum-graecum*
- *Withania somnifera*
- *Woodfordia fruticosa*
- *Zingiber officinale*

Antiinflammatory agents: arthritis and rheumatism
- *Andrographis paniculata*
- *Azadirachta indica*
- *Boswellia serrata*
- *Curcuma longa*
- *Cyperus rotundus*
- *Mucuna pruriens*
- *Paederia foetida*
- *Phyllanthus emblica*
- *Semecarpus anacardium*
- *Woodfordia fruticosa*
- *Zingiber officinale*

Muscle relaxant
- *Gymnema sylvestre*

Anticonvulsants (incl. antiepileptics)
- *Acorus calamus*
- *Fumaria indica*
- *Piper nigrum*
- *Ricinus communis*

Memory and learning enhancers
- *Bacopa monniera*
- *Withania somnifera*

Antiparkinsonian agent
- *Mucuna pruriens*

Antipsychotic
- *Fumaria indica*

Anxiolytics
- *Azadirachta indica*
- *Bacopa monniera*
- *Zingiber officinale*

Antistress agents
- *Boerhaavia diffusa*
- *Ocimum sanctum*
- *Tinospora cordifolia*
- *Withania somnifera*

Adaptogens
- *Asparagus racemosus*
- *Withania somnifera*

Aphrodisiacs: male
- *Mucuna pruriens*
- *Tribulus terrestris*

CNS stimulants
- *Mucuna pruriens*
- *Ricinus communis*

CNS depressants
- *Azadirachta indica*
- *Swertia chirata*

Antidiabetic agents

Hypoglycaemics
- *Acacia catechu*
- *Aegle marmelos*
- *Andrographis paniculata*
- *Azadirachta indica*
- *Caesalpinia bonducella*
- *Curcuma longa*
- *Eucalyptus globulus*
- *Ficus religiosa*
- *Fumaria indica*

- *Gymnema sylvestre*
- *Holarrhena antidysenterica*
- *Mangifera indica*
- *Momordica charantia*
- *Mucuna pruriens*
- *Nigella sativa*
- *Ocimum sanctum*
- *Phyllanthus emblica*
- *Phyllanthus niruri*
- *Plantago ovata*
- *Plumbago zeylanica*
- *Punica granatum*
- *Ricinus communis*
- *Swertia chirata*
- *Syzygium cumini*
- *Tamarindus indica*
- *Tinospora cordifolia*
- *Trigonella foenum-graecum*
- *Zingiber officinale*

Malignant disease

Anticancer activity: cytotoxics and supportive therapies

- *Abrus precatorius*
- *Acacia catechu*
- *Allium sativum*
- *Asparagus racemosus*
- *Azadirachta indica*
- *Boswellia serrata*
- *Carica papaya*
- *Cedrus deodara*
- *Embelia ribes*
- *Eucalyptus globulus*
- *Euphorbia hirta*
- *Ficus religiosa*
- *Glycyrrhiza glabra*
- *Gossypium herbaceum*
- *Mangifera indica*
- *Momordica charantia*
- *Ocimum sanctum*
- *Paederia foetida*
- *Phyllanthus emblica*
- *Piper nigrum*
- *Plumbago zeylanica*
- *Rubia cordifolia*
- *Semecarpus anacardium*
- *Terminalia arjuna*
- *Terminalia chebula*
- *Tinospora cordifolia*
- *Withania somnifera*

Chemoprevention

Immunomodulators

- *Abrus precatorius*
- *Aegle marmelos*
- *Allium sativum*
- *Andrographis paniculata*
- *Asparagus racemosus*
- *Azadirachta indica*
- *Boswellia serrata*
- *Centella asiatica*
- *Curcuma longa*
- *Euphorbia hirta*
- *Holarrhena antidysenterica*
- *Mangifera indica*
- *Ocimum sanctum*
- *Phyllanthus emblica*
- *Picrorrhiza kurroa*
- *Piper longum*
- *Plumbago zeylanica*
- *Ricinus communis*
- *Semecarpus anacardium*
- *Tamarindus indica*
- *Terminalia chebula*
- *Tinospora cordifolia*
- *Withania somnifera*
- *Woodfordia fruticosa*
- *Zingiber officinale*

Free radical scavengers and antioxidants

- *Aegle marmelos*
- *Allium sativum*
- *Bacopa monniera*
- *Carica papaya*
- *Commiphora mukul*
- *Curcuma longa*
- *Eucalyptus globulus*
- *Glycyrrhiza glabra*
- *Gymnema sylvestre*
- *Mangifera indica*
- *Ocimum sanctum*
- *Phyllanthus emblica*
- *Phyllanthus niruri*
- *Piper nigrum*
- *Plumbago zeylanica*
- *Ricinus communis*
- *Rubia cordifolia*
- *Tamarindus indica*
- *Terminalia belerica*
- *Terminalia chebula*
- *Tinospora cordifolia*
- *Trigonella foenum-graecum*
- *Withania somnifera*
- *Zingiber officinale*

Antimutagenic agents

- *Curcuma longa*
- *Punica granatum*
- *Terminalia chebula*

Anticlastogen

- *Phyllanthus niruri*

Infections and infestations

Antibacterials

- *Abrus precatorius*
- *Acorus calamus*
- *Adhatoda vasica*
- *Allium sativum*
- *Asparagus racemosus*
- *Cyperus rotundus*
- *Eucalyptus globulus*
- *Euphorbia hirta*
- *Ficus religiosa*
- *Gardenia gummifera*
- *Gossypium herbaceum*
- *Holarrhena antidysenterica*
- *Leptadenia reticulata*
- *Piper longum*
- *Ricinus communis*
- *Tamarindus indica*
- *Terminalia arjuna*
- *Terminalia chebula*
- *Trachyspermum ammi*
- *Zingiber officinale*

Antibiotic resistance modifier

- *Plumbago zeylanica*

Anticaries or antiplaque agents

- *Embelia ribes*
- *Gymnema sylvestre*
- *Syzygium cumini*

Antifungal agents

- *Acacia catechu*
- *Allium sativum*
- *Azadirachta indica*
- *Boswellia serrata*
- *Carica papaya*
- *Cedrus deodara*
- *Embelia ribes*
- *Euphorbia hirta*
- *Fumaria indica*
- *Leptadenia reticulata*
- *Ricinus communis*
- *Tamarindus indica*
- *Trachyspermum ammi*

Antitubercular drugs

- *Adhatoda vasica*
- *Centella asiatica*

Antivirals

- *Allium sativum*
- *Andrographis paniculata* (common cold)
- *Azadirachta indica*
- *Caesalpinia bonducella*
- *Centella asiatica*
- *Curcuma longa*
- *Ficus religiosa*
- *Glycyrrhiza glabra*
- *Gossypium herbaceum*
- *Gymnema sylvestre*
- *Mangifera indica*
- *Momordica charantia* (HIV)
- *Phyllanthus emblica*
- *Phyllanthus niruri*
- *Punica granatum*
- *Tamarindus indica*
- *Terminalia arjuna*
- *Terminalia chebula*
- *Trachyspermum ammi* (hepatitis C)
- *Withania somnifera*
- *Woodfordia fruticosa*
- *Zingiber officinale*

Antiprotozoals

- *Andrographis paniculata* (leishmania, malaria)
- *Asparagus racemosus*
- *Azadirachta indica* (malaria)
- *Berberis aristata* (leishmania, chlamydia)
- *Caesalpinia bonducella* (malaria)
- *Carica papaya*
- *Cyperus rotundus* (malaria)
- *Euphorbia hirta*
- *Ficus religiosa*
- *Holarrhena antidysenterica*
- *Phyllanthus niruri* (malaria)
- *Ricinus communis*
- *Semecarpus anacardium*
- *Swertia chirata* (leishmania)
- *Terminalia chebula*
- *Zingiber officinale*

Insecticides

- *Abrus precatorius*
- *Adhatoda vasica*
- *Azadirachta indica*
- *Cedrus deodara*
- *Gardenia gummifera*
- *Ocimum sanctum*
- *Ricinus communis*
- *Trachyspermum ammi*

Insect repellent

- *Zingiber officinale*

Anthelmintics

- *Allium sativum*
- *Andrographis paniculata*
- *Caesalpinia bonducella*
- *Carica papaya*
- *Embelia ribes*
- *Ficus religiosa*
- *Gardenia gummifera*
- *Momordica charantia*
- *Nigella sativa*
- *Paederia foetida*
- *Punica granatum*
- *Ricinus communis*
- *Semecarpus anacardium*
- *Zingiber officinale*

Molluscicides

- *Abrus precatorius*
- *Asparagus racemosus*
- *Momordica charantia*
- *Solanum nigrum*
- *Tamarindus indica*

- *Trachyspermum ammi*
- *Zingiber officinale*

Reproductive and urinary systems

Antifertility agents: pre- and postcoital contraceptives

- *Abrus precatorius*
- *Adhatoda vasica*
- *Azadirachta indica*
- *Carica papaya*
- *Embelia ribes*
- *Euphorbia hirta*
- *Gossypium herbaceum*
- *Momordica charantia*
- *Nigella sativa*
- *Plumbago zeylanica*
- *Ricinus communis*
- *Solanum xanthocarpum*
- *Terminalia arjuna*

Antioxytocic

- *Nigella sativa*

Oestrogenic drugs

- *Caesalpinia bonducella*
- *Curcuma longa*
- *Cyperus rotundus*
- *Ricinus communis*

Galactagogues (induce or enhance milk production)

- *Asparagus racemosus*
- *Euphorbia hirta*
- *Leptadenia reticulata*
- *Ricinus communis*

Oxytocics and uterine stimulants

- *Caesalpinia bonducella*
- *Salmalia malabarica*

Spermatogenesis enhancers

- *Allium sativum*
- *Mucuna pruriens*

Spermicide

- *Trachyspermum ammi*

Prostate hypertrophy inhibitor

- *Crataeva nurvala*

Urolitholytic agents: kidney and bladder stones

- *Crataeva nurvala*
- *Tribulus terrestris*

Allergies

Antiallergic drugs

- *Abrus precatorius*
- *Curcuma longa*
- *Tinospora cordifolia*

Antianaphylactic

- *Terminalia chebula*

Complement inhibiting

- *Boswellia serrata*

Injuries

Bone-healing promoter

- *Cissus quadrangularis*

Wound-healing promoters

- *Adhatoda vasica*
- *Carica papaya*
- *Centella asiatica*
- *Curcuma longa*

Glossary

Abortifacient An agent which causes abortion

Adenocarcinoma Carcinoma derived from glandular tissue or in which the tumour cells form recognisable glandular structures

Adrenalectomise To excise one or both adrenal glands

Alexipharmic An antidote or remedy for poisoning

Alopecia Baldness; loss of the hair from skin areas where it normally is present

Alterative An agent which gradually restores healthy bodily functions

Amenorrhoea Absence or abnormal stoppage of the menses

Amoebicidal Kills amoebae

Anabolic A substance which helps in constructive metabolic processes

Analgesia Alleviation of pain without causing loss of consciousness

Angina Spasmodic, choking or suffocating pain; now used only to denote angina pectoris

Anodyne An agent that relieves pain

Anorexia Lack or loss of appetite for food

Anthelmintic Destructive to worms

Anthrax An infectious bacterial zoonotic disease

Antiamoebic Destroys or suppresses the growth or reproduction of amoebae

Antibacterial Destroys bacteria or suppresses their growth or reproduction

Antichlamydial An agent that destroys bacteria of the family Chlamydiaceae

Anticonvulsant Prevention or relief of convulsions

Antidiabetic A substance that alleviates symptoms of diabetes

Antidiarrhoeal Effective in combating diarrhoea

Antidote A remedy for counteracting a poison

Antifungal Destroys fungi or suppresses their growth or reproduction

Antihistamine An agent that counteracts the effects of histamine

Antihypercholesterolaemic Decreases high levels of cholesterol in the blood

Antihyperglycaemic Reduces excessively high blood glucose levels

Antihypertensive An agent that reduces high blood pressure

Antiinflammatory Counteracting or suppressing the inflammatory process

Antileishmanial Effective against leishmania

Antimalarial An agent that is therapeutically effective against malaria

Antimicrobial Kills microorganisms or suppresses their multiplication or growth

Antineoplastic An agent that inhibits the development and proliferation of malignant cells

Antioxidant A substance that significantly delays or prevents oxidation

Antioxytocic An agent that prevents the evacuation of the uterus by causing relaxation of the myometrium

Antiperiodic Prevention of periodic recurrence of symptoms, such as in malaria

Antiphlogistic An agent that counteracts inflammation and fever

Antipyretic An agent that reduces fever

Antirheumatic Prevention or alleviation of rheumatism

Antiseptic A substance that inhibits the growth and development of microorganisms without necessarily killing them

Antispasmodic An agent that relieves spasm, usually of smooth muscle

Antituberculotic Therapeutically effective against tuberculosis

Antitumour An agent that inhibits or prevents the development of tumour or the maturation and proliferation of malignant cells

Antiviral An agent that destroys viruses or suppresses their replication

Aperient A mild or gentle purgative

Aperitive Stimulating the appetite

Aphrodisiac A drug that arouses the sexual instinct

Aphthae Small oval or round ulcers, usually with a greyish exudate

Apoplexy Sudden neurologic impairment due to a cerebrovascular disorder

Appetiser An agent that increases desire, especially the natural and recurring desire for food

Arista Traditional preparation made by mixing a decoction of the drug with a sugary solution for a period of time, during which it ferments, generating alcohol which facilitates the extraction of active principles and serves as a preservative

Arthritis Inflammation of the joints

Asava Traditional medicinal preparation made by soaking the drug, in powder form, in a similar manner to the production of an *arista* (qv)

Ascites Effusion and accumulation of serous fluid in the abdominal cavity

Astringent Causing contraction, usually by external application; styptic

Babesiosis A group of tick-borne diseases caused by infection with Babesia protozoa

Bactericide An agent that destroys bacteria

Bacteriostatic An agent that inhibits the growth or multiplication of bacteria

Bloat	Distension of the stomach or caecum
Bradycardia	Slowing of heart beat (and pulse rate) to less than 60 beats/min
Bronchitis	Inflammation of the bronchi
Cachexia	A profound wasting state; generally ill health and malnutrition
Carcinoma	A malignant growth of epithelial cells which tend to infiltrate surrounding tissues and give rise to metastases
Cardiotonic	An agent that has a tonic effect on the heart, improving strength of beat
Caries	Decay or death of a bone in which it becomes softened, discoloured and porous; particularly applied to dentition
Cariostatic	An agent that prevents the formation of dental caries
Carminative	A medicine that relieves flatulence and assuages pain
Catarrh	Inflammation of a mucous membrane, with discharge; especially of the respiratory passages and sinuses
Chemotherapeutic	Treatment of disease by chemical agents, particularly of infections and cancers
Choleretic	An agent that stimulates the flow of bile into the duodenum
Cholinergic	A term applied to sympathetic and parasympathetic nerve fibres which release acetylcholine at synapses when a nerve impulse passes
Cicatrisation	The formation of a scar (or cicatrix) during the healing of a wound
Conjunctivitis	Inflammation of the conjunctiva of the eye; hyperaemia associated with discharge
Constipation	Infrequent or difficult evacuation of the faeces
Copraemia	Poisoning due to faecal material in the blood
Counterirritant	An agent which causes a superficial irritation, intended to relieve pain in another or deeper part of the body
Cystitis	Inflammation of the urinary bladder
Debility	Lack or loss of strength
Decoction	A herbal formulation prepared by boiling the plant parts in water
Decongestant	An agent that reduces congestion or swelling
Demulcent	A soothing, mucilaginous or oily formulation which allays irritation of inflamed or abraded surfaces
Dental caries	Localised destruction of the enamel and calcified tissue of the teeth, leading to cavity formation
Dental plaque	A soft, thin film of food debris, mucin and dead epithelial cells deposited on the teeth, providing a medium for the growth of bacteria
Dentifrice	A preparation used with a toothbrush for cleaning the surfaces of the teeth
Deobstruent	An agent preventing obstruction or blocking
Depurative	Purifying or cleansing
Detoxification	Reduction or removal of poisonous properties
Diaphoretic	Promotion of perspiration
Diuretic	An agent that promotes the excretion of urine and may therefore reduce blood pressure
Dosha	A principle or 'humour' which governs biological and psychological functions of the mind, body and consciousness
Dropsy	Oedema, usually caused by cardiac insufficiency
Dysmenorrhoea	Painful menstruation
Dyspepsia	Impairment of digestion; usually applied to epigastric discomfort following meals
Dysphonia	Any impairment of voice or difficulty in speaking
Dystocia	Abnormal or difficult labour
Dysuria	Painful or difficult urination
Ecbolic	Oxytocic, causing contraction of the uterus
Eczema	A pruritic papulovesicular dermatitis, characterised in the acute stage by erythema, oedema associated with serous exudation, vesiculation, crusting and scaling
Emaciation	Excessive leanness; a wasted condition of the body
Emetic	A substance causing vomiting
Emmenagogue	An agent that induces menstruation
Emollient	An agent which softens or soothes irritated skin or a mucous membrane
Endometritis	Inflammation of the endometrium, the inner mucous membrane of the uterus
Enteritis	Inflammation of the intestine, particularly the small intestine
Enterorrhagia	Haemorrhage from the intestine
Enterotoxin	A toxin produced by a microbe affecting the intestinal mucosa, causing vomiting and diarrhoea
Epilepsy	A group of syndromes characterised by paroxysmal transient disturbances of brain function which may manifest as episodic impairment or loss of consciousness, abnormal motor or sensory phenomena
Epistaxis	Haemorrhage from the nose
Erysipelas	An acute superficial form of cellulitis, often caused by infection with streptococci, and characterised by a spreading hot, bright red, oedematous rash and a circumscribed plaque with a raised indurated border
Expectorant	Promotes the ejection of mucus or fluid from the lungs and trachea

Febrifuge An agent that reduces body temperature in fever

Fecundity Ability to produce offspring rapidly and in large numbers

Fibrosarcoma A malignant tumour composed of cells and fibres which produces collagen but otherwise lacks cellular differentiation

Fistula An abnormal passage between two internal organs or from an internal organ to the surface of the body

Flatulence Excessive amounts of air or gases in the stomach or intestine leading to distension

Foot and mouth disease (aphthous fever) An acute, highly contagious viral disease of hoofed animals, characterised by formation of vesicles and erosions on the mucous membranes and skin

Free radical A highly reactive molecule with an unpaired electron that causes damage to tissues

Galactagogue An agent that promotes the flow of milk

Galactopoietic Induction of milk secretion

Gastralgia Gastric spasm or colic

Gastritis Inflammation of the stomach

Gastrosis Any disease of the stomach

Gingivitis Inflammation of the gingivae (gums)

Glossitis Inflammation of the tongue

Glycosuria Presence of glucose in the urine

Guna The attributes of various substances in Ayurveda, representing the attributes of earth, water, fire, air and ether

Guru Heavy (one of the *gunas*, qv); that which is digested slowly and increases *kapha*

Haematuria Blood in the urine

Haemorrhagic Pertaining to or characterised by haemorrhage (excessive bleeding)

Haemostat An agent that checks bleeding; styptic

Hepatitis Inflammation of the liver

Hyperdipsia Intense thirst of relatively brief duration

Hypermetropia Long-sightedness, where light rays are brought to a focus behind the retina, as a result of the eyeball being too short

Hypocholesterolaemic Pertaining to abnormally diminished levels of blood cholesterol

Hypoglycaemic An agent that lowers the level of glucose in the blood

Hypolipidaemic An agent that reduces serum lipid concentrations

Hypotensive Lowering of blood pressure

Hypothermia A low body temperature, due to environmental exposure or a state of decreased metabolism

Immunomodulator An agent that specifically or non-specifically augments or diminishes immune responses

Implantation The initial stage of reproduction after fertilisation; attachment of the blastocyst to the epithelial lining of the uterus and embedding in the endometrium

Influenza An acute viral infection involving the respiratory tract, marked by inflammation of the nasal mucosa, pharynx and conjunctiva, headache and generalised myalgia

Infusion The steeping of a herb in water to extract its medicinal principles; a 'tea'

Inotropic Affecting the force or energy of muscular contractions, especially of the heart

Insecticide Any substance selectively poisonous to insects

Jaundice A syndrome characterised by deposition of bile pigments in the skin, mucous membranes and sclera, resulting in a yellow appearance of the patient

Kapha One of the three *dosha* (qv), responsible for maintaining bodily resistance

Kaphavatashamak A substance which relieves *kapha* and *vata dosha*

Kasaya Astringent, producing clarity, stiffness, traction in the tongue and the throat, dryness in the mouth, pain in the cardiac region and heaviness. Increases *vata*

Katu Pungent (one of the *rasas*, qv); stimulant, mouth cleansing, anthelmintic, promotes bleeding. Used in dyspepsia, cardiac and skin disorders

Lactogenic Stimulation of milk production

Laghu Light (one of the *gunas*, qv); easy to digest. Increases *vata* and *pitta*, decreases *kapha*

Larvicidal Destructive to insect larvae

Laryngitis Inflammation of larynx, attended with dysphagia, dryness or soreness of the throat

Laxative Promotion of evacuation of the bowel

LD_{50} Median lethal dose

Leucoderma Acquired cutaneous depigmentation produced by a substance or dermatosis

Leucorrhoea A whitish, viscid discharge from the vagina or uterine cavity

Lithiasis The formation of calculi or 'stones' in the kidney or gall bladder

Lumbago Pain in the lumbar (lower back) region

Madhur Sweet (one of the six *rasas*, qv); pleasing, healing, beneficial for thirst, burning sensations, poisoning. Increases *kapha*, decreases *pitta*

Maggots Larvae of an insect, especially when living in decaying flesh

Malignant Pertaining to tumours, meaning invasive or metastatic

Masticatory A remedy to be chewed but not swallowed

Mastitis Inflammation of mammary gland or breast

Menorrhagia Excessive uterine bleeding, the period of flow being as usual

Metritis Inflammation of the uterus

Metrorrhagia Uterine bleeding, usually of variable amount, occurring at irregular but frequent intervals, the period of flow being sometimes prolonged

MTD Maximum tolerated dose at which no adverse effect is observed

Myocardial infarction A 'heart attack'; the formation of an area of necrosis in the muscle of the heart due to local ischaemia resulting from obstruction, commonly by a thrombus or embolus

Myopia Near or short-sightedness, an error of refraction in which rays of light are brought to a focus in front of the retina, as a result of the eyeball being too long from front to back, or an increased strength in refractive power of the eye

Neuralgia Pain extending along the course of one or more nerves

Neuroleptic A term referring to the effects on cognition and behaviour of antipsychotic drugs, producing a state of apathy, lack of initiative, limited range of emotions and in psychotic patients a reduction in confusion and agitation

Nidation Implantation of the fertilised ovum in the endometrium

Oedema The retention of abnormally large amounts of fluid in the tissues of the body

Oestrogenic Having the properties of an oestrogen; producing oestrus in animals

Ophthalmia Severe inflammation of the conjunctiva or deeper structures of the eye

Orchitis Inflammation of the testis, marked by pain and swelling

Ossification The formation of bone; the conversion of fibrous tissue or cartilage into bone

Osteoarthritis Non-inflammatory degenerative joint disease characterised by painful degeneration of cartilage, hypertrophy of bone at the margins and changes to the synovial membrane

Otorrhoea Discharge from the ear, especially if purulent

PAF Platelet-activating factor

Pharyngitis Inflammation of the pharynx

Phthisis Tuberculosis, especially of the lungs

Piscicidal Poisonous to fish

Pitta One of the *doshas* (qv) concerned with balance of potential and kinetic energies and involving digestion

Placebo A dummy medical treatment given solely for its psychophysiological effects

Polyuria The passage of an unnaturally large volume of urine, a characteristic of diabetes

Proctitis Inflammation of the rectum

Prolapse The detachment or falling down of an organ, particularly the uterus

Purgative Causing rapid evacuation of the bowels

Rasa The initial taste of a substance; sweet, sour, salt, pungent, bitter or astringent

Rasayana A rejuvenator or adaptogen which alleviates symptoms of ageing and promotes vitality

Refrigerant An agent reducing bodily heat or fever

Restorative Capable of restoring health or strength

Reticuloendothelial system A group of cells including specialised endothelial cells and reticular cells of lymphatic tissues (macrophages) and bone marrow (fibroblasts) with the ability to take up and sequester inert particles

Rubefacient An agent that reddens the skin by increasing blood flow

Ruksha Unctuous (one of the *gunas*, qv)

Rumination The regurgitation and multiple chewing of food, as in cattle

Scabies A contagious dermatitis caused by the mite *Sarcoptes scabiei*, characterised by intense itching and a papular eruption over tiny, raised sinuous burrows (cuniculi) produced by the egg-laying female mite

Scrofula Former name for a type of tuberculous lymphadenitis

Sedative An agent that allays excitement

Septicaemia Systemic disease associated with the presence of pathogenic microorganisms or toxins in the blood; blood poisoning

Shita Cold (one of the *gunas*, qv)

Sinusitis Inflammation of a sinus, either purulent or not, acute or chronic

Snigdha Oily (one of the *gunas*, qv)

Spasmolytic Alleviating spasm; antispasmodic

Splenitis Inflammation and painful enlargement of the spleen, usually produced by pyaemia

Splenomegaly Enlargement of the spleen

Sterilant A sterilising agent destroying microorganisms

Stimulant An agent that produces stimulation, of the central nervous system or by causing tension on muscle fibres

Stomachic A medicine which enhances the functional activity of the stomach

Stomatitis Inflammation of the oral mucosa which may involve the palate, tongue, floor of the mouth and gingivae

Styptic An astringent and haemostatic remedy

Tachycardia	Excessively rapid heart beat; applied to an adult rate above 100 beats per minute
Teratogenic	Producing anomalies of the foetus
Tetanus	Acute, often fatal disease caused by the anaerobic bacillus *Clostridium tetani*
Thermogenic	Producing heat
Tikshna	Hot, fast acting, sharp (one of the *gunas*, qv)
Tikta	Bitter (one of the *gunas*, qv). Overshadows all other tastes. Appetiser and mouth cleanser, blood purifier and antipyretic, removes pus, toxins, serous discharge, increases *vata* and *pitta*
Tonic	A term used for medicinal preparations believed to have the power of restoring normal tone or function to tissues
Tonsillitis	Inflammation of the tonsils
Tridosha	The basic forces of the universe. The combination of the five elements gives the *doshas* (qv); the *tridosha* influences all mental and physical processes. From ether and air comes *vata*. From fire and water comes *pitta*. From earth and water comes *kapha*. The balance of the *doshas* determines body type, temperament and predisposing illnesses
Tympanites	A type of indigestion in cattle and sheep, marked by an abnormal collection of gas in the first stomach; also called bloat
Unctuous	Greasy or oily; oleaginous
Urethritis	Inflammation of the urethra
Urticaria	A reaction, usually transient, involving a rash or blistering of the upper dermis, localised oedema caused by dilation and increased permeability of the capillaries
Ushna	Hot (one of the *gunas*, qv)
Uterotonic	An agent that increases the tonus of uterine muscle
Vaginitis	Inflammation of the vagina; it is marked by pain and by a purulent discharge
Vata	One of the *doshas* (qv), mainly concerned with the nervous system and all bodily movement
Veerya	The potency of the drug, either heating or cooling
Vermifuge	An agent expelling worms or intestinal animal parasites; anthelmintic
Vertigo	A sense that either the environment or one's own body is revolving or falling; resulting from disease of the inner ear or a disturbance of the vestibular pathways in the central nervous system
Vesicant	Causing blisters
Vipaka	A postdigestive effect of the drug related to its taste: sweet, sour or pungent

Index

Page numbers in **bold** refer to major discussions in the text and usually include history, habitat, botanical description, parts used, traditional/modern uses, major chemical constituents, medicinal/pharmacological activities, safety profile, dosage and Ayurvedic properties.

A

aam **178–181**
aamra **178–181**
abdominal complaints, *Cyperus rotundus* 122
abhiru **51–55**
abortifacients
  Abrus precatorius 9
  Aegle marmelos 26
  Aristolochia indica 48
  Carica papaya 88
  Leptadenia reticulata 175
  Plumbago zeylanica 239
  Ricinus communis 254
Abrus precatorius .... **6–12,** Plate 1
Acacia catechu .... **13–15,** Plate 2
Acanthaceae 20, 40
Acorus aromaticus **16–19**
Acorus calamus .... **16–19,** Plate 3
adaptogens 337
  Asparagus racemosus 52
  Withania somnifera 322
Adhatoda vasica .... **20–24,** Plate 4
Adhatoda zeylanica **20–24**
adosa **20–24**
adrak (dried) **329–333**
Aegle marmelos .... **25–29,** Plate 5
aflatoxin inhibition, *Euphorbia hirta* 143
aged garlic extracts (AGE) 32
ageing, Hayflick system 32
aglycones, *Asparagus racemosus* 52
agnivardhana **306–310**
air, element 1
ajowan **306–310**
ajwain **306–310**
aldose reductase inhibition, *Phyllanthus niruri* 217
aliphatic alcohols, *Ficus religiosa* 146
alkaloids
  Abrus precatorius 7
  Adhatoda vasica 21
  Aegle marmelos 26
  Aristolochia indica 47
  Asparagus racemosus 52
  Bacopa monniera 65
  Berberis aristata 70
  Carica papaya 89
  Crataeva nurvala 114
  Embelia ribes 130
  Fumaria indica 151
  Holarrhena antidysenterica 173
  Mucuna pruriens 191
  Nigella sativa 197
  Paederia foetida 207
  Phyllanthus niruri 216
  Piper longum 226
  Piper nigrum 232
  Punica granatum 248
  Ricinus communis 252
  Solanum xanthocarpum 271
  Symplocos racemosa 278
  Tinospora cordifolia 303
  Trigonella foenum-graecum 316
  Withania somnifera 322
alkanes, *Euphorbia hirta* 142
allergies 341
  see also antiallergic drugs
Allium sativum .... **30–39,** Plate 6
amides
  Piper longum 226
  Piper nigrum 232
aminoacids
  Allium sativum 31
  Caesalpinia bonducella 84
  Centella asiatica 103
  Ficus religiosa 146
  Gossypium herbaceum 164
  Mucuna pruriens 191
  Piper nigrum 232
  Plumbago zeylanica 240
  Salmalia malabarica 261
  Tamarindus indica 284
  Trigonella foenum-graecum 316
amla **210–214**
amlaki **210–214**
amlika **283–289**
amrita **302–305**
anabolic activity, *Mucuna pruriens* 193
Anacardiaceae 178
analgesics 336
  Acorus calamus 17
  Bacopa monniera 66
  Boswellia serrata 80
  Embelia ribes 131
  Fumaria indica 151
  Mucuna pruriens 193
  Nigella sativa 198
  Ocimum sanctum 203
  Ricinus communis 252
  see also antinociceptive activity
anar **247–250**
Andrographis paniculata .... **40–45,** Plate 7
angarvelli **182–189**
anjawar **244–246**
anthelmintics 340
  Allium sativum 36–37
  Andrographis paniculata 41
  Caesalpinia bonducella 85
  Carica papaya 88, 93
  Embelia ribes 129, 130
  Ficus religiosa 147
  Gardenia gummifera 155
  Momordica charantia 185
  Mucuna pruriens 190
  Nigella sativa 198
  Paederia foetida 208
  Phyllanthus niruri 217
  Punica granatum 248
  Ricinus communis 252–253, 254
  Semecarpus anacardium 265
  Zingiber officinales 331

anthocyanins
Abrus precatorius 7
Polygonum aviculare 244
Punica granatum 248
Symplocos racemosa 277
Woodfordia fruticosa 327
anthraquinones
Aegle marmelos 26
Polygonum aviculare 244
Woodfordia fruticosa 327
antiageing activity, *Allium sativum* 32
antiallergic drugs 341
Abrus precatorius 9
Curcuma longa 118
Tinospora cordifolia 303
antiamoebic activity
Carica papaya 94
Euphorbia hirta 142
Punica granatum 248
Ricinus communis 254
Semecarpus anacardium 265
Terminalia chebula 299–300
antianaphylactics 341
Terminalia chebula 299
antiarthritics
Boswellia serrata 80
Commiphora mukul 110
Curcuma longa 117
Paederia foetida 207–208
Semecarpus anacardium 265
antiasthmatics 336
Abrus precatorius 7
Adhatoda vasica 21
Boswellia serrata 81
Curcuma longa 120
Euphorbia hirta 143
Ficus religiosa 147
Ocimum sanctum 203
Picrorrhiza kurroa 221–222
Piper longum 226–227
Solanum xanthocarpum 272
see also broncholytics
antiatherosclerotics 335–336
Allium sativum 36
Andrographis paniculata 42
Azadirachta indica 58
Commiphora mukul 111
antibacterials 339
Abrus precatorius 10
Acorus calamus 18
Adhatoda vasica 21–22
Allium sativum 33–34
Asparagus racemosus 52
Azadirachta indica 57–58
berberine 73
Cyperus rotundus 124
Eucalyptus globulus 136
Euphorbia hirta 142–143
Ficus religiosa 147
Gossypium herbaceum 165
Holarrhena antidysenterica 173
Leptadenia reticulata 176
Piper longum 227
Ricinus communis 252
Tamarindus indica 286
Terminalia arjuna 291–292
Terminalia chebula 299
Trachyspermum ammi 309
antibiotic resistance modifiers 339
Plumbago zeylanica 241
anticancer activity 338
Abrus precatorius 7
Acacia catechu 14
Allium sativum 34–35
Asparagus racemosus 52
Azadirachta indica 59
Boswellia serrata 80
Carica papaya 94
Cedrus deodara 100
Embelia ribes 131
Eucalyptus globulus 137
Euphorbia hirta 142
Ficus religiosa 147
Glycyrrhiza glabra 159
Gossypium herbaceum 165
Mangifera indica 180
Momordica charantia 183–184
Ocimum sanctum 203
Paederia foetida 208
Piper nigrum 233
Plumbago zeylanica 240
Rubia cordifolia 258
Semecarpus anacardium 263
Terminalia arjuna 291
Terminalia chebula 299
Tinospora cordifolia 303
Withania somnifera 324
Woodfordia fruticosa 327
see also antineoplastic activity
anticaries agents 339
Gymnema sylvestre 169
antichlamydial activity, *Berberis aristata* 70
anticlastogens 339
Phyllanthus niruri 217
anticoagulants 335
Plumbago zeylanica 242
Polygonum aviculare 245
anticonvulsants 337
Acorus calamus 17–18
Fumaria indica 151
Piper nigrum 233
Ricinus communis 254
anticytotoxic activity *see* cytoprotective activity
antidermatophytic activity, *Allium sativum* 34
antidiabetics 337–338
Azadirachta indica 58
Momordica charantia 182
Nigella sativa 197
Punica granatum 248–249
Trigonella foenum-graecum 316–317
see also hypoglycaemics
antidiarrhoeals 334
Abrus precatorius 10
Aegle marmelos 27
Andrographis paniculata 41
berberine 71–72
Caesalpinia bonducella 85
Euphorbia hirta 142
Holarrhena antidysenterica 173
Plantago ovata 237
Punica granatum 247
Syzygium cuminii 281

antidysentery agents 334
Holarrhena antidysenterica 172, 173
Piper longum 225
Punica granatum 247
antidyspepsia agents
Adhatoda vasica 22
Aegle marmelos 26
Andrographis paniculata 40
Cissus quadrangularis 106
Cyperus rotundus 122
Fumaria indica 150
Gardenia gummifera 154
Phyllanthus emblica 212
antiemetics 334
Cyperus rotundus 123
Zingiber officinales 330
antiepileptics 337
see also anticonvulsants
antifertility activity 341
Abrus precatorius
females 8–9
males 8
Adhatoda vasica 22
Aristolochia indica 47–48
Azadirachta indica 59–60
Carica papaya 89–91, 94
Euphorbia hirta 143
Gossypium herbaceum 164
Momordica charantia 185
Nigella sativa 198
Plumbago zeylanica 240
Solanum xanthocarpum 272
antifibrinolytics 335
Boerhaavia diffusa 77
Symplocos racemosa 278
antifibrotic activity, *Polygonum aviculare* 245
antifilarials
Andrographis paniculata 43
Caesalpinia bonducella 85
Ricinus communis 254
antifungals 339
Acacia catechu 14
Allium sativum 34
Azadirachta indica 57–58
Boswellia serrata 81
Carica papaya 94
Cedrus deodara 100
Embelia ribes 129
Euphorbia hirta 143
Fumaria indica 151
Leptadenia reticulata 176
Tamarindus indica 286
Trachyspermum ammi 308–309
antigenotoxic agents, *Momordica charantia* 185
antihaemorrhagics
Holarrhena antidysenterica 172
Mucuna pruriens 192
Polygonum aviculare 244
antihaemorrhoidals, *Plantago ovata* 237
antihepatotoxic activity *see* hepatoprotective agents
antihyperglycaemic agents *see* hypoglycaemics
antihypertensives 335
Allium sativum 36
Andrographis paniculata 43
Carica papaya 92
Cyperus rotundus 123
Eclipta alba 127
Eucalyptus globulus 137
Fumaria indica 151
Leptadenia reticulata 176
Ocimum sanctum 203
Phyllanthus niruri 216
Polygonum aviculare 245
Terminalia belerica 295
Trachyspermum ammi 307–308
Withania somnifera 324
see also calcium channel antagonists; diuretics
antiinflammatory agents 336
Abrus precatorius 9
Acacia catechu 14
Acorus calamus 17
Aegle marmelos 27
Andrographis paniculata 40
Azadirachta indica 59
berberine 72
Boswellia serrata 80
Caesalpinia bonducella 86
Commiphora mukul 111
Crataeva nurvala 115
Curcuma longa 118
Cyperus rotundus 123
Eclipta alba 127
Eucalyptus globulus 137
Euphorbia hirta 142
Fumaria indica 151
Glycyrrhiza glabra 160
Mangifera indica 179, 180
Mucuna pruriens 193
Nigella sativa 197–198
Ocimum sanctum 203
Paederia foetida 207
Phyllanthus emblica 213
Picrorrhiza kurroa 222
Piper longum 227
Piper nigrum 233
Plumbago zeylanica 240–241
Polygonum aviculare 245
Ricinus communis 253
Semecarpus anacardium 265
Solanum nigrum 269
Swertia chirata 275
Syzygium cuminii 281
Tamarindus indica 285
Terminalia belerica 296
Trigonella foenum-graecum 317
Woodfordia fruticosa 327
Zingiber officinales 330
antilarval activity, *Centella asiatica* 104
antileishmanial drugs
berberine 72
Swertia chirata 275
antilipolytics, *Momordica charantia* 185
antimalarials
Aegle marmelos 26
Andrographis paniculata 41
Azadirachta indica 58
Caesalpinia bonducella 85
Cyperus rotundus 123
Phyllanthus niruri 217
antimicrobials
Aegle marmelos 27
Berberis aristata 70

antimicrobials (*contd*)
Carica papaya 94
Centella asiatica 104
Curcuma longa 118–119
Embelia ribes 131
Glycyrrhiza glabra 159
Mangifera indica 179
Momordica charantia 185
Nigella sativa 197
Ocimum sanctum 203
Phyllanthus emblica 212
Phyllanthus niruri 216–217
Piper nigrum 232
Plumbago zeylanica 241
Polygonum aviculare 245
Punica granatum 248
Semecarpus anacardium 265
Swertia chirata 275
Symplocos racemosa 278
Terminalia belerica 295
Tribulus terrestris 312
Trigonella foenum-graecum 317
Withania somnifera 324
antimutagenic agents 339
Allium sativum 35
Curcuma longa 119
Glycyrrhiza glabra 160
Gossypium herbaceum 165
Punica granatum 249
Terminalia arjuna 291
Terminalia belerica 296
Terminalia chebula 299
antineoplastic activity
Semecarpus anacardium 264
Tinospora cordifolia 303
see also anticancer activity
antinociceptive activity
Azadirachta indica 58
Eclipta alba 127
Phyllanthus niruri 217
see also analgesics
antiobesity agents 334
Commiphora mukul 111
Cyperus rotundus 123
Terminalia belerica 295–296
antioestrogenic activity
Aristolochia indica 48
Caesalpinia bonducella 85
antioxidants 339
Allium sativum 35–36
Bacopa monniera 66
Carica papaya 94–95
Curcuma longa 119
Eucalyptus globulus 136
Glycyrrhiza glabra 159
Gymnema sylvestre 169
Mangifera indica 179
Phyllanthus emblica 212
Phyllanthus niruri 217
Piper nigrum 233
Plumbago zeylanica 241
Ricinus communis 254
Rubia cordifolia 258
Tamarindus indica 285
Terminalia belerica 295
Terminalia chebula 299–300
Tinospora cordifolia 303
Trigonella foenum-graecum 317–318
Withania somnifera 324
Zingiber officinales 331
antioxytocics 341
Nigella sativa 198
antiparasitic activity
Allium sativum 34
berberine 73
see also anthelmintics; antiamoebic activity; antileishmanial drugs; antimalarials; antiprotozoals; antischistosomal drugs
antiparkinsonian agents 337
Mucuna pruriens 190, 191–192
antiplaque agents 339
Embelia ribes 131
Syzygium cuminii 281
antiplatelet agents 335
Abrus precatorius 9
Allium sativum 36
Andrographis paniculata 41–42
Berberis aristata 70
Berberis aristata (berberine) 72
Rubia cordifolia 258
Trachyspermum ammi 307
Zingiber officinales 330
antiprotozoals 340
Asparagus racemosus 52
Ficus religiosa 147
antipsychotics 337
Fumaria indica 151
antipyretics 336
Andrographis paniculata 42
Azadirachta indica 58
Cyperus rotundus 123
Mucuna pruriens 193
Phyllanthus emblica 213
Woodfordia fruticosa 327
Zingiber officinales 330
antischistosomal drugs
Ricinus communis 254
Zingiber officinales 331
antiseptics
Eucalyptus globulus 135
Gardenia gummifera 154, 155
antispasmodics 334
Acorus calamus 17
Adhatoda vasica 21
Bacopa monniera 66
Cedrus deodara 100
Centella asiatica 103
Curcuma longa 119
Euphorbia hirta 142
Gardenia gummifera 155
Paederia foetida 208
Phyllanthus niruri 208
Symplocos racemosa 278
antispermatogenic agents, *Ocimum sanctum* 204
antistress agents 337
Boerhaavia diffusa 77
Ocimum sanctum 202–203
Tinospora cordifolia 303
Withania somnifera 322
antithrombotic agents 335
see also antiplatelet agents
antitubercular drugs 340
Adhatoda vasica 22
Centella asiatica 104

antitussives 336
Asparagus racemosus 52
antiulcer agents 334
Abrus precatorius 6
Acorus calamus 17
Aegle marmelos 26
Asparagus racemosus 52–53
Azadirachta indica 58, 60
Carica papaya 93
Centella asiatica 103
Curcuma longa 119
Cyperus rotundus 122
Ficus religiosa 147
Glycyrrhiza glabra 158–159
Ocimum sanctum 201
Solanum nigrum 269
Swertia chirata 275
Terminalia belerica 295
Tinospora cordifolia 303
Withania somnifera 324
Zingiber officinales 329
antiurolithiasis activity, *Phyllanthus niruri* 217
antivirals 340
Allium sativum 34
Andrographis paniculata 41
Azadirachta indica 57–58
Caesalpinia bonducella 85
Centella asiatica 104
Curcuma longa 119
Ficus religiosa 147
Glycyrrhiza glabra 159
Gossypium herbaceum 165
Gymnema sylvestre 169
Mangifera indica 179–180
Momordica charantia 185
Phyllanthus emblica 211
Phyllanthus niruri 216
Punica granatum 248
Tamarindus indica 286
Terminalia arjuna 291–292
Terminalia chebula 299
Trachyspermum ammi 308
Withania somnifera 324
Woodfordia fruticosa 327
Zingiber officinales 331
anxiolytics 337
Azadirachta indica 59
Bacopa monniera 65–66
aphrodisiacs
male 337
Mucuna pruriens 190, 193
Tribulus terrestris 311
Apiaceae 102, 263
Apocynaceae 172
Araceae 16
ardhrakam **329–333**
Aristolochiaceae 46
Aristolochia indica **46–50,** Plate 8
arjun **290–293**
arjuna **290–293**
arjun myrobalan **290–293**
arthritis treatment 337
see also antiarthritics; antiinflammatory agents
asagandh **321–325**
β-asarone 17
Asclepiadaceae 167, 175
ashwagandha **321–325**
ashwakarnabeez **236–238**
ashwattha **145–149**
asparagus, wild **51–55**
Asparagus racemosus **51–55,** Plate 9
Asteraceae 126
asthisandhani **106–109**
asthma treatment *see* antiasthmatics
astringents, *Aegle marmelos* 25
atherosclerosis, protection against *see* antiatherosclerotics
atmagupta **190–195**
Australian fever tree **134–140**
ayaskrti, Gymnema sylvestre 167
Ayurveda
history xii–xiii
principles **1–5**
Azadirachta indica **56–63,** Plate 10

B

babri **126–128**
bacillary dysentery, *Aegle marmelos* 26
Bacopa monniera **64–68,** Plate 11
bacterial infections, treatment *see* antibacterials
bahera **294–297**
bahupatra **215–219**
bael **25–29**
Balsamodendron mukul **110–114**
barambhi **64–68**
barna **114–116**
barun **114–116**
bel **25–29**
beleric myrobalan **294–297**
Bengal quince **25–29**
Berberidaceae 69
berberine 71–73
Berberis aristata **69–75,** Plate 12
Berberis chitria **69–75**
Berberis floribunda **69–75**
bhaira **294–297**
bhallataka **263–267**
bhangra **126–128**
bhilawa **263–267**
bhringaraja **126–128**
bhuinanvalah **215–219**
bhumyaamlaki **215–219**
bhunimba **40–45, 274–276**
bibhitaki **294–297**
bilharzia tapeworm, *Abrus precatorius* 7
bilva **25–29**
bio-availability enhancement
Piper longum 227
Tamarindus indica 286–287
bird's foot **315–320**
bishop's weed **306–310**
bitter gourd **182–189**
bitter melon **182–189**
black catechu **13–15**
black cumin **196–200**
black nightshade **268–270**
black pepper **231–235**
bladder stones 341
blond psyllium **236–238**
blue gum tree **134–140**
Bombax malabaricum **261–262**
bonduc nut **83–87**
bone-healing promoter 341
Cissus quadrangularis 106, 107–108
bone marrow enhancement, *Ocimum sanctum* 203

bone resorption inhibition, *Boerhaavia diffusa* 77
bone setter **106–109**
Boerhaavia diffusa **76–78,** Plate 13
Boerhaavia procumbens **76–78**
Boerhaavia repens **76–78**
Boswellia serrata **79–82,** Plate 14
bo-tree **145–149**
brahmi **64–68**
broken horn 14
broncholytics 336
  Adhatoda vasica 21
  Bacopa monniera 66
  see also antiasthmatics
bufadienolides, *Tamarindus indica* 284
bulk laxatives 334
Burseraceae 79, 110

C

Caesalpinia bonduc **83–87**
Caesalpinia bonducella **83–87,** Plate 15
Caesalpinia crista **83–87**
calcium channel antagonists 335
  Boerhaavia diffusa 77
caltrops **311–314**
cancer, supportive therapies 338
  see also anticancer activity
Capparidaceae 114
carbohydrates
  Abrus precatorius 7
  Mucuna pruriens 191
  Syzygium cuminii 280
  Trigonella foenum-graecum 316
carcinogens, *Acorus calamus* 18
cardenolide, *Tamarindus indica* 284
cardioprotectants 335
  see also cardiovascular activity
cardiotonics 335
  see also cardiovascular activity
cardiovascular activity 335–336
  Aegle marmelos 27
  Andrographis paniculata 42
  Azadirachta indica 59
  Salmalia malabarica 262
  Terminalia arjuna 290, 291
  Terminalia chebula 299
  Tribulus terrestris 312
  Zingiber officinales 330–331
Caricaceae 88
Carica papaya **88–98,** Plate 16
caries, treatment/prevention 339
  Gymnema sylvestre 169
carotene, *Paederia foetida* 207
carotenoids
  Carica papaya 89
  Mangifera indica 179
Carum copticum **306–310**
cassane diterpenes, *Caesalpinia bonducella* 84
castor bean **251–256**
castor oil plant **251–256**
Cedrus deodara **99–101,** Plate 17
cell differentiation induction, *Andrographis paniculata* 42
Centella asiatica **102–105,** Plate 18
central nervous system 1, 336–337
  depressants 337
    Azadirachta indica 59
    Swertia chirata 275
  stimulants 337
    Mucuna pruriens 193
    Ricinus communis 253
chavica roxburghii **225–230**
chemopreventative agents 338–339
chido **122–125**
Chinese flower **206–209**
chirayita **274–276**
chirbhita **88–98**
chiretta **274–276**
chitra **239–243**
chitraka **239–243**
chitravalli **257–260**
Chlamydia psittaci, antichlamydial activity, *Berberis aristata* 70
cholagogues 335
  Adhatoda vasica 22
  Curcuma longa 117
choleretics 335
cholesterol-lowering activity *see* hypocholesterolaemics
choti katheri **271–273**
chromones, *Mangifera indica* 179
cirrhosis, protection against 334–335
  see also hepatoprotective agents
Cissus quadrangularis **106–109,** Plate 19
coagulation inhibition *see* anticoagulants
cognitive function, *Bacopa monniera* 65
collagenase inhibition, *Eucalyptus globulus* 137
Combretaceae 290, 294, 298
Commiphora mukul **110–114,** Plate 20
complement inhibiting drugs 341
  Boswellia serrata 80
conessi **172–174**
consciousness 1
constipation, *Ocimum sanctum* 204
contraceptives
  Embelia ribes 130–131
  postcoital 341
  precoital 341
  Punica granatum 249
  Ricinus communis 254
cosmic energy 1
cotton **163–166**
coughing, prevention 336
  Asparagus racemosus 52
coumarins
  Aegle marmelos 26
  Ficus religiosa 146
  Glycyrrhiza glabra 158
  Ricinus communis 252
  Trigonella foenum-graecum 316
coumestan derivatives, *Glycyrrhiza glabra* 158
cowhage **190–195**
cowitch **190–195**
crab's eye **6–12**
Crataeva magna **114–116**
Crataeva nurvala **114–116,** Plate 21
Crataeva religiosa **114–116**
creat **40–45**
Cucurbitaceae 182
cucurbitacin glycosides, *Picrorrhiza kurroa* 220
cumbi-resin **154–156**
Curcuma domestica **117–121**
Curcuma longa **117–121,** Plate 22
cutch tree **13–15**
Cyperaceae 122
Cyperus rotundus **122–125,** Plate 23
cytokinins, *Phyllanthus emblica* 211

cytoprotective activity
  Acorus calamus 17
  Cyperus rotundus 123
  Phyllanthus niruri 217
cytotoxic agents *see* anticancer activity
cytotoxins 338
  Nigella sativa 198
  Phyllanthus emblica 211–212
  Tribulus terrestris 313

D

Dabur Research Foundation (DRF) viii–ix
  activities viii
  background viii
  contact information ix
  facilities ix
  manpower viii
  networking ix
  objectives viii
dadim **247–250**
daruhaldi **69–75**
daru haridra **69–75**
dashmool, *Aegle marmelos* 26
datura poisoning, *Andrographis paniculata* 41
dental caries, treatment/prevention 339
  Gymnema sylvestre 169
deodar **99–101**
dermatitis
  Mangifera indica 180
  Nigella sativa 198
  see also skin disorders
devadaru **99–101**
dhai **326–328**
dhataki **326–328**
dhatoora *(datura)* poisoning, *Andrographis paniculata* 41
dhatus 3–4
diabetes, prevention/treatment *see* antidiabetics
diallyl sulphide (DAS) 32
diarrhoea
  Adhatoda vasica causing 22
  chronic, *Aegle marmelos* 25
  poultry, *Andrographis paniculata* 41
  ruminants
    Acacia catechu 14
    Aegle marmelos 26
diarrhoea treatment *see* antidiarrhoeals
dietary supplementation, *Ficus religiosa* 147–148
digestive activity
  Aegle marmelos 25
  animals, *Aegle marmelos* 26
  Gardenia gummifera 155
  Plumbago zeylanica 242
dikamali **154–156**
dikamali **154–156**
disease, treatment 4
diterpenes, *Tinospora cordifolia* 303
diuretics 335
  Allium sativum 36
  Boerhaavia diffusa 77
  Carica papaya 92
  Eucalyptus globulus 137
  Gymnema sylvestre 167
  Phyllanthus niruri 216
  Ricinus communis 254
  Syzygium cuminii 281
  Tribulus terrestris 311
dori **175–177**
doshas 1
drug adsorption *see* bio-availability enhancement
drug biotransformations, *Piper longum* 227–228
dudhi **141–144**
dugadhika **141–144**
dyer's madder **257–260**
dysentery, prevention/treatment *see* antidysentery agents
dysentery, bacillary, *Aegle marmelos* 26
dyspepsia, treatment/prevention *see* antidyspepsia agents

E

earth, element 1
Eclipta alba **126–128**, Plate 24
Eclipta prostrata **126–128**
elements, five 1
embelia fruit **129–133**
Embelia ribes **129–133**, Plate 25
Embolica officinalis **210–214**
embolic myrobalan **210–214**
emmenagogues
  Abrus precatorius 7
  Carica papaya 88
  Commiphora mukul 110
  Gossypium herbaceum 163
endi **251–256**
endocrine system 1
Entamoeba histolytica, effect of berberine 73
enzymes, *Carica papaya* 89
epilepsy, animals, *Bacopa monniera* 65
eranda **251–256**
essential oils
  Acorus calamus 17
  Adhatoda vasica 21
  Cedrus deodara 100
  Centella asiatica 103
  Cyperus rotundus 122–123
  Eucalyptus globulus 135
  Mangifera indica 179
  Ocimum sanctum 202
  Paederia foetida 207
  Zingiber officinales 330
esters, *Piper longum* 226
ether (space) 1
Eucalyptus globulus **134–140**, Plate 26
Eugenia cumini **279–282**
Eugenia jambolana **279–282**
Euphorbiaceae 141, 210, 215, 251
Euphorbia hirta **141–144**, Plate 27
eye disorders
  Abrus precatorius 7
  ruminants, *Acorus calamus* 17
  Terminalia belerica 296

F

Fabaceae 6, 315
false daisy **126–128**
fatty acids
  Adhatoda vasica 21
  Berberis aristata 70
  Caesalpinia bonducella 84
  Embelia ribes 130
  Mangifera indica 179
  Momordica charantia 183
  Mucuna pruriens 191
  Ocimum sanctum 202
  Paederia foetida 207
  Phyllanthus emblica 211

fatty acids (*contd*)
- *Ricinus communis* 252
- *Salmalia malabarica* 261
- *Syzygium cuminii* 280
- *Tamarindus indica* 285
- *Trachyspermum ammi* 307

females, antifertility activity, *Abrus precatorius* 8–9
fenugreek **315–320**
fertility
- inhibition *see* antifertility activity
- potentiation, *Tribulus terrestris* 312

fever, treatment *see* antipyretics
fever nut **83–87**
fibrinolytic activity
- *Commiphora mukul* 112
- *see also* antifibrinolytics

Ficus religiosa **145–149,** Plate 28
filaricidal activity *see* antifilarials
fire, element 1
fire-flame bush **326–328**
fixed oil
- *Nigella sativa* 197
- *Semecarpus anacardium* 264
- *Terminalia belerica* 295

flavanols, *Trigonella foenum-graecum* 316
flavone derivatives, *Centella asiatica* 103
flavones
- *Allium sativum* 32
- *Tamarindus indica* 284
- *Woodfordia fruticosa* 327

flavonoid glycosides, *Nigella sativa* 197
flavonoids
- *Abrus precatorius* 7
- *Acacia catechu* 14
- *Adhatoda vasica* 21
- *Asparagus racemosus* 52
- *Bacopa monniera* 65
- *Berberis aristata* 70
- *Carica papaya* 89
- *Cedrus deodara* 100
- *Crataeva nurvala* 115
- *Eclipta alba* 127
- *Eucalyptus globulus* 135
- *Euphorbia hirta* 142
- *Gardenia gummifera* 155
- *Glycyrrhiza glabra* 158
- *Gossypium herbaceum* 164
- *Leptadenia reticulata* 176
- *Ocimum sanctum* 202
- *Phyllanthus niruri* 216
- *Polygonum aviculare* 244
- *Punica granatum* 248
- *Ricinus communis* 252
- *Semecarpus anacardium* 264
- *Symplocos racemosa* 277
- *Syzygium cuminii* 280
- *Terminalia arjuna* 291
- *Tribulus terrestris* 312

flavonols
- *Allium sativum* 32
- *Tamarindus indica* 284

fluoride toxicity 286
free radical scavengers 339
- *see also* antioxidants

Fumariaceae 150
Fumaria indica **150–154,** Plate 29
Fumaria parviflora **150–154**
Fumaria vallantii **150–154**
fumitory **150–154**
fungal infections, prevention/treatment *see* antifungals
furanoditerpenes, *Caesalpinia bonducella* 84

G

GABA, *Boerhaavia diffusa* effect 77
gadahpurna **76–78**
galactagogues 341
- *Asparagus racemosus* 53
- *Cissus quadrangularis* 107
- *Euphorbia hirta* 143
- *Leptadenia reticulata* 176

gandhaprasarini **206–209**
Gardenia gummifera **154–156,** Plate 30
garden nightshade **268–270**
garlic **30–39**
gastric irritation, *Picrorrhiza kurroa* 222
gastrointestinal tract, *Piper nigrum* 232–233
Gentianaceae 274
Giardia lamblia, effect of berberine 73
ginger **329–333**
glucosinolates, *Carica papaya* 89
glycans, *Curcuma longa* 118
glycosides
- *Allium sativum* 31
- *Trachyspermum ammi* 307

Glycyrrhiza glabra **157–162,** Plate 31
gokhru **311–314**
gokshura **311–314**
golmirch **231–235**
gonorrhoea, *Abrus precatorius* 7
Gossypium herbaceum **163–166,** Plate 32
gotu kola **102–105**
Gratiola monnieria **64–68**
green chiretta **40–45**
growth regulatory activity, *Azadirachta indica* 60
guggul **110–114**
guggulu **110–114**
gulancha tinospora **302–305**
guluchi **302–305**
Gunas (twenty attributes) 3
gunja **6–12**
gurmar **167–171**
guruchi **302–305**
Gymnema sylvestre **167–171,** Plate 33

H

hadjora **106–109**
haldi **117–121**
harad **298–301**
haridra **117–121**
haritaki **298–301**
Hayflick system, ageing 32
heat stroke, *Mangifera indica* 178
hepatic enzyme induction, *Piper nigrum* 233
hepatitis, protection against *see* hepatoprotective agents
hepatoprotective agents 334–335
- *Acacia catechu* 14
- *Allium sativum* 33
- *Andrographis paniculata* 42
- *Azadirachta indica* 59
- berberine 71
- *Berberis aristata* 70–71

Boerhaavia diffusa 77
Curcuma longa 119
Eclipta alba 127
Fumaria indica 151
Glycyrrhiza glabra 159
Gymnema sylvestre 169
Mangifera indica 180
Momordica charantia 185
Nigella sativa 197
Paederia foetida 208
Phyllanthus emblica 212
Phyllanthus niruri 215, 216
Picrorrhiza kurroa 221
Piper longum 227
Polygonum aviculare 245
Ricinus communis 253–254
Rubia cordifolia 258
Solanum nigrum 269
Swertia chirata 275
Terminalia arjuna 291
Terminalia belerica 295
Tinospora cordifolia 304
Withania somnifera 324
Zingiber officinales 330
hepatotoxic effects, *Punica granatum* 249
Herpestis monniera **64–68**
Himalaya cedar **99–101**
Holarrhena antidysenterica **172–174**, Plate 34
holy basil **201–205**
'honey urine,' *Gymnema sylvestre* 167
houseflies, *Acorus calamus* 17
human constitution *(prakruti)* 2–3
humours, three *(tridosha)* 1–2
hydrocarbons
Adhatoda vasica 21
Berberis aristata 70
Caesalpinia bonducella 84
Cedrus deodara 100
Ficus religiosa 146
Mangifera indica 179
Woodfordia fruticosa 327
Hydrocotyle asiatica **102–105**
hypercholesterolaemia 335–336
see also antiatherosclerotics
hyperlipidaemia 335–336
see also antiatherosclerotics
hypersensitivity reactions, *Plantago ovata* 237
hypertension 335
see also antihypertensives
hypocholesterolaemics
Boswellia serrata 80
Curcuma longa 120
Piper longum 227
Plantago ovata 237
Semecarpus anacardium 265
Trigonella foenum-graecum 317
hypoglycaemics 337–338
Acacia catechu 14
Aegle marmelos 27
Andrographis paniculata 42
Azadirachta indica 59
Caesalpinia bonducella 85
Curcuma longa 119
Eucalyptus globulus 137
Ficus religiosa 146–147
Fumaria indica 151–152
Gymnema sylvestre 168
Holarrhena antidysenterica 173
Mangifera indica 180
Momordica charantia 184–185
Mucuna pruriens 192
Ocimum sanctum 203
Phyllanthus emblica 212
Phyllanthus niruri 216
Plantago ovata 237
Swertia chirata 275
Syzygium cuminii 280–281
Tamarindus indica 285–286
Terminalia belerica 296
Tinospora cordifolia 304
Trigonella foenum-graecum 304
see also antidiabetics
hypolipidaemics
Allium sativum 32–33
Caesalpinia bonducella 85
Carica papaya 92
Commiphora mukul 111–112
Ficus religiosa 146–147
Gymnema sylvestre 169
Ocimum sanctum 203
Phyllanthus emblica 211
Plumbago zeylanica 241
Tamarindus indica 285
Terminalia arjuna 291
Terminalia belerica 295
Zingiber officinales 331
hypoprolactinaemics, *Mucuna pruriens* 192
hypotensive agents *see* antihypertensives
hypothermics, *Gardenia gummifera* 155

I

imli **283–289**
immune system 1
immunomodulatory activity 338
Abrus precatorius 7–8
Aegle marmelos 28
Allium sativum 32
Andrographis paniculata 43
Asparagus racemosus 53–54
Azadirachta indica 60
Boswellia serrata 80
Centella asiatica 104
Curcuma longa 119–120
Euphorbia hirta 143
Holarrhena antidysenterica 173
Mangifera indica 180
Ocimum sanctum 202
Phyllanthus emblica 212
Picrorrhiza kurroa 221
Piper longum 226
Plumbago zeylanica 241
Ricinus communis 253
Semecarpus anacardium 264
Tamarindus indica 285
Terminalia chebula 299
Tinospora cordifolia 303–304
Withania somnifera 322–324
Woodfordia fruticosa 327
Zingiber officinales 331
Indian barberry **69–75**
Indian bdellium tree **110–114**
Indian birthwort **46–50**

Indian blackberry 279–282
Indian gooseberry 210–214
Indian liquorice 6–12
Indian madder 257–260
Indian olibanum tree 79–82
Indian pennywort 102–105
indigestion, *Cissus quadrangularis* 106
infections, treatment 339–341
infestations, treatment 339–341
inflammatory activity
  Rubia cordifolia 258
  see also antiinflammatory agents
injuries *see* wound-healing promoters
inknut 298–301
insecticides 340
  Abrus precatorius 9
  Adhatoda vasica 22
  Azadirachta indica 60
  Cedrus deodara 100
  Embelia ribes 131
  Eucalyptus globulus 137
  Gardenia gummifera 155
  Ocimum sanctum 201
  Solanum xanthocarpum 272
  Trachyspermum ammi 308
insect repellents 340
  Eucalyptus globulus 135, 137
  Zingiber officinales 331
interceptive activity, *Aristolochia indica* 48
intestinal worms, *Mucuna pruriens* 190
iridoid glucosides
  Paederia foetida 207
  Picrorrhiza kurroa 220
iridoids
  Rubia cordifolia 258
  Salmalia malabarica 262
  Swertia chirata 274
irritable bowel syndrome, *Aegle marmelos* 27
irritants, *Mucuna pruriens* 193
isapghul 236–238
isharmul 46–50
isoflavones, *Caesalpinia bonducella* 84
isoflavonoids
  Abrus precatorius 7
  Eclipta alba 127
  Glycyrrhiza glabra 158
isosarone 17
ispaghula 236–238

J

jambu 279–282
jambul 279–282
Jammu xii
jamun 279–282
jaundice, *Andrographis paniculata* 40
java plum 279–282
jequirity 6–12
jivanti 175–177
Justicia adhatoda 20–24
Justicia paniculata 40–45

K

kakamachi 268–270
kakubha 290–293
kalajaji 196–200
kalajira 196–200
kalmegh 40–45
kalmirch 231–235
kalonji 196–200
kankarej 83–87
kantkari 271–273
kapas 163–166
kapha 1, 2
  constitution 3
  disorders 4
  morbidity
    Aristolochia indica 46–47
    Gossypium herbaceum 164
karavellaka 182–189
karela 182–189
kateli 271–273
katikaranja 83–87
katukarohini 220–224
kavach 190–195
khadira 13–15
khair 13–15
khetpapra 150–154
kidney stones 341
kirat 274–276
kirata-tikta 274–276
knotgrass 244–246
kuberakshi 83–87
kula kudi 102–105
kurchi 172–174
kutaja 172–174
kutaki 220–224
kutki 220–224

L

lactation inducing drugs 341
lactation promotion 341
  buffaloes, *Asparagus racemosus* 51
  see also galactagogues
laghu kantkari 271–273
Lamiaceae 201
larvicides
  Allium sativum 36
  Eucalyptus globulus 137
lasan 30–39
lasuma 30–39
laxatives
  bulk 334
  Glycyrrhiza glabra 158
  Picrorrhiza kurroa 222
  Plantago ovata 237
  Ricinus communis 253
  stimulant 334
learning ability enhancers 337
  Bacopa monniera 65
  see also memory enhancers
Leguminoceae 6
Leguminosae 13, 83, 283
Leishmania treatment *see* antileishmanial drugs
leptadenia 175–177
Leptadenia reticulata 175–177, Plate 35
leukaemia, *Acacia catechu* action 14
lice, treatment in birds, *Acorus calamus* 17
lignans
  Boerhaavia diffusa 76
  Commiphora mukul 111
  Phyllanthus niruri 216
  Piper longum 226
  Tribulus terrestris 312
Liliaceae 51

Liliaceae 30
limonoids, *Azadirachta indica* 57
lipid peroxidation activity, *Polygonum aviculare* 245
lipids
Cissus quadrangularis 107
Commiphora mukul 111
see also hypocholesterolaemics
lipolytic activity 252
liquorice **157–162**
liver protectants *see* hepatoprotective agents
lodh **277–278**
lodhra **277–278**
long pepper **225–230**
Lysimachia monnieria **64–68**
Lythraceae 326

M

machoti **244–246**
madhuka **157–162**
madhu meha, Gymnema sylvestre 167
majeeth **257–260**
makoi **268–270**
malabar nut **20–24**
malaria treatment *see* antimalarials
males, antifertility activity, *Abrus precatorius* 8
malignant disease, herbs active against 338
see also anticancer activity
Malvaceae 163, 261
mandukparni **102–105**
Mangifera indica **178–181**, Plate 36
mango tree **178–181**
manjista **257–260**
manjit **257–260**
margosa **56–63**
maricha **231–235**
marking-nut tree **263–267**
medicinal preparations 4
melanocyte proliferation, *Piper nigrum* 233
Meliaceae 56
memory enhancers 337
Bacopa monniera 65
Withania somnifera 322
Menispermaceae 302
Menispermum cordifolium **302–305**
meshasringi **167–171**
metabolic activity, *tridosha* 2
methi **315–320**
methika **315–320**
minerals
Allium sativum 32
Carica papaya 89
Ficus religiosa 146
Piper nigrum 232
Syzygium cuminii 280
Tamarindus indica 285
molluscicides 340–341
Abrus precatorius 9
Asparagus racemosus 54
Cedrus deodara 100
Solanum nigrum 269
Tamarindus indica 286
Trachyspermum ammi 308
Zingiber officinales 331
Momordica charantia **182–189**, Plate 37
Moniera cunefolia **64–68**
monoterpenes, *Curcuma longa* 118
monoterpenoids
Allium sativum 31
Carica papaya 89
Syzygium cuminii 280
Tamarindus indica 285
Trachyspermum ammi 307
Moraceae 145
moral disposition 3
morphine tolerance inhibition, *Withania somnifera* 324
motha **122–125**
mouth disorders, *Syzygium cuminii* 279
mucosa protection, *Plantago ovata* 237
Mucuna pruriens **190–195**, Plate 38
Muldera multinervis **231–235**
mulethi **157–162**
murabbas, Aegle marmelos 25
muscle relaxants 337
Cyperus rotundus 123
Gymnema sylvestre 169
mustaka **122–125**
mutagenicity, protection *see* antimutagenic agents
Mycobacterium, agents active against *see* antitubercular drugs
myocardial necrosis, *Phyllanthus emblica* 212
myrobalan **298–301**
Myrobalanus bellirica **294–297**
Myrsinaceae 129
Myrtaceae 134, 279
myrtle flag **16–19**
Myrtus cuminii **279–282**

N

nadi-hingu **154–156**
naphthalene derivatives, *Plumbago zeylanica* 240
nasomali **244–246**
necrotising pancreatitis, *Phyllanthus emblica* 212
neem **56–63**
neem tree **56–63**
nephroprotective activity, *Tribulus terrestris* 312
Newcastle disease, *Andrographis paniculata* 41
Nigella sativa **196–200**, Plate 39
nilgiri **134–140**
nim **56–63**
nimba **56–63**
nirabarhmi **64–68**
nitrogenous compounds
Abrus precatorius 7
Gymnema sylvestre 168
nutgrass **122–125**
nutsedge **122–125**
Nyctaginaceae 76

O

obesity prevention *see* antiobesity agents
Ocimum sanctum **201–205**, Plate 40
oedema 335
see also diuretics
oestrogenic drugs 341
Cyperus rotundus 123
Ficus religiosa 147
omum **306–310**
ophthalmic delivery, *Tamarindus indica* 286
oral contraceptives, *Abrus precatorius* 7
organic acids
Phyllanthus emblica 211
Tamarindus indica 284
oxytocics 341
Salmalia malabarica 262

P

Paederia foetida 206–209, Plate 41
Paederia scandens 206–209
Paederia tomentosa 206–209
pain management *see* analgesics; antinociceptive activity
palatal taste response inhibition, *Gymnema sylvestre* 168–169
papaya 88–98
Papilionaceae 157, 190
papita 88–98
parasites, prevention/treatment *see* anthelmintics; antiamoebic activity; antileishmanial drugs; antimalarials; antiprotozoals; antischistosomal drugs
parasympatholytic activity, *Ficus religiosa* 147
Parkinson's disease, management *see* antiparkinsonian agents
parpata 150–154
pawpaw 88–98
peepal 145–149
peepul 145–149
peptic ulcers, prevention/treatment *see* antiulcer agents
peptides, *Allium sativum* 32
periploca of the wood 167–171
pharmacological activities, *Plantago ovata* 237
phenanthrene derivatives, *Aristolochia indica* 47
phenolic acids, *Ricinus communis* 252
phenolic compounds
  Semecarpus anacardium 264
  Zingiber officinales 330
phenolics
  Caesalpinia bonducella 84
  Mangifera indica 179
  Picrorrhiza kurroa 220
  Syzygium cuminii 280
phenols, *Phyllanthus niruri* 216
phenylpropanoids
  Commiphora mukul 111
  Curcuma longa 118
Phyllanthus amarus 215–219
Phyllanthus emblica 210–214, Plate 42
Phyllanthus fraternus 215–219
Phyllanthus niruri 215–219, Plate 43
Phyllanthus sellowianus 215–219
phytosterols
  Adhatoda vasica 21
  Berberis aristata 70
  Caesalpinia bonducella 84
  Centella asiatica 103
  Cissus quadrangularis 107
  Gardenia gummifera 155
  Glycyrrhiza glabra 158
  Leptadenia reticulata 176
  Punica granatum 248
  Ricinus communis 252
  Tamarindus indica 284
  Tribulus terrestris 311
  Withania somnifera 322
  Woodfordia fruticosa 327
Picrorrhiza kurroa 220–224, Plate 44
pigmentation, *Cyperus rotundus* 123
pigweed 76–78
Pinaceae 99
pipal 145–149
Piperaceae 225, 231
Piper latifolium 225–230
Piper longum 225–230, Plate 45
Piper nigrum 231–235, Plate 46
Piper sarmentosum 225–230
Piper tritoicum 231–235
pippala 145–149
pippali 225–230
pitpapra 150–154
pitta 1, 2
  constitution 3
  disorders 4
  morbidity
    Aristolochia indica 46
    Gossypium herbaceum 164
Plantaginaceae 236
Plantago ovata 236–238, Plate 47
Plumbaginaceae 239
Plumbago zeylanica 239–243, Plate 48
poisoning
  Abrus precatorius 6, 10
  dhatoora *(datura), Andrographis paniculata* 41
  Gymnema sylvestre 167
  Polygonum aviculare 245
Polygonaceae 244
Polygonum aviculare 244–246, Plate 49
polypeptides, *Gymnema sylvestre* 168
polyphenolics
  Berberis aristata 70
  Polygonum aviculare 244
polyphenols
  Eucalyptus globulus 135
  Euphorbia hirta 142
  Ocimum sanctum 202
  Phyllanthus emblica 211
  Phyllanthus niruri 216
  Solanum xanthocarpum 272
  Terminalia arjuna 291
  Terminalia belerica 295
  Terminalia chebula 299
polysaccharides
  Azadirachta indica 57
  Plantago ovata 236
  Tamarindus indica 284
pomegranate 247–250
postcoital contraceptives 341
prakruti (human constitution) 2–3
prasarini 206–209
precoital contraceptives 341
principles of *Ayurveda* 1–5
prostate hypertrophy inhibitor 341
prostrate knotweed 244–246
proteins
  Abrus precatorius 7
  Momordica charantia 183
  Mucuna pruriens 191
  Ricinus communis 252
psychological disposition 3
psychoneurological activity, *Centella asiatica* 104
punarnava 76–78
Punicaceae 247
Punica granatum 247–250, Plate 50

Q

quinones
  Abrus precatorius 7
  Aristolochia indica 47
  Embelia ribes 130
  Paederia foetida 207
  Rubia cordifolia 258

R

radioprotective effect, *Ocimum sanctum* 203
rajas 3
rakta-pushpa **261–262**
Ranunculaceae 196
rasayanas 102
rasonam **30–39**
rati **6–12**
reproductive system
  herbs active on 341
  increased egg yield 176
respiratory activity 336
  Adhatoda vasica 20
  Solanum xanthocarpum 272
respiratory complaints, animals
  poultry, *Andrographis paniculata* 41
  ruminants, *Adhatoda vasica* 21
rheumatism, treatment 337
  see also antiarthritics; antiinflammatory agents
Ricinus communis **251–256,** Plate 51
rotenoids, *Boerhaavia diffusa* 76
Rubiaceae 154, 206, 257
Rubia cordifolia **257–260,** Plate 52
Rubia mungisth **257–260**
Rubia munjista **257–260**
Rubia secunda **257–260**
Rutaceae 25

S

sacred basil **201–205**
sacred fig **145–149**
salai **79–82**
sallaki **79–82**
Salmalia malabarica **261–262,** Plate 53
saponins
  Abrus precatorius 7
  Bacopa monniera 65
  Eclipta alba 126–127
  Gymnema sylvestre 167–168
  Mangifera indica 179
  Nigella sativa 197
  Paederia foetida 207
  Tribulus terrestris 311
  Trigonella foenum graecum 316
satavari **51–55**
satva 3
scorpion bite, *Cyperus rotundus* 122
Scrophulariaceae 64, 220
sedge weed **122–125**
Semecarpus anacardium **263–267,** Plate 54
semul **261–262**
sesquiterpenes
  Aristolochia indica 47
  Curcuma longa 118
  Gossypium herbaceum 164
sexual dysfunction, *Tribulus terrestris* 312–313
shatavari **51–55**
shatter stone **215–219**
shiranjitea **326–328**
Shiva, Lord 25
Shiva, tree of ('*shivadruma*') 25
'*shivadruma*' 25
Siddha medicine 107
silk cotton tree **261–262**
sison ammi **306–310**
skin disorders
  Abrus precatorius 6
  Cedrus deodara 100
  Leptadenia reticulata 175
  see also dermatitis
small fennel **196–200**
snakebite
  Abrus precatorius 7
  Aegle marmelos 26
  Gymnema sylvestre 167
snakeweed **141–144**
Solanaceae 268
Solanaceae 271, 321
Solanum americanum **268–270**
Solanum nigrum **268–270,** Plate 55
Solanum surattense **271–273**
Solanum xanthocarpum **271–273,** Plate 56
sonth (fresh) **329–333**
sparrow-grass **51–55**
spasmogenic activity, *Leptadenia reticulata* 176
spasmolytic activity *see* antispasmodics
spermatogenesis enhancers 341
  Allium sativum 33
  Mucuna pruriens 192–193
spermatozoa, motility reduction, *Abrus precatorius* 8
spermicides, *Trachyspermum ammi* 309
spogel **236–238**
spreading hogweed **76–78**
steroidal glycoalkaloids, *Solanum nigrum* 269
steroidal glycosides, *Asparagus racemosus* 52
steroidal saponins
  Caesalpinia bonducella 84
  Solanum nigrum 269
steroid lactones, *Withania somnifera* 322
sterols
  Commiphora mukul 111
  Ficus religiosa 146
  Momordica charantia 183
  Mucuna pruriens 191
  Nigella sativa 197
  Ocimum sanctum 202
  Solanum xanthocarpum 271
  Syzygium cuminii 279
stilbene derivatives, *Cissus quadrangularis* 107
stimulant laxatives 334
stimulants, *Piper longum* 226
stone breaker **215–219**
stress, management *see* antistress agents
sugars
  Boswellia serrata 80
  Tamarindus indica 284
sulphur compounds, *Allium sativum* 31
sunanda **46–50**
surasa **201–205**
sweetening agents, *Abrus precatorius* 9–10
sweet flag **16–19**
sweet sedge **16–19**
Swertia chirata **274–276,** Plate 57
switradilepa, *Andrographis paniculata* 41
Symplocaceae 277
symplocos bark **277–278**
Symplocos racemosa **277–278,** Plate 58
Syzygium cuminii **279–282,** Plate 59

T

tailparna **134–140**
tamarind **283–289**

Tamarindus indica **283–289**, Plate 60
tamas 3
tannins
  Acacia catechu 14
  Aegle marmelos 26
  Crataeva nurvala 114
  Eucalyptus globulus 135
  Euphorbia hirta 142
  Ficus religiosa 146
  Phyllanthus niruri 216
  Punica granatum 248
  Salmalia malabarica 261
  Symplocos racemosa 278
  Terminalia chebula 299
  Woodfordia fruticosa 326–327
taste response inhibition, *Gymnema sylvestre* 168–169
tekarajah **126–128**
tellicherry **172–174**
temperament 3
teratogens
  Boerhaavia diffusa 77
  Solanum nigrum 269
Terminalia arjuna **290–293**, Plate 61
Terminalia belerica **294–297**, Plate 62
Terminalia chebula **298–301**, Plate 63
Terminalia cuneata **290–293**
terpenes
  Aristolochia indica 47
  Azadirachta indica 57
  Commiphora mukul 111
terpenoids, *Momordica charantia* 183
terra japonica **13–15**
thermogenic activity
  Piper nigrum 233
  Zingiber officinales 331
three-leaved caper **114–116**
thyme-leaved gratiola **64–68**
Tinospora cordifolia **302–305**, Plate 64
Tinospora glabra **302–305**
tintiri **283–289**
toxicity concerns xiii
Trachyspermum ammi **306–310**, Plate 65
trailing eclipta **126–128**
tranquillising effect, *Cyperus rotundus* 123
Tribulus terrestris **311–314**, Plate 66
Trichomonas vaginalis, effect of berberine 73
tridosha (three humours) 1–2
  metabolic activities 2
Trigonella foenum-graecum **315–320**, Plate 67
triterpene glycosides, *Eclipta alba* 126–127
triterpenes
  Adhatoda vasica 21
  Aegle marmelos 26
  Bacopa monniera 65
  Boswellia serrata 79–80
  Crataeva nurvala 115
  Cyperus rotundus 123
  Euphorbia hirta 142
  Gardenia gummifera 155
  Gymnema sylvestre 167–168
  Mangifera indica 179
  Mucuna pruriens 191
  Ocimum sanctum 202
  Phyllanthus niruri 216
  Plumbago zeylanica 240
  Punica granatum 248
  Swertia chirata 274
  Symplocos racemosa 277
  Syzygium cuminii 280
  Tamarindus indica 284
triterpene saponins, *Glycyrrhiza glabra* 158
triterpenoid glycosides, *Terminalia chebula* 299
triterpenoids
  Abrus precatorius 7
  Centella asiatica 103
  Eucalyptus globulus 135
  Leptadenia reticulata 176
  Paederia foetida 207
  Rubia cordifolia 258
  Terminalia arjuna 291
  Terminalia belerica 295
trypsin inhibition, *Embelia ribes* 131
tulsi **201–205**
tundakesi **163–166**
turmeric **117–121**
twenty attributes *(gunas)* 3

U

ugragandha **16–19**
ulcers, prevention/treatment *see* antiulcer agents
Umbelliferae 102, 263, 306
Unani medicine 129
  Allium sativum 31
Uncaria gambier 13
urinary disorders
  Adhatoda vasica 20
  ruminants, *Boerhaavia diffusa* 76
urinary system, herbs active on 341
urolitholytic agents 341
  Crataeva nurvala 115
  Tribulus terrestris 312
uterine stimulants 341
  Caesalpinia bonducella 85–86
  Plumbago zeylanica 241–242
uterotonic agents 341
  Adhatoda vasica 22
  Carica papaya 91–92
  see also uterine stimulants

V

vacha **16–19**
vanari **190–195**
varuna **114–116**
varunadi ghrtam, Gymnema sylvestre 167
varunadi kasayam, Gymnema sylvestre 167
vasaka **20–24**
vasicine 21
vata
  constitution 2–3
  disorders 4
  morbidity
    Aristolochia indica 46
    Gossypium herbaceum 164
vibeekaka **294–297**
vibitaki **294–297**
vidanga **129–133**
viranga **129–133**
virus infection prevention/treatment *see* antivirals
viswabhesaja **329–333**
Vitaceae 106
vitamin C, *Paederia foetida* 207

vitamins
- *Allium sativum* 32
- *Carica papaya* 89
- *Ficus religiosa* 146
- *Mangifera indica* 179
- *Piper nigrum* 232
- *Syzygium cuminii* 280
- *Tamarindus indica* 285
- *Trachyspermum ammi* 307

Vitis quadrangularis **106–109**

volatile constituents
- *Momordica charantia* 183
- *Tamarindus indica* 285

volatile oils
- *Glycyrrhiza glabra* 158
- *Nigella sativa* 197
- *Piper longum* 226
- *Piper nigrum* 232

vomiting
- *Adhatoda vasica* causing 22
- prevention *see* antiemetics

vrinda **201–205**

W

water, element 1
white leadwort **239–243**
wild asparagus **51–55**
winter cherry **321–325**
wireweed **244–246**
Withania somnifera **321–325,** Plate 68
Woodfordia floribunda **326–328**
Woodfordia fruticosa **326–328,** Plate 69
wound-healing promoters 341
- *Adhatoda vasica* 22
- *Carica papaya* 93–94
- *Centella asiatica* 103–104
- *Curcuma longa* 117

wounds, ruminants, *Acacia catechu* 14

X

xanthones
- *Boerhaavia diffusa* 76
- *Mangifera indica* 179
- *Swertia chirata* 274

Y

yashtimadhu **157–162**
yavanika **306–310**
yellow-berried nightshade **271–273**
yellow gentian **220–224**

Z

Zingiberaceae 117, 329
Zingiber officinales **329–333,** Plate 70
Zygophyllaceae 311